PHARMACY EXPOSED

1,000 Things That Can Go Deadly Wrong At the Drugstore

Dennis Miller, R.Ph.

ATTENTION: IMPORTANT NOTE TO READERS

This book should not be used as a substitute for professional medical advice or care. The reader should consult his or her physician in matters relating to his or her health. In particular, the reader should consult his or her physician before acting on any of the information or advice contained in this book.

Stopping a medication can be very dangerous. Every reader must consult with his or her physician before starting, stopping, or changing the dose of any medication.

Nothing in this book should be interpreted as stating or implying that the reader should ever discontinue a drug or take it differently from how it was intended by his or her physician. This could have devastating health consequences. For example, discontinuing a blood pressure medication could cause a heart attack or stroke. Many drugs are absolutely essential and even life-saving. NO ONE should EVER stop taking any medication without careful consultation with a physician and medical supervision. Even potentially dangerous drugs can be essential for health.

Part of the reason for writing this book is to encourage patients to have discussions with their physicians about the risks and benefits of drugs, and about whether there may be (sometimes major) lifestyle or dietary changes that might lessen the need for some drugs. This book is about prevention. This is not a book that advocates taking drugs differently from how they were prescribed by a physician. This book describes the author's opinion about issues relating to pharmacy, pharmacists, and pharmaceuticals. Other pharmacists may have different opinions. The reader is encouraged to seek a wide range of opinions on all the issues discussed in this book.

One of the risks in writing a book about drugs is that some readers may misinterpret the author's intentions and then do something contrary to his or her health. Indeed, such fear sometimes keeps pharmacists from frankly discussing the pros and cons of drugs with our customers. We live in a very litigious society in which sometimes it seems to be impossible to have a mature and intelligent conversation about the risks and benefits of drugs without fear of a lawsuit.

This book is intended to provide information about pharmacy issues in general, but not provide specific professional advice to any particular reader. Accordingly, any such information is not intended to replace or substitute for professional medical advice or the labeling recommendation of any given product. Readers are advised to consult their own physicians, with whom they can consider individual health needs and concerns, for specific medical advice and treatment. The author shall not be liable or responsible for any loss or damage incurred allegedly as a consequence of the use and application of any information or suggestions contained in this book.

The author is not engaged in rendering professional advice or services to the individual reader. The ideas and suggestions contained in this book are not intended as a substitute for consulting with your physician. All matters regarding your health require medical supervision. The author specifically disclaims any responsibility for any liability, loss, or risk, personal or otherwise, which is incurred as a consequence, directly or indirectly, of the use and application of any of the contents of this book.

Stopping some drugs abruptly may cause sudden rebound or withdrawal effects. If multiple drugs are being taken, stopping one drug can sometimes change the effects of another. If you stop taking a drug or take it differently from how your physician intended it to be taken, that is ABSOLUTELY CONTRARY to the purpose of this book.

This book is meant to help reform the system, not to scare you out of taking medications. Suddenly halting the use of a drug can be deadly. Please do not do it. As Stephen Fried wrote in his classic book *Bitter Pills*, "Drug companies and doctors often make decisions based on the assumption that we are too dumb to understand the medications we're given. Don't prove them right." (Stephen Fried, *Bitter Pills: Inside the Hazardous World of Legal Drugs,* New York: Bantam Books, 1998, front matter/disclaimer)

The author believes that many drugs are absolutely essential and even lifesaving. Trying to decide which drugs are essential and which are optional is something that should be done between patients and doctors. For consumers interested in trying to cut down on the number of medications they take, this should be done only in consultation with a physician. This is not a do-it-yourself project. This is NOT analogous to Home Depot where "do-it-yourself" is encouraged.

Should Americans be wary of taking drugs? Should Americans be skeptical of the honesty of the pharmaceutical industry? Should Americans wonder about the safety and effectiveness of drugs? Should Americans wonder whether the FDA is doing an adequate job in keeping unsafe drugs off the market? Should Americans wonder whether physicians are sufficiently aware of the potential adverse effects of drugs?

Furthermore, should health professionals be afraid to write books about these issues because of the possibility of being sued if someone decides on his or her own to stop taking a critical medication and then suffers some horrific consequence like a heart attack or stroke? Does our litigious society keep health professionals from discussing these issues publicly? Does the immense legal and political clout of the medical-industrial complex intimidate health professionals from speaking out?

The possibility of adverse effects from a drug or drugs should not cause the reader to overlook the benefits of medication. A reader concerned about adverse effects of medication should discuss with his or her doctor the benefits as well as the risks of taking the medication. The author is certainly not the first to suggest that Americans may be overmedicated or that drugs carry potential risks. Here are some examples of prominent experts who have spoken out on these issues:

> **"I find it hard to imagine that a system this corrupt can be a good thing, or that it is worth the vast amounts of money spent on it."**—Marcia Angell, M.D., former editor, *New England Journal of Medicine* (*The Truth About the Drug Companies: How They Deceive Us and What To Do About It,* New York: Random House, 2004, pp. 169-170)

I find it hard to imagine that a system this corrupt can be a good thing, or that it is worth the vast amounts of money spent on it. But in addition, we have to ask whether it really is a net benefit to the public to be taking so many drugs. In my view, we have become an overmedicated society. Doctors have been taught only too well by the pharmaceutical industry, and what they have been taught is to reach for a prescription pad. Add to that the fact that most doctors are under great time pressure because of the demands of managed care, and they reach for that pad very quickly. Patients have also been well taught by the pharmaceutical industry's advertising. They have been taught that if they don't leave the doctor's office with a prescription, the doctor is not doing a good job. The result is that too many people end up taking drugs when there may be better ways to deal with their problems. (Marcia Angell, M.D., *The Truth About the Drug Companies: How They Deceive Us and What To Do About It*, New York: Random House, 2004, pp. 169-170)

"There is no such thing as a 'safe' drug."
George Lundberg, M.D., former editor, *Journal of the American Medical Association* (*Severed Trust: Why American Medicine Hasn't Been Fixed*, New York: Basic Books, 2000, p. 152)

We are in genuine danger of overmedicating ourselves in this country, at great cost and often with questionable benefit. It has been found, for example, that overuse of pain medication can rebound and cause the very pain the mediation was designed to control. When people overuse products like Excedrin, Tylenol, and Advil, for instance, to control headaches—and some people take as many as fifteen tablets per day—the medication itself can cause headaches, yet another paradox in medicine.

People also encounter trouble with prescribed products designed to control conditions that may be better addressed by diet or exercise. Many patients have a strong desire to resolve all their health problems with a drop, a pill, or a plaster. That desire goes back to the days of nostrums and elixirs, only now the medications come with all kinds of scientific assurances. Think of those splashy magazine ads with great graphics and large type on one page, followed by another page of dense type with warnings, precautions, and listings of adverse reactions. The glamour is on one page, and the science is on the other. What looks easy in one place suddelnly looks terribly complicated and difficult in another. How come? The answer is simple: there is no such thing as a 'safe' drug.

(George Lundberg, M.D., *Severed Trust: Why American Medicine Hasn't Been Fixed*," New York: Basic Books, 2000, p. 152)

U. S. pharmaceutical companies remain a world model for creating devious methods to get physicians and patients to do what the companies want, whether or not it is in the best interest of the patient. (George Lundberg, M.D., *Severed Trust: Why American Medicine Hasn't Been Fixed*, New York: Basic Books, 2000, p. 145)

"I'm a therapeutic nihilist. My philosophy is the fewer drugs people take, the better off they are."—Former FDA Commissioner (1980-81) Jere Goyan (quoted in Philip J. Hilts, *Protecting America's Health: The FDA, Business, and One Hundred Years of Regulation*, New York: Knopf, 2003, p. 207)

In one of his first press conferences as commissioner, [Goyan] said frankly "our society has become overmedicated. We have become too casual about the use of drugs, and I'm referring to legitimate prescription and nonprescription drugs, not illicit drugs.... Too many people are taking too many drugs without proper understanding of their potential harmful effects.... I'm a therapeutic nihilist. My philosophy is the fewer drugs people take, the better off they are." He added, "I have a strong belief in the patient's right to know. My philosophy on this makes doctors and some of my colleagues uneasy, but in the best interests of public health, it should be mandated."

He believed drug companies tend to emphasize the selling of drugs, not conveying information about them. He believed as well that doctors are inattentive and often give the wrong drug at the wrong time in the wrong amounts, without regard to cost. At one meeting of doctors he said bluntly, "I staunchly refuse to accept the notion that any physician, merely because he graduated from medical school and is currently a card-carrying member of his or her county medical society, is great, or good, or even tolerably competent. Too much of drug therapy has been atrociously irrational." [Former FDA Commissioner (1980-81) Jere Goyan, quoted in Philip J. Hilts, *Protecting America's Health: The FDA, Business, and One Hundred Years of Regulation*, New York: Knopf, 2003, p. 207]

> **"...it's hard to find a drug that *doesn't* have a problem"**—David
> Flockhart, M.D., Georgetown University
> **"...most doctors don't have a clue"**—Raymond Woosley, M.D.,
> Georgetown Univerisity
> (quoted in Stephen Fried, *Bitter Pills: Inside the Hazardous World of
> Legal Drugs*, New York: Bantam, 1998, p. 102)

"You know, in the field we're in," Flockhart said, "it's hard to find a drug that *doesn't* have a problem–"

"And most doctors don't have a clue," Woosley shot in. "In clinical pharmacology, we have an attitude about drugs. We think drugs could be part of the problem. Doctors in practice just don't have that attitude. They *never* think about their drugs. They just think drugs are all wonder drugs, silver bullets–"

"Well, *that's* a disservice," Flockhart interrupted. "They're aware of the drugs you get blood levels on, and they know *why*. It's just that the information those doctors receive about drugs is heavily biased toward the pharmaceutical industry."

"No, it's all about how *great* this drug is, how *great* that drug is," Woosley Insisted. "It's never 'Oh, don't forget to check the EKG, don't forget that this drug might cause your patients to act crazy!' You know, we have a lot of good doctors in this country, but they've sold out to the drug industry–"

"Well, it's not so much that they've sold out," Flockhard tried to break in. "It's just the information they get–"

"They're out on the circuit, giving talks about how great drugs are because *that's what the drug companies pay them to do!*" Woosley said. "We need docs whose livelihoods don't depend on the drug industry and who are willing to stand up and say there's something wrong with a drug!"

> A former high-ranking FDA official had recently looked me straight
> in the eye and insisted that "the amount of preventable harm done by
> the misuse of drugs and the lack of properly identifying drug side ef-
> fects exceeds the sum total of all occupational and environmental haz-
> ards in the United States." (Stephen Fried, *Bitter Pills: Inside the
> Hazardous World of Legal Drugs,* New York: Bantam Books, 1998, p. 122)

Keep in mind that there are many medications that are absolutely critical and even life-saving. Not all drugs are good, and not all drugs are bad. Americans like black and white answers to every question. Americans do not like nuance. The author of this book is ABSO-LUTELY NOT saying that all drugs are bad.

Pharmacy Exposed is certainly not the first book that discusses the safety and effectiveness of pharmaceuticals, whether Americans are overmedicated, and whether our medical system gives incredibly short shrift to prevention. See, for example, the following:

1. **Overdosed America**: *The Broken Promise of American Medicine* by John Abramson, M.D.
2. **Prescription for Disaster**: *The Hidden Dangers in Your Medicine Cabinet* by Thomas J. Moore
3. **Bitter Pills**: *Inside the Hazardous World of Legal Drugs* by Stephen Fried
4. **The Truth About the Drug Companies**: *How They Deceive Us and What to Do About It* by Marcia Angell, M.D.
5. **Powerful Medicines**: *The Benefits, Risks, and Costs of Prescription Drugs* by Jerry Avorn, M.D.
6. **Natural Causes**: *Death, Lies, and Politics in America's Vitamin and Herbal Supplement Industry* by Dan Hurley
7. **Selling Sickness**: *How the World's Biggest Pharmaceutical Companies Are Turning Us All into Patients* by Ray Moynihan and Alan Cassels
8. **The $800 Million Pill**: *The Truth behind the Cost of New Drugs* by Merrill Goozner
9. **The Big Fix**: *How the Pharmaceutical Industry Rips Off American Consumers* by Katharine Greider
10. **Protecting America's Health**: *The FDA, Business, and One Hundred Years of Regulation* by Philip J. Hilts
11. **Top Screwups Doctors Make and How To Avoid Them** by Joe and Teresa Graedon
12. **Inside the FDA**: *The Business and Politics Behind the Drugs We Take and the Food We Eat* by Fran Hawthorne
13. **The Whistleblower**: *Confessions of a Healthcare Hitman* by Peter Rost, M.D. (Sep 10, 2006)
14. **Big Pharma**: *Exposing the Global Healthcare Agenda* by Jacky Law
15. **On The Take**: *How Medicine's Complicity with Big Business Can Endanger Your Health* by Jerome Kassirer, M.D.

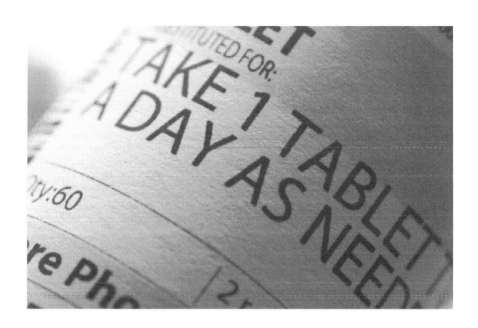

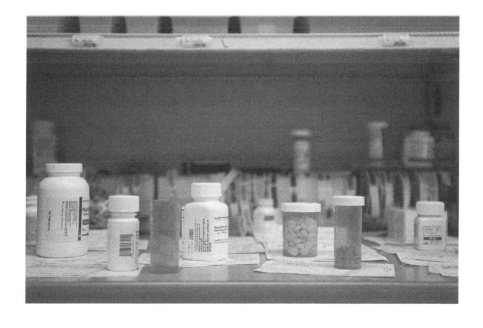

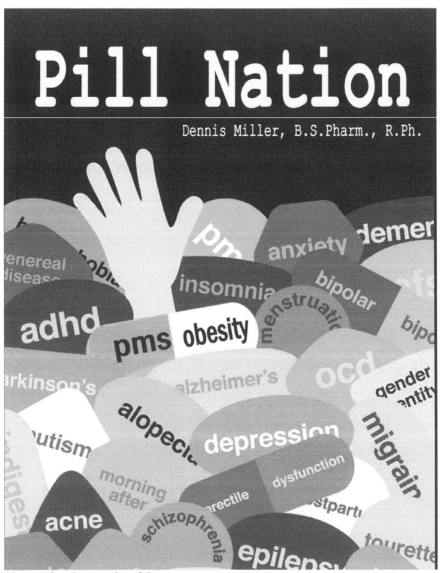

The author's next book?

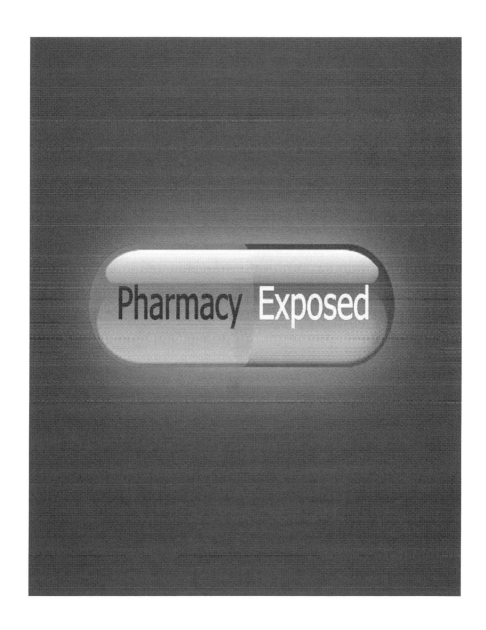

PHARMACY EXPOSED

DENNIS MILLER, B.S.PHARM., R.PH.

All the Shocking Secrets About Pharmacists and Chain Drugstores

FOREWORD BY JOE GRAEDON
BESTSELLING AUTHOR OF
THE PEOPLE'S PHARMACY

Alternate book cover #1

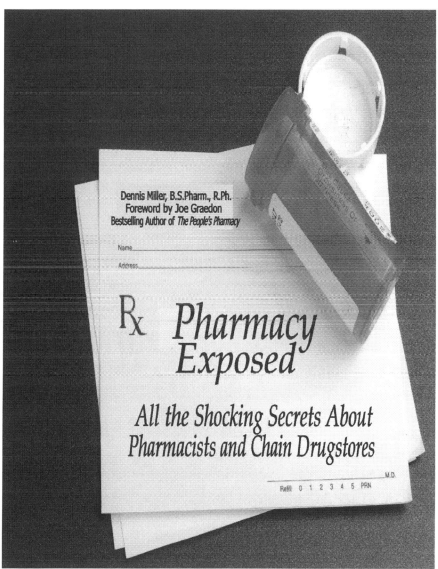

Dennis Miller, B.S.Pharm., R.Ph.
Foreword by Joe Graedon
Bestselling Author of *The People's Pharmacy*

Name

Address

℞ *Pharmacy Exposed*

All the Shocking Secrets About Pharmacists and Chain Drugstores

M.D.

Refill 0 1 2 3 4 5 PRN

Alternate book cover #2

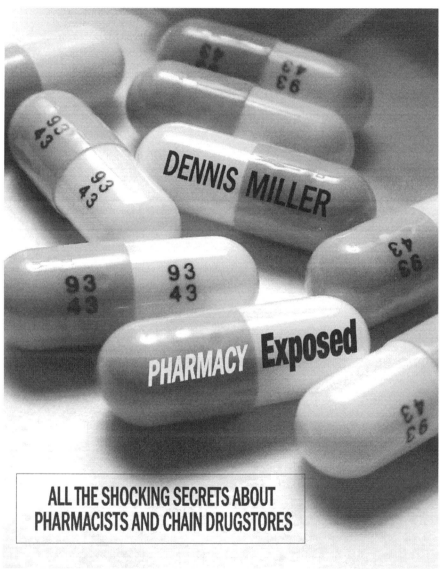

Alternate book cover #3

All the Shocking Secrets About Pharmacists and Chain Drugstores

Pharmacy Exposed

Dennis Miller, B.S.Pharm., R.Ph.

Foreword by Joe Graedon

Bestselling Author of The People's Pharmacy

Alternate book cover #4

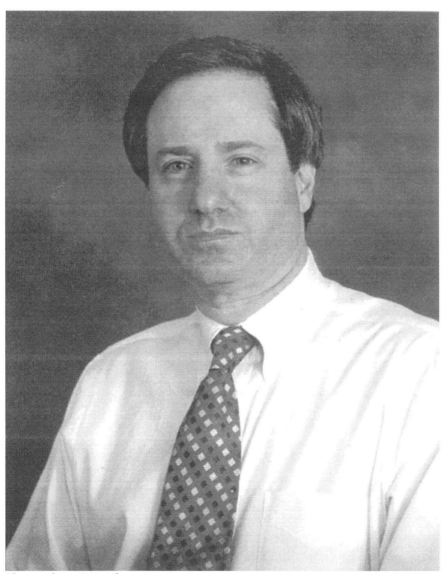

The author several years ago

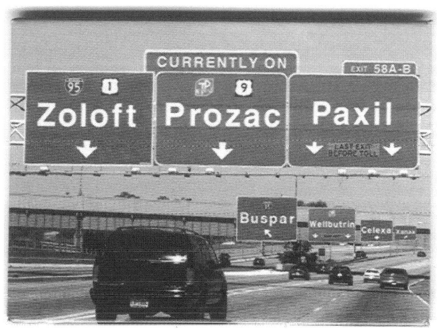

Antidepressant highway

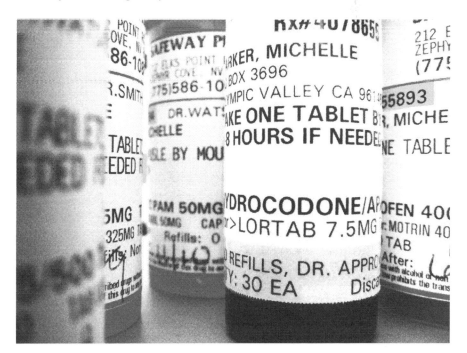

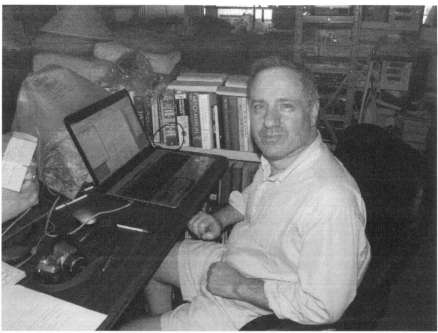

The author writing this book

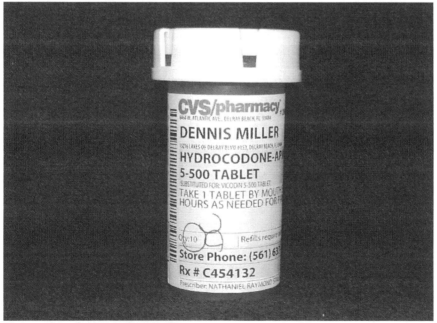

The author fractured a tooth

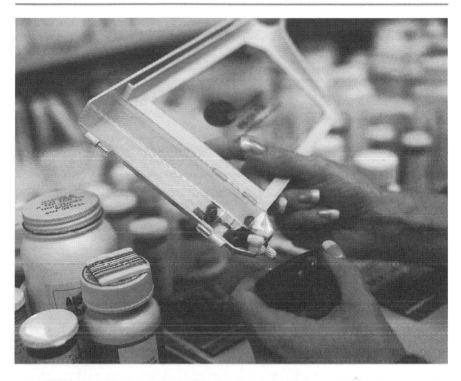

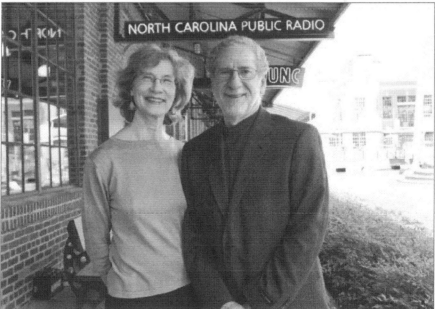

Joe and Teresa Graedon outside North Carolina Public Radio

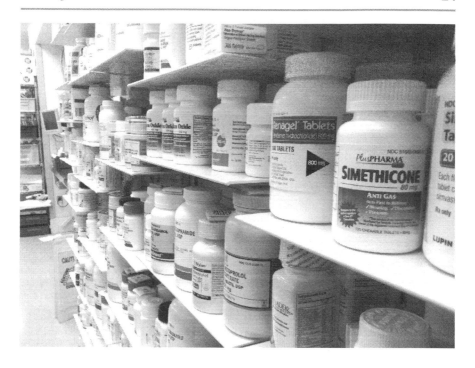

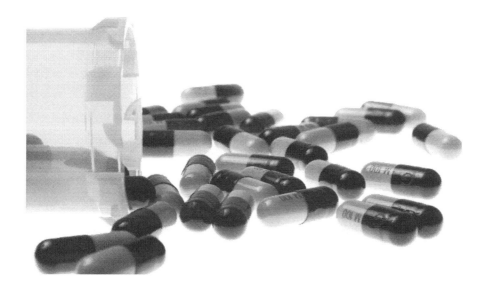

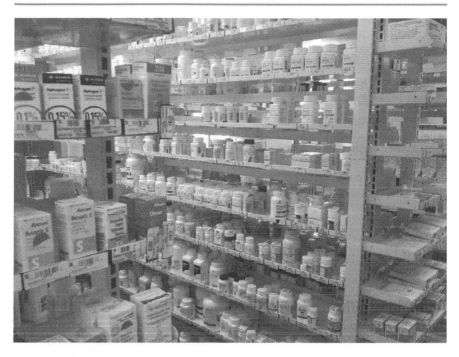

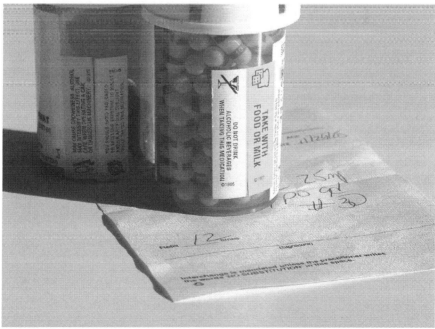

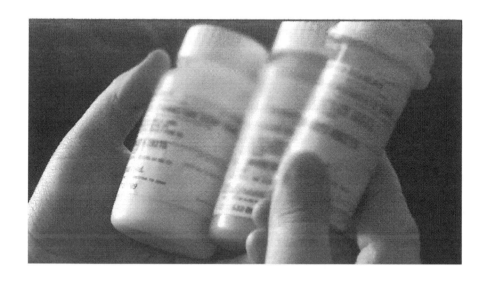

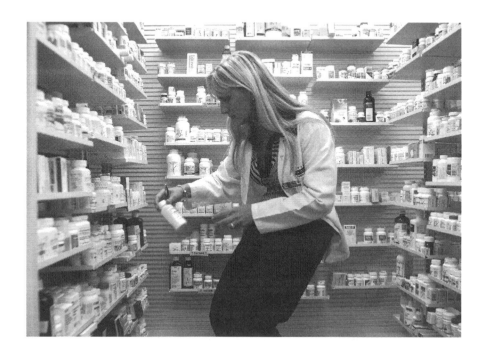

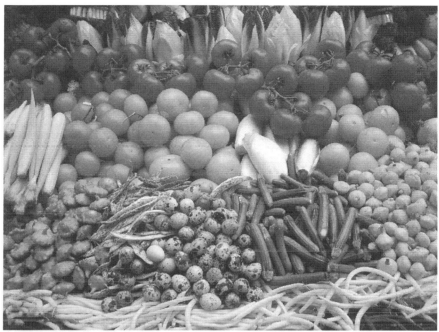

Eating whole foods as they exist in nature can help prevent disease

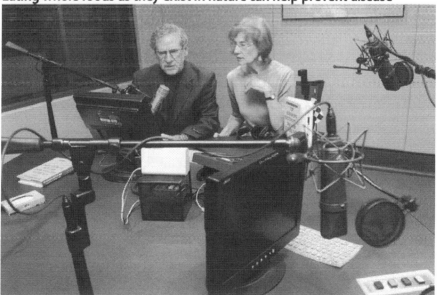

Joe and Teresa Graedon on the radio discussing their new book "Top Screwups Doctors Make And How To Avoid Them"

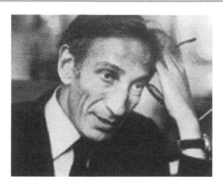

Ivan Illich (above and next page) was the author of *Medical Nemesis: The Expropriation of Health* (New York: Pantheon Books, 1976). This book was published one year after I graduated from pharmacy school. No book has has influenced my views on modern medicine more than *Medical Nemesis*.

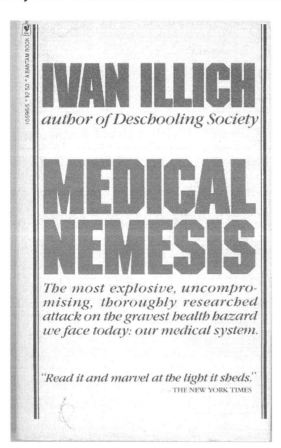

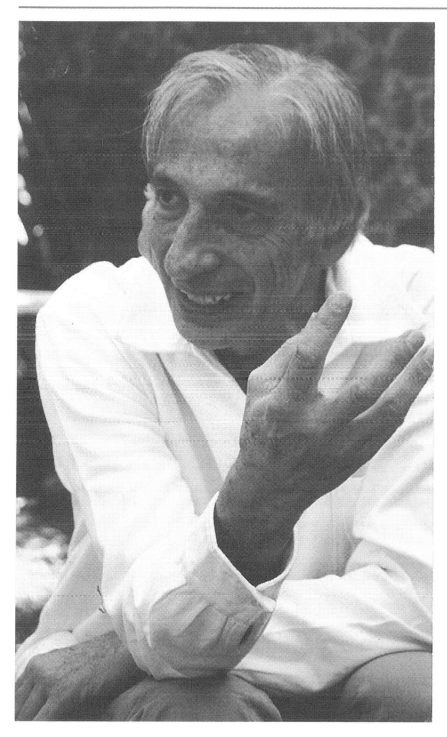

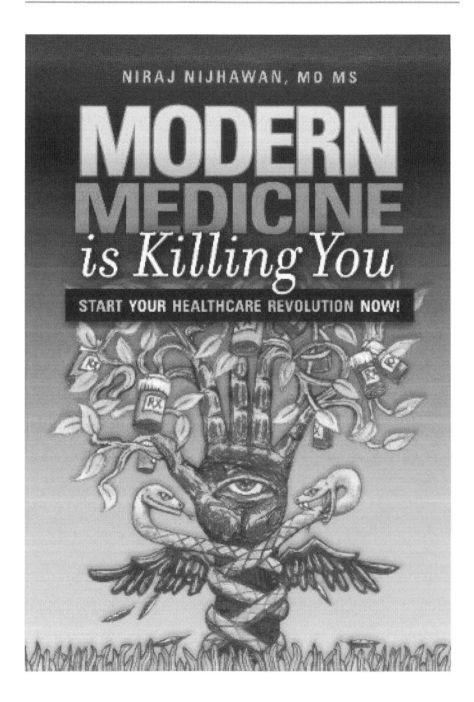

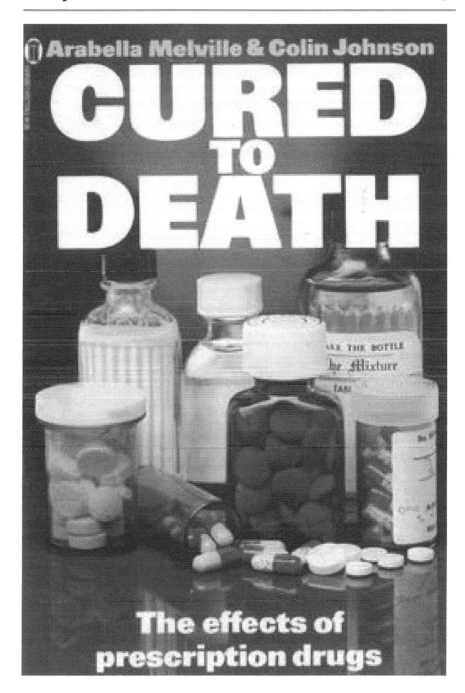

Arabella Melville & Colin Johnson

CURED TO DEATH

The effects of prescription drugs

HOW THE WORLD'S
BIGGEST PHARMACEUTICAL
COMPANIES ARE TURNING
US ALL INTO PATIENTS

SELLING SICKNESS

RAY MOYNIHAN
ALAN CASSELS

RAY D. STRAND, M.D.

DEATH BY PRESCRIPTION

THE SHOCKING TRUTH BEHIND AN OVERMEDICATED NATION

- An adverse drug reaction is five times more likely to *kill* you than an automobile accident or AIDS

- Don't become the FDA's guinea pig . . . the use of newly released drugs could be potentially life-threatening

- The use of prescription medication is the third leading cause of death in the U.S.

- Discover the *deadly* partnership formed by the U.S. Congress between the FDA and pharmaceutical companies

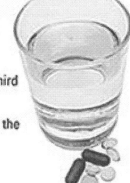

U.S. News
& WORLD REPORT

AUGUST 26, 1996

Danger

AT THE drugstore

Pharmacists are
your last defense
against risky drug
interactions. Too
many are blowing it

INVESTIGATIVE REPORT

U.S. News & World Report cover story, August 26, 1996

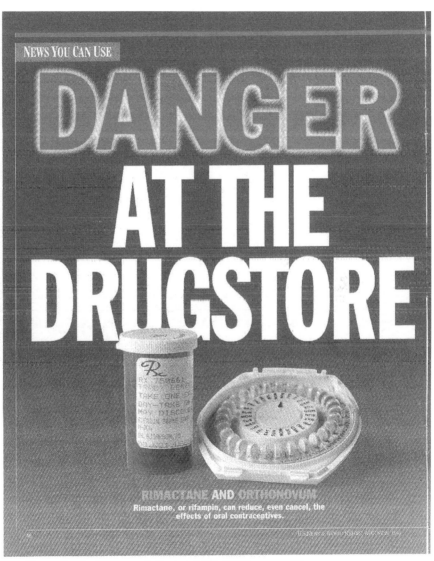

U.S. News & World Report, August 26, 1996, page 46

ACCUTANE • ADVIL • ALBUTEROL • AMOXICILLIN • ASPIRIN • COUMADIN • DARVON • HALCION

PRESCRIPTION for DISASTER

THE HIDDEN DANGERS IN YOUR MEDICINE CABINET

- Why you're ten times more likely to be hospitalized by a prescription drug than by an automobile accident.
- The risks of Prozac, Aleve, Ritalin, Seldane, Premarin, Zocor, Halcion, and many other drugs.
- Why most doctors tell their patients nothing about the adverse effects of their medication.
- How you can reduce your risks.

THOMAS J. MOORE

PREMARIN • PRILOSEC • PROCARDIA XL • PROPRANOLOL • PROVENTIL • PROZAC • REDUX • RELAFEN

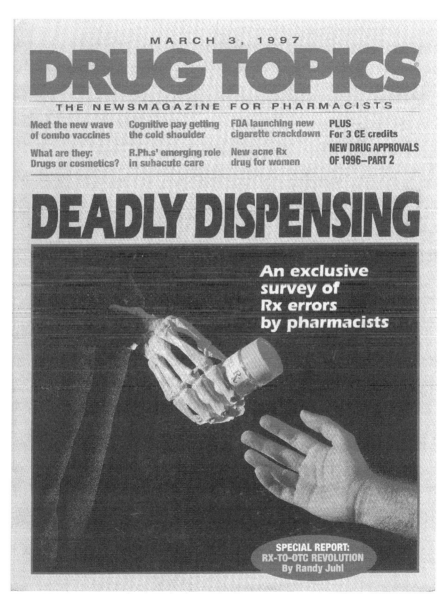

MARCH 3, 1997

DRUG TOPICS

THE NEWSMAGAZINE FOR PHARMACISTS

Meet the new wave of combo vaccines	Cognitive pay getting the cold shoulder	FDA launching new cigarette crackdown	PLUS For 3 CE credits
What are they: Drugs or cosmetics?	R.Ph.s' emerging role in subacute care	New acne Rx drug for women	NEW DRUG APPROVALS OF 1996–PART 2

DEADLY DISPENSING

An exclusive survey of Rx errors by pharmacists

SPECIAL REPORT: RX-TO-OTC REVOLUTION By Randy Juhl

Drug Topics cover story March 3, 1997 on pharmacy mistakes

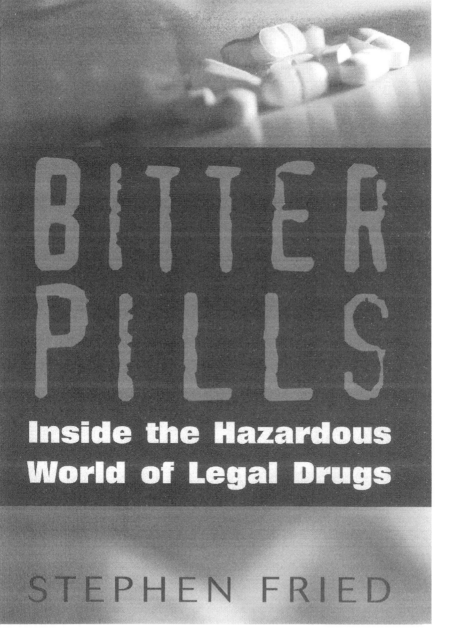

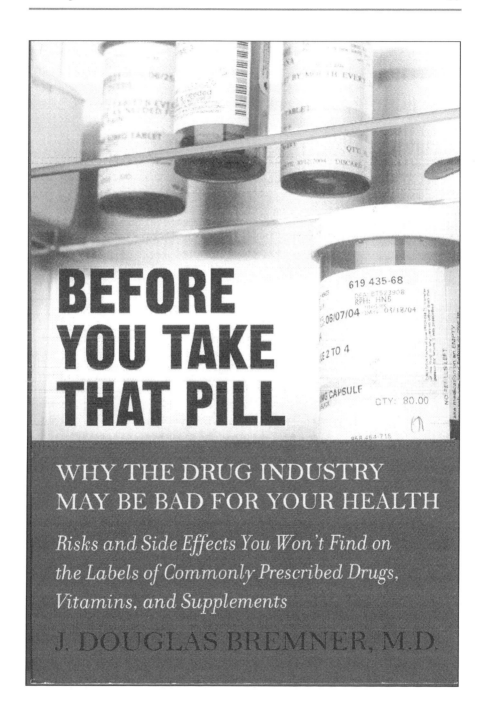

BEFORE YOU TAKE THAT PILL

619 435-68
DEA: BT523908
RPH: HN6
06/07/04   03/18/04
E 2 TO 4
MG CAPSULE
QTY: 80.00

WHY THE DRUG INDUSTRY
MAY BE BAD FOR YOUR HEALTH

*Risks and Side Effects You Won't Find on
the Labels of Commonly Prescribed Drugs,
Vitamins, and Supplements*

J. DOUGLAS BREMNER, M.D.

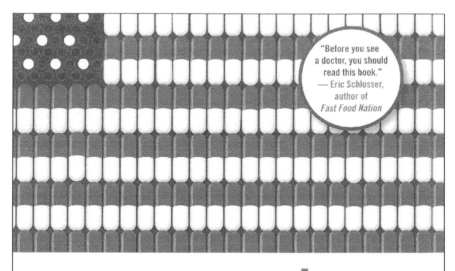

"Before you see a doctor, you should read this book."
—— Eric Schlosser, author of *Fast Food Nation*

OVERDO$ED

AMERICA

THE BROKEN PROMISE OF AMERICAN MEDICINE

How the Pharmaceutical Companies Distort Medical Knowledge, Mislead Doctors, and Compromise Your Health

JOHN ABRAMSON, M.D.

ROBERT S. MENDELSOHN, M.D.

CONFESSIONS
OF A
MEDICAL
HERETIC

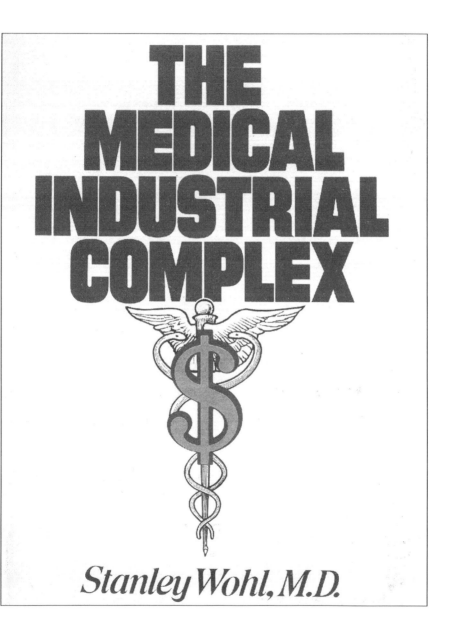

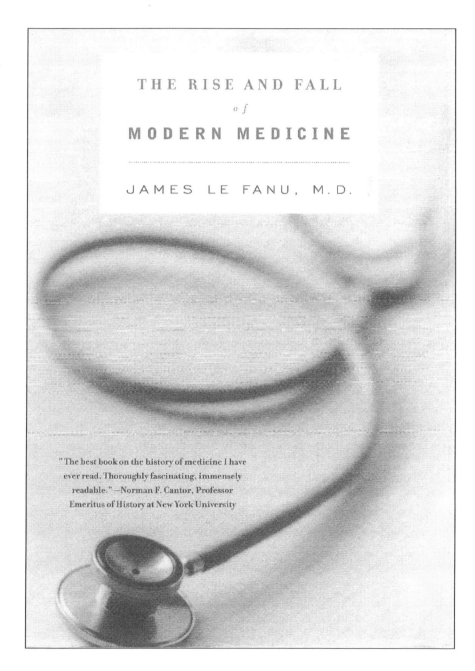

THE RISE AND FALL

of

MODERN MEDICINE

JAMES LE FANU, M.D.

"The best book on the history of medicine I have
ever read. Thoroughly fascinating, immensely
readable." —Norman F. Cantor, Professor
Emeritus of History at New York University

CHECK HERE BEFORE YOUR NEXT CHECKUP

WHAT DOCTORS DON'T TELL YOU

THE TRUTH ABOUT THE DANGERS OF MODERN MEDICINE

SHOULD YOU AGREE TO:
• STEROIDS FOR ASTHMA? • CHOLESTEROL-LOWERING DRUGS?
• ANGIOPLASTY? • HORMONE REPLACEMENT THERAPY?
• ANY TREATMENT YOU DON'T KNOW ENOUGH ABOUT?

LYNNE McTAGGART

How the Pharmaceutical Companies Transformed
Themselves into Slick Marketing Machines
and Hooked the Nation on Prescription Drugs

OUR
DAILY
MEDS

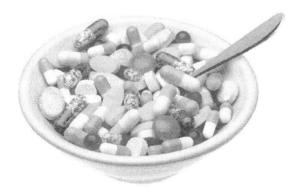

MELODY PETERSEN

POWERFUL MEDICINES

The Benefits, Risks,
and Costs of
Prescription Drugs

JERRY AVORN, M.D.

The Truth About the Drug Companies

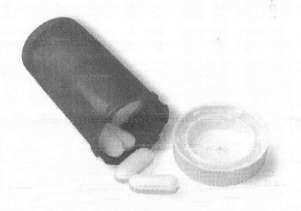

HOW THEY DECEIVE US
AND WHAT TO DO ABOUT IT

MARCIA ANGELL, M.D.

Former editor in chief of The New
England Journal of Medicine
Winner of the Polk Award

DON'T BE A STATISTIC

TOP SCREWUPS DOCTORS MAKE AND HOW TO AVOID THEM

- Top 10 Doctor Errors • Top 10 Pharmacist Errors
- Diagnostic Disasters • Preventing Hospital Screwups

JOE GRAEDON, MS, AND TERESA GRAEDON, PhD

Bestselling authors of *The People's Pharmacy*

PiLLS THAT WORK

PiLLS THAT DON'T

•

DEMANDING AND GETTING THE BEST AND SAFEST
MEDICATIONS FOR YOU AND YOUR FAMILY

Includes the Proven 12-Week Action Plan
for Eliminating and Replacing
Unnecessary, Unsafe, and Inappropriate
Prescription Medications

GIDEON BOSKER, M.D.

"The sharpest critique of the medical establishment in a decade."—*The Utne Reader*

DISEASE-MONGERS

How Doctors, Drug Companies, and Insurers Are Making You Feel Sick

LYNN PAYER

Author of *Medicine and Culture*

A PHARMACIST'S
GUIDE TO AVOIDING
DANGEROUS DRUG
INTERACTIONS,
REACTIONS AND
SIDE-EFFECTS

Every year more than **700,000 trips to the ER** are caused by adverse drug reactions — **make sure you're not one of them**

ARE YOUR MEDS MAKING YOU SICK?

This handy reference guide could save your life or the life of a loved one. Read it before starting multiple meds. If you're already taking them, read it today.

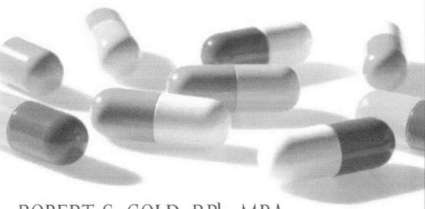

ROBERT S. GOLD, RPh, MBA

How to Prevent
Dangerous Interactions,
Avoid Deadly Side Effects, and
Be Healthier with Fewer Drugs

ARE YOUR PRESCRIPTIONS KILLING YOU?

Armon B. Neel, Jr., PharmD, CGP,
and Bill Hogan

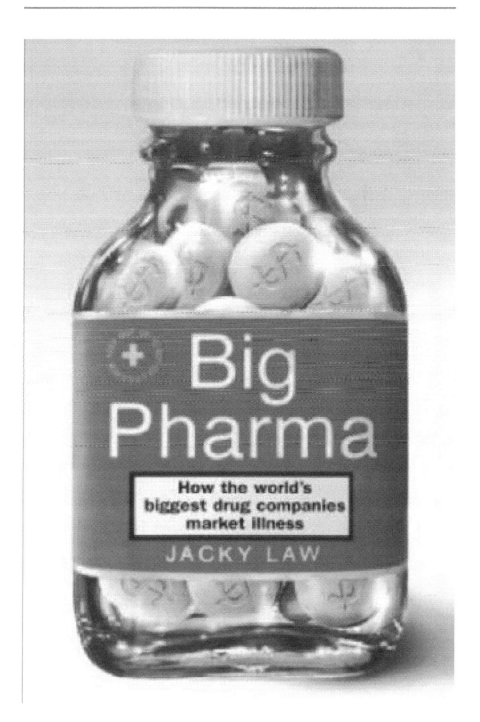

CONTENTS

FOREWORD

For decades the mysterious world of pharmacy has escaped public attention. I say mysterious because what goes on behind the counter has been largely invisible to patients. A prescription is written by a physician and transmitted either the old-fashioned way on a piece of paper or, increasingly, by fax or electronically (known as "e-prescribing"). The patient picks up a bottle of pills a short time later, frequently from a clerk or a pharmacy technician.

What happens behind the counter remains secretive. Mail order pharmacy practice is even more obscure. That said, the profession of pharmacy continues to be held in very high esteem by the public. According to the Gallup poll, people consistently rank pharmacists above most other professions, including physicians, when it comes to honesty and ethics.

Despite routinely providing pharmacists superb scores for professional standards, most people are clueless about the number of mistakes that happen in pharmacies across the country every year. That is why *Pharmacy Exposed* is such an unusual and important book. To my knowledge, this is the first time a pharmacist has revealed in such extraordinary detail what happens behind the counter. More important, Dennis Miller makes clear who should be held accountable for the harm that results from unsafe working conditions. When employers cut staffing levels and technicians are hired to save money, there are increasing risks for patients.

Although this book focuses primarily on problems in the pharmacy, important questions are also raised about physicians' responsibilities, as well as the risks and benefits of the medications they prescribe. Although I do not agree with everything Dennis Miller says about the "best and worst drugs in the pharmacy," I recognize that regulators, physicians and even other pharmacists have ignored his perspective for much too long. Mr. Miller raises important questions about drug safety and effectiveness and about the controversy surrounding the quality of generic drugs, something I have been concerned about for several years.

Dennis Miller is fed up with the status quo. He has become the biggest whistle-blower in the history of his profession. His goal is to overhaul a system that has accepted a high number of mistakes as the price for doing business—mistakes that can jeopardize their customers' health. After reading *Pharmacy Exposed* patients will not look at their neighborhood pharmacy in the same light again.

Rather than being mainly concerned with how long it takes to fill their prescriptions, customers should realize how high the stakes are at the pharmacy. It is deeply regrettable that understaffing as a result of cost-cutting often means that pharmacists don't have nearly as much time as they would like to answer questions from customers. Realizing this, customers should be sure to check their prescriptions carefully, ask questions about anything they don't understand or that doesn't look right, and possibly save their own lives. Keep in mind that the best pharmacist is not necessarily the fastest pharmacist. Quality takes time.

Joe Graedon

ACKNOWLEDGEMENTS

For several years, I lived in Oxford, North Carolina which is about thirty miles from Joe Graedon's home in Durham. We used to get together every few months and argue whose perspective on Pharma and modern medicine was more accurate. Occasionally we would meet for lunch at one of the restaurants in Durham. During one phone conversation in which we were discussing where to meet, Joe suggested a particular restaurant and I said, "I'd rather meet at your house so that I can yell at you." He laughed because he knew exactly what I was saying. Our get-togethers usually involved both of us forcefully arguing that our perspective was correct. I want to thank Joe for giving me constant encouragement, criticism, and suggestions as I sought his advice on this book. I first met Joe sometime around 1980. We seldom went more than a few months without speaking on the phone, exchanging e-mails, and yelling at each other. Suffice it to say that Joe doesn't agree with everything I've written in this book. The year is now 2012 and Joe (later joined by his wife and co-author Terry) has now published fifteen books. In other words, the Graedons have published fifteen books essentially in the time span that it took me to complete this book. Joe's most frequent criticism of my writing has been that I tend to repeat important points. For example, he says that I use the fast food metaphor too often. In fact, the McDonald's-ization of pharmacy is one of the major themes in this book.

I would like to thank my brother Jeff for patiently reading most of the chapters in this book and providing criticism. My first drafts of this book way back in the early 1980s were so horrible that Jeff told me he would be embarrassed to let anyone see it. Jeff loves grammar and punctuation and spelling. (He's a math teacher and amateur linguist who maintains several websites, including one titled "Word Oddities and Trivia.") His grammatical suggestions have been invaluable and I am very grateful for his criticisms of the manuscript. All remaining grammar, punctuation, and spelling errors are my fault, not his. I always told Jeff I wanted his "brutally honest" assessment as I e-mailed him each successive chapter. His comments ranged from "terrible," to "not interesting," to "okay" to "very good." Sometimes he said I was including too much detail for a book aimed at a general audience, but I often protested that the pharmacists who read this book may be interested in more detail. So I have included some material that my brother suggested I omit, because I'm hoping it will be of interest to pharmacists.

I want to thank Janice Zoeller who was then editor-in-chief at *American Druggist*. Many years ago, I sent her some of my typewritten pages on the origins of drug brand names and asked whether she was interested in publishing it. When I followed up with a phone call, she said she liked the material and was willing to publish it with a few changes. I was so shocked that I asked her, "Are you serious?" She could plainly see that I was a rookie as a writer. That was back in early 1999 and it became the first article I ever had published. Since she received a lot of favorable mail from pharmacists, she published a second article nearly a year later on an entirely different collection of drug brand names. I was looking forward to writing more articles for *American Druggist* because Janice seemed to be the kind of editor who liked edgy articles written by pharmacists, i.e., just the kind of thing I was interested in. But, unfortunately, *American Druggist* ceased publication shortly after my second article was published in that magazine. I believe I was not to blame.

I looked for another pharmacy magazine that might be willing to publish articles written by a pharmacist with an "attitude." I want to thank Harold Cohen, R.Ph., who was then the editor-in-chief at *Drug Topics*. He subsequently approved several of my "Viewpoint" editorials. When Harold became the editor-in-chief at *U.S. Pharmacist*, Judy Chi moved up to the position of editor-in-chief at *Drug Topics*. I want to thank Judy for continuing to publish more of my Viewpoints over the years. (Judy's mantra: "condense, condense, condense.") When *Drug Topics* moved from New Jersey to Ohio a few years ago, a new editorial staff took over the magazine. I want to thank Julia Talsma (editor-in-chief) and Julianne Stein (managing editor) for publishing one of my Viewpoints from the current editorial offices in Ohio. I have now had a total of seventeen "Viewpoints" published in *Drug Topics*.

I want to thank Carol Ukens who was a senior editor at *Drug Topics* before retiring a few years ago. Carol is an extremely intelligent person who was one of the most perceptive pharmacy writers for many years. I used to call her every few months to run ideas past her. She was always extremely friendly, helpful, and professional. It was rare that there was a pharmacy subject about which she was uninformed. Pharmacy journalism is not the same today without her wisdom and insight.

Each time an article is published, it gives an aspiring author a little more confidence and a little more courage. I gained a little confidence when *Good Housekeeping* magazine used me as a major source for an article on pharmacy mistakes (June 2005). And I gained a little more confidence when James O'Donnell asked me to write a chapter on pharmacy mistakes for the second edition (2005) of his book *Drug Injury: Liability, Analysis, and Prevention.*

I would not have had the courage to continue with this book without the encouragement and criticism I received from these people over the thirty years that I worked on this book. A constant (and, at times, overwhelming) worry during this period was that this book would never see the light of day.

For those pharmacists who feel strongly about pharmacy issues and are yearning to see their words in print, my advice is to keep at it, be persistent, keep improving your writing, and don't be completely discouraged by rejection. I've certainly had my fair share of rejections and discouragements over the last thirty years.

Dennis Miller

INTRODUCTION

It is my hope that *Pharmacy Exposed* becomes a paradigm shifting book. This very controversial book will upset a lot of people in positions of power in the world of pharmacy, particularly those at the highest levels of the big chain drugstores, but also those at the state boards of pharmacy and at this nation's many schools of pharmacy. While readers of this book will not agree with everything I say, I hope to make a very compelling case that the status quo in pharmacy today is completely unacceptable and is, in fact, a prescription for disaster.

I advocate a major overhaul in pharmacy toward one that serves patients' needs rather than corporate interests, and toward one that places the health and well-being of pharmacy customers ahead of corporate profits. I have attempted to say what many pharmacists passionately believe but are afraid to verbalize out of fear of jeopardizing their employment. Too many pharmacists today feel that the chain drugstore model has been disastrous for the public safety and for the profession of pharmacy. So it is not surprising that many pharmacists are not recommending pharmacy as a career for their children.

The pharmacy of today that I describe is one controlled by the bottom line, in which cost-cutting is the core guiding principle. This singular obsession with profits causes the big chains to cut pharmacy staffing to levels that are a threat to the public safety. The chains have embraced the fast food model with disastrous consequences in a system that rewards quantity over quality. This is a system where pharmacists are forced to fill prescriptions as if they were working at McDonald's, Burger King, or Wendy's. It is a system where pharmacists too often don't have enough staffing to adequately answer questions from customers. It is a system that cuts costs by hiring more technicians to do tasks formerly done by pharmacists. It is a system in which insurance companies erect an ever-increasing number of obstacles to dampen utilization while at the same time making policyholders' and pharmacists' lives more complicated. It is a system in which pharmacy mistakes are a horrific yet predictable and inevitable consequence of the chains' obsession with the bottom line.

The pharmacist's daily reality too often consists of arrogant doctors with some or all of the following traits: 1) notoriously illegible handwriting, 2) inadequate knowledge of drug interactions and a rude or dismissive attitude toward pharmacists who call about those potential drugs interactions or questionable doses, and 3) receptionists who too often have a very poor understanding of drug names yet routinely phone prescription orders to the pharmacy. The pharmacist's daily reality also consists of corporate bean counters who only care about numbers, and about how fast pharmacists can fill prescriptions. Pharmacists feel that their speed in filling prescriptions is much more highly valued by the chains than the pharmacist's knowledge of drugs. The pharmacist's daily reality consists of impatient customers who only care about how long they will have to wait for their prescriptions to be filled, and who seem to have no understanding of the potential hazards in the pharmacy and how common pharmacy mistakes are.

A huge number of pharmacists are deeply disgusted with state boards of pharmacy for being too intimidated by the legal and political clout of the chains, and for being too timid to at least try to pass regulations that address the understaffing that is endemic to chain pharmacies. Pharmacists feel that understaffing is at the heart of the epidemic of pharmacy mistakes in America. Pharmacists believe that state boards of pharmacy are doing a breathtakingly poor job in protecting the public safety by failing to mandate staffing levels that are adequate for the safe filling of prescriptions.

Many pharmacists feel that pharmacy schools have grossly misrepresented what conditions are like in the real world. Many pharmacists say they would like to bring a class action lawsuit against the schools of pharmacy for promoting a sugar-coated view of pharmacy, and for promoting a professional model for which the big chains have complete and utter disdain. Pharmacy schools promote a model of the pharmacist as drug expert, but the big chains want nothing to do with that model. The big chains expect pharmacists to fill an ever-increasing number of prescriptions with the same or even decreasing levels of staffing. The big chains seem to have a huge preference for fast pharmacists over knowledgeable or helpful pharmacists.

Ours is a nakedly profit-driven health care system in a culture that demands a quick-fix pill for every ill. It is a culture that prefers pills instead of prevention. It is a culture in which the public has been well-conditioned by pharma advertising to salivate for the latest wonder drug. It is a culture of fast food in which pharmacy drive-thru windows are a threat to the public safety by creating an expectation for service that is as speedy as McDonald's.

It is my hope that *Pharmacy Exposed* serves as an urgently-needed antidote to this madness, showing readers how they can protect themselves and avoid becoming a casualty of a system that is in crisis.

Please note: As is customary, brand name drugs are capitalized and generic names are in lower case.

PART I

DANGER AT THE DRUGSTORE

Chapter 1

Memorable misfills

Every pharmacist has his own horror stories that are seared into his brain. Here are some that stand out in my mind from twenty-five years as a pharmacist.

1. A pharmacist, upon discovering his own error, closed the store and rushed to the customer's house to retrieve the wrong medication.

In North Carolina, the state in which I worked for most of my career, it has been the law that a drugstore cannot be open without a pharmacist on duty unless the pharmacy is barricaded in such a way that there is no access by the public. This is to prevent unauthorized persons from having access to the drugs in the pharmacy.

A pharmacist told me the following anecdote. He discovered one day that he mistakenly dispensed prednisone to someone instead of phenobarbital. It's easy to see how this can happen. Both of these are small white tablets. Prednisone is a powerful drug similar to cortisone. Phenobarbital is a totally unrelated drug, usually used (years ago) to prevent seizures. Taking the prednisone instead of the phenobarbital meant this customer could have had a seizure while, for example, driving a car. The results could have been disastrous.

In horror, this pharmacist told me that he locked the doors to the entire store and went to that person's home to retrieve the incorrect pills. I don't recall this pharmacist's description of the reaction from the customer when the pharmacist arrived at that customer's home. But I assume the customer must have been at least surprised. This pharmacist is a smooth talker so I assume he made up some innocuous reason for asking for the pills back.

Let me assure you that closing the entire store (as required by law if the pharmacy cannot be barricaded) is not a minor event. Closing the doors of the store in the middle of the day is a major violation of company policy. Nevertheless, being sued by a customer is even more highly frowned upon. If our supervisors found out about this incident, they would be unhappy that this pharmacist closed the store, but they would agree that he made the right decision under the circumstances.

2. I lied to a customer about my mistake.

Here is a mistake that I made myself which I lied my way out of. In 1976, I had been out of pharmacy school for about a year. I mistakenly filled a prescription for V-Cillin-K liquid instead of Keflex liquid. These are both antibiotics that were very popular at that time under their brand names. They are usually filled generically now. At that time, they were both packaged in boxes that were nearly identical: a white box with some green trim. The prescription was for a child.

For some reason, I happened to be looking back through the pile of prescriptions I had filled that morning and I happened to realize my error. I came upon a prescription in the pile that called for Keflex, but I realized that I had not dispensed any Keflex that morning. I remembered dispensing V-Cillin-K.

I called the child's mother and proceeded to lie to her. I made up the following story. I said that I happened to notice on the box in which the product was packaged that the date code indicated that the product was nearing its expiration. I told her that it was still good, that it was not out of date, but that I would feel more comfortable if she returned to the pharmacy so that I could give her a fresher bottle.

This was all a big lie. My error had nothing to do with expiration dates. I had simply dispensed the wrong drug.

As I had hoped, the customer was understanding and in fact seemed to appreciate my efforts to assure that her child was getting fresh medication. She seemed to be grateful and appreciative that I would go to these lengths to assure that the medication was fresh. As I said, this was all a big lie, a pretext to get her to bring the incorrect medication back. I had the correct medication ready when she returned and I think she was really proud of me for being so concerned that the medication was fresh. But it was all a big lie.

3. A pharmacist, terrified, called her husband and told him to go to a customer's house to get a prescription filled incorrectly.

A pharmacist told me this story: She had several prescriptions on the counter. One was for Mepergan Fortis, a powerful narcotic pain reliever. Another was for cephalexin 500 mg, an antibiotic. Both of these drugs are capsules that look nearly identical when viewed through the amber pill container. This pharmacist gave the customer Mepergan Fortis instead of the cephalexin. In describing this incident to me, she said that she had been interrupted by phone calls and various other distractions which resulted in her switching the medications. The customer had already left the pharmacy with the wrong medication when the pharmacist realized her mistake.

In absolute horror she called her husband who was at home. Knowing the customer's address from our computer, she told her husband to go to that person's house and retrieve the medication. She told me that she cried into the phone to her husband: "GO GET IT! GO GET IT!" Her voice broke as she relayed this story to me.

4. We'd like to ram that stopwatch up his ass!

An error occurred when my partner dispensed the antibiotic doxycycline 100 mg instead of the antidepressant Doxepin 100 mg.

The circumstances surrounding this error are interesting. In 1993, my employer held what they called a contest to see whether pharmacists were following corporate procedures. Supervisors came around to each store with a clipboard and a list of procedures to see whether we were following guidelines. The chain said that the store with the highest score in each district would win a prize.

One of the parameters checked was the time it took the pharmacist to fill each prescription. Incredibly, each supervisor had a stopwatch. The supervisor reset the stopwatch with each prescription. When the pharmacist first touched the prescription, the supervisor started the stopwatch. When the pharmacist finally put the medication in the bag, the stopwatch was stopped. Other criteria checked were things like how many times the phone rang before the pharmacist answered, whether or not the pharmacist returned to any calls on hold every 30 seconds to tell the caller the status of his call, whether technicians wasted time chatting on the phone with friends, etc.

What happened in this case was that the pharmacist was so distressed by the experience of being timed with a stopwatch that he inadvertently dispensed the antibiotic doxycycline 100 mg instead of the antidepressant Doxepin 100 mg. Let me emphasize that this so-called contest was held on actual prescriptions for actual customers in the middle of an actual business day. It was not held at some special contest site. The chain had the nerve to subject us to this stressful indignity as if it were no more disruptive of our work routine than a wart on our hand.

Enough pharmacists eventually complained so vociferously that management was forced to drop the stopwatch. But the rest of this "contest" (actually a productivity test) remained in subsequent stores that were tested. Most pharmacists say it was the most demeaning thing they've experienced since graduating from pharmacy school. I think it's an indication of the powerlessness of chain pharmacists, the wage-labor nature of our job, and the fact that pharmacy is now less a profession and more an assembly line. Like most workers in America, pharmacists today are piece-work, assembly line workers who are closely monitored.

5. My partner was sued for this error

A local doctor called one day and said to me that one of his patients was in his office and "he's dying." The doctor said that we
mistakenly dispensed carbamazepine 200 mg (an anti-seizure medication) instead of theophylline 200 mg (an anti-asthma medication).
The doctor said that seizures were not one of the patient's medical
conditions. The doctor said that the patient indeed has asthma and
that it was out of control the last few days when he was taking the
anti-seizure medication while expecting it to be the anti-asthma
medication. Even though I don't know for sure, I suspect that the
patient was sitting across the desk from the doctor and that the doctor made the call to me in the presence of the patient to emphasize to
the patient that it was not the doctor's fault that the patient's asthma
was out of control.

I said to the doctor, "Are you serious that the patient is dying?"
The doctor's reply was that no, the patient wasn't dying, but that he
was pretty damn mad for suffering with uncontrolled asthma for the
last few days. The doctor, who has a reputation in town for frequently having an arrogant attitude, implied that the patient had
grounds for a malpractice suit against us.

Further into the conversation (when it was clear that the patient
would be okay), I asked the doctor the question that was uppermost
on my mind from the beginning: "Which pharmacist's name is on
the label?" The doctor was criticizing me as if I had filled the prescription and I didn't enjoy being on the receiving end of his anger if
another pharmacist had filled the prescription. The law in my state
requires us to put on the label at least the last name and first initial of
the pharmacist who filled the prescription. The doctor read out my
partner's name. I breathed a huge sigh of relief to myself. This took
a little wind out of the doctor's sails, as it was apparent he was
blaming the wrong person.

I called my partner at home and told him what had happened.
My partner said that he didn't know whether he should call the patient and apologize because, by admitting error, the likelihood of a
malpractice claim might increase. It turns out that my partner did call
the patient and apologize. My partner says that the patient appreci-

ated the apology. But it turns out that the patient sued my partner and our employer anyway. I don't know the dollar amount of the settlement given to the patient because lawsuits are not something that pharmacists like talking about. And I'm afraid that my partner would tell me, "It's none of your business."

The issue of whether pharmacists should admit an error and apologize to the customer is one of considerable controversy. In 1993, at a day-long meeting of about two dozen of the chain's pharmacists in the local district, our supervisors said that we should admit errors to customers and apologize. There was a great deal of discussion of this point. I have come to the conclusion that it was a corporate decision that the pharmacist responsible for the error should apologize to the customer.

During our lunch break that day, the half dozen pharmacists sitting around my table discussed this idea of admitting our error and apologizing to the customer. A couple of older pharmacists said they had never done it that way before and they didn't want to start now. They implied that the best way to handle errors was to try to obfuscate the whole thing either by lying or saying something to the customer like the drug is a generic equivalent or that it's the same drug from a different manufacturer. Of course, we tailor our smoke screen to the specific circumstances. If the customer is in danger, obviously we've got to take more direct action.

One of these older pharmacists said that most auto insurers recommend that policyholders not admit fault. I went home and checked my State Farm car insurance policy and, sure enough, on the back of my wallet card are these exact words: "Do not admit fault. Do not discuss the accident with anyone except State Farm or Police."

So why would my employer (one of the largest drug chains in the country) suggest that we admit fault to the customer and apologize? At our table, we concluded that the corporation was trying to protect itself by isolating us as the bad apple. In other words, we concluded that they were trying to isolate us on a limb and then, if necessary, cut off that limb. We figured that the chain would endeavor to get rid of us through various means if the case received widespread publicity in our community. As a result, most pharmacists I know are not eager to admit fault and apologize to customers.

How did this error occur?

It so happens that carbamazepine is the generic for Tegretol. In the alphabetical system that most pharmacies use to stock drugs, the generic product is stocked beside the brand name product. So, in this case the carbamazepine is stocked in the "T" section as is the theophylline. In the case of this particular pharmacy, the carbamazepine was shelved directly above the theophylline.

There's nothing unusual about this. What was unusual was that we happened to stock the generic carbamazepine and the generic theophylline from the same generic manufacturer. It so happens that this manufacturer's containers all look alike. The size of the bottle, the color of the label, the color of the container, the printing on the bottle, etc., all look identical. The only difference, of course, is that the names of the pills in the bottles are different. Many manufacturers try to vary the size of the containers, the colors of the labels, etc., for this very reason, to make it easier for the hurried pharmacist to distinguish products quickly. What happened was that my partner inadvertently picked up the identical-looking bottle above the theophylline. The customer ended up getting carbamazepine (for seizures) instead of theophylline (for asthma). As a consequence, my partner and our employer were sued.

6. A pharmacy gave my stepfather the wrong medication

A pharmacy gave my stepfather a diabetes medicine (Glucophage) by mistake, instead of his blood pressure medicine (Toprol XL). My stepfather has never had diabetes.

In April of 1998, my stepfather was on Toprol XL for blood pressure. One morning, as he prepared to take one of his Toprol tablets, he said to me, "Why do some of these pills look different?" He proceeded to pour the contents of his prescription bottle onto the kitchen table.

I was amazed at what I saw. A scenario I know all-too-well was happening in my own family. It was instantly obviously that an error had been made by his pharmacy. The label indicated that the bottle contained Toprol XL, but it was clear that approximately half of the tablets in the bottle were not Toprol XL. I was initially unsure what the other tablets were. All the tablets were round and white but half of them were a little larger than the other half. Then I remembered that the other tablets looked like Glucophage 500 mg because of the markings BMS 500. (BMS stands for Bristol-Myers Squibb, the manufacturer.)

I told my stepfather that somehow the pharmacy had placed a diabetes medicine in the same bottle with his blood pressure medicine. He was not overly concerned but he was eager to go to the pharmacy to ask what had happened.

I told him that I would like to accompany him just as an observer, not mentioning to the pharmacist there that I, too, am a pharmacist. As we drove to the pharmacy (a large national chain), I told him to prepare for what I call the "minimization routine" in which the pharmacist downplays the significance of the error.

This pharmacy is one of the busiest community pharmacies I have ever seen, judging by the number of white coats (pharmacists, technicians, and cashiers) in the pharmacy. I counted thirteen. I figure they must do over 600 prescriptions per day based on the personnel levels I've seen in the pharmacies I've worked in. They may even do considerably more than that.

My stepfather asked for the pharmacist-in-charge. That pharmacist poured the contents of the bottle onto a tray and said simply "Hmm."

My stepfather asked the pharmacist "What are these other pills?"

The pharmacist could not identify the Glucophage 500 by seeing the imprint BMS 500 on the pills. Rather than show the pills to his coworkers (which is what I would have done), he proceeded to examine reference material that identifies pills by their markings (i.e., letters and numbers imprinted on the pill). He was finally able to determine that BMS stood for Bristol-Myers Squibb, so he called that manufacturer. He was told that BMS 500 is their diabetes medicine Glucophage.

The pharmacist told my stepfather, "This other medicine is Glucophage, a diabetes medicine." The pharmacist then asked my stepfather, "Have you ever had diabetes or been on Glucophage?"

My stepfather: "No."

The pharmacist: "Hmm. I don't know how this could have happened."

My stepfather: "What would have happened if I took those wrong pills?"

The pharmacist: "It may have lowered your sugar a little bit."

My stepfather: "Could that have hurt me?"

The pharmacist: "Only if you had taken a whole bunch of 'em."

The pharmacist then chose his words carefully, as I do in situations like this. He said, "Sorry for the inconvenience. We will refund the price of the prescription to you." The pharmacist then replaced the Glucophage with Toprol XL and gave my stepfather a slip for a refund.

My stepfather and I then proceeded to the refunds and exchanges counter in another part of this store. The pharmacy is only one department in this huge store. We had an authorization from the pharmacy for a refund of approximately thirty dollars.

On the way home from the store, I asked my stepfather how he felt about the situation. He wasn't very upset. He said, "Accidents happen. I'll only get mad if it happens again."

My stepfather is a very nice person and doesn't get upset easily yet I feel that his attitude about this incident reflects the attitude I see from customers whenever I have to explain (or explain away) an error. The public does not seem to understand the significance of these events. In most cases, no harm is done by our errors. But the possibility of an absolute catastrophe is much greater than you know.

Note that the pharmacist chose his words carefully by saying "I'm sorry for the inconvenience" rather than saying "I'm sorry for the error." We pharmacists try to avoid using the word "error," fearing a lawsuit. "Inconvenience" is a much less scary word than "error."

My employer, too, refunds the price of the prescription whenever there has been an error.

7. I erroneously typed "Take one tablet three times a day" on a sleeping pill prescription. Sleeping pills are obviously taken at bedtime.

A short time after the sleeping pill Halcion was introduced onto the market, I received a prescription for this drug in which the doctor specified the directions "Take one tablet three times a day." Obviously, sleeping pills are not taken three times a day. They are taken at bedtime.

Believe it or not, pharmacists may not necessarily be aware of the indications (approved uses) for a new drug or the number of times per day that it is usually administered. With so many new drugs being introduced these days (at least in part because the FDA is under pressure from Congress and the drug industry to relax standards for approvals—according to some critics), it becomes more difficult for pharmacists to keep up. We have a learning curve with each drug. And don't forget that there are a few thousand drugs on pharmacy shelves.

Of course, it is inexcusable that a pharmacist would dispense a drug for which he doesn't know the indications or how many times daily it's usually taken, but this is what actually happens sometimes in the real world. Certainly I was negligent in not checking the official prescribing information before I dispensed this drug. But the doctor made the original error and I didn't catch it.

Pharmacists are very busy people with very hectic lives and families to raise, etc. Finding the time to keep on top of the flood of new drugs is something to which we should give a high priority, but, in the real world, lots of drugs are dispensed in this country that pharmacists are not "on top of."

Part of the problem may be the circus atmosphere surrounding new drugs and pharmacists' feeling that drug companies are leading us around by the nose, forcing us to learn about their latest wonder drug.

Allow me to digress for a minute. It is a fact that a large fraction of the new drugs introduced each year are simply "me-too" or "copy-cat" drugs. For a detailed explanation of "me-too" drugs, see *The Truth About the Drug Companies* (NY: Random House, 2004) by

Marcia Angell, M.D. Angell is a former editor-in-chief at *The New England Journal of Medicine.* In essence, each pharmaceutical company wants to have a "player" in a "hot" field (blood pressure, depression, cholesterol, type-2 diabetes, etc.), whether or not that player is any better than existing players. In many cases, the new drugs are no better and, in some cases, they're worse than existing drugs. The FDA does not require that new drugs be safer or more effective than existing drugs. New drugs must be sufficiently different to qualify for a patent. Drug companies want to get their share of any lucrative disease market. In my opinion, it is quite possible that pharmacists' skepticism toward the flood of copy-cat drugs contributes to a relaxed attitude toward learning about these new products. At least that attitude has affected me.

Back to the Halcion error. How was this error discovered? One day the physician who wrote the prescription called. I happened to be on duty at that time. He said something like "Somebody there typed 'three times a day' on a sleeping pill prescription I wrote." Apparently the patient had brought it to the doctor's attention.

Of course, this is an extremely uncomfortable situation for any pharmacist to be in. It's our worst nightmare. The pharmacist's immediate reaction is to hope that it may have been our partner or a fill-in pharmacist who filled the prescription. So, before we let the doctor chew us out, we delay things momentarily by saying something like "Let me pull the actual prescription from our files."

It turns out that my initials were on the prescription, so I was the pharmacist who had filled the prescription and made the error. But wait a minute! I see that the doctor specifically wrote "TID" on the prescription (the Latin abbreviation for "three times a day"). I said to the doctor, "I have your prescription in my hand and it clearly says 'TID'. You are welcome to stop by the pharmacy and examine it if you like."

The doctor's attitude softened. Somewhat surprisingly, he did not question the fact that he had mistakenly specified "TID." But he asked, "Why would you type 'three times a day' on a sleeping pill prescription?" I didn't have a good answer, but neither did he have a good answer for his mistake. So we were basically even (we had both screwed up) and the conversation then ended. Thank God.

There could have been tremendous liability involved if, for example, the patient didn't know this was a sleeping pill. A huge number of our customers are in a complete fog as to the precise purpose of each medication they swallow. So, if, for example, this customer had indeed taken it three times a day (not knowing it was a sleeping pill) and then he had been involved in a car accident, the potential liability for me and my employer could have been tremendous.

In this example, what percent of the fault belonged with me and what percent belonged with the physician? The doctor made a mistake and I didn't catch it. Luckily, as far as I know, the patient suffered no ill effects. But this could have been an absolute disaster.

8. "Is it even Claritin?"

In one store, a customer walked up to the pharmacy counter and said to me, "There are only fourteen tablets in this bottle but there's supposed to be thirty." The day before, another pharmacist had miscounted the tablets. The prescription was for Claritin, a non-sedating antihistamine used for allergy symptoms. (Claritin is now available without a prescription. At the time of this incident, it required a prescription.) This customer said that the pharmacist who dispensed the medication the day before was very busy: "He had four other customers waiting." The customer then asked me, "Is it even Claritin?"

When a customer asks something like "Is it even Claritin?" pharmacists know that we'd better have a good answer because we're talking to someone who knows enough to realize that pharmacists do indeed make mistakes. This is the type of question that pharmacists can't bullshit their way out of. A customer like this is essentially saying, "I trusted this pharmacist to fill my prescription correctly and I'm wondering if he did indeed fill it correctly."

Claritin is a very common-looking white pill. It is not a pill that is easily distinguished because of a distinctive color or shape. I went to our shelves and grabbed our stock bottle of Claritin, intending to show her that what we had in our stock bottle labeled Claritin was identical to what she had in her bottle. I asked her if she could read the numbers on the pills in her bottle. She said, "My eyesight isn't too good but it looks like 453 or 458." I was thankful that her eyesight was good enough to see that. I knew that I would be able to satisfy her since she was able to read the number. I showed her that the tablets in our stock bottle were numbered "458" and she seemed to be satisfied. Satisfying customers after an error is not always so easy, as the next anecdote will illustrate.

9. A customer goes ballistic because we forgot to tell him that a medication needed to be refrigerated and shaken before each use.

Here is an incident that was extremely uncomfortable for me. One morning a man approached the pharmacy and asked me to look in our computer and refill his mother's prescription for the antibiotic Duricef. This antibiotic was being used for a skin infection. He commented to me that since his mother had Alzheimer's disease, she needed the liquid form because she could not swallow capsules.

When I refilled the prescription and handed it to him, I told him to be sure to refrigerate it and to shake it well before each use. The man went ballistic. He told me that no one had ever told him to shake it or to refrigerate it. He emphasized that his mother had already finished two courses of this drug without shaking or refrigerating the container. He said that there were no SHAKE WELL or REFRIGERATE stickers on the bottle. He told me that the bottle had been kept on the kitchen table during both prior courses and that he had not shaken the bottle before giving her each dose. He asked me if the medication had lost its potency because it was not refrigerated. He wondered whether failing to refrigerate the drug was the reason it was not curing his mother's skin infection.

I decided to call the manufacturer, Bristol-Myers Squibb, while he was standing in front of me. I wanted to get a precise answer to his question and I wanted to show him that I took his concerns seriously. The person with whom I spoke at Bristol-Myers Squibb told me that their studies show that Duricef is stable at room temperature for ten days. What that means is that the active ingredient itself is stable for ten days. However, the person at Bristol-Myers Squibb was unable to guarantee that no microbial growth had taken place, contaminating the contents.

I told the customer that the manufacturer said it was probably still stable, but I did not tell him the second part of the message. I was afraid he would go into an absolute rampage if I told him about the possibility of contamination. He was already ballistic over the fact that we had failed to tell him that the medication was supposed to be refrigerated and that it needed to be shaken before each use.

He said he would call his doctor to see what harm may have occurred.

I gave him this refill at no charge. He told me that he felt that we should refund the price of the two previous courses. We did. Anything to please this man!!! I would have given him all the money in my wallet if I thought it would calm him down.

It appears that a pharmacy student had omitted a SHAKE WELL and REFRIGERATE sticker both times. The pharmacist with whom she was working evidently did not catch her omission. Upon my mentioning this incident to the pharmacy student later, she did not claim that she must have applied these stickers. The pharmacist-in-charge at this store said to her, "We've got to remember to put on those stickers!"

I was just filling in at this store so I don't know whether there were any further developments like a lawsuit. But the fact remains that I was placed in this extremely uncomfortable situation as a result of sloppy work done by others (i.e., the tech's omission of the stickers and the pharmacist's failure to catch that omission).

In my experience, when situations like this occur with a substitute pharmacist, that substitute pharmacist is sometimes blamed for not being able to defuse the situation quickly. Full-time pharmacists who have an assigned store (substitute pharmacists float between stores) sometimes seem to feel they can defuse any situation in their pharmacy in short order. So, despite my best efforts, I stood the chance of being accused (by the pharmacist for whom I was filling in) of doing a poor job in handling this irate customer.

10. A pharmacy student typed the wrong directions, instructing a customer to take four Lasix per day, rather than one per day as the doctor specified.

This error occurred when a pharmacy student typed the label directions for Lasix 40 mg (a diuretic): "Take one tablet 4 times a day." The student should have typed: "Take one tablet daily." The pharmacist who was on duty at that time was supposed to check this prescription, but that evidently did not happen. I blame the high volume of prescriptions done at this store, plus poor physician handwriting on the prescription, plus the use of Latin abbreviations.

The Latin abbreviation for "Take 1 tablet 4 times a day" is "1 qid." The Latin abbreviation for "Take 1 tablet daily" is "1 qd." If doctors would discontinue the practice of using Latin abbreviations on prescriptions and instead write out this stuff in plain English, there would be a lot fewer errors made by pharmacists who have difficulty reading doctors' handwriting.

When I was given this bottle of the diuretic Lasix to refill, I happened to look at the directions. That's something many or most pharmacists usually don't have time to do—we assume the directions are typed correctly initially. But for some reason I happened to look at the directions. What I noticed bothered me. I knew from experience that a smaller dose is far more commonly prescribed. I went to our prescription files and looked up the doctor's original prescription. Sure enough, it said, "Take one tablet daily" rather than what the pharmacy student typed on the label, "Take 1 tablet 4 times a day."

I then called my partner at home and told her what had happened. My partner hadn't caught the error made by our pharmacy student. My partner said to me, "Ask the customer how he's actually taking it. Maybe he's been on it before and maybe he knows he should just take one tablet daily instead of four times a day." So I asked the customer how he had been taking the Lasix. It turns out that this customer is a very nice man but he doesn't seem to be very intelligent. He laughed and said, "I noticed that the bottle said to take four a day but I knew that was wrong. I told my doctor and he said, 'Boy, they're really trying to dry you out!' [Diuretics like Lasix are used to remove excess fluid.] I've just been taking one a day."

Once again, I felt the weight of the world lifted from my shoulders. The customer did not know that our pharmacy student had screwed up, nor did the customer know that my partner had failed to catch the error. The customer never seemed to hold this error against us even though I certainly would have been upset and would tend to lose confidence in a pharmacist if a similar error had happened to me if I were the patient. And I'm surprised we never got an angry call from this customer's doctor.

11. A pharmacist told me that she discovered "at least a half dozen major errors" in a month. She said, "And I don't mean minor errors!"

I once worked briefly with a pharmacist who had only been licensed for three or four months. One day she told me that, soon after graduation from pharmacy school, she was placed in an extremely busy store in which she felt totally overwhelmed. She told me that in the month she worked there, she discovered "at least a half dozen major errors" that had been made by other pharmacists filling in at that store. Our district supervisor hadn't been able to find a permanent replacement for that store so there were a large number of pharmacists filling in there in the meantime. This young pharmacist told me, "And I don't mean minor errors!" She told me that she came to work early each day and left late and that she was still unable to handle the workload.

There are disagreements about what should be termed a "major error." "Major errors" do not necessarily mean "major harm." In fact, most major errors do not cause major harm. But some of them do. Getting Drug X instead of Drug Y at your drugstore can be a major mistake, but that doesn't necessarily mean that you will suffer major—or any—harm. If you get an anti-depressant like Prozac instead of an anti-arthritis drug like Celebrex, that is a major mistake by the pharmacy, but you are unlikely to suffer major harm.

12. A tech told me that a pharmacist she works with "doesn't check shit."

There's no doubt that the error rate among pharmacists spans the entire spectrum. Some pharmacists very rarely make mistakes. Other pharmacists scare me a great deal. The pharmacy tech at one store told me that one of the male pharmacists she works with "doesn't check shit." In other words, for example, once the pills are put in the bottle, this pharmacist doesn't usually look back a second time to see if they're the right pills or that the right directions are on the label, etc. She said that he makes lots of errors when he's talking to his new girlfriend on the phone. She said that he does things like putting medications for two completely unrelated people in the same bag.

I know this pharmacist and I can vouch for the fact that he does indeed make lots of errors. But so far none of the errors has been serious enough to jeopardize his job or reputation. From my perspective, he seems to think he can bullshit his way through anything in life—even a serious prescription error.

13. A pharmacist who was filling in for me dispensed the wrong eye drops to a child. As a result, the child's eye doctor was unable to perform an examination as planned.

Less than a year after graduation from pharmacy school, I was working in a pharmacy in Summersville, West Virginia. This is a town with a population of only a few thousand. The pharmacy was open only from 9 AM to 5 PM so I was the only pharmacist assigned to this store. My days off were infrequent in this pharmacy, yet one day off is especially memorable. On that day a relief pharmacist had the misfortune of filling a child's prescription with the wrong eye drops. The eye drops were intended to prepare the child's eyes for an upcoming eye exam. The drops were to be applied in the morning on the day that the parents were to make an hour's drive to the child's eye doctor in Charleston, West Virginia. The eye drops that this relief pharmacist mistakenly dispensed did not prepare the child's eyes properly. As a result, the eye doctor was unable to perform the exam as planned. This forced the parents to take off another day from work in order to make a second trip to Charleston.

As I said, I had been out of pharmacy school less than a year so I was unprepared for the task of handling this error. Even though I didn't make the error myself, I felt some responsibility because it happened in the store in which I was the only full-time pharmacist. I assumed that my employer (Rite Aid) would want me to try do anything I could to avoid a lawsuit.

It so happens that one of the technicians in that store had a very loose acquaintance with the parents of this child. I asked this technician to accompany me one evening to visit the family at their home. Luckily this technician has a very friendly personality and she's able to make conversation with people easily. I asked the tech to "do all the talking" herself because I was very uncomfortable with the entire situation. Even though I felt that visiting the parents at their home was a nice gesture, I dreaded it. I asked the tech to basically tell the parents that we were concerned about the error and that we regretted the hassle that it put them through, i.e., lost wages from taking time off from work to go a second time to the eye doctor in Charleston. My tech did what I felt was a great job in showing compassion for the family and regret for the error.

Over the years, I have learned that errors like this are so commonplace that having a pharmacist visit a family at home is highly unusual. But this was a small town and I feared that word would get around about this error and customers would be reluctant to have their prescriptions filled in this pharmacy.

During our visit the parents told me that they felt they deserved compensation for the ordeal, including travel expenses and lost wages. I was never told the dollar amount that was agreed upon, but I do know that my boss gave them a check.

14. Two people with the same name

At one store where I worked for a few years, my partner discovered that, to our dismay, there are two customers with the same rather uncommon name. I filled a prescription for Xanax for anxiety for one of these customers. The day before, my partner had filled a prescription for another customer with the same name. That prescription was for methocarbamol, a muscle relaxant. The next day, unknown to both of us, both customers' prescriptions were in the same bin, alphabetized by last name, ready to be picked up.

You guessed it. The prescription I filled for Xanax was picked up by the customer who was supposed to get the methocarbamol. My partner told me that this customer realized something was amiss when she got home and read the drug leaflet that we include with each prescription. It was only when she returned to the pharmacy with the wrong pills that my partner realized that there were two customers with the same name at this store. This was before we had computers which help us catch things like this.

Luckily, this customer seemed to be very understanding and there was no other fallout from this incident. My partner refunded the price of the incorrect medication and gave her the correct medication at no charge. This is company policy whenever a mistake is made.

15. Naproxen instead of Naprelan

A customer called from home and asked, "Is my prescription for Naprelan ready?" I went over to the area where we keep finished prescriptions to check to see if there was a bag for this customer. Indeed there was, but the label on the bag stated naproxen, not Naprelan. These are two very similar drugs used for pain and inflammation. The difference is that naproxen is taken two (or more) times a day whereas Naprelan is taken once a day.

I told the customer on the phone that her prescription was ready and then hurried to correct the medication before she arrived at the store. This error was easy to fix. Had I first noticed the error when the customer was standing in front of me at the pharmacy, it would have taken a little quick thinking to make up an excuse to correct it without the customer realizing that I had discovered an error at that instant. I usually say something innocuous like "Hold on just a minute and let me check one thing." The customer is usually oblivious to what I'm doing because most customers seem to think that errors in the pharmacy are impossible. Quite wrong.

16. Switched drugs: Entex PSE and PCE 500

A tech filled two prescriptions as follows. One was for the antibiotic PCE 500 mg (erythromycin), taken twice a day. The other was for Entex PSE, a drug used for colds, also taken twice a day. The tech filled both prescriptions correctly in every detail except one. She put the PCE 500 in the Entex PSE bottle. And she put the Entex PSE in the PCE 500 bottle. So the medications that the patient would have received were correct but they were in the wrong bottles. In this case, it would likely have resulted in no harm since both tablets are taken twice a day.

17. Monopril instead of minoxidil

At one store where I worked, my partner dispensed Monopril on a prescription that called for minoxidil. Notice that both drug names look and sound somewhat alike. The customer brought back the bottle and asked, "Why do these pills look different from the ones I've been on?" I am not proud of this fact but I lied to this customer in explaining this error made by my partner. I told the customer that the unfamiliar pill was a generic equivalent for the drug the customer had been getting.

We pharmacists often feel that if no harm seems to have occurred, why should we tell the customer that, yes, we screwed up? Of course we correct the error but we don't necessarily admit to the customer what has happened.

In my twenty-five year career as a pharmacist, enforcement fluctuated regarding the policy that we report all errors to corporate headquarters. Sometimes pharmacists were strongly encouraged to report errors to management. At other times, we didn't hear much from our bosses about the need to report errors. Even when the policy of reporting errors was being tightly enforced, many (perhaps most) pharmacists didn't report errors. Pharmacists often felt that since the chain expected us to fill prescriptions so quickly, it was inevitable that mistakes would occur. It was kind of an "us versus them" (pharmacists versus management) attitude. The chains want us to fill prescriptions much more quickly than we're comfortable in doing, so why should we as pharmacists serve up our heads on a platter in our litigious society? Management screws us, so we're just getting even.

In this case with Monopril and minoxidil, both drugs are used for blood pressure. The customer seemed to be doing okay (admittedly a leap of faith on my part) so rather than open a huge can of worms by admitting my partner had given her the wrong drug, I lied to her. I did, of course, give her the correct pills in refilling the prescription.

It is situations like this that most pharmacists dread. Our attitude becomes: *What harm is done by lying ourselves out of a very embarrassing situation that could lead to a lawsuit? If management gave us adequate support staff, errors like this wouldn't happen nearly as often.*

18. A pharmacist was incredibly negligent in adding rubbing alcohol to a child's antibiotic rather than distilled water

Rubbing alcohol is a very toxic substance if swallowed. Some pharmacists routinely use this substance as a disinfectant to clean their prescription counter. These pharmacists often transfer this rubbing alcohol from the manufacturer's stock container into a rubber squeeze container, thus making it easier to spray on the counter. Here's a brief story illustrating what can happen when a floater pharmacist fills in at a pharmacy for another pharmacist's day off (or for sick days, vacation days, jury duty, etc.).

Most children's antibiotics arrive at the pharmacy as a dry powder. When the pharmacist fills a prescription for such an antibiotic, we add distilled water and then shake the container to dissolve the powder and make a nice suspension. For convenience, some pharmacists transfer distilled water from gallon—or larger—containers to smaller containers that are much easier to handle.

I was working for Rite Aid in Hurricane, West Virginia. One day all the pharmacists at neighboring Rite Aid pharmacies were gossiping about how a local relief pharmacist had added rubbing alcohol to the dry powder rather than distilled water. The gossip among pharmacists regarded his incredible negligence in not first ascertaining the contents of the plastic squeeze bottle before adding it to the dry powder. This floater pharmacist assumed that the plastic squeeze container held distilled water. In fact, it contained rubbing alcohol.

Luckily the mother of the child for whom the antibiotic was intended immediately questioned the smell of the medication. Rubbing alcohol has a fairly strong and distinctive odor that should be easy to detect. The child's mother returned the medication to the drugstore before giving a dose to her child. So the child was not harmed in any way.

Though this incident is quite scary, like most errors it did not result in any discipline to the pharmacist responsible. I doubt that most employers would fire a pharmacist for such a mistake, even though our bosses might indeed feel that this pharmacist demonstrated spectacular stupidity in not first determining the contents of the squeeze bottle. This pharmacist simply assumed that it must contain distilled water.

For a better understanding of the potential seriousness of this incident, here's a snippet from *FDA Consumer* that discusses a FDA recall from a manufacturing plant in Puerto Rico. The plant's error is very similar to this pharmacist's mistake. The plant mistakenly attached labels indicating distilled water to containers that actually held rubbing alcohol. (Tom Cramer, "Recall retrieves rubbing alcohol labeled as distilled water," *FDA Consumer*, December 1991. http://findarticles.com/p/articles/mi_m1370/is_n10_v25/ai_11767821 Accessed Nov. 3, 2006)

Thousands of bottles labeled "Agua Destilada" (distilled water) were pulled from pharmacy shelves in Puerto Rico and the Virgin Islands after FDA investigators discovered that a number of the bottles contained rub-

bing alcohol, not distilled water. Five days after the labeling error was discovered, the manufacturing plant responsible was closed and has not reopened. The labeling mix-up could have killed or injured hundreds of children, since the distilled water was labeled for use in preparing infant formula and medicines. An infant can die after consuming formula containing less than half an ounce of rubbing alcohol. However, no injuries were reported in connection with the incident.

OTHER PHARMACISTS' MOST MEMORABLE MISFILLS

A highly abbreviated version of this chapter was published as an editorial that I wrote for *Drug Topics* ("Memorable Misfills of a Retail Pharmacist," April 16, 2007, p. 44). With each editorial I write for this magazine, my e-mail address is included in case any readers care to comment. Several pharmacists e-mailed me with their own most memorable misfills. Here's a sample:

Pharmacist dispenses chili peppers instead of diabetes medication

When I had my pharmacy in West Los Angeles during the 80's, filling 300 to 500 prescriptions per day in a heavily Jewish neighborhood, I had, as an employee pharmacist, one of the fastest and most accurate Rx fillers. I'll call him JT. He could clear the counter in a nanosecond. There was a hot dog stand connected to the outside of my building and JT had the habit of taking a 20 dram vial and filling it with chili peppers so he could snack on them while filling prescriptions. Anyway, JT worked every other day for me so one day, after he had worked, I received an absolutely frantic call from one of my best and oldest customers. She was sobbing, knowing that the story she was about to tell me would be hard to believe. She had picked up her prescription the day before. But when she went to take her prescribed medication that morning, she opened her 20 dram vial to find, not her medication, but eleven chili peppers. "How could this be?" she asked, her voice trembling, for she had paid a hefty price for her medications. At first, I could not believe her and was a bit dismissive. But all of a sudden, in the back of my mind, I remembered JT's habit of filling a vial with chili peppers. What could I say but to convince her that someone had broken into her house in the middle of the night, stole her diabetes medications and replaced it with chili peppers? It took almost an hour and one-half on the phone with her and in the meantime, her prescription was filled correctly and sent out. I was still on the phone with her when my delivery person arrived, and she was so thankful. I was her hero that day and I am ashamed.—[Pharmacist D. S.]

Pharmacist dispenses diet pill with directions "four times a day" instead of "once a day"

My most memorable error was on the typed sig [directions] on a Dexamyl Spansules prescription, a popular diet pill by SK&F (Dextroamphetamine/Amobarbital). Of course, the sig was one a day. I typed four times a day. Gadzooks. The poor woman didn't eat a thing for 2 days. She did not sleep either. When she came in, I confessed and made the correction. This was around 1968. She continued to trade with us. Acted as if nothing had happened.—[Pharmacist J. P.]

Customer requests repeat of pharmacist's mistake in dose of antidepressant

Back in 1988 in Puerto Rico a lady came to the pharmacy to get her Pamelor refilled for the third time. She left and then came back to tell me that I had given her the wrong medicine. I looked at it and I had indeed filled it correctly (Pamelor 10mg). She said "But the one you gave me last month was such and such color." We had given her 25mg Pamelor the previous month! I explained the filling error to her. She then looked at me and said "Look, I have not felt this good for a long time. You have got to misfill it again!" I explained to her that I could not do that. Later that week we got a call from her doctor for a new prescription for Pamelor 25mg!—[Pharmacist P. V.]

Pharmacist dispenses wrong type of alcohol, causing permanent scar on face of young lady

About 1957 when I was a young owner, I employed a much older pharmacist. He supplied isopropyl alcohol on a open call for rubbing alcohol. (Alcohol USP means ethyl alcohol.) The young lady squeezed a zit, dabbed on alcohol, took a nap, and woke up with a burn on the temple area the size of a quarter. My insurance adjuster said juries are very sympathetic to young ladies with scars but he would settle in such a manner that we would keep the customer. Six hundred dollars for plastic surgery did just that and the family remained patients for 42 more years. When I saw the girl, now a grandmother, in the Shop-Rite last year, the scar was still there.—Name withheld by request

---

Pharmacist dispenses gabapentin 600 mg instead of 100 mg

After my editorial titled "When efficiency is all that matters" appeared in Drug Topics *(February 2011, p. 56), I received an email from a Rite Aid pharmacist in Buffalo. In his email he discussed Rite Aid's new fifteen minute guarantee. Customers would be given a five dollar coupon if their prescriptions were not ready within fifteen minutes. This fifteen minute guarantee resulted in a tremendous amount of pharmacist anger directed at Rite Aid in the pharmacy blogosphere from pharmacists working in all settings, including Rite Aid pharmacists. This fifteen minute guarantee puts a tremendous amount of stress on pharmacists and techs, increasing the chance of a serious pharmacy mistake. This pharmacist and I subsequently exchanged a few emails. In one of those emails, I asked him whether he had ever made a serious pharmacy error. He replied:*

A few weeks ago you asked me if I had ever had a serious error. Ironic... Yesterday my DM [district manager] called to tell me I had dispensed a Rx for 100 mg gabapentin as 600 mg. [Gabapentin, the generic for Neurontin, is an antiseizure drug that is also used to treat various neuropathies/neuralgias. It is available in strengths from 100 mg to 800 mg.] I researched it and found that the tech had input [entered into the pharmacy computer] 600 mg and I, on checking, let it get by me. The lady took it for 2 weeks and is in the hospital being weaned off it. I feel like crap!! This is the scenario... It was in hour 10 of a 13 hour day. I had not eaten a thing all day. We had a stack of 35 baskets to input and did 398 Rx's that day. One pharmacist [on duty] all day. At the time of the error [there were only] one input tech and one cashier [on duty]. Put that in your book next to a picture of a pharmacist throwing up. That's my picture.

The other sick part is I tell my DM how much of my day had now been destroyed and she says, "Don't worry, you will get a call from our insurance company. Tell them what happened. I make calls like this all the time. You are not a repeat offender like many are." Didn't make me feel better but what a bunch of crap that is. Interestingly I had a conversation with her about 4 weeks ago about the $5 fiasco [coupon given to customers who have to wait more than fifteen minutes] and told her that someday it will cause a big problem and the story will end up on the front page of the local newspaper and at that point you can kiss Rite Aid business in Buffalo goodbye. I hope I am not that story!!—[Pharmacist in Buffalo]

Two errors posted on "The Student Doctor Network"

Hospital pharmacist misses neonatologist's error in dose of antibiotic vancomycin

I am an overnight pharmacist at a 450-bed hospital. It can get VERY busy. I only have one tech and the nursing staff at my hospital is horrible. I spend 90% of my night answering the most retarded questions. Anyhoo, I have been here a year and I made my first error. I received an antibiotic order from the nursery. The order was for vanco [vancomycin], Claforan and a TPN. I started working on it immediately. Checking doses, volumes, concentrations, etc. Within 2 minutes the nurse calls me, "We just scanned you an order that is super stat!!!! We need it right away!! Did you get it!?" I was slightly annoyed but understood the urgency. Obviously the call distracted me. I told the nurse we would have everything ready in 30 minutes. Three minutes later another nurse calls, "I know we already called you but this really needs to get up here sooner than 30 minutes. The doctor is standing right here, blah blah blah...." So now I am officially pissed and I told the nurse that this is the second interruption I have had trying to process this order. I kindly asked her to not call me anymore. I hung up and ironically I said to my tech "See, this is how mistakes happen!" Long story short, the neonatologist wrote for 100mg/kg of vanco, not 10mg/kg. I missed it too, with all the phone calls I probably bypassed the alert on the computer. The baby was fine when all was said and done but the part that gets me is that they didn't hang the drug until 2 hours later because there was no line access. I know this wasn't entirely my fault but I hate when stuff like this slips past me.

My hospital won't have CPOE [computerized physician order entry] until later this year. So everything is still paper. When I was informed of the error, my director was very explicit that she wasn't blaming me. I am very grateful that I work at an institution that doesn't believe in the "blame and shame" approach to handling errors. For my defense, I simply explained that the excessive phone calls from nursing, in this example and many others, needs to stop. One pharmacist can't process orders and pick up the phone every 2 minutes to be harassed by poorly trained nurses. I am surprised I haven't made any other errors in the past! —**Pharmacist, Miami Beach, Florida** (The Student Doctor Network, Accessed March 27, 2012 http://206.82.221.135/showthread.php?p=12314689)

> ### Pharmacy student explains how patient received
> ### 40 mg of cholesterol-lowering drug lovastatin
> ### for three weeks—instead of 10 mg

My worst error resulted from me trusting the system too much. The days I'm scheduled, I'm the only intern/tech pulling and labeling meds. Usually, there are orders to be filled from 2-3 PM lying around along with the new admissions, so I end up filling about 150 orders in a 4 hour shift by myself. When I get into a groove of filling the orders, I have a tendency to overlook some things.

This particular error, the order was for a card of lovastatin 10 mg. I went to the box of lovastatin 10 mg cards, pulled it, labeled it, and threw it into the basket to be checked. It got checked and sent to the patient, and no one realized the error until 3 weeks later. The patient received lovastatin 40 mg instead of lovastatin 10 mg. The tech who makes all the cards and packs them onto the boxes on the shelves placed the 40 mg cards in the 10 mg box. **—Pharmacy student, Franklin Square, New York** (The Student Doctor Network, http://206.82.221.135/showthread.php?p=12314689 Accessed Mar. 27, 2012)

Chapter 2

The hidden epidemic of pharmacy mistakes in America

Most people view the pharmacist's job as fairly straightforward, uneventful, and even boring. Doctors write prescriptions and pharmacists fill those prescriptions. What could be simpler? Too often, the reality is quite different. Due to competitive pressures in the marketplace, pharmacy has been transformed into a high-speed, high-stress, high-stakes enterprise in which powerful prescription drugs are just a blur on a hamburger assembly line. The big drugstore chains have embraced the McDonald's fast food model with disastrous consequences.

I quit pharmacy after twenty-five years because I was so fed up with slinging out prescriptions as fast as my hands and feet would allow. I am trying to expose the fact that mistakes are far more common in drugstores than patients and physicians realize. Powerful prescription drugs are dispensed across America in a system that is guaranteed to produce errors. The big chain drugstores don't want you to know that pharmacies are purposely understaffed to increase productivity and profitability.

A huge number of pharmacists are disillusioned with the profession and are not recommending pharmacy as a career for their children. A huge number of pharmacists say that they would never have chosen pharmacy as a career if they had known what conditions are like in what we sarcastically refer to as "McPharmacy." This is a reckless system that treats powerful and potentially deadly prescription drugs as if they were no different from any other consumer product in America. The big drugstore chains run their operations as if pharmacists were dispensing nothing more hazardous than a Big Mac at McDonald's or a Slurpee at 7-Eleven.

Many pharmacists feel that the chains have made the cold calculation that it is more profitable to sling out prescriptions at lighting speed and pay customers harmed by mistakes than it is to provide adequate staffing so that mistakes are a rarity rather than a predictable occurrence. Understaffing sometimes forces pharmacists to take educated guesses rather than call doctors to clarify illegible prescriptions. Understaffing sometimes causes pharmacists to override potentially significant drug interactions rather than phone the doctor who prescribed the drugs.

The chain drugstores' obsession with speed increases the occurrence of pharmacy mistakes. Pharmacists are under tremendous pressure to fill prescriptions at unsafe speeds. Drive-thru windows increase mistakes by creating the expectation among customers that prescriptions should be filled as quickly as McDonald's fills burger orders. It is a fact that the speed with which pharmacists fill prescriptions is one of the primary criteria used by chain management in determining whether pharmacists are doing a satisfactory job.

Pharmacists go home at night crossing their fingers and wondering whether all the prescriptions they filled (and supervised techs in filling) that day were filled properly. They say to themselves something like, "Mrs. Jones was in today but I don't even remember checking her prescriptions."

Pharmacists desperately hope that the public will become so enraged as to demand that the chains provide adequate staffing for the safe filling of prescriptions. Understaffing increases pharmacy profitability but it also increases the frequency of serious pharmacy mistakes. Don't allow yourself to become a pharmacy statistic. Let chain management know that the current system is entirely unacceptable. I can state with certainty that the public has no idea how common pharmacy mistakes are today.

As of today, I have written seventeen editorials for *Drug Topics*. I include my e-mail address (dmiller1952@aol.com) with each editorial in case any pharmacists care to comment. A huge number of pharmacists have pleaded with me to try to reach an audience beyond the pharmacists who read that magazine. Pharmacists desperately hope that the general public will be enraged by the common occurrence of pharmacy mistakes. Pharmacists desperately hope that the public will demand that safe staffing levels be given priority over the bottom line.

What would your reaction be if someone told you that there are **OVER FIFTY MILLION MISTAKES IN AMERICA'S PHARMACIES EACH YEAR?** Would you say that's impossible? The reality is that a large study of pharmacy mistakes estimates that "51.5 million errors occur during the filling of 3 billion prescriptions each year." (Eliz. Flynn, et. al., "National Observational Study of Prescription Dispensing Accuracy and Safety in 50 Pharmacies," *Journal of the American Pharmaceutical Assoc.*, March/April 2003, pp. 191-200) Some of the errors are trivial; others are deadly.

Margaret Mulligan, then the editor-in-chief at *Drug Topics*, wrote in the July 2009 issue, "While even one error is one too many, errors happen—to the tune of four errors per 250 scripts filled per day. The chance that a retail customer will receive an incorrectly filled prescription is approximately one in 30; the chance that an error will be clinically important is one in 1,000. How is this still happening in 2009?" (Margaret Mulligan, "System Breakdown: 4 Med Errors, 250 Scripts/Day," *Drug Topics*, July 2009, p. 22)

The following pages describe several very serious pharmacy mistakes that I found in various pharmacy magazines and web searches. Search Google for *pharmacy mistakes* and you will probably be shocked by what you discover. I have included over a dozen cases in which pharmacy mistakes appear to be the direct cause of patient deaths. The cases below are arranged by the size of the monetary award or settlement. I have arbitrarily placed the incidents involving patient deaths together near the middle of this chapter.

Carol Ukens, then a senior editor at *Drug Topics*, described three instances in which pharmacists killed themselves as a result of pharmacy mistakes. (Carol Ukens, "Compounding case leads to R.Ph. suicide," *Drug Topics*, May 6, 2002, pp. 44, 49)

A California pharmacist committed suicide in 2002 after a compounding error was blamed for three deaths. The pharmacist was not present when the error occurred in 2001, but he was a co-owner of the pharmacy where the compounding took place.

Jamey Phillip Sheets, 32, apparently could not accept the punishment meted out by the California pharmacy board for a fatal outbreak of meningitis from a drug compounded in the pharmacy he co-owned. A looming license suspension, five years on probation, and a hefty fine were more than the despondent pharmacist could bear. Late last month, he attached 500 mg of fentanyl patches to his neck and chest and lay down to die.

The Sheets suicide is not an isolated incident. For example, about a year ago, an Oregon pharmacist took her life after an error killed a patient. And about five years ago, a Kentucky pharmacist involved in a fatal error was on his way to the pharmacy board to surrender his license. Instead, he stopped his car and stepped in front of a semitrailer barreling down the Interstate.

Incidents involving pharmacy mistakes seem to be adequately reported by local newspapers and local television stations, but the national media has not, in my opinion, given this subject the coverage that it deserves. A noteworthy exception was a 16-minute segment on ABC News' *20/20* in which Brian Ross went undercover to report on pharmacy mistakes. The segment was titled, "Pharmacy Errors: Unreported Epidemic?" In my opinion that title accurately describes the problem except that the question mark should have been replaced by an exclamation point.
[http://abcnews.go.com/Video/playerIndex?id=2997449 (June 13, 2007)]

Most of the cases described below involve mistakes made at drugstores. A few cases involve mistakes made at hospitals and nursing homes. Notice that the blood thinner Coumadin (warfarin) is involved in a large number of these cases with huge settlements. Since Coumadin is prescribed most commonly in the 5 mg tablet, if your doctor prescribes any dose other than 5 mg, be extra careful that your pharmacy gets it right. Oral drugs for Type II diabetes are also involved in many cases. Used improperly, Type II diabetes drugs can cause seriously low blood sugar levels, sometimes resulting in brain damage.

A study published in 2011 in *The New England Journal of Medicine* by Dr. Dan Budnitz found that blood thinners and diabetes drugs cause most emergency hospital visits for drug reactions among people over 65 in the United States. Most of the hospital emergency visits were for things like unintended overdoses, adverse effects, or allergic reactions. The study does not have a separate category for hospital emergency visits resulting from pharmacy mistakes. Nevertheless, the drugs that cause the most hospitalizations in the Budnitz study are quite similar to the drugs involved in huge awards in pharmacy mistake lawsuits. Anahad O'Connor describes the Budnitz study in *The New York Times*. (Anahad O'Connor, "Four Drugs Cause Most Hospitalizations in Older Adults," *The New York Times*, November 23, 2011 http://well.blogs.nytimes.com/2011/11/23/four-drugs-cause-most-hospitalizations-in-older-adults/):

Just four medications or medication groups—used alone or together—were responsible for two-thirds of emergency hospitalizations among older Americans, according to the report. At the top of the list was warfarin, also known as Coumadin, a blood thinner. It accounted for 33 percent of emergency hospital visits. Insulin injections were next on the list, accounting for 14 percent of emergency visits.

Aspirin, clopidogrel and other antiplatelet drugs that help prevent blood clotting were involved in 13 percent of emergency visits. And just behind them were diabetes drugs taken by mouth, called oral hypoglycemic agents, which were implicated in 11 percent of hospitalizations.

All these drugs are commonly prescribed to older adults, and they can be hard to use correctly. One problem they share is a narrow therapeutic index, meaning the line between an effective dose and a hazardous one is thin.

…Some require blood testing to adjust their doses, and a small dose can have a powerful effect. Blood sugar can be notoriously hard to control in people with diabetes, for example, and taking a slightly larger dose of insulin than needed can send a person into shock. Warfarin, meanwhile, is the classic example of a drug with a narrow margin between therapeutic and toxic doses, requiring regular blood monitoring, and it can interact with many other drugs and foods. ...

One thing that stood out in the data, the researchers noted, was that none of the four drugs identified as frequent culprits are typically among the types of drugs labeled "high risk" for older adults by major health care groups. The medications that are usually designated high risk or "potentially inappropriate" are commonly used over-the-counter drugs like Benadryl, as well as Demerol and other powerful narcotic painkillers. And yet those drugs accounted for only about 8 percent of emergency hospitalizations among the elderly.

Major pharmacy mistakes

How do chain pharmacists react when they read about huge settlements in pharmacy mistake cases? In my experience, many chain pharmacists seem to react positively, figuring that the only thing that will get the attention of chain management is million dollar jury awards. I've heard several pharmacists comment something like, "Well I hope that the media coverage embarrasses the chains into providing adequate staffing so that pharmacy mistakes aren't inevitable."

[Please note: Throughout this book, brand name drugs are capitalized and generic names are in lower case.]

---

1. Walgreen's pharmacist dispensed diabetes drug glipizide instead of gout drug allopurinol, leading to renal failure, stroke and death—$31.3 million award in Illinois

---

A Cook County, Illinois jury awarded $31.3 million to the estate of **Leonard Kulisek**, a Schaumburg man who died in 2002 after becoming ill the previous year when a Walgreens pharmacist gave him the wrong medication. Kulisek was supposed to pick up his gout medication but was given glipizide, a drug used to treat diabetes. The drug dropped his blood sugar to dangerously low levels and triggered a string of health problems, including a stroke in May 2001. ("Wal-

greens to appeal $31 million med-error award," *Drug Topics*, Nov. 6, 2006
http://www.drugtopics.com/drugtopics/article/articleDetail.jsp?id=38 2507&pageID=2)

---

2. Thrifty-Payless drugstore dispensed 100 mg of phenobarbital to girl instead of 15 mg prescribed—brain damage— $30.6 million award in California

A California jury awarded $30.6 million to the family of a girl who suffered brain damage following a phenobarbital dispensing error at a Thrifty Payless drugstore in Costa Mesa in 1994. The jury concluded that **Bryn Cabanillas** suffered brain damage after a Thrifty Payless drugstore dispensed 100 mg of phenobarbital instead of the 15 mg prescribed. The jury decided that the girl, who was born with cerebral palsy, should be paid $5.3 million for past damages and $25.3 million to cover medical costs and other living expenses during her projected 50-year lifespan. The panel found that the error took 20 years off her life. (Carol Ukens, "A jury awards $30 million in Rx error lawsuit," *Drug Topics*, August 3, 1998, p. 15)

---

3. Walgreens dispensed blood thinner warfarin in 10 times the dose prescribed, causing cerebral hemorrhage— $25.8 million award in Florida

A jury awarded $25.8 million to the family of a cancer patient who was given a wrong prescription, had a stroke and died several years later, lawyers said on Aug. 17, 2007. **Beth Hippely** was prescribed warfarin, a blood thinner, in 2002 to treat breast cancer. The prescription filled at a Walgreens pharmacy was 10 times what her doctor prescribed, court documents said. The Polk County [Florida] Circuit Court jury found the prescription error caused a cerebral hemorrhage resulting in permanent bodily injury, disability and physical pain. The mother of three died in January 2007 at the age of 46. A 19-year-old pharmacy technician, with little training, misfilled the prescription, according to court documents. "Beth Hippely died unnecessarily because this tenfold overdose with warfarin by the pharmacy she trusted caused her cancer to come back with a vengeance and it interrupted all of her cancer treatments," her lawyer Chris Searcy said. (Associated Press, Bartow, Florida, Aug. 18, 2007, http://www.cbsnews.com/stories/2007/08/18/business/main318097 9.shtml)

---

4. Walgreens dispensed adult diabetes drug glipizide to infant girl instead of anti-seizure drug phenobarbital— $21 million judgment in Illinois

A prescription medicine Tracey Gehrke got from a Walgreens in Illinois was supposed to prevent seizures in her infant daughter, who had been born prematurely. The pharmacy instead filled **Alexandra Gehrke**'s prescription with an adult diabetes drug. A Cook County jury awarded $21 million to the Gehrke family, of Elgin. (Michael Higgins, "A $21 Million Judgment Against Walgreens in the Case of a Paralyzed Elgin Girl Points Up Potential Dangers in 3 Million Annual Pharmacy Errors," chicagotribune.com, August 11, 2004)

---

5. Pharmacist prepared contaminated chemotherapy, causing paralysis—$18.5 million jury award in New Jersey

A New Jersey Superior court jury awarded $18.5 million to a man who was paralyzed from the waist down after he received contaminated chemotherapy treatment for leukemia. The jury found Eun Mi Jhun, the pharmacist who prepared the contaminated medication, responsible for the paralysis. The contaminated dose was injected into the spine of **Anton Weck** in 2001, resulting in his paralysis. Weck had previously been undergoing chemotherapy for three years and was receiving his final dose at the time he was paralyzed. (http://www.totalinjury.com/verdicts_medical_injury.asp)

---

6. Rite Aid pharmacist dispensed adult diabetes drug Glynase to young girl instead of Ritalin—brain damage—$16 million award

A young girl who suffered brain damage as a result of a dispensing error by a Rite Aid pharmacist was awarded $16 million in damages under a jury verdict. Instead of Ritalin to treat the child's attention deficit disorder, the pharmacist dispensed Glynase—a drug used to reduce blood sugar levels in diabetics. ("Newsbites," *Drug Store News*, November 4, 1996, p. 15.)

7. Pharmacy dispensed anti-asthma drug theophylline to nursing home patient instead of pain killer Darvocet— $15 million settlement

A pharmacist phoned a nursing home to inform the staff that the wrong drug had been sent to one of the home's patients. He explained that pharmacy technicians mistakenly filled a prescription for the pain killer Darvocet with the anti-asthma drug theophylline. The patient deteriorated, and he ultimately died. The patient's family sued, claiming the wrong drug caused seizures, a reversal in his recovery, and ultimately, his death. On the eve of the defendant's motion to dismiss the wrongful death action, the parties settled for $15 million. (Health Providers Service Organization–HPSO. (1999). Pharmacy. Medical Malpractice, Verdicts, Settlements, and Experts, 18(7), 41
http://www.hpso.com/newsletters/1-2000/pharm2.shtml#lesson)

8. Baby died after hospital pharmacy error caused fatal dose of IV sodium chloride—$8.25 million settlement in Illinois

Born 15 weeks premature, **Genesis Burkett** survived despite weighing just 1 pound, 8 ounces. But the little boy couldn't survive a medication mistake made at a suburban hospital that gave him the wrong IV dosage and took his life when he was 40 days old. Advocate Lu-

theran General Hospital in Park Ridge has agreed to settle his parents' wrongful-death lawsuit for $8.25 million—the largest such settlement ever in Illinois, according to the parents' lawyers. Fritzie and Cameron Burkett, of Chicago, are relieved the hospital acknowledged the error that killed their only child, their attorney said Thursday. "They're grateful the hospital recognized their significant loss," Patrick Salvi said. "They hope it never happens again." Genesis Burkett died at the hospital on Oct. 15, 2010, after receiving a fatal dose of sodium chloride in an IV administered to him after heart surgery. The suit claimed an error made by the hospital pharmacy resulted in Genesis getting a dose 60 times the amount that was prescribed by the boy's doctor, causing the infant to go into cardiac arrest and die. "The pharmacy made a critical mistake," Salvi said. A hospital investigation showed the mistake occurred because the dosage for the boy's IV "had been incorrectly entered into the machine that mixes IV solutions," Lutheran General spokesman Greg Alford said. Since his death, the hospital has changed procedures to prevent similar mistakes, according to Alford, who said, "We have taken comprehensive steps . . .to ensure this type of tragedy does not happen again." (Dan Rozek, "Couple whose baby died from wrong IV dose gets $8.25 million," *Chicago Sun Times*, April 5, 2012
http://www.suntimes.com/news/metro/11730830-418/couple-whose-baby-died-from-wrong-iv-dose-gets-825-million.html)

---

9. Thrift Drug pharmacist dispensed double the maximum allowable dose of Rocaltrol—$8 million award in Pennsylvania

A Pittsburgh jury awarded **Michael Brown** $8 million in a drug error lawsuit against J. C. Penney, parent of Thrift Drug. The suit alleged that a Thrift pharmacist mistranscribed a telephone prescription for Rocaltrol, synthetic vitamin D. As a result, Brown, then 17, received a dosage that was double the maximum allowable. He went into hypercalcemic crisis and is totally disabled by seizures. ("Jury awards $8 million in drug error suit," *Drug Topics*, October 7, 1996, p. 7.)

> ## 10. Pharmacy error causes kidney transplant patient to take 1,250 mg of prednisone daily for 3 days, instead of 250 mg daily—loss of kidney—$7.7 million award in South Carolina

Late in 2006, a jury delivered a verdict ordering Eckerd Corporation to pay Ms. **Tiffany Phillips** $7.7 million for a pharmacy error which resulted in the loss of the young woman's new kidney. CVS, also a named defendant in the action, reached a confidential settlement with Phillips for an undisclosed amount. In 2002, plaintiff Tiffany Phillips went to the Eckerd pharmacy in Lancaster, South Carolina, to get a prescription filled for an anti-rejection drug (prednisone) in connection with a recent kidney transplant. The Lancaster Eckerd didn't have enough of the medication on site, so a pharmacy technician called a Lancaster CVS pharmacy to fill the entire prescription. However, an apparent miscommunication between the two stores occurred, resulting in Ms. Phillips being instructed to take 1250 milligrams a day of the drug for three days, over four times the intended amount of 250 milligrams. After taking the drug dispensed to her, Phillip's new kidney failed and she underwent a second kidney transplant. [*The Charlotte Observer*, Dec. 21, 2006, Page 1B. See also grossmanjustice.com (Law Offices of Scott. D. Grossman, LLC, Freehold, New Jersey, posted on March 28, 2007 by Scott Grossman), http://injurylaw.grossmanjustice.com/2007/03/articles/pharmacy-error/pharmacy-error-case-results-in-8-million-verdict/]

> ## 11. Pharmacy failed to dilute adult medication—infant received massive overdose of high blood pressure drug enalaprilat— $7.1 million award in Massachusetts

A Suffolk County, Mass. jury awarded $7.1 million in damages to the family of **Joey Rice**, a 4-year old Newton boy who, as a premature infant, received a massive overdose of the high blood pressure drug enalaprilat after pharmacists at Children's Hospital in Boston failed to dilute an adult medication. The dose had more than 100 times the proper amount. (Anne Barnard, "Family Awarded $7.1m for Overdose, *The Boston Globe,* March 28, 2002)

12. Death of two-year-old Ohio girl after pharmacy improperly compounded intravenous solution—$7 million settlement

An Ohio grand jury has indicted pharmacist Eric Cropp for manslaughter and reckless homicide in the death of a two-year-old child, which resulted from an improperly compounded IV solution. Both charges carry penalties of up to five years in prison. The medical error occurred in 2006 at Rainbow Babies & Children's Hospital where the child, **Emily Jerry**, was a patient undergoing chemotherapy. According to testimony presented before the Ohio board of pharmacy, the prescription for etoposide with a base solution of 0.9% sodium chloride was instead compounded by a technician with a base solution of 23.4% sodium chloride. Three days after receiving the medication, the child died. The grand jury declined to indict the technician, Katie Dudash. (Reid Paul, "Former pharmacist indicted for manslaughter after med error," *Drug Topics*, Sept. 17, 2007, p. 10. See also the Emily Jerry Foundation emilyjerryfoundation.org and http://emilyjerryfoundation.org/man-seeks-nationwide-law-after-toddlers-death/)

13. Walgreens dispensed female hormone Cycrin to a male rather than the prescribed blood thinner Coumadin— $6 million settlement in Florida

The insurance carrier for Walgreens agreed to pay $6 million to settle a dispensing error lawsuit in Daytona Beach, Fla. A Walgreens pharmacy dispensed Cycrin, a female hormone, to the plaintiff, **E. Nathan Johnson**, instead of the Coumadin prescribed. He took the wrong drug for eleven days before his wife discovered the error. Two days later, he suffered a stroke and subsequently a heart attack that left him in a coma. He now resides in a special care facility. "Walgreen settles Rx suit," *Drug Topics*, October 7, 1996, p. 7.)

---

14. Thirty-one year-old high school wrestling coach dies from interaction between tramadol and methadone— Walgreen's in Arizona—$6 million award

Most prescription errors don't cause major health problems, but the outcomes occasionally can be catastrophic. Walgreens has lost three trials involving deaths caused by drug mistakes since September 2006. Verdicts in the cases totaled more than $61 million. The cases include the 2002 death of **Eric Warren**, a 31-year-old Arizona high school wrestling coach. He died from an interaction between tramadol and methadone, painkillers dispensed at different times by a Walgreens pharmacy in Flagstaff, Ariz. A jury awarded his family $6 million in October 2007 after hearing evidence that Walgreens pharmacist Al Salembier neither warned Warren about the potential drug interaction nor double-checked the second prescription with his doctor. Walgreens is appealing the case. (Kevin McCoy and Erik Brady, "Speed, High Volume Can Trigger Mistakes," *USA Today*, 2/11/08, http://www.usatoday.com/money/industries/health/2008-02-11-pre-scrption-errors_N.htm   Accessed March 16, 2008)

15. Pharmacy dispensed .025 mg of the synthetic thyroid hormone Synthroid to 71-yr-old man instead of .125 mg— $5 million settlement in Texas

A 71-year-old man was given a prescription for .125 mg Synthroid #100. His pharmacy filled it with .025 Synthroid #100. Due to the error, the patient suffered respiratory distress and weakness. The man sued and the case was settled for $5 million plus taxable costs. (Health Providers Service Organization–HPSO. Staff. 1998. Pharmacy. Medical Malpractice, Verdicts, Settlements, and Experts, 14(8), 54. http://www.hpso.com/newsletters/6-99/pharm1.html#court)

---

16. Amphotericin ordered for child with infection following appendectomy prepared in adult dosage, instead of child dosage—Cardiac arrest and renal failure—$3.85 million settlement includes $200,000 to child's sister, who witnessed arrest

The plaintiff, age nine, was taken to a hospital in August 2006 due to an infection after the removal of her appendix. The antifungal drug, Amphotericin, was prescribed, but the hospital's pharmacy prepared an adult dose rather than one for a child. Shortly after taking the drug intravenously, the child went into cardiac arrest and renal failure with her seven year-old sister watching. She was resuscitated after being given blood transfusions and then transferred to another hospital for a six-week stay. The child suffers post-traumatic stress disorder, but has no physical sequella from the incident. According to a published account a $3.85 million settlement was reached, which included $200,000 to the sister who witnessed the arrest.
(April 2010 Legal Case Study, HPSO—Healthcare Providers Service Organization
http://www.hpso.com/case-studies/casestudy-article/328.jsp)

17. Dilaudid prescription filled with dexamethasone—Cushing's Syndrome and depression—$2.5 million verdict

The plaintiff had rheumatoid arthritis and obtained a prescription for Dilaudid from her physician in November 2006. She took it to the pharmacy to be filled. The plaintiff was dispensed dexamethasone. After a couple of weeks the plaintiff noted that her pain continued. She returned to the pharmacy and was told that the prescription was correct. She continued to have pain and went to her physician, who immediately realized the error. The plaintiff was referred to another physician who gave her a prescription to taper the dosage of the dexamethasone to wean her off gradually. The plaintiff, however, suffered depression, psychiatric disorders, brain damage, cognitive damage, exacerbation of her previous medical problems and Cushing's

Syndrome. The plaintiff declined from an active lifestyle to wheelchair confinement. The plaintiff alleged negligence in dispensing the medication. The defendant admitted negligence, but disputed any long-term, permanent injuries. According to the *Jury Verdict Reporter,* a $2.5 million verdict was returned. (July 2010 Legal Case Study, HPSO—Healthcare Providers Service Organization, http://www.hpso.com/case-studies/casestudy-article/331.jsp)

---

18. Pharmacy confusion caused patient to consume 320 mg of prednisone daily for weeks instead of 80 mg daily— $2.5 million award in North Carolina

---

The defendant physician intended to prescribe an 80 mg daily dose of prednisone for the plaintiff's loss of kidney function. The pharmacist who received the prescription claimed that it indicated that 80 mg be taken 4 times a day, for a daily total of 320 mg. After receiving the first refill, the patient went to the emergency room and was diagnosed with thrush. He continued taking the 320 mg of prednisone daily for 23 days, until a follow-up visit with the physician revealed the dosage error. The plaintiff contracted a bacterial infection of the lungs and aspergillosis, a fungal infection of the brain, resulting in numerous operations and hospital stays. The plaintiff suffered permanent kidney failure and will require dialysis for the rest of his life. He sued the physician and the clinic for negligently writing the prescription and the pharmacy chain for negligence in dispensing the drug. Following the trial against the pharmacy chain, the jury awarded the plaintiff $2.5 million in compensatory damages. The appellate court upheld the verdict. (Larry M. Simonsmeier, JD, RPh, "The Dosage Was Too High, No Matter Where the Rx Was Filled," *Pharmacy Times,* December 2002 http://www.pharmacytimes.com/Article.cfm?Menu=1&ID=288 Accessed March 9, 2006)

19. Medication error in child with Urea Cycle Syndrome results in excessive blood ammonia levels and brain damage— $2.5 million settlement in New Jersey

At the age of two and four months, the child experienced severe hyperammonemia requiring hospitalization. The correct protocol was ordered, but prepared in an incorrect concentration by the hospital pharmacist. The patient's nurse then elevated an IV bag containing the prepared formula, but failed to compare the label on the bag (prepared by the pharmacist) with the written order from the physician. As a result, the patient received only twenty-five percent of the required medication over a period of nineteen hours. This undermedication situation resulted in escalating and dangerously high blood ammonia levels. When the error was discovered, the hospital failed to timely perform hemodialysis to remove the high levels of ammonia from the blood. The patient went into coma and was airlifted to another hospital for treatment. He suffered permanent brain injury as a result of the medication error. Eight years old at the time of settlement, the child is permanently disabled and has a seizure disorder. The case settled tor $2,500,000. ("Medication Error in Child With Urea Cycle Syndrome Results in Excessive Blood Ammonia Levels and Brain Damage—$2.5 Million Settlement in New Jersey," January 2003 Legal Case Study, Healthcare Providers Service Organization, http://www.hpso.com/case/cases_prof_index.php3?id=70&prof=Ph armacist Grecco v. Unnamed Hospital, Essex County, New Jersey, Superior Court)

20. Death: Wal-Mart pharmacist dispensed Ziac instead of Zaroxolyn—$1.27 million award

The Arkansas Supreme Court upheld a $1.27 million jury award for a woman whose husband died after a Wal-Mart pharmacist gave him the wrong prescription medication, which he took for two and a half months before his death. Wal-Mart's lawyers had appealed the earlier verdict, saying there was insufficient evidence of the cause of his death and that the award to his widow and daughter was excessive. The man died in 1997 after a Wal-Mart R.Ph. in Arkansas filled his prescription for Zaroxolyn, a diuretic, with Ziac, a high blood pressure medication. The drug allowed fluid to accumulate in his body and caused severe weight gain. He died of congestive heart failure. ("Court upholds jury award in Wal-Mart death case," *Drug Topics,* July 14, 2003 http://www.drugtopics.com/be_core/d/templates/issue/show_article. jsp?stylesheet=/be_core/d/stylesheets/xslt/view_free_pages.xsl&file-name=/be_core/d/online_only_content/free_pages/latehot.xml&sho wPoll=no)

---

21. Pregnant woman's prescription for Medrol filled with dexamethasone—Child born with multiple problems— $1.1 million settlement

---

The plaintiff mother was prescribed Medrol in a two-milligram dose for a pulmonary problem in May 2005 when she was five months pregnant. The plaintiff claimed that the defendant's pharmacist filled the prescription with Dexamethasone, which should not be taken during pregnancy and that the four-milligram dose was twenty times the normal amount for that drug. The woman's son was born prematurely, weighing two pounds and suffers from severe growth retardation, impaired speech, motor weakness and esophagitis as a result of the pharmacy error. The woman continued to take the wrong drug until March 2006, when her physician made an investigation after she developed swelling problems. The defendant claimed that the pharmacy error was caused by the woman's physician and that the child's problems were due to the mother's pre-eclampsia. According to a published account, a $1.1 million settlement was reached, most of which was placed into a structured settlement for the child. ("Pregnant woman's prescription for Medrol filled with dexamethasone—Child born with multiple problems—$1.1 million settlement," Health Providers Service Organization, January 2011 Legal Case Study, http://www.hpso.com/case-studies/casestudy-article/339.jsp)

---

22. K-Mart's labeling instructed 20 mg of the blood thinner Coumadin per day instead of 5 mg per day— Overdose caused complications from hip surgery— $1.05 million verdict in Indiana

Dr. Alan Glock, then age fifty-nine, had been an orthopedic surgeon since the middle 1960's. In the fall of 1997, severe osteoarthritic changes necessitated a hip replacement which was performed on October 2, 1997 by Dr. Jeffrey Pierson. On October 5, 1997, Dr. Glock was discharged from the hospital with a prescription for Coumadin, a blood-thinning drug. He was advised to take one pill daily. The prescription was filled at K-Mart and store employees indicate Dr. Glock was advised to take one five milligram pill per day. Despite this warning, K-Mart's labeling instructed that the five milligram pills should be taken four times daily. As a result of the excessive Coumadin intake, the plaintiff's recovery from the hip surgery was prolonged for an additional three months, which otherwise would not have occurred. The plaintiff continues to report additional complex symptoms, all resulting from the overdose of Coumadin, and he has been unable to return to the practice of medicine. The problems include intra-cranial bleeding, with resulting vision and hearing problems, and a compartment syndrome in his hip. ("Instructions for Coumadin Written on Bottle Incorrectly—Overdose Causes Complications From Hip Surgery—$1,052,461 Verdict in Indiana," June 2002 Legal Case Study, Healthcare Providers Service Organization http://www.hpso.com/case/cases_prof_index.php3?id=63&prof=Ph armacist Alan Glock and Carolyn Glock v. K-Mart, U.S. District Court, District of Indiana at Indianapolis, Case No.99 CV 1184)

---

23. Patient given 900 mg of anti-seizure drug Dilantin daily for several days instead of 300 mg daily—Dilantin toxicity blamed for acceleration of dementia—$1 Million verdict in Alabama

The plaintiff, a seventy-seven year-old man, alleged that the staff at the defendant Birmingham hospital overmedicated him with anti-seizure medication so severely in 1999 that his dementia was accelerated, and he suffered additional brain damage and damage to his sense of balance. He claimed that during a May 26 through June 1, 1999 hospitalization at Baptist Medical Center Montclair, after a fall at his home, he was given more than three times the dose of Dilantin than what his physician prescribed. Robert Ferguson testified that he was able to drive, hunt, fish, and walk on his own prior to the hospitalization. But the overdose left him with severely altered memory, and dependent on a cane and wheelchair. ("Nurse and Pharmacy Staff Err in Administering Treble Dose of Dilantin—Dilantin Toxicity Blamed for Acceleration of Dementia and Damage to Balance—$1 Million Verdict in Alabama," August 2003 Legal Case Study, Healthcare Providers Service Organization http://www.hpso.com/case/cases_prof_index.php3 Robert Ferguson v. Baptist Health System d/b/a Baptist Medical Center, Montclair. Jefferson County, Alabama.)

---

24. Plaintiff claims improper pharmacy directions caused him to ingest 100 mg of prednisone daily for 17 days (instead of for 5 days)—$1 million New York settlement

---

In January 1995, the defendants dispensed the steroid prednisone to the plaintiff, a thirty-six-year-old electrician. The plaintiff claimed that the defendants failed to properly label the prescription, which should have instructed him to ingest 100 milligrams of prednisone daily for five days only. The plaintiff ingested 100 milligrams for nearly seventeen days, and he then required additional prednisone for a gradual taper from the medication. The plaintiff claimed that defendants also altered the strength of the tablets prescribed—instead of dispensing fifty tablets, each containing ten milligrams, defendants dispensed fifty tablets, each containing fifty milligrams, resulting in the plaintiff ingesting an additional 1670 milligrams of prednisone than was intended by his oncologist. He subsequently developed avascular necrosis of the hips, which, he claimed, was a direct result of the excess medication ingested. The plaintiff requires bilateral hip replacements. According to The New York Jury Verdict Reporter, this action settled for $1,000,000 during trial. ("Improper Labeling of Prescription—Overdose of Prednisone—Bilateral Avascular Necrosis of the Hips—$1

Million New York Settlement," June 2000 Legal Case Study, Healthcare Providers Service Organization, http://www.hpso.com/case/cases_prof_index.php3?id=19&prof=Ph armacist   John and Rose Marie Oliver v. Evkin Pharmacy Corp., Ralph Ekstrand and Vincent Conte, Nassau County (NY) Supreme Court, Index No. 18963/97)

---

25. Pharmacy mistake results in patient taking 1800 mg of the bipolar disorder drug lithium daily (instead of the prescribed 900 mg daily)—Failure to notice signs of lithium toxicity lead to death—$1 Million settlement

---

A pharmacy error and the failure to notice signs and lithium toxicity lead to the death of 51 year-old woman. The decedent was a mentally retarded woman who died from lithium toxicity on May 13, 2002. She had been a resident at the defendant residential home from 1992 until her death in 2002. On April 13, 2002, the defendant pharmacy and pharmacist incorrectly filled the decedent's lithium prescription, dispensing lithium carbonate 300 mg capsules instead of the prescribed lithium carbonate 150 mg capsules. This mistake resulted in decedent consuming 1800 mg of lithium carbonate daily, instead of the prescribed 900 mg daily dosage, prior to her death. The case was settled for one million dollars during litigation with the pharmacy, pharmacist and residential home defendants. The case remains ongoing against the primary care physician and psychiatrist regarding failure to notice signs of lithium toxicity. ("$1M settlement for medication error, lithium toxicity," 2006 Medical Malpractice Settlement Report, Medical Malpractice Attorneys Lubin & Meyer PC, 100 City Hall Plaza, Boston, MA 02108, http://www.lubinandmeyer.com/cases/lithium.html)

---

26. Death of cancer patient in Ohio—Pharmacist indicted for allegedly dispensing an overdose of chemotherapy drugs

---

An Ohio pharmacist was indicted by a grand jury for allegedly dispensing an overdose of chemotherapy drugs that led to the death of a cancer patient. Daniel Scott, 41, a longtime pharmacist at Riverside Mercy Hospital in Toledo, was charged with one count of involuntary manslaughter in the death of **Lyle Ganske** on July 11, 2000. Prosecutors charged that Scott quadrupled the dosages of Adriamycin (doxorubicin HCl, Pharmacia) and vincristine he dispensed at the Riverside Mercy Home Pharmacy Services outpatient facility. The chemotherapy error was triggered when a nurse rewrote the physician's original order, said James Brazeau, an attorney who represented Scott before the pharmacy board. He said that the physician's order called for only one dose spread out over four days, but, in a phone call, a nurse indicated that the dose was to be "times four days," Brazeau said. The pharmacist interpreted that to mean a dose for each of four days. (Carol Ukens, "Ohio pharmacist indicted in Rx error death," *Drug Topics*, November 19, 2001, p. 22)

---

27. Death of 8-year-old Virginia girl after Demerol (meperidine) prescription filled with Roxanol (morphine)

Two days after getting her tonsils out, 8-year-old **Megan Colleen McClave** told her father in a raspy voice that her throat was aching. So Mike McClave went over to the kitchen cupboard and got out a bottle of prescription medicine he had filled at a local pharmacy. He mixed a couple of teaspoons into a glass of cherry-flavored 7-Up, remembering that Megan earlier had spit out the pain killer because it was bitter and "yucky." This time she slowly sipped about half the mixture. She felt sick and drowsy, but she watched a movie on television, made Jell-O with her dad and took a few more sips of the 7-Up mixture before crawling into bed for the night. The next morning, Megan never woke up. Because of a horrible mistake by a Newport News pharmacist, Megan was not given the standard pain-dulling medication her doctor had prescribed, but a powerful morphine-based compound typically used to comfort terminally ill cancer patients. ("Pharmacist's Mistake Costs 8-Year-Old Hampton Girl Her Life," *The Virginian-Pilot*, October 31, 1994, page B5, Source: Associated Press, Dateline: Hampton, Va.   http://scholar.lib.vt.edu/VA-news/VA-Pilot/issues/1994/vp941031/10310070.htm)

28. Death of Connecticut woman—Lawsuit filed alleging pharmacy caused fatal mix-up by dispensing opium tincture instead of paregoric. Opium tincture contains 25 times as much morphine as paregoric.

The family of a Connecticut woman filed a lawsuit alleging that she died because a community pharmacist dispensed opium tincture instead of camphorated opium tincture, which is commonly known as paregoric. **Donna Marie Altieri**'s physician wrote a prescription for one teaspoon of "tincture of opium camphorated" for her chronic diarrhea on June 15, 2001. The 51-year-old grandmother took the prescription to a CVS drugstore in Southington, where it was filled. However, the script was misfilled with opium tincture, which contains 25 times as much morphine as paregoric. The next day, she took one dose then complained of feeling weak, tired, and achy and went to sleep. She never woke up. An emergency room physician said Altieri probably died of a heart attack. One of her two sons found that hard to believe and became suspicious. He asked for an autopsy. Two months later, the coroner ruled her death was due to accidental morphine intoxication. (Carol Ukens, "Lawsuit alleges fatal paregoric mix-up," *Drug Topics*, March 18, 2002, http://www.drugtopics.com/drugtopics/article/articleDetail.jsp?id=116571)

29. Death of 5-year-old Virginia boy after 500 mg of imipramine dispensed (for bedwetting) instead of 100 mg

A five-year-old Virginia boy died as a result of an order entry and compounding error that was not caught by the usual check system. In this case, imipramine was dispensed in a concentration five times greater than prescribed. Imipramine is a tricyclic antidepressant used to treat adults, but it is also used to treat childhood enuresis (bedwetting). A technician entered the concentration into the computer as 50 mg/mL instead of 50 mg/5mL, along with the prescribed directions to give 2 teaspoonfuls at bedtime. He then mixed the solution using the incorrect concentration on the label and placed the prescription in a holding area to await a pharmacist's verification. The high work-load made it impossible for the pharmacist to check the prescription right away. When the child's mother came in to pick up the prescription, the clerk was unaware that it had not been checked and gave it to the mother without telling a pharmacist. At bedtime, the mother gave the child two teaspoons of the drug (500 mg instead of the intended 100 mg) and found him dead the next morning. An autopsy confirmed imipramine poisoning. (Institute for Safe Medication Practices, "Tragic community pharmacy error—one year after owner talks about workload stresses to *NY Times*," August 23, 2000 http://www.ismp.org/MSAarticles/Tragic.html)

---

30. Death of man given wrong directions on insulin—
Ten times the prescribed dose

The decedent went to the doctor to obtain some insulin for his diabetes. Several days after seeing the doctor, the decedent overdosed from the prescribed insulin. The decedent was in a coma in a nursing home and on a ventilator for two months prior to his death. The plaintiff claimed that the prescription given to the decedent was a different brand from what the decedent had been using. The plaintiff also claimed that the prescription was written for twenty units in the morning and ten units in the evening, but the pharmacy filled the prescription for 200 units in the morning and 100 units in the evening. (Healthcare Providers Service Organization, January 2007 Legal Case Study, http://www.hpso.com/case/cases_prof_index.php3?id=118&prof=Pharmacist)

---

31. Death of baby girl after dose of zinc
dispensed is one thousand times larger than
neonatologist ordered at Las Vegas hospital

It was a simple miscalculation. Yet the error slipped through the hands of three pharmacists and several nurses at a Las Vegas hospital, leading to the death of a premature baby girl. The error leading to the death of three-week-old **Alyssa Shinn** on Nov. 9, 2006 certainly served as a wake-up call to Summerlin Hospital Medical Center, the facility where the mistake occurred. The breakdown that resulted in Alyssa Shinn's death began with the mishandling of the infant's prescription by hospital pharmacist Pamela Goff. In her testimony to the pharmacy board, Goff tearfully admitted she selected the wrong unit of zinc for the infant's TPN IV bag, choosing 330 mg rather than 330 mcg—a dose 1,000 times larger than Shinn's neonatologist had ordered. ("Infant death leads to changes at Las Vegas hospital," Michael Barbella, *Drug Topics*, Sept. 3, 2007, p. 18)

---

32. Death in Michigan is apparently caused by tenfold analgesic dosage error

---

Tenfold drug administration errors are common and pernicious in healthcare systems, but they could be almost entirely eliminated. They occur when a decimal placement is written incorrectly or misread. Decimal errors can result in a 10-fold, 100-fold, or even 1,000-fold overdose or underdose. Combine dosage danger with the fact that the cure can sometimes be worse than the dilemma, and you have the sad case of what appears to have happened at Botsford General Hospital in Farmington Hills, Mich. A recent lawsuit alleges that a hospital patient received a 10-fold overdose of an analgesic, which resulted in a dangerous drop in blood pressure. As a result of an attempt to treat that condition, the patient became paralyzed and died. But it was the decimal error that apparently killed him. (Martin Sipkoff, *Drug Topics*—Health-System Edition, Aug. 21, 2006 http://www.drugtopics.com/drugtopics/article/articleDetail.jsp?id=36 5727)

---

33. Three deaths attributed to colchicine compounded by Texas pharmacy

---

The Oct. 12, 2007 issue of *Morbidity & Mortality Weekly Report* describes three deaths attributed to a Texas compounding pharmacy error resulting from an eightfold overdose in patients seeking off-label treatment with IV colchicine for back pain. Toxicology reports showed the colchicine vials contained 4 mg/ml instead of the 0.5 mg/ml indicated on the label; therefore, the intended 2-mg dose was actually 16 mg. Bonnel et. al. (*J Emerg Med*, 2002) showed that deaths have been reported with cumulative doses of colchicine as low as 5.5 mg. According to *MMWR*, the deaths underscore the potentially fatal ramifications of errors by compounding pharmacies, which generally are not subject to the same oversight and manufacturing practices as pharmaceutical manufacturers. In response to the incident, the Texas State Board of Pharmacy, in cooperation with the FDA, issued a recall of all colchicine that had been sold or produced by the compounding pharmacy within the past year. ("*MMWR* reports on colchicine deaths due to compounding error: Three deaths determined to be result of colchicine toxicity," October 15, 2007, *Drug Topics* Daily News www.drugtopics.com/drugtopics/article/articleDetail.jsp?id=465163)

---

34. Three deaths blamed on compounded betamethasone— California pharmacist commits suicide

Jamey Phillip Sheets, 32, apparently could not accept the punishment meted out by the California pharmacy board for a fatal outbreak of meningitis from a drug compounded in the pharmacy he co-owned. A looming license suspension, five years on probation, and a hefty fine were more than the despondent pharmacist could bear. In 2002, he attached 500 mg of fentanyl patches to his neck and chest and lay down to die. The downward spiral that ended in Sheets' suicide began in 2001 when a meningitis outbreak was traced to betamethasone compounded in a pharmacy he co-owned. The contaminated drug mixed in Doc's Pharmacy in Walnut Creek was blamed for three deaths and 13 hospitalizations. The meningitis outbreak triggered a heavy media barrage and public outrage aimed at the pharmacy and the practice of compounding. And that put the pharmacy board under heavy pressure to discipline those responsible for the contamination. (Carol Ukens, "Compounding case leads to R.Ph. suicide," *Drug Topics*, May 6, 2002, pp. 44, 49)

---

35. Death after Maryland pharmacy allegedly dispensed wrong strength of Humulin—Wal-Mart settles wrongful death suit due to insulin overdose

On December 13, 2005, **Keith Scofield** visited a Wal-Mart pharmacy in Frederick, Maryland, and ordered over-the-counter Humulin R (U-100). Instead, he was allegedly given Humulin R (U-500), a prescription drug that contains five times the insulin of the requested medication. He injected the insulin on December 20, 2005, lapsed into a diabetic coma, and died on January 2, 2006, according to a lawsuit filed by his family. The suit was settled during mediation without admission of liability or fault. (Linda von Wartburg, "Wal-Mart Settles Wrongful Death Suit Due to Insulin Overdose," *Diabetes Health*, Aug 7, 2007 http://www.diabeteshealth.com/read/2007/08/07/5361.html Source: *Business Week*, July 2007)

---

36. Pharmacy failed to dispense correct number of Risperdal tablets for psychosis—Child commits suicide due to lack of drug—$875,000 gross verdict

The decedent, age twelve, was discharged from the hospital in September 2002 with a diagnosis of psychosis no.5./schizophrenia. She was discharged with a prescription for a thirty-day supply of Risperdal, consisting of ninety .025 milligram tablets. Her mother filled the prescription on the day after discharge at a pharmacy. On the tenth day there was only one tablet remaining and the mother contacted the pharmacy about the shortage. The child went without medication for four days and committed suicide by hanging herself with a jump rope. A verdict for $875,000 was returned with the mother being found twenty-five percent contributorily negligent in not noticing any shortage earlier. ("Failure to Dispense Correct Number of Pills for Prescription for Risperdal—Child Commits Suicide Due to Lack of Drug—$875,000 Gross Verdict," September 2006 Legal Case Study, Healthcare Providers Service Organization,

http://www.hpso.com/case/cases_prof_index.php3?id=114&prof=P
harmacist)

**37. Three-year-old dies after pharmacist prepares
over ten times prescribed dose of arginine—
$850,000 settlement in Florida**

ORLANDO, Fla. (AP)–Edna Irizarry, a pharmacist who filled a prescription that led to the death of a Florida boy, faced disciplinary action from the Florida Board of pharmacy for processing a prescription for 3-year-old **Sebastian Ferrero**, who died in October 2007. Ferrero died at a Shands hospital in Gainesville, two days after a routine test was supposed to help doctors determine why the boy's growth was below average. Instead of receiving the prescribed dose of 5.75 grams of the amino acid arginine, officials said the Shands Medical Outpatient Pharmacy gave him more than 60 grams. Hospital workers at Shands administered the arginine, and did not realize the dosing error even when the Ferreros asked them to check their son, who developed a headache and appeared to be in extreme pain. Shands admitted its errors caused Sebastian's death. Luisa Ferrero and her husband, Horst, received an $850,000 settlement from Shands Healthcare at the University of Florida. ("Pharmacist fined for role in 3-year-old's death." Sarah Larimer, Associated Press, Aug. 13, 2008 http://hosted.ap.org/dynamic/stories/F/FL_MEDICATION_ERROR _FLOL-?SITE=FLTAM&SECTION=US

**38. Fatal overdose—K-Mart Pharmacy dispenses 5 mg of
blood thinner Coumadin instead of 2 mg prescribed—
$810,000 Illinois verdict**

On May 30, 1995, a K-Mart pharmacy misfilled and mislabeled a prescription for decedent's blood thinner, dispensing five milligram pills instead of the two milligram pills for approximately one year, and the May 30 bottle in question was labeled as containing two milligram pills. Ingestion of the Coumadin overdose caused decedent, a seventy-six year old man, to develop an intracranial hemorrhage. On June 14 his wife found him soaked in blood which was coming from his mouth, rectum and ears. He was taken to St. James Hospital, where he died June 15, 1995. K-Mart contended decedent was contributorily negligent for failing to seek medical attention for blood in his urine on June 13, and that the effects of a Coumadin overdose could have been reversed in a matter of hours with no residual effects. According to the Cook County Jury Verdict Reporter, the jury returned a $900,000 verdict against K-Mart, reduced by ten percent to $810,000 for contributory negligence. (K-Mart Pharmacy Misfills Coumadin Prescription, Resulting In Fatal Overdose—$810,000 Illinois Verdict," August 1999 Legal Case Study, Healthcare Providers Service Organization, http://www.hpso.com/case/cases_prof_index.php3?id=17&prof=Ph armacist Estate of Ernest Van Hattem, deceased v. K-Mart Corp., d/b/a K-Mart Pharmacy No. 7289, Cook County (IL) Circuit Court, Case No. 95L-1322 1)

---

39. Pharmacy fills tramadol (Ultram) prescription with Avinza—Death—$750,000 Settlement

The plaintiff's decedent, age seventy-four, took a prescription for tramadol to the pharmacy, but it was filled with high-dosage tablets of Avinza. She was found by her home health aide unconscious in December 2007. She was taken to a hospital, where she died of pneumonia a week later. The plaintiff claimed that the high level of opiates in her blood led to respiratory suppression and pneumonia. The pharmacy maintained that the Avinza did not cause the death, but that the decedent might have fallen following ingestion of the Avinza and that she had pneumonia before the accident. According to a published account, a $750,000 settlement was reached. ("Tramadol Filled With Avinza—Death—$750,000 Settlement," Healthcare Providers Service Organization, March 2011 Legal Case Study, http://www.hpso.com/case-studies/casestudy-article/341.jsp

---

40. Walgreen's mistakenly fills 1 grain thyroid prescription with 2 grains—Man develops increased circulation problems in leg—Below-knee amputation of leg— $691,179 net verdict in Colorado

The plaintiff, age fifty-six, was diagnosed with severe peripheral vascular disease in his right leg in May 1996. The plaintiff had been on thyroid replacement hormone since 1970. In early November 1996 a Walgreen pharmacy mistakenly refilled the plaintiff's one grain prescription with two-grain medication. The plaintiffs alleged that within one week of starting to take the double-dose medication, the plaintiff had symptoms of thyroid excess, including pain in the right leg and a sore on the right toe which would not heal. Testing in late December 1996 revealed that the plaintiff's blood flow was fifty-seven percent of normal, which was further reduced than testing done in April 1996. In early February 1997 the plaintiff had an arteriogram due to continued pain. The test results and tissue oxygen results were markedly low. The plaintiff was hospitalized in February 1997 and his right leg was amputated below the knee. While hospitalized, the hospital pharmacist discovered the medication error. The plaintiff claimed that the hormone excess caused the right leg to burn oxygen faster than it could be supplied and caused acceleration of the plaintiff's peripheral vascular disease and poor wound healing. The defendant admitted negligence in filling the prescription but denied that the error caused the amputation. The defendant claimed that the plaintiff lost his leg as a natural progression of his peripheral vascular disease and contended that the plaintiff did not properly follow the recommendations of his physicians. According to Jury Verdict Reporter of Colorado a $1,141,179 verdict was returned for the plaintiff and his wife was awarded $50,000. The judgment was reduced to $691,179 based on the applicability of the Health Care Availability Act. ("Thyroid Replacement Hormone Filled With Excessive Dosage–Man Develops Increased Circulation Problems in Leg--Below-Knee Amputation of Leg–$691,179 Net Verdict in Colorado," March 2005 Legal Case Study, Healthcare Providers Service Organization, http://www.hpso.com/case/cases_prof_index.php3?id=96&prof=Pharmacist)

> ### 41. Compounding pharmacist prepares T3 capsules of varying dosages for Wilson's Syndrome patient, causing thyrotoxicosis—$650,000 settlement in North Carolina

The plaintiff, age forty-five, had a history of cardiac palpitations and shortness of breath. She presented to a physician seeking medical treatment for weight loss. The physician diagnosed her with Wilson's Syndrome, a disorder of peripheral conversion of thyroxin to T3 and ordered thyroid studies. Though he initially ruled out Wilson's Syndrome, the physician reconsidered based on the plaintiff running an average temperature below 98.6. The physician prescribed T3, to be prepared by the defendant compounding pharmacist. The plaintiff began taking the T3, and four days later began suffering thyrotoxicosis, with symptoms of tachycardia, lightheadedness, insomnia, and itching. Analysis of the T3 capsules prepared by the defendant pharmacist revealed wildly varying dosages between capsules, with some containing thousands of times the prescribed dosage. The plaintiff continued to experience tachycardia and shortness of breath after being discharged, and was later diagnosed with post traumatic stress disorder. According to published accounts, the case settled for $650,000. ("Compounding Pharmacist Prepares T3 Capsules of Varying Dosages for Wilson's Syndrome Patient, Causing Thyrotoxicosis–$650,000 Settlement in North Carolina," September 2005 Legal Case Study, Healthcare Providers Service Organization http://www.hpso.com/case/cases_prof_index.php3?id=102&prof=Pharmacist)

> ### 42. CVS pharmacy refilled Haldol prescription with ten times the correct dosage—Man with Tourette's Syndrome suffers overdose—Jury awards $383,300

Plaintiff, a thirty-eight year old maintenance supervisor at the time of this incident on August 4, 1995, suffers from Tourette's syndrome. He claimed that defendant CVS store in Tottenville negligently filled his prescription of Haldol, and dispensed a refill that was ten times the correct dosage. Plaintiff testified that his prescription was for .5 milligrams of Haldol, to be taken four times a day as needed. He contended that defendant dispensed a refill of Haldol containing five milligram tablets. On September 1, 1995, plaintiff took three Haldol pills and suffered an overdose. He testified that he felt as if he was having a heart attack and then blacked out. Plaintiff testified that as his neighbor was driving him to the hospital, he jumped out of the car and began rolling on the road shoulder screaming. Defendant CVS conceded liability after testing samples of the medication that it had dispensed, but contended that plaintiff was contributorily negligent in the manner in which he took the medication. Plaintiff argued that the medication that defendant dispensed was a generic brand and that the pills he took were the same color and shape as the correct dosage of Haldol. Plaintiff claimed he suffered post-traumatic stress disorder with depression, nightmares, and a sixty-pound weight loss. Plaintiff also claimed that his Tourette's syndrome has worsened. He testified that he now takes antidepressants and tranquilizers. According to The New York Jury Verdict Reporter, the jury awarded plaintiff $358,300, and plaintiff wife $25,000. ("Haldol Prescription Was Ten Times the Proper Dosage—Man With Tourette's Syndrome Suffers Overdose—Post-Traumatic Stress Disorder—New York Court Directs Verdict for Plaintiff on Liability—Jury Awards $383,300" November 2000 Legal Case Study, Healthcare Providers Service Organization, http://www.hpso.com/case/cases_prof_index.php3?id=37&prof=Pharmacist Anthony and Toniann Davi v. Hook-Superx, Inc. d/b/a Revco Drug Center, n/k/a CVS Pharmacy, Richmond County, New York, Supreme Court, Index No. 12856/96)

---

43. Pharmacy dispensed 5 mg of blood thinner Coumadin instead of 1 mg, resulting in stroke—Speech and right-side weakness necessitate move to nursing home— $374,400 net verdict

---

The plaintiff, age eighty-two, took a prescription for Coumadin to the pharmacy to be filled. The prescription was for one milligram pills, but she was dispensed five milligram pills. The plaintiff stopped

taking the drug after noticing that the pills were the wrong color. A large black-purple hematoma then developed on her shoulder due to the excessive anti-coagulant. The plaintiff suffered a stroke twenty-three days after filling the prescription, causing her severe speech impairment and right-sided weakness. The plaintiff had been living independently in her own home, but had to reside in a nursing home after the stroke. The plaintiff's doctor's records indicated that he recommended that she resume taking Coumadin about a week after receiving the excessive dosage. The plaintiffs own notes stated that the physician had taken her off the anticoagulant, but warned her that she could suffer a stroke. The defendant pharmacy claimed that even though the prescription had been mistakenly filled, it was corrected soon thereafter and the physician's doctor was called. The defendants maintained that the stroke was not connected to the Coumadin and that it was due to the plaintiff's actions in failing to resume her Coumadin once her condition was stabilized. According to a published account the jury found the pharmacy fifty-two percent at fault and assigned forty-eight percent fault to the plaintiff. The verdict was for $720,000, but the net amount was $374,400. ("Woman dispensed wrong pills for Coumadin prescription resulting in stroke—Speech and right-side weakness necessitate move to nursing home—$374,400 net verdict." Health Providers Service Organization, June 2011 Legal Case Study
http://www.hpso.com/case-studies/casestudy-article/349.jsp)

---

44. Prescription for the acid-reflux drug Prilosec filled with the anti-depressant Prozac—Infant hospitalized for five days—$350,000 verdict

---

The plaintiff child, age eleven months, was treated by her pediatrician for stomach complaints and was prescribed Prilosec. Her physician called in the prescription to the defendant pharmacy. The prescription was filled with Prozac instead of Prilosec. The child became severely ill and was hospitalized for five days as a result of ingesting Prozac. The defendant admitted liability and the matter was tried on the issue of damages only. The plaintiffs alleged that the child suf-

fered permanent injuries from the incident, while the defendant contended that the plaintiff made a good recovery. ("Prilosec Prescription Filled With Prozac–Infant Hospitalized for Five Days–$350,000 Verdict," June 2007 Legal Case Study, Healthcare Providers Service Organization
http://www.hpso.com/case/cases_prof_index.php3?id=124&prof=Pharmacist)

---

45. Leukeran dispensed instead of prescribed leucovorin— Man claims increased risk of developing leukemia— $350,000 settlement

---

The plaintiff, age sixty-five, was undergoing treatment for peripheral neuropathy which was causing foot pain. The physician prescribed leucovorin, which was intended to lessen the side effects the plaintiff was experiencing with his medication. The defendant pharmacy, however, dispensed the drug Leukeran, which is usually prescribed to treat certain leukemias or malignant lymphomas. Leukeran can lead to the development of leukemia in a cancer-free individual. The plaintiff took the drug for about eleven months, during which time he experienced severe flu-like symptoms and depression, leading him to retire from employment earlier than planned. The pharmacy's error was discovered when the plaintiff changed providers for his prescription medications and was dispensed the correct medication. After alerting his prescribing physician of the error, the plaintiff was referred to an oncologist, who advised him of the potential of Leukeran to cause leukemia. The plaintiff alleged negligence in dispensing the wrong drug and maintained that he had an increased risk for developing leukemia. According to a *Verdict Reporter*, a $350,000 settlement was reached. (April 2009 Legal Case Study, HPSO–Health Providers Service Organization,
http://www.hpso.com/case-studies/article/260.jsp)

---

46. Prescription for the ADHD drug Adderall filled with diabetes drug glipizide—Five year-old boy experiences seizures and severe hypoglycemia—$325,000 Massachusetts settlement

The plaintiff, a five year-old boy, was prescribed Adderall for ADHD (Attention-Deficit Hyperactivity Disorder). His aunt had an Adderall prescription for him filled at the defendant pharmacy and began administering the medication for the child the following day, according to posted dose instructions as labeled by the pharmacy. After three days, the plaintiff began to experience seizures and severe hypoglycemia. He was admitted to the hospital, where it was determined that the prescription, although labeled as Adderall, was actually filled incorrectly with Glipizide, a glucose-lowering drug for diabetes. Liability was admitted and the case proceeded on the issue of damages only. The plaintiff alleged that, as a result of taking the wrong medication, he suffered a deterioration in his behavioral and cognitive functions. At the onset of seizures, he experienced tonic-clonic seizures with severe hypoglycemia. The defendant, however, contended the plaintiff's behavioral and cognitive difficulties were not related to taking the wrong medication, but were tied to residual effects of the pre-existing ADHD disorder, and the fact that he had been previously abandoned and abused. According to Massachusetts, Connecticut, Rhode Island Verdict Reporter, this case was settled for $325,000 (with half of the proceeds allocated to special needs trust, and the remaining half to be paid via a structured settlement with guaranteed payout of $410,000). ("Adderall Prescription Filled With Glipizide— Five Year-Old Boy Experiences Seizures and Severe Hypoglycemia— $325,000 Massachusetts Settlement," November 2004 Legal Case Study, Healthcare Providers Service Organization, http://www.hpso.com/case/cases_prof_inde)

---

47. Pharmacist dispenses Calan instead of Lasix—Woman rushed in near-coma to emergency room—$305,000 award

In February 1997, the plaintiff, a fifty year-old licensed vocational nurse who suffered from polymyositis—a chronic inflammatory dis-

ease of the muscle tissue-and hypertension, was hospitalized for one week with congestive heart failure. She was discharged on various medications, including the diuretic Lasix, and Calan, a calcium channel blocker used to treat hypertension. On April 27, 1997, the plaintiff's son picked up a prescription that was intended by her physician's prescription to be Lasix, filled for the plaintiff at the Thrifty Pharmacy in Long Beach, California. On May 1, 1997, the plaintiff's daughter found her mother in a near-coma condition. The plaintiff was rushed to the hospital, where she was diagnosed with pneumonia, hypoxia, congestive heart failure, and a polymyositis flare-up. She was hospitalized for five days. Shortly after discharge, she checked her medication and discovered Thrifty's error in filling the prescription. The plaintiff alleged that as a result of the pharmacy error, the pills she had taken from the bottle labeled Lasix were actually Calan. So, for four days she received no Lasix, and she received an apparent overdose of Calan. This medication mix-up caused the May 1997 health crisis, leading to her hospitalization, and this permanently aggravated her polymyositis, and may have caused brain damage with resulting cognitive deficits. The defendant argued the plaintiff was given the correct medication and she was either confused or untruthful. All of the plaintiff's medical problems were attributable to natural causes and not to any alleged drug mix-up. The defendant maintained the plaintiff's claims of brain damage and/or cognitive defects were false. The jury awarded a gross damages verdict of $305,000. ("Lasix Prescription Filled With Calan—Woman Rushed In Near-Coma Condition to Emergency Room," July 2001 Legal Case Study, Healthcare Providers Service Organization http://www.hpso.com/case/cases_prof_index.php3?id=49&prof=Pharmacist
Ivis Higgins v. Thrifty Payless/Rite Aid, Los Angeles County Superior Court Case No. NC 023 050)

---

48. Eckerd Drug dispenses clonazepam instead of clonidine— $250,000 Pennsylvania settlement

---

In Sloan v. Eckerd Drug (Pennsylvania), the patient went to her Eckerd pharmacy to fill a prescription for clonidine, a drug she used to

control hypertension or high blood pressure. The pharmacy filled the prescription with clonazepam, a medicaiton which poses a risk of dependency. The patient took the medication for 3 weeks and experienced headaches, memory loss, and depression. She became addicted to the drug and required outpatient psychiatric treatment. She sued the pharmacy and her pharmacist and the case settled before trial for $250,000. (Attorney Dan Frith from the Frith Law Firm in Roanoke, Virginia, "Pharmacy Mistakes Kill," February 13, 2008. Accessed February 28, 2008.
http://roanoke.injuryboard.com/medical-malpractice/pharmacy-mistakes-kill.php?googleid=14934)

---

49. Blind man dispensed 50 microgram Fentanyl patches, instead of the prescribed 25 microgram patches—Overdose blamed for worsening of sleep apnea—$200,000 settlement

The plaintiff, who is blind and uses a seeing-eye dog, brought a prescription for two boxes of 25 microgram Fentanyl patches to the defendant pharmacy. The pharmacy dispensed the plaintiff two boxes of 50 microgram Fentanyl patches. The plaintiff was unable to detect the dosage error before using the medication. The plaintiff applied the narcotic patches over the course of a week as prescribed and suffered a debilitating overdose. In addition to extreme discomfort, confusion, nausea and lethargy, the overdose caused permanent worsening of the plaintiffs sleep apnea, necessitating numerous sleep studies and supplemental oxygen therapy during sleep. The pharmacy admitted the error, but disputed the damages. A $200,000 settlement was reached, according to a published account. (March 2010 Legal Case Study, HPSO—Healthcare Providers Service Organization
http://www.hpso.com/case-studies/casestudy-article/326.jsp)

---

50. Wal-Mart pharmacist dispenses anti-fungal Grifulvin to four month-old child, rather than expectorant guiafenesin—$175,000 immediate settlement, plus agreement to pay for any future treatment

---

On November 4, 1998, the parents of **Taylor Lang** went to the Wal-Mart in Charleston, Missouri to have a prescription filled for their infant daughter. Their pediatrician had prescribed guaifenesin, an expectorant, for the infant, who had developed croup/cough. The pharmacist instead, by error, dispensed Grifulvin, an anti-fungal agent used to treat ringworm. After reading the medication literature included with the packaging, the parents called the pharmacy the next morning to verify that Taylor had been given the correct prescription. The pharmacist assured the Langs that the prescription was correct, and should be taken as directed, and that the information on a printed insert with a medication does not always reflect the purpose for which that medication was prescribed. Her explanation was that medications often have multiple uses. For twenty days, four month-old Taylor, who weighed thirteen pounds, was given doses of Grifulvin that would have been inappropriate even for a full-weight adult. She developed severe diarrhea, stomach cramps and pain, and general lethargy. When the mistake was finally verified, after the parents took the still-ill child along with the medication back to the pediatrician's office, Taylor was tested for liver damage, a potential side-effect of Grifulvin. Initially, Taylor had elevated liver enzymes, but a short time later, after the drug was withdrawn, her enzyme levels returned to normal. After four years of further development, she appears to have no permanent liver damage. The plaintiff alleged the Wal-Mart pharmacist departed from the standard of care in two instances—once when the incorrect medication was dispensed and secondly, when the pharmacist informed the parents by phone that Grifulvin was the correct drug, and to take it as directed on the labeling. The parties reached a settlement of $175,000, with an additional $500,000 available if Taylor should develop liver damage prior to age twenty. ("Wal-Mart Pharmacist Gave Four Month-Old Child Anti-Fungal Agent Rather Than Expectorant—Severe Diarrhea, Stomach Pain and Lethargy—Elevated Liver Enzymes—$175,000 Immediate Settlement, Plus Agreement to Pay for Future Treatment Provision in Missouri," Sept. 2004 Legal Case Study, Healthcare Providers Service Organization http://www.hpso.com/case/cases_prof_index.php3)

---

51. Lawsuit alleges Walgreen's dispensed chemotherapy drug Matulane to pregnant woman instead of prenatal vitamin Materna, leading to miscarriage

Walgreen Co. has been sued by a Missouri woman and her husband who claim she had a miscarriage after a prescription for prenatal vitamins was filled with a chemotherapy drug carrying a similar brand name. Walgreens failed to properly supervise pharmacy personnel who dispensed the medicine to **Chanda Givens** instead of what her doctor prescribed, lawyers for Givens and her husband, Courtenay, said in a complaint filed in federal court in St. Louis. Givens had a miscarriage after taking the drug for less than a month. Givens received a prescription for Materna, a prenatal vitamin, on March 6, 2007. The pharmacist at her local Walgreens instead gave her Matulane, used to treat Hodgkin's disease. The drug is designed to interfere with the growth of cells by blocking their ability to split and reproduce, the complaint states. (Bloomberg News: "Suit: Chemo drug led to miscarriage," chicagotribune.com, October 19, 2007 www.chicagotribune.com/business/chi-fri_brief2_1019oct19,0,6644474.story)

---

52. Pharmacist dispenses anti-arthritis Arava instead of anti-hypertensive Avapro—Confidential settlement

The plaintiff began to experience high blood pressure, weight loss, extreme headaches, uncontrollable diarrhea, blurred vision, and changes in her mental state in April 1999. Her treating physician was unable to diagnose the cause of her illness—and in particular could not understand why the patient's blood pressure medication which he had prescribed, Avapro, was no longer working. One month later, the plaintiff noticed that the contents of her medication bottle were listed as Arava—a rheumatoid arthritis drug. She telephoned the national pharmacy chain where she had picked up her prescription, but she was not able to speak to the pharmacist who filled the order. The plaintiff discovered that the night pharmacist who had filled the plaintiff's medication had misfilled forty-five prescriptions between June 1997 and November 2000 at that pharmacy. Other pharmacists at this same store averaged one error per year. The plaintiffs also discovered that the defendant pharmacist frequently worked ten-hour shifts seven nights in a row. After the error in this case became known to his supervisor, he was transferred to a different pharmacy in another town. But the regional supervisor did not tell his new on-site supervisor about his pattern of errors. The district supervisor also disclosed during discovery that she had never fired a pharmacist for incompetence, and she has been with the company since 1994. The plaintiffs also discovered that the pharmacy does not have a nationwide written policy requiring prescription misfills to be tracked. According to a published account, after the plaintiffs filed their negligence case in district court, a confidential settlement was reached shortly before trial. ("Overworked And Error-Prone Pharmacist Misfills Prescription—Confidential Settlement," June 2006 Legal Case Study, Healthcare Providers Service Organization http://www.hpso.com/case/cases_prof_index.php3?id=111&prof=Pharmacist)

---

53. Pharmacist dispenses Tobradex eye drops for one-month old infant instead of Tobrex—causing steroid-induced glaucoma

A pediatric ophthalmologist prescribed Tobrex (tobramycin) 0.3% ophthalmic drops for a one-month-old infant with a blocked tear duct (one drop 3 times a day to the left eye). The physician indicated this drug by checking off a space on a preprinted prescription order form which listed 12 different ophthalmic drops including Tobradex (tobramycin and dexamethasone) which appeared on the line above Tobrex. Somehow, the pharmacist misread the prescription order and erroneously dispensed Tobradex. Compounding the error, the pharmacist refilled the prescription with Tobradex when the initial supply was exhausted. When the infant's eye continued to worsen, the mother returned to the ophthalmologist. Under general anesthesia for a complete examination, the physician made a diagnosis of non-congenital, steroid-induced (dexamethasone) glaucoma. Surgery may be required. ("Child suffers glaucoma from inadvertent use of corticosteroid-containing eye drops," Institute for Safe Medication Practices, June 30, 1999 newsletter http://www.ismp.org/Newsletters/acutecare/articles/19990630.asp?p tr=y)

---

54. Pill splitting leads to rhabdomyolysis and renal failure, setting stage for legal trouble

Patient compliance is always a tricky issue, but adding a complicated dosing regimen to the mix—such as pill splitting—can compound the problem, setting the stage for legal trouble. The following is a case illustrating the potential for medication errors with pill splitting.

A 59-year-old man who had undergone heart transplant was prescribed simvastatin (Zocor, Merck) at a dose of 20 mg. His cholesterol was slightly elevated (208 mg/dL), so the nurse practitioner increased his prescription for simvastatin from 20 mg to 40 mg at bedtime. When the patient took his simvastatin prescription to the pharmacy, the pharmacist filled it with an 80-mg tablet, with instructions for the patient to take one "half tablet at bedtime." The pharmacist did not contact the prescriber or the patient's clinic to divulge this information.

Six months later, the patient's cholesterol had risen slightly. He explained to the nurse practitioner that he was taking "half a tablet." She noted that the patient had previously been prescribed a 40-mg tablet and, thus, she assumed that he was taking 20 mg simvastatin as the half-tablet. The nurse practitioner told the patient to take "a whole tablet" from then on with the belief that he would then be taking 40 mg at bedtime. In actuality, the patient was now taking 80 mg per day—double the dose intended by the prescriber.

A few weeks later, the patient began to experience leg pain and was hospitalized. Physicians discovered that he had developed rhabdomyolysis, a serious muscle disease that can cause kidney failure. Fortunately, the patient survived the ensuing renal failure. The simvastatin was discontinued.

When confronted with the facts, the nurse practitioner and the lawyers for the clinic blamed the pharmacist for changing the prescription from a 40-mg tablet to one-half of an 80-mg tablet. They contended that the overdose, which led to the rhabdomyolysis, would not have occurred if the pharmacist had advised the nurse practitioner and the clinic of the dosage shift. The lawyers for the pharmacy (a managed care pharmacy group) defended the pill splitting, stating that it was a routine, cost-effective practice. The pharmacy denied any wrongdoing in the matter.

This case is about communication. The prescriber did not know that the pharmacy was changing the prescription to take advantage of pill splitting. The nurse practitioner assumed that the patient was taking a certain dose, without examining the prescription bottle and without calling the pharmacy to verify what dose he was taking. Such assumptions can cause serious health problems for the patient—and increased liability for the pharmacy. (James O'Donnell, PharmD, "Pill Splitting Leads to Rhabdomyolysis And Renal Failure, Setting Stage for Legal Trouble," *Pharmacy Practice News*, Issue: 2/2004, Volume: 31:02 http://www.pharmacypracticenews.com/index.asp?section_id=51&show=dept&issue_id=74&article_id=3515)

---

55. Walgreen's pharmacist dispenses Risperdal instead of Pediapred—Baby permanently injured

---

NEW PORT RICHEY, Florida—An alleged pharmacy mix-up that sent a 5-month-old to the emergency room and on to intensive care has prompted a negligence lawsuit against Walgreens and one of its pharmacists. The baby, adopted by plaintiffs Sandra and Charles Watts, was poisoned after ingesting "a potent psychotropic drug prescribed to adults for the treatment of schizophrenia," the lawsuit states. Identified in the lawsuit only by initials, the child spent five days in intensive care at All Children's Hospital in St. Petersburg with unspecified injuries following the incident Jan. 4, 2005, according to the lawsuit. According to the lawsuit, the incident began Jan. 3, 2005, when the 5-month-old was diagnosed with an upper respiratory infection and prescribed drugs including amoxicillin and the

steroid Pediapred. When the Wattses took the handwritten prescriptions to the pharmacy at 7020 Massachusetts Ave. later that day, an employee asked for and noted the patient's date of birth, July 21, 2004, and then entered the prescriptions into the store's computer system, the lawsuit states. However, the employee entered Risperdal instead of Pediapred and "the computer generated a label in the minor's name listing Risperdal instead of Pediapred as the minor's prescribed medication," the lawsuit states. The next day, Sandra Watts administered the first dose of Risperdal before taking the baby to day care, the lawsuit states. Soon after, Watts got a call from day care personnel advising her the child was limp. A doctor at River's Edge Pediatrics, where the baby was a patient, quickly diagnosed the problem, and the child was rushed to Community Hospital of New Port Richey and then to All Children's, the lawsuit states. The complaint does not detail the baby's injuries but states they are permanent. ("Walgreens Named In Prescription Lawsuit," David Sommer, *The Tampa Tribune*, May 13, 2007
http://pasco.tbo.com/pasco/MGBYTO5HM1F.html)

---

56. Walgreen's mistake results in 5-year-old taking male hormone testosterone for 2 months rather than Inderal prescribed for hand tremors and hyperactivity

---

When Tabitha Jones picked up her stepson's medicine at a Walgreens store near Nashville in 2004, she had no way to know the pharmacy was so busy that its manager had asked for more staffing months earlier to "decrease the pharmacist's stress."

She also had no idea the drug Walgreens gave her that day was a steroid never intended for children and not the blood pressure drug prescribed to treat **Trey Jones**' hand tremors and hyperactivity. Walgreens refilled the prescription four times, eventually at double the adult dosage, before the error was caught. The 5-year-old not only went into premature puberty but also erupted in rages.

Trey's parents sued Walgreens, fearing the steroid could stunt the boy's growth or cause liver damage. "We don't know what could happen later on down the road," his father, Robert Jones Jr., said in a 2006 pretrial deposition.

Trey Jones ate three meals a day like a typical 5-year-old until he started taking Methitest, a synthetic hormone for older males whose bodies aren't producing enough testosterone. Afterward, he "would eat a plate full of food and come back and get seconds, and 10 minutes later, he would want thirds," his father, Robert, said in his deposition. The boy's wall-kicking rages made it difficult for him to focus on schoolwork. "You couldn't tell him to do anything," his father said.

Trey's hands continued to shake, so his doctor doubled the initial 10-milligram dose of Inderal. Walgreens again misfilled the prescription, this time with a higher dosage of the steroid. Trey began experiencing genital pain, his father said.

When Walgreens caught the error, the pharmacist told Tabitha Jones only to contact Trey's doctor, court records show. Trey's parents halted the steroid use soon afterward. Trey, now 8, gets regular growth and liver tests. Natasha Leibel, a Columbia University pediatric endocrinologist not involved with the case, says steroid use by a child "could, in theory, ... compromise adult height." Liver disease is a rarer effect of long-term use, she says.

Trey's parents filed a complaint with the Tennessee pharmacy board and sued Walgreens. Robert Jones knew the challenges would be hard but says keeping drug errors "from happening to someone else" was reason enough to fight.

Pretrial discovery in the Jones case showed the Springfield, Tenn., pharmacy where the errors began was busy: Trey's prescription was among 477 filled by two pharmacists on Sept. 30, 2004.

Months earlier, pharmacy manager Jill Brown had written in an internal report that the store had surpassed its goal of averaging 350 prescriptions a day and "could use a third pharmacist to ... decrease the pharmacist's stress." But she said in a pretrial deposition that Walgreens guidelines say a store must average 550 prescriptions a day to get a third pharmacist.

David Work, a former North Carolina Board of Pharmacy executive director tapped as an expert witness by the Jones family, wrote in a report filed in court that the store's prescription volume and staffing represented "a breach of Walgreens' (safety) obligation."

U.S. District Court Judge Aleta Trauger, who presided over the Jones case, wrote in a 2007 pretrial ruling, "Although the defendant denies that there is any connection between number of prescriptions processed per day and mistakes, common sense and at least one purported expert argue in favor of the opposite conclusion." Trauger said she would let a jury decide whether the prescription volume amounted to recklessness, a finding that could have exposed Walgreens to punitive damages.

But the case never went to trial. Walgreens acknowledged in a pretrial conference in March 2007 that it had violated the standard of care owed to Trey. The parties reached a late-December 2007 settlement that includes a confidentiality order barring Walgreens and Trey's family and attorneys from discussing the financial terms and other details.

Tennessee's pharmacy board conducted its own investigation. In 2005, it imposed a $500 fine on Walgreens pharmacist Avani Sindhal for violating state rules that require pharmacists to keep health and safety as their top concern. She said in a 2006 deposition that she thought Trey's prescription called for the steroid. Sindhal, who still works for Walgreens, also said she didn't recall seeing Trey's birth date on the prescription.

(Kevin McCoy and Erik Brady, "Speed, High Volume Can Trigger Mistakes," *USA Today*, February 11, 2008. Accessed March 16, 2008. http://www.usatoday.com/money/industries/health/2008-02-11-prescription-errors_N.htm#uslPageReturn)

57. Safeway pharmacist accidentally gives abortion drug to pregnant woman instead of antibiotic

FORT LUPTON, Colo.—Having a baby should be a joyous time in one's life, but a 19-year-old Fort Lupton woman is filled with fear and uncertainty about her unborn child.

A pharmacist at a Fort Lupton Safeway at 1300 Dexter gave the wrong drug to the mother-to-be.

It's a potent drug that could harm or even kill her child.
"This will be our first baby. Yah, it'll be my first baby," says **Mareena Silva** and her boyfriend Christopher Castillo.

Silva is 6 weeks pregnant.

She was supposed to get antibiotics at the Safeway pharmacy, but the pharmacist accidentally gave her a prescription for another woman with a similar name.

"I didn't notice it didn't have my name on it because the lady's name is really similar to mine. It's Maria and mine is Mareena," she says. The two women share the same last name.

And that mistaken prescription was for methotrexate, a medication used to treat cancers.

The pharmacist told her to bring back the medicine. When she arrived, he told her to throw up the pill.

It had been about 25 minutes since she'd taken it.

"My doctor called immediately and said you need to get to an ambulance. I'm sending one to Safeway," she says.

Silva later learned methotrexate can cause birth defects in an unborn baby. She said that the drug is also used to cause abortions in troubled pregnancies.

The manufacturer warns that some people have died after taking this medication every day by accident.

"That's my biggest worry…is the baby being healthy and my baby surviving through this whole thing," says Silva.

Safeway's Public Affairs Director Kris Staaf released this statement:

We are "….very concerned about how this happened and we are conducting a full and complete investigation. Safeway has pharmacy systems and processes in place to prevent this kind of occurrence. We have a well-earned reputation for reliability and safely filling prescriptions and we will continue to work diligently to ensure our procedures and polices are being followed at each of our pharmacies."

"I'm angry. But there's not much I can do about it. I just wish I caught it sooner," says Silva.

The CU School of Pharmacy says it teaches its students to confirm with customers their street address or date of birth. That way, they make sure they are giving the right medicine to the right person. Silva says the pharmacist did not ask her these questions.

She says the pharmacist even told her the drug he was giving her was not good for a pregnant woman. And she said that's what the hospital prescribed. So, it must be okay.

"But I thought he was talking about the antibiotic," she says. Safeway says it is sorry for the mistake and it will pay for Silva's medical expenses.

(Tammy Vigil, "Pharmacist gives pregnant woman wrong prescription," KDVR-TV, Feb. 5, 2011,
http://www.kdvr.com/news/kdvr-pregnant-woman-giving-wrong-meds-20110204,0,5536174.story)

---

58. Thirteen prescriptions affected with CVS mix-up involving dispensing tamoxifen tablets (for breast cancer) to children instead of fluoride tablets (for prevention of tooth decay)

Between December 2011 and February 2012, a CVS pharmacy in Chatham, N.J., dispensed tamoxifen tablets instead of 0.5 mg chewable fluoride pills. The mix-up could have affected as many as 50 children, but only 13 prescriptions definitely were found to be affected, according to a CVS statement.

Michael J. DeAngelis, a spokesperson for CVS, stated that all families that could have received the wrong medication were contacted as soon as the mix-up was uncovered. "Fortunately, most of the families we spoke to informed us that their children did not receive any incorrect pills," he stated. "We will continue to follow up with families who believe that their children may have received incorrect medication. Thankfully, no negative effects have been reported."

DeAngelis said that the incident involved only a few tamoxifen pills mixed in with the fluoride tablets and that it was due to a "single medication restocking issue" at the Chatham pharmacy. The problem was brought to the pharmacy's attention by a parent, according to DeAngelis.

The consumer affairs division of New Jersey's attorney general's office has called for CVS to provide information on how the switch occurred, along with all communications about the problem. Company representatives will have to appear for questioning. CVS is conducting its own investigation. "We are also cooperating fully with the New Jersey attorney general's office," CVS's DeAngelis said.

(Valerie DeBenedette, "CVS mix-up of tamoxifen, fluoride tablets affects 13 prescriptions," *Drug Topics*, March 7, 2012)

---

59. Lawyer says hospital patient mistakenly injected with "extremely poisonous" green clothing dye instead of fluorescent dye used for angiograms

The attorney for Elijah Goodwin claims he was injected with a green dye normally used for dyeing clothing while at Northwestern Memorial Hospital in Chicago. Labeling the procedure as "a fiasco," the lawyer said he could not comprehend how no one in the operating room questioned the injection.

During a post-operative angiogram, doctors accidentally used "Brilliant Green dye" which is typically used to color silk, wool and other fabrics, according to the lawsuit. And moreover, this dye is "extremely poisonous." The hospital is alleged to have the dye in the pharmacy because it is "on occasion used in medicine as a topical anesthesia." The attorney said the consequences of the procedure were "really bad." These "really bad" consequences allegedly include: permanent damage to his lungs caused by permanent scarring, a seizure disorder that shuts down his kidneys for a time, and coughing spells in the middle of the night.

The lawyer said that "the drug they administered didn't have any FDA packaging" on it. The drug that the doctors wanted to use is called "IC Green," a florescent dye used in angiograms. According to the attorney, IC Green comes in powder form, while the chemical dye for coloring clothing comes in a liquid form. He concludes that "it was a really, really horrible mistake." (Atty. Stephen Alexander, "Lawyer Says Patient Injected With Green Clothing Dye," Technorati.com, April 8, 2012
http://technorati.com/women/article/lawyer-says-patient-injected-with-green/)

How do customers react when they discover pharmacy mistakes?

Even though many mistakes remain undiscovered, customers do sometimes detect the pharmacist's error. One day a lady handed me her prescription container and told me that I refilled her prescription with the wrong drug. Sure enough, the day before I had given her the wrong antidepressant. I dispensed Paxil 20 mg instead of Prozac 20 mg. She looked at me with an expression implying that I was a sloppy or incompetent pharmacist, that I should be ashamed of myself, and that the community would be better off if I worked somewhere else. She did not know that I try extremely hard to be accurate. I think it would be fair to say that I made fewer errors during my 25-year career than most pharmacists. I assume she would not have been impressed if I had tried to assure her about my error rate. Auto accidents, for example, are statistically uncommon, but if you are involved in one, statistics are of little comfort. This customer knew nothing of my deep concern for accuracy. Her expression made me feel an inch tall. She seemed to wonder how I still had a license to be a pharmacist.

This incident occurred over fifteen years ago, but it is seared deeply into my brain. Immediately after the incident occurred, I asked myself how I could have made this mistake. Most likely, this error occurred because both drug names begin with the letter "P", both drugs are in the same class of antidepressants known as SSRI's, and both are available in 20 mg. strengths. Apparently my subconscious verified several relevant factors, but obviously not all. Fatigue, workload, and distractions may also have played a role.

One of the biggest surprises for me during my career as a pharmacist is that most customers do not become angry when they discover a pharmacy mistake. Most customers return to the pharmacy oblivious to the fact that the error implies a complete breakdown in the pharmacy. The number one job of the pharmacist is to dispense the right drug to the right customer. I would probably lose confidence in a pharmacist if he dispensed the wrong drug to me or a member of my family. Most customers seem to be much more forgiving or else they don't understand the significance of pharmacy errors. Most customers don't realize that pharmacist errors can be anywhere from trivial to fatal.

Here are two examples from Complaints.com and one from ComplaintNow.com in which pharmacy customers did indeed understand the significance of pharmacy mistakes.

Today I submitted a prescription to my usual Rite-Aid Pharmacy in Concord NH. The prescription was for 200mg of Serzone. I picked up the prescription just in time to pop one of the pills in which I was an hour behind in taking. Serzone is a mild anti-depressant anxiety drug.

As I was ready to put the pill in my mouth, I noticed it looked nothing like the Serzone pills I had been taking in the past.

It was stamped with Seroquel. I thought that was strange. Was it a generic for Serzone, or did my therapist change my drug without telling me? I called the pharmacy and the girl who answered said Seroquel worked the very same way and did not seem to think there was a mistake.

I asked her to go check the original prescription, because I didn't trust her untrained opinion.

Sure enough! They gave me the wrong drug.

She said again that they work very much the same. On further investigation on the net, I found that they are two very different drugs! Seroquel is a drug to treat schizophrenia! With some serious side effects. I can't believe they did this.

I almost started to take this drug. I see now how people die from pharmacists' sloppiness. There is a lesson to be learned here.
—Rebecca Spencer, "Rite-Aid Pharmacy in Concord, New Hampshire— Prescription filled with wrong drug," Complaints.com, Feb. 1, 2002 http://www.complaints.com/february2002/complaintoftheday.february2.5.htm   (Accessed August 16, 2005)

After a recent trip to a Walgreen's store, I feel compelled to tell you how unhappy I was with the pharmacy. Let me tell you why I was dissatisfied.

I have been to the store twice to have a prescription filled and both times they were filled incorrectly.

The first time was a dosage error. The second time was the wrong medication. While the medication given was not life threatening, it frightens me to think that if this has happened to me 100% of the time, how many other people are walking out of Walgreen's with an incorrect prescription?

The next customer may be a heart patient. Will someone have to die before this is taken seriously?

I am a new customer of Walgreen's. As a result of this experience, I definitely will not shop there again. Since word of mouth is the most effective form of advertising, I definitely will also tell others about this experience.

I hope Walgreen's is committed to customer service and I am confident they will want to resolve this issue quickly and thoroughly.

Again, you can be sure my dissatisfaction will be voiced to others.
—Rod Faulkner, "Pharmay Error: Walgreen's," Complaints.com, Dec. 2, 2000 http://www.complaints.com/complaintofthedaydecember32000.11.htm (Accessed August 16, 2005)

The pharmacy at my local Winn Dixie filled the prescription for my 5 day old 7 week premature twins wrong. They had the dosage way too high to where if I would have given it to them, it would have caused them to quit breathing. I have actually spoken to the DM [district manager] for the pharmacy and he said that he got all the proper paperwork filed and turned it over to the legal dept, and that they would be in contact with me. That was over a week ago and I still have not heard anything. I understand that they don't see the gravity of the situation. They feel like I caught their mistake so no harm came to my infant, but I feel differently. I was on medication and recovering from a C-section. What if I had been resting and my husband or someone had went to give them the medicine and just read the directions on the bottle!!! I am very upset over this matter.
—Chelle1205, ComplaintNow.com, Apr. 13, 2012
http://www.complaintnow.com/Winn-Dixie-Stores-Inc./complaint/complaints/thread/print/160147/173959

| **HOW TO PROTECT YOURSELF** |
| **FROM SERIOUS PHARMACY MISTAKES** |

There are several practical things that pharmacy customers can do to protect themselves from harm.

In the last few years, several websites have become available that greatly simplify the process of identifying tablets and capsules, whether they are brand name drugs or generics. Search Google for pill identifier and you will find several websites such as **1) drugs.com, 2) rxlist.com, 3) healthline.com, 4) healthtools.aarp.org, and 5) webmd.com.**

Identifying your tablets or capsules on these websites is usually surprisingly simple. All you have to do is enter the numbers or letters or words that are stamped or imprinted on your pills. I grabbed several different pills at random to see how accurate the the drugs.com website is in identifying pills. I entered the numbers, letters, and words into the appropriate fields and was quickly given the precisely correct identity for each pill. Here is the information I entered and the results.

54 543	Correctly identified as Roxicet
SP 4220	Correctly identified as Niferex-150
Endo 602	Correctly identified as Endocet
INV 276 10	Correctly identified as prochlorperazine 10 mg
M 15	Correctly identified as generic Lomotil
Watson 349	Correctly identified as generic Vicodin
KU 108	Correctly identified as generic Levbid
MP 85	Correctly identified as generic Septra DS
OC 20	Correctly identified as Oxycontin 20 mg

Even though all of these pills were identified quickly and accurately, obviously these pill identifier websites have no way of determining whether the pills in your bottles are actually what your doctor prescribed. For example, many drugstores print a short physical description of your pill on the prescription label or on an "auxiliary" label attached to the side of the vial. These descriptions can be very helpful in verifying that the pills in your bottle match the brand or generic name on the label. But keep in mind that if your pharmacist or tech misreads your doctor's handwriting and enters the wrong drug into the computer, you may have an accurate description of the wrong pill.

In the last few years, several websites have become available that offer free drug interaction checkers. Search Google for drug interaction checker. On most of these websites, you can enter up to a dozen or more drugs and receive very helpful information about potential drug interactions.

A few years ago, *USA Today* reported the case of a 31-year-old high school wrestling coach who died from an interaction between tramadol and methadone, painkillers dispensed at different times by a pharmacy in Flagstaff, Arizona. A jury awarded the patient's family six million dollars after hearing evidence that the pharmacist neither warned the patient about the potential drug interaction nor double-checked the second prescription with his doctor. (Kevin McCoy and Erik Brady, "Speed, High Volume Can Trigger Mistakes," *USA Today*, Feb. 11, 2008)

In this tragic case, if the patient had used one of the online drug interaction checkers available today, he would have seen that the **AARP.org** checker labels this interaction as "severe." He would have seen that the **medscape.com** checker describes this interaction with the words "serious" and "monitor closely." He would have seen that the **drugs.com** checker states "Comcommitant use of tramadol and other opoids should be avoided in general."

If the size, shape, or color of your pills change when you have your prescriptions refilled, call your pharmacist and ask why. In most cases, the answer is that you have received a generic made by a different company. But that is not always the case.

William Winsley, executive director of the Ohio State Board of Pharmacy, comments on this tendency to freely use the "It must be a generic" explanation ("Are All Drug Errors System Errors?" *Drug Topics*, April 15, 2002, pp. 18, 20). He says that several cases of severe patient harm have resulted from using this explanation too freely:

When a patient calls the pharmacy and asks if the medication he just received is correct since it has a different color or shape than what he was

expecting, the prudent pharmacist reviews the prescription, the patient record, and asks for the color, shape, and identifying marks on the dosage form received by the patient. In several cases this board [the Ohio State Board of Pharmacy] has dealt with, the pharmacist did none of these steps. Instead, he told the patient that the dosage form must have been a generic equivalent and should be safe to take. Several cases of severe patient harm have resulted, followed by board hearings, due primarily to the pharmacist's carelessness.

Pharmacy customers need to become actively involved in learning as much as they can about the drugs their doctors prescribe. With so many potent pills on the market today, you cannot afford to be a passive consumer. Passivity is a dangerous posture in our medical system that seems to value speed over accuracy and quantity over quality.

In the following chapters, you will learn in much greater detail about the infinite number of things that can go deadly wrong at the drugstore, and practical things you can do to protect yourself.

PART II

DOCTORS

Chapter 3

Why doctors' handwriting is no laughing matter

You've heard all the jokes about physicians' illegible handwriting. I challenge you to name another activity in our society in which such critical information is conveyed in such a reckless manner. There's no question that illegible handwriting causes some people to get the wrong drug, the wrong dose, and/or the wrong directions. A hurried pharmacist is forced to occasionally make educated guesses. By the time the pharmacist gets through the busy phone number to the receptionist or nurse, or by the time he locates a doctor who is away from his office or has gone home for the day, the pharmacist is causing other customers to get upset from having to wait.

When a pharmacist calls a doctor's office and talks to the doctor himself, the doctor's tone often implies something like "What kind of a pharmacist are you that you can't read prescriptions?" If the drug name and directions are bad, the signature is even worse. I have had prescriptions in which not only were the drug or directions unclear but it was impossible to identify which doctor, among several in the group practice, actually wrote the prescription. Calling the office then becomes a demeaning experience because I don't even know which doctor's office to request the receptionist connect me with. One time I ended up describing the doctor's signature to the nurse/receptionist as we tried to figure out which doctor had actually written the prescription. I had to be pleasant because obviously it's taboo to be rude to doctors (and their staff) but I usually feel like saying "Why can't that guy write like someone who got past the first grade?"

Physicians are not people who inherently write poorly. They did not have courses in medical school on how to write poorly. In my opinion, illegible handwriting is an expression of ego, a statement of the doctor's position in the power hierarchy of modern medicine. Illegible handwriting is an ongoing affirmation of medicine's dominance over pharmacy.

Imagine this scenario: Say a physician were to be sued for malpractice and the judge were to tell the doctor, "Write out your defense in your own handwriting." In this imaginary scenario, I bet that the physician's handwriting would be perfectly legible.

When a pharmacist receives a prescription that is not entirely plain, his attitude is often, "If the doctor doesn't care enough to write plainly and if he doesn't show me enough respect to write plainly, why should I show more than an equal amount of concern for the prescription?" This is the attitude that frequently contributes to the possibility that the pharmacist will make an educated guess rather than call the doctor's office.

An illegible prescription can mean only one thing: the doctor doesn't really care enough to ensure that there is absolutely no chance of an error in reading the prescription. In one town in which I worked, a pediatrician known for his arrogance called my partner and chewed her out for mentioning to a child's parents that the tetracycline he was prescribing could leave their child's teeth permanently discolored with a very unattractive gray tint. Yet this physician has some of the most illegible handwriting in town. After my partner told me about this, I wanted to call the doctor and say that if he cared so much about the well-being of his patients, why couldn't he write legibly enough to make sure that his patients got what he wanted. It is my feeling that his illegible handwriting says something about his basic concern for his patients.

When my father was discharged from a hospital several years ago, his physician handed him a prescription. I was standing next to my father and looked at the prescription as the doctor momentarily turned away. A few seconds later, I asked the doctor "Do you want...?" I was immediately interrupted by the doctor who said, "Don't worry about it. The pharmacist can read it." I felt like saying, "I've been a pharmacist for twenty-five years and I can't read it." But that would have upset my father who prefers to avoid confrontations. As it turned out, the pharmacist in my father's home town filled the prescription with what we both guessed was the proper medication. It made sense from the diagnosis. It was one of those borderline prescriptions where we were right at the edge of uncertainty. An extra millimeter and the doctor would have been phoned.

Has there been a deliberate effort to create a mystery around the handwritten prescription?

It never ceases to amaze me the way in which customers laugh and smile when I tell them that I can't read their doctor's handwriting. They seem to have the feeling that a prescription is a statement of the doctor's intellectual brilliance and that "Wow, it's so brilliant that even the pharmacist can't read it!" Instead, customers should be repulsed by illegible handwriting. If customers only knew the endless opportunities for disaster that can result from a poorly written prescription, they would demand that doctors write legibly.

I often feel that an illegible prescription is part of the mystique that physicians intentionally cultivate for themselves. It's part of the placebo effect inherent in the doctor's prescription. Several years ago, *FDA Consumer* published an article that said that, historically, physicians intentionally cultivated such a mystery around the prescription. Ask pharmacists whether they feel this effort to create mystery has ended. Prescriptions were originally made up of all kinds of symbols and Latin to intentionally create a mystery. There was, in fact, a conspiracy.

In an effort to keep the knowledge of medicine and pharmacy from the general public, physicians used strange alchemic symbols to designate the materials and processes to be used in compounding medications.

"The effect on the appearance of the prescription may be readily imagined," one medical historian has written, "and it is evident that the physician succeeded perfectly in making his preparation a mystery to the patient." Keeping the patient in the dark and creating an aura of mystery and magic are precisely the reasons given by medical historians to explain the use of Latin in prescription writing as late as 1900.

Ask any pharmacist whether he believes this ended in 1900. Latin abbreviations are in common use today even though, in most cases, an English abbreviation could be written just as quickly. It is obvious that this deliberate effort to create a mystery is still very much alive today.

According to another issue of *FDA Consumer* (March 1979, p. 12), English physicians were forbidden to teach their patients about medicines four hundred years ago: "Back in 1555 England's Royal College of Physicians advised the profession thus: 'Let no physician teach the public about medicines or even tell them the names of medicines...'." The article goes on to say "That attitude persists to some extent to this day, but change is coming." I can only say that change is not coming very fast. In my opinion, the creation of mystery is still a large part of the prescription.

Illegible handwriting combined with Latin abbreviations facilitate the creation of a fog of mystery surrounding the prescription. Patients are endlessly impressed that doctors use Latin abbreviations. In reality, most doctors use fewer than a dozen Latin abbreviations in their practices. The average prescription contains maybe two or three of these abbreviations, such as: *po* (by mouth), *qd* (daily), *bid* (twice a day), *tid* (three times a day), *qid* (four times a day), *ac* (before meals), *pc* (after meals), *q4h* (every 4 hours), and *hs* (at bedtime). Doctors and pharmacists certainly do not need to be able to read formal Latin as such. We simply need to know a few dozen Latin abbreviations. In less than an hour, most people could memorize (or at least become familiar with) all the Latin abbreviations used in prescriptions.

Jesse Vivian, a pharmacist, attorney, and professor at Wayne State University College of Pharmacy, writes: "Practitioners of any vocation in any sector of the universe have communication shortcuts, abbreviations, and foreign phrases or languages that are known only to those inside the occupation. In fact, there is a notion that professionals intentionally use words or phrases that are unknown to the general populace as a mechanism of keeping lay people from getting to know too much about any given profession." ("In Pari Delicto," *U.S. Pharmacist*, January 2007, p. 88)

Doctors have been slow in adopting computers in their prescribing and for transmitting these prescriptions to pharmacies. If the use of computers by doctors becomes routine someday and the handwritten prescription becomes history, I wonder whether this will contribute to a cultural shift in medicine. Will the demise of doctors' illegible scrawl eliminate the feeling of mystery and aura that has been such an important part of the handwritten prescription for so long? Have doctors been slow in embracing electronic prescribing partly because they have known intuitively that the mystique created by their illegible handwriting is a powerful tool in their armamentarium? Handing a patient an illegibly written prescription is certainly more awe-inspiring than telling the patient "I'm going to transmit the prescription to the pharmacy." When the prescription leaves the realm of mystery and enters the realm of commerce as a simple commodity, the magical and placebo aspects of the process are diminished. There is more magic when a prescription comes directly from the hands of a god than from a computer.

Should we as pharmacists welcome the predicted demise of the handwritten prescription and the magical/mystical aura associated with it? Should we view this as a sign of medicine's embrace of science and rejection of snake oil? Every pharmacist knows that the placebo effect can be powerful. Placebos can lessen pain, lower blood pressure, ease depression, etc. Should the placebo effect be ridiculed? Is it dishonest for a health professional to marshal whatever recuperative powers he can? When prescribing a drug, a doctor may say to the patient, "This is a highly effective drug." Such comments have been shown to increase the likelihood that the patient will experience benefits from the drug. On the other hand, when a doctor says to the patient, "I'm not sure whether this drug will work, but let's give it a try," the likelihood of patient benefit is diminished to some extent. This is the power of suggestion. The placebo effect is closely associated with the ritual involved in prescribing drugs. It's part of the whole authoritarian figure, white coat, dangling stethoscope scene that doctors intentionally cultivate.

Our customers seem to think that their doctor's handwritten prescription is far more than a simple note telling the pharmacist what drug to dispense, in what quantity, with what directions, etc. Many of our customers view the prescription as a personalized directive from a god. Of course, doctors do little to dissuade their patients from viewing them as gods.

Two lawsuits based on doctors' illegible handwriting

Illegible handwriting has been a sore spot with pharmacists for many years. It seems that whenever a pharmacist misreads an illegible prescription and consequently dispenses the wrong drug, the pharmacist gets all the blame. But things may be changing. Physicians were named in two lawsuits in the late 1990s because of illegible handwriting.

An illegible prescription that allegedly triggered a fatal medication error resulted in a physician being named as a defendant in a liability lawsuit in Texas. (Carol Ukens, "Fatal Vision, "*Drug Topics*, Sept. 1, 1997, p. 32) A lawsuit was filed against a cardiologist, a pharmacist, and a chain pharmacy in Odessa, Texas, on behalf of the widow and three children of a man who died following the medication error.

The suit alleged, in effect, that the cardiologist who wrote the illegible prescription handed the pharmacist a loaded gun. The pharmacist then pulled the trigger by failing to contact the prescriber and by failing to catch an excessive dosage.

The case began when a man in his 40s was discharged from the hospital by the cardiologist who had been treating him for heart problems. The physician wrote a prescription for the anti-angina drug Isordil. The suit alleged that when presented with the illegible prescription, the pharmacist made no attempt to contact the physician for clarification. The pharmacist read the prescription as the antihypertensive drug Plendil. The patient took the medication for one day. The following morning he suffered a heart attack, and he died several days later.

The plaintiff's attorney, Kent Buckingham, said, "The physician screwed up by writing illegibly. The pharmacist screwed up by not calling."

The pharmacist was named in the suit because he did not question the illegible prescription or the high dose of Plendil. The pharmacy was named in the suit because it failed to incorporate controls that could have prevented the error. For example, the pharmacy computer did not catch the excessive dose. And the physician was named in the suit for writing illegibly. According to the Institute for Safe Medication Practices, naming physicians in dispensing error lawsuits has been uncommon. ("Handwriting on the wall?" ISMP Medication Safety Alert, Institute for Safe Medication Practices, July 16, 1997)

On October 14, 1999 the jury found the physician liable for poor penmanship. The cardiologist, Albertson's pharmacy, and the pharmacist were ordered to pay $450,000 to the relatives of the deceased man. The physician was ordered to pay $225,000. Albertson's and the pharmacist were ordered to pay the other $225,000, but the pharmacy settled with the plaintiffs earlier for an undisclosed amount without admitting fault. ("Jury Punishes Poor Rx Penmanship," *Drug Topics*, November 1, 1999, p. 8)

I had hoped that this jury award would send a message to the medical profession that doctors need to learn basic penmanship. Alas, nothing has changed. But I am sure that pharmacists continue to hope that physicians are held accountable for their handwriting. Common sense says that it is almost impossible that this error would have occurred if the prescription had been typewritten or generated by a computer.

In a New York case, a plaintiff sought to recover damages from a pharmacy and pharmacist after ingesting the antihypertensive drug Dynacirc, which was erroneously dispensed instead of the prescribed antibiotic Dynacin. Subsequently, the pharmacy and pharmacist filed a suit against the prescriber, alleging negligence based on the physician's failure to write the prescription clearly and legibly. The pharmacy was found liable for the damages resulting from the dispensing error, and its attempt to shift liability to the physician failed. (Larry M. Simonsmeier, "Pharmacy Blames Physician's Handwriting," *Pharmacy Times*, June 1997, p. 21)

Who should be liable when an injury results from a prescription error allegedly caused by physicians' poor handwriting? Pharmacists are usually irate when they are held liable for misreading a poorly written prescription, while the physician goes blameless.

I propose that all patients who receive poorly legible prescriptions tell their doctors that they are concerned that the pharmacist will have difficulty reading it. If enough people begin doing this, doctors will get the message. The public should be offended by prescriptions that are poorly legible. Patients should request that each letter in each word is plainly written and that each number is plainly written. Doctors cannot justify their poor handwriting. If the public demands it, physicians will be forced to take more time with their handwriting, or, better yet, adopt computer-based prescribing and computer link-ups with community pharmacies.

Illegible handwriting wastes too much time. It wastes the pharmacist's time having to decipher the scrawl. It wastes the doctor's staff's time when the pharmacist calls. It wastes the doctor's time resolving the confusion. And, of course, it inconveniences our (frequently impatient) customers.

The magazine *Pharmacy Times* has a regular section each month titled "Can You Read These Rx's?" I have noticed that some pharmacists approach this section (and illegible handwriting in general) as a fun game. Rather than be amused or entertained or challenged by poorly written prescriptions, pharmacists should be offended. The stakes are simply too high.

Here are a few more things that I wish the public would encourage their doctors to do, in order to cut down on errors from poorly written prescriptions. I wish doctors would always write the purpose of the medication on the prescription. For example, doctors should write, "Take one tablet daily for blood pressure" rather than "Take one tablet daily." This helps both the pharmacist and patient verify that the right medication is being dispensed.

Doctors should write out instructions rather than use abbreviations. For example, they should write "daily" rather than "QD." "QD" is too easily interpreted as QID (four times a day). Several years ago, a pharmacy intern at our store typed "Take one tablet four times a day" on a prescription for the diuretic Lasix for which the doctor had written "1 QD" (one tablet daily). We didn't discover the error until the customer returned for a refill. In this case, no harm occurred because the customer had been taking this drug for several months. We asked him about it and he said, "Yeah, I saw your directions, but I knew I was just supposed to take one a day. I mentioned it to my doctor and he said, 'Wow, they're really trying to dry you out!'" In other circumstances, the results could have been disastrous.

Nurses can't read doctors' handwriting

Nurses, like pharmacists, have trouble reading doctors' handwriting. Both nurses and pharmacists are often reluctant to check with the doctor, often because of the doctor's attitude. Here is an anecdote from a caring physician, David Hilfiker, M.D., that accurately describes the trouble illegible handwriting can cause (*Healing the Wounds: A Physician Looks at His Work*, New York: Pantheon, 1985, pp. 156-157).

Angie (I don't even know her last name) lays her own work aside and starts to copy the orders for Mrs. Dimmerling. "Who the hell does he think he is?" she mutters to herself. "I can hardly read this." I continue to write, but I'm listening, almost without knowing it, to Angie's angry comments to herself.

"Beth," Angie says as she walks over to an older nurse on the other side of the nurses' station, I can't even read this. What's Oberdorfer want here?"

"Hmm. I'm not sure. Looks like two teaspoons of Maalox every two hours."

"Yeah, I guess you're right. Two teaspoons. Wait a minute! Oberdorfer never orders two teaspoons of antacid. Remember him getting on that poor intern for not ordering enough? He said you always order at least two tablespoons. Remember him quoting that Journal article about antacid efficacy? He can't have meant two teaspoons."

"Yeah, but he sure didn't write two tablespoons. That's got to be two teaspoons. Why don't you page him and ask."

"Oh, sure, page Oberdorfer and tell him he blew it. 'Dr. Oberdorfer,'" Angie mimics herself in a singsong Southern drawl, "'I think you just made a mistake. You didn't really mean two teaspoons of Maalox, did you?' Come on, Beth, remember when Tricia tried to correct him? He just laid into her and ripped her apart. He wrote 'two teaspoons' and Mrs. Dimmerling's getting two teaspoons."

"I suppose so. It won't hurt Mrs. Dimmerling any, and maybe it'll teach Oberdorfer a lesson. I wouldn't count on that, though."

Angie and Beth return to their work and I try to return to mine. I can hardly believe what I've just heard.

I can't read this prescription: Does the doctor want Pediaprofen? Pediapred? No! He wants Pediazole.

Several years ago I received a poorly legible prescription from a local doctor. It was a Saturday morning when a lady brought in a prescription for her young son. I couldn't tell whether the doctor wanted Pediaprofen or Pediapred. The directions were clearly written: "Take 2 teaspoonsful every 12 hours." I called the doctor's office and got his answering service. I was told that this doctor was not on call this weekend. His partner was on call. The doctor who had actually written this prescription a couple of days earlier was at the beach this weekend. I asked the answering service to have the on-call partner call me at the pharmacy.

An hour or so later, the partner finally called. I explained the situation to him. I said, "It looks like either Pediaprofen or Pediapred." Then the doctor asked me, "How old is the child?" We had the child's age in the computer from a previous visit. Based solely on the child's age and his partner's directions, the doctor determined that the prescription couldn't be for Pediaprofen. He concluded that it had to be Pediapred. So he said, "Make it Pediapred."

It turns out that the customer was not coming back until later in the day, so I kept the prescription on the counter and kept looking at it. I was uncomfortable with the way that the partner had come to his decision without checking the patient's records.

About three hours later (the child's mother still hadn't come back), I looked at the prescription again and, eureka! it occurred to me: It's not Pediapred or Pediaprofen. It's Pediazole!!!

So I double-checked the recommended dosage for Pediazole. The *Physicians' Desk Reference* says that Pediazole should be given three or four times per day, not every twelve hours as the doctor had clearly written.

I called the doctor's on-call partner and told him that I thought the prescription was not for Pediaprofen or Pediapred. I said it looks like Pediazole. The doctor then said that I should fax the prescription to their office—where he would be in an hour—so that he could look at it. He told me that he also wanted to show his partner how much of a problem this illegible handwriting was causing.

We get a ton of prescriptions from these two doctors so I didn't want to make either of them mad at us. So I said jokingly that I wished he wouldn't make his partner mad at us for this incident. (I know from past experience that the out-of-town partner can be a first class jerk.) He said, "If he gets mad, that's his problem." Hopefully, my joking eased the tension in this situation because the partner with whom I was speaking was becoming mildly irritated over the situation.

I faxed the prescription to their office. About three hours later, having received no return call, I called their office and asked whether he received my fax. He said, "Yeah, and it looks like Pediazole." This made him look negligent for jumping to the conclusion earlier that the prescription was for Pediapred.

The doctor asked whether I had the mother's phone number handy because he wanted to call her to see exactly what the child's problem was in order to determine which drug had been prescribed.

I gave the doctor the patient's home phone number. A few minutes later, the doctor called back and said that he had spoken with the child's mother and that, based on the child's symptoms, the prescription had to be for Pediazole even though he couldn't figure out why his partner had prescribed it every twelve hours.

In summary, this is what happened. I initially called this doctor and told him that his partner apparently was prescribing either Pediaprofen or Pediapred. The partner jumped to the conclusion that the prescription had to be for Pediapred. It turns out that it was neither. It was for Pediazole.

Situations such as this occur far too frequently. It's time that pharmacists take a stand and it's time that the public realizes the absurdity of jokes about doctors' illegible handwriting. Illegible handwriting is no laughing matter.

Note: Just because all three of these drug names start with *pedia* doesn't mean they're used for the same thing. They certainly are not. They are all entirely different. Pediaprofen (now, Children's Motrin) is used for pain, fever, and inflammation. Pediapred is a prednisone-like drug that is used for a long list of disorders (endocrine, rheumatic, collagen, skin, allergies, respiratory, blood disorders, cancers, etc.). Pediazole is an antibiotic. *Pedia* in each case stands for "pediatric." What these three drugs do have in common is that they're all used in kids.

Is it harder to read male doctors' handwriting?

The existence of physicians' poor penmanship has been acknowledged for a long time. But I have never heard anyone ask the obvious question: "*Why* do physicians write so poorly?" Probably the most frequently cited explanation is that doctors are very busy people. But this explanation isn't very convincing because lots of people in our society are very busy. Is illegible handwriting proportional to how busy one is, or are there other considerations?

A study in the *British Medical Journal* [Berwick DM and Winick-off, DE, "The truth about doctors' illegible handwriting: a prospective study," *BMJ* 1996 Dec 21-28;313(7072):1657-8] found that significantly lower legibility than average was associated with being an executive and being male, rather than being a doctor per se.

It might be interesting to ask pharmacists whether they feel that female physicians are less likely to have illegible handwriting. What percent of calls to doctors' offices for prescription clarification are to female physicians? As I look back on my career as a pharmacist, my impression is that calls to doctors' offices to clarify illegible handwriting are overwhelmingly to male doctors.

Of course, it would be wrong to associate illegible handwriting completely with ego. One of the most arrogant physicians in one town I used to work in had absolutely beautiful handwriting. I never recall having any difficulty in reading his prescriptions. Yet, whenever he called the pharmacy, it was clear that he expected us to genuflect to him. We were only pharmacists and he was the doctor and God help us if we forgot that.

In fairness to doctors, it occurs to me that there are lots of pharmacists who also write poorly. Is poor handwriting by pharmacists any less dangerous than poor handwriting by doctors? I can recall many instances in which I have had questions about a phoned-in prescription that was transcribed by another pharmacist. It wouldn't be so bad if all pharmacists filled all their "doctor phone-ins" themselves before they leave their shift. However, in many instances, pharmacists leave a pile of these "doctor phone-ins" for the pharmacist on the next shift. But there is a significant difference here. When the illegible handwriting is from another pharmacist, I can usually contact that pharmacist more easily than a doctor. And the pharmacist's attitude is usually more understanding and less arrogant, so I am less reluctant to call the pharmacist.

Chapter 4

Mistakes when doctors phone, fax, and e-prescribe drugs

Mistakes when doctors talk too damn fast
while phoning prescriptions to the pharmacist

I once worked with a pharmacist who had recently graduated from pharmacy school. He had been licensed for only a few weeks. One day he made the comment to me that he was sometimes having difficulty keeping up with doctors when they phoned in prescriptions. This pharmacist asked me if I knew any way to slow the doctors down. In the real world, telling the doctors "Slow down!" is not a great option. Doctors are busy people who seem to do everything in a hurry, including speaking with pharmacists.

This young pharmacist has a very legitimate concern. Doctors often phone the pharmacy with anywhere from one to five prescriptions for a single patient. The pharmacist must write down the patient's name, the drug name, the number of pills, how often the pills are to be taken (once a day, three times a day, every 4 hours, etc.), and the number of refills. Each piece of info is critically important, so pharmacists are rightfully concerned with writing down everything accurately. The more prescriptions the doctor phones in, the greater the chances that pharmacists will write down something incorrectly.

Early in my career, I, too, experienced this problem with speedy doctors. On more than one occasion, I had to call back to the doctor's office and ask the receptionist/nurse/office manager, "Dr. Smith just called me with a prescription for Bob Williams and I'm not sure how many Vicodin he wants Mr. Williams to have. Could you ask Dr. Smith?" Obviously this is an uncomfortable conversation and it is time consuming.

Some pharmacists think they can remember the doctor's instructions as if somehow our brain records everything and lets us mentally rewind and replay the phone conversation after the doctor has hung up. But most pharmacists do try to write down everything as the doctor speaks, rather than rely on our memory. Sometimes I write down the info so quickly that I can't decipher my own handwriting after the doctor has hung up.

You ask: Why not read each prescription back to the doctor? Reading everything back to the doctor when the doctor finishes is a good idea but it is sometimes quite uncomfortable because the doctor's impatience is palpable. Reading everything back to the doctor might imply that I am a rookie pharmacist who's not confident and competent in my job. Pharmacists sometimes like to impress doctors by our ability to keep up with them. An experienced pharmacist doesn't have to ask the doctor to repeat anything. After writing down everything the doctors says, the experienced pharmacist immediately says to the doctor simply "Thank you." We as pharmacists are saying to the doctor: *Doctor, you think you're good at what you do. Well I'm just as good at what I do.*

In answering this young pharmacist's question regarding a method to slow down doctors on the phone, I told him what worked for me: "To slow the doctor down, every few seconds I interject an *okay* into the conversation. Sometimes I say *okay* quickly. Other times I drag out my *okay* for as long as I can. The pharmacist needs a way to break the doctor's stride when he's off to the races. Only a doctor who's a first class jerk will run over your *okays*. Inserting the word *okay* forces the doctor to pause momentarily or else appear to be a complete asshole who's totally unconcerned with avoiding mistakes."

Clearly, most phone calls from doctors are not what I would describe as being at a leisurely pace. I once witnessed a pharmacist answer the phone line reserved for incoming calls from doctors (our so-called "doctors' line").   After a few moments, the pharmacist said, "Doctor, can you hold on for a second? You caught me with my pants down." The pharmacist couldn't find a pen or prescription pad to write down the doctor's prescription. This could be viewed as a friendly and human way to ask the doctor to wait for a few seconds, but I admit I felt a little uncomfortable hearing the pharmacist express it that way.

Mistakes when prescriptions are phoned to drugstores by doctors' nurses or receptionists

A not uncommon source of error is when a nurse or receptionist phones the pharmacy with a prescription. Young pharmacists are surprised that doctors so often allow inexperienced staff with very little knowledge of drug names to phone prescriptions to the pharmacist. It's as if the nurse or receptionist is doing nothing more critical than phoning the local sub shop with a lunch order.

When the nurse or receptionist calls the pharmacist, it is not uncommon for us to hear her ask for help in deciphering a drug name. Pharmacists commonly hear her say: "You'll have to help me with this one" or "This one looks like" or "I'll need to spell this one for you." Pharmacists are not only amazed that doctors allow such inexperienced people to relay prescriptions to the pharmacy, but we are often worried that we can be blamed if an error occurs.

The nurse or receptionist can misread the doctor's prescription but, if an error occurs, that nurse or receptionist can claim "I phoned in the right medication! The pharmacist must have written it down wrong!" Obviously, we as pharmacists don't have proof (a handwritten prescription in our files) that the nurse or receptionist made a mistake.

I was filling in at a pharmacy in Durham, North Carolina, for a week for a pharmacist's vacation. One day I came to work and the other pharmacist said to me that I had taken a phoned-in prescription from a doctor's office in which I wrote down Prilosec, when, in fact, the prescription was for Prozac. Apparently the patient had questioned the medication received, called the doctor's office, asked the nurse or receptionist what had happened, and then, apparently, that same nurse or receptionist claimed to have called in the right medication.

Of course, it is very possible that I did indeed write down the wrong drug. Both Prilosec and Prozac can sound very similar on the phone, especially when there's background noise in the pharmacy: another phone ringing, technicians jabbering, customers talking and complaining, etc.

So, I could have made the error, or the nurse or receptionist may have misread the doctor's prescription. It's possible that I misunderstood the drug name. Perhaps I had just filled a prescription for Prilosec and consequently I had that drug on my mind.

When the other pharmacist informed me that the nurse or receptionist claimed I simply wrote down the wrong drug, I had no way of proving otherwise. The nurse or receptionist may have misread the doctor's handwriting and she may have been covering up for her own error.

On another occasion, a different nurse or receptionist phoned me with a prescription for Inderal LA 40 mg. Inderal is used for conditions like hypertension, angina, or migraine. I didn't recall that this sounded like a strength that was available so I asked the nurse or receptionist to repeat the drug name and strength. She said again, "Inderal LA 40mg." I said, "Could you hold on just a second?" I wanted to take a quick look at our shelves to see whether we had such a strength. We didn't but this doesn't necessarily mean that it is not on the market. We were extremely busy at that time, so I didn't have the opportunity to check the appropriate reference material to see whether it was indeed on the market. So I returned to the phone and repeated again, "Inderal LA 40 mg." The nurse or receptionist again said "Yes." When I finally had time to look it up, I discovered what I suspected. The drug is not available in that strength. The long-acting form of Inderal (known as Inderal LA) is available only in the following strengths: 60 mg, 80 mg, 120 mg, and 160 mg. I called back and asked to speak with the same nurse or receptionist with whom I had spoken previously. I said to her, "Inderal LA 40 mg is not listed." She said, "Hold on and let me check." She returned a few minutes later and said, "It's supposed to be Inderal LA 160 mg." I told my partner about this incident and she commented, "If people only knew how many mistakes are made in doctors' offices!" The bottom line is that this nurse or receptionist called in a dose that was one-fourth of the intended dose. Under other circumstances, this could have been a dangerous mistake.

Here is an example of a nurse calling a pharmacy about a commonly prescribed drug. In this case, the nurse was apparently inadequately familiar with the drug to be able to prevent an obvious misinterpretation of a doctor's directions. Examples like this happen all the time in pharmacies across America. This example involves the anti-diarrheal drug Imodium which is available as 2 mg capsules. A fancy term for "diarrhea" is "unformed stools." Hospital pharmacist Steve Timmerman writes in *Drug Topics* ("Strange Rx Stories: Now That's a Smart Stool," July 1, 2002, p. 42):

It's not unusual to receive orders for Imodium as "two capsules now and then one after each loose stool." One evening, a nurse called and told me she needed Imodium 4 mg for an initial dose and then 2 mg for every time there was an "informed stool." I repeated this order back to her and questioned the "informed" part. She was confident the order read "informed stool." I brought the initial dose to the patient care area and picked up the copy of the order. The physician had actually written for 2 mg to be given after each "unformed" stool.

The point is that the system is absolutely fraught with the potential for errors from the time a doctor decides to prescribe a drug until that medication is picked up at the drugstore.

Mistakes when prescriptions are faxed to drugstores from doctors' offices

Prescriptions faxed from doctors' offices can be another significant source of errors. Here are three separate incidents involving prescriptions faxed to pharmacies. The first incident involved Neurontin, the second incident involved Monopril, and the third incident involved lisinopril/hctz.   (Kate Kelly, PharmD, and Allen J. Vaida, PharmD, "'Fax Noise' Can Result in Medication Errors," *Pharmacy Times*, July 2004, p. 28)

Most health care practitioners would agree that facsimile (fax) machines have facilitated communication of prescriptions. There are, however, inherent problems associated with this technology. In fact, a recent article in the *Journal of Managed Care Pharmacy* found that prescriptions received by fax required a greater number of clarification calls than those received by other methods of communication.

We received a report from a longterm care facility about a patient who had been receiving Neurontin (gabapentin) 600 mg tid [three times a day]. An order had been faxed to the pharmacy that the pharmacist thought read to change the Neurontin dose to "300 mg 1 tab qid [four times a day]." The change was made, and the new dose was sent to the facility.

Later, when the pharmacist received the original order and compared it with the faxed order, he realized that the physician had actually requested a change to "800 mg 1 tab qid." The left side of the order had been cut off during the fax transmission, making the "8" look like a "3." Fortunately, because the pharmacist had been sent the original order for comparison, he quickly realized the mistake. Unfortunately, not all outpatient pharmacies receive the original prescription for comparison.

In another report, a faxed prescription was received at a pharmacy for what appeared to be for Monopril (fosinopril) "10 mg #90 one tablet daily." Despite the fact that the fax machine created a definite vertical streak that ran between the drug name and the strength, the pharmacist felt confident in her interpretation of the prescription. Unfortunately, the prescription was actually for "40 mg." The streak had run through the "4" in "40 mg," making it look like "10 mg" instead.

A prescription was faxed to a mail-order pharmacy... for "lisinopril/hctz." (Note: Institute for Safe Medication Practices does not condone the use of the abbreviation "hctz.") The pharmacist interpreted this order as "20/25 mg." What the prescriber had actually written, however, was "20/12.5 mg." A subtle vertical gap in the faxed copy (which also can be seen "breaking" the circles around "3 months supply") had obliterated the

"1" in "12.5." In addition, the pharmacist reading the order had misinterpreted the decimal point as one of many stray marks.

Mistakes when prescriptions are transmitted electronically from doctors to drugstores

Much has been written lately about how transmitting prescriptions electronically to pharmacies can drastically cut down on errors. Many articles imply that this technology can virtually eliminate errors caused by doctors' illegible handwriting. But few of these articles explain that electronic prescriptions (e-prescribing) can introduce a new set of problems. Pharmacists have many stories about problems that can result from the use of this technology. For example, here is a post from the Internet discussion group sci.med.pharmacy by a pharmacist who goes by rxempress (rxempress@mmchsi.com) (Subject: What do you think about medication errors? Newsgroups: sci.med.pharmacy, Sept. 16, 2004)

I have caught quite a few errors on electronic prescriptions. Our local doctors are using palm pilots which involve a touch sensitive screen. I have seen a couple cases where they selected the wrong drug (touched the wrong one). Last week one was sent to me with the directions "one tablet 4 times daily". This was 4 times the regular dose. Dr keyed in QID (4 times daily) and meant QD (once daily). This is exactly the type of error that these systems are supposed to prevent. (It is very easy to misread a handwritten QID and a QD). The mistakes are still being made... it's just easier to read the mistake. It's catching the mistake that's the tough part and in this case contacting the doctor and explaining the mistake took about a week to do.

There are advantages and disadvantages to having doctors transmit prescriptions electronically to the pharmacy. One pharmacist sent me an e-mail in which he stated one advantage:

Electronic prescriptions seem to be increasing all the time. Depending on the store I think they are about 10% of the total. One positive way to

look at these prescriptions is that in the past each one would have been the phone ringing. The telephone ringing in my ear has a Pavlov's dog reaction in me. I am sure the sound raises my pressure a bit each time. The phone is such an intrusion on what you are doing at the moment.

Here is a disadvantage of electronic prescriptions. This is a case from the Institute for Safe Medication Practices in which a hospitalized patient died from respiratory arrest after a physician entered drug orders electronically under the name of the wrong patient. ("Oops, Sorry, Wrong Patient!: A Patient Verification Process is Needed Everywhere, Not Just at the Bedside," Institute for Safe Medication Practices—ISMP Medication Safety Alert! Acute Care Edition, posted May 17, 2011,
http://www.medscape.com/viewarticle/742372?src=mp&spon=30)

A dehydrated lung cancer patient was admitted to the emergency department for IV hydration. Another patient from a motor vehicle accident (MVA) was awaiting intubation and transfer to a local trauma center. The same physician was caring for both patients. The physician gave verbal orders for vecuronium and midazolam for the MVA patient, but he inadvertently entered the medication orders electronically into the cancer patient's record. The nurse caring for the cancer patient went on break, and a covering nurse administered the paralytic and sedative to the cancer patient even though he was not intubated. The patient experienced a respiratory arrest and died.

Here is another case from the Institute for Safe Medication Practices. In this case a doctor's error on an electronic prescription was made worse when a pharmacist edited the prescription in an attempt to correct that doctor's error. The patient suffered respiratory arrest as a consequence of the pharmacist's error in the process of correcting the doctor's error. The patient was fortunately resuscitated. ("Keeping patients safe from iatrogenic methadone overdoses," Institute for Safe Medication Practices—ISMP Medication Safety Alert! Acute Care Edition, Feb. 14, 2008
http://www.ismp.org/newsletters/acutecare/articles/20080214.asp)

ISMP received a report about a 17-year-old patient with a traumatic brain injury who received 25 mg of methadone BID [twice a day] instead of methylphenidate. Using the hospital's computerized prescriber order entry system, the physician had increased the patient's methylphenidate dose from 20 to 25 mg, but he accidentally selected a 2.5 mg tablet strength, which was available in the hospital (1/2 tablets of the 5 mg strength were routinely packaged by the pharmacy). During the order verification process, the pharmacist edited the order to indicate that 10 mg strength tablets should be used, but he accidentally changed the order from methylphenidate to methadone. The mnemonics for these drugs were almost identical: methadone 10 mg = METH10, and methylphenidate 10 mg = METH10T. The computer system did not alert the pharmacist that he had inadvertently changed the ordered medication, rather than the strength of tablets used to prepare the dose. The patient suffered a respiratory arrest after taking two doses of methadone; fortunately, he was resuscitated.

When pharmacist Joe Laborsky was the publisher at *Drug Topics*, he maintained a "Publisher's Blog" in which he invited feedback from pharmacists. During one period in the latter part of 2007, Laborsky's blog dealt with electronic prescribing. Several pharmacists posted comments questioning the accuracy of e-prescribing. ("Publisher's Blog: E-prescribing—Pharmacy Pays To Play," *Drug Topics*, Sept. 13, 2007). Here is a sample:

Kelly / Pflugerville, Texas / Posted Oct 31, 2007 **It has been my experience thus far that the chance of errors in prescribing is much greater with electronic prescribing than traditional methods. Those who tout e-prescribing as safer obviously haven't worked much in a pharmacy to observe the system in actual practice. Their interests are self-serving in trying to sell technology for the sake of technology and their profits, without any practical advantages whatsoever. It is so much easier to erroneously click on the wrong button than to write out the wrong drug. I have spent much more time contacting doctors in the past several months to clarify electronic prescriptions (wrong drug, strength, directions) than I have in the last several years with traditional prescriptions.**

Ken / Mendham, New Jersey / Posted Oct 16, 2007 **Accuracy? I have found more errors by e-prescribers than with written Rxs. The difference is that when the error is made, the e-script makes it look appropriate. ...As for improved accuracy "studies", who's paying for these studies?**

Frustrated R.Ph. / Iowa / Posted Oct 17, 2007 **I agree with others. I have seen horrible errors with electronic generated prescriptions.**

Drug Topics publisher Joe Laborsky, R.Ph. comments / Nov. 7, 2007:
Thanks to all of you who took the time to respond to my e-prescribing blog. ...I have to tell you that I was surprised to hear from many of you about mistakes M.D.s have made using this technology. This alarms me even more in that one of the primary advantages of this technology is that it should be a more accurate and reliable means of communicating the prescriber's choice of medication(s) to the pharmacy.

Harold E. Cohen, R.Ph, Editor-in-Chief at *U.S. Pharmacist,* offers his perspective on electronic prescriptions ("The e-ffective Pharmacist," *U.S. Pharmacist,* Feb. 2008, p. 2):

There is much discussion lately about how e-prescribing is the answer to all of pharmacy's woes, particularly drug errors. In fact, a spokesperson for General Motors was quoted in the *Detroit News* as saying, "The benefits of ePrescribing are overwhelming in terms of reducing medication errors." I'm not so sure. There is little doubt that e-prescribing will certainly all but eliminate prescription errors caused by sloppy physician handwriting, but it does nothing for prescriptions that are written incorrectly in the first place, and that seems to be a far bigger issue than illegible handwriting. One New York pharmacist recently wrote me that she has personally witnessed several errors with prescriptions that were electronically transmitted. She recalled one instance in which a very legible electronically transmitted prescription had the wrong drug prescribed on it. The pharmacist caught the mistake because the prescription was not consistent with her patient's medical and drug history. Other problems she's encountered are prescriptions containing "strengths which do not exist, directions which are terminated before the prescription was sent electronically [she thinks the directions may have been too long and didn't entirely fit into that data field], and no indication of whether the physician pre-scribed a generic or brand." She has also received prescriptions for pa-tients who normally do not get their prescriptions filled in her store. She said that several times patients have arrived to pick up an electronically transmitted prescription that was not yet transmitted. In such cases, she must then call the doctor and get the prescription over the phone. The electronic prescription generally arrives after the patient has already left the store with the filled prescription in hand. That wouldn't be so bad if it weren't for the fact that she is paying a transmission fee for every e-pre-scription she receives. She concludes: "I haven't found electronic trans-missions to have decreased mistakes or saved time; it just changed the nature of mistakes being committed and causes me to call the physician for a different reason. Adding insult to injury, my pharmacy is paying for these mistakes to be transmitted."

Estimates vary regarding the precise frequency at which prescrip-tions are transmitted electronically from doctors to pharmacies. Eighteen percent of prescriptions were being sent electronically in 2010, up from six percent in 2008, according to a National Progress Report on e-prescribing released by SureScripts, which operates an e-prescription network. SureScripts says that e-prescribing was used by one in four prescribers in 2010. SureScripts also says that the federal government's leadership and incentive structures are part of the rea-son for this increase. ("E-Prescribing Nearly Tripled in 2009: Re-port," *U.S. Pharmacist*, September 2010, p. 59)

Why have doctors been slow in embracing computer-based pre-scribing? Perhaps a big reason is the cost and complexity of comput-erizing a medical practice. Perhaps doctors fear what happens when their system crashes in the middle of a very hectic day. Of course, one of the biggest reasons for doctors continuing to embrace hand-written prescriptions is that they're so handy.

Perhaps computers make the doctor feel that the computer is in charge, not the doctor. That's certainly how I feel in the drugstore. The computer is the nerve center of the pharmacy nowadays. Phar-macy has become largely a data entry enterprise in which the ability to type fast is a major asset for technicians and pharmacists. But computers are very humbling and egalitarian.

I'm speculating but perhaps doctors don't want to become servants to computers wherein their large egos are subsumed by the strict dictates of this technology. Perhaps doctors see the computer as a threatening cultural shift in medicine that moves the emphasis toward technology and away from the view that the doctor is the center of the universe. Perhaps doctors would like their patients to believe that the prescription is too magical and mysterious for something as pedestrian as a computer. Perhaps doctors view computers as appropriate for data-entry, bookkeeping, billing, and scheduling, but inadequate for perpetuating the belief that doctors are gods.

According to a study supported by the federal Agency for Healthcare Research and Quality and the Harvard Risk Management Foundation, e-prescriptions are just as error-prone as paper scripts. (Robert Lowes, "E-Prescriptions Just as Error-Prone as Paper Scripts," *Medscape Medical News*, July 1, 2011. *J Am Med Inf Assn.* Published online June 29, 2011 www.medscape.com)

Government and the healthcare industry have placed big bets on digital technology, and electronic prescribing in particular, for the sake of patient safety, but a new study reports that the error rate with computer-generated prescriptions in physician offices roughly matches that for paper scripts: about 1 in 10.

However, results from the study, published online June 29 in the *Journal of the American Medical Informatics Association*, are not as damning as they may initially appear. Error rates varied widely depending on the type of e-prescribing software used, with some programs outperforming pen and paper. In addition, software improvements could eliminate more than 80% of the mistakes, most of them involving omitted information.

In 2010, an estimated 190,000 physicians were electronically prescribing, the technical term for transmitting scripts directly to a pharmacy computer, according to a pharmacy industry group called Surescripts. That number does not include physicians who create a prescription with computer software and then either fax it to the pharmacy or give patients a printout.

Since 2009, the federal government has been paying hundreds of millions of dollars in Medicare bonuses to physicians and other clinicians who electronically prescribe. The government operates an even pricier incentive program for electronic health records, and e-prescribing is one of the prerequisites for earning a 6-figure bonus.

The new study study examined nearly 3900 computer-generated prescriptions received by a pharmacy chain in 2008 in Florida, Massachusetts, and Arizona, regardless of whether they were faxed or electronically transmitted to pharmacies or were printed out. Of those prescriptions, 11.7% contained at least 1 error. Researchers did not ascertain whether errors were corrected by the pharmacy chain or whether they led to an actual adverse drug event. Lead author Karen Nanji, MD, MPH, writes that the 11.7% figure is "consistent with the literature on manual handwritten prescription error rates."

Roughly one third of the errors represented potential adverse drug events, none of them life-threatening.

Software Improvements Must Be Physician-Friendly

Omitted information such as drug dose, duration, and frequency accounted for almost 61% of the errors detected by the authors. The rest of the errors stemmed from unclear, conflicting, or clinically incorrect information.

Software improvements, Dr. Nanji and coauthors write, could eliminate the vast majority of these mistakes. E-prescribing programs can incorporate so-called forcing functions that would prevent physicians from completing a prescription unless they enter required information, including complete drug names and proper abbreviations. Likewise, decision-support tools can issue alerts about a wrong drug dose or frequency. However, the authors note, physicians may rebel against e-prescribing software if antierror safeguards make it too slow or annoying to use.

Some e-prescribing programs included in the study appeared to give users a technological edge. The error rate associated with one such program was only 5.1% compared with a whopping 37.5% for another. However, the study did not assess whether the root cause was system design or how well or poorly the systems were implemented in physician offices. Training physicians and staff on new software systems, the authors note, is often given short shrift.

Chapter 5

Getting prompt answers from doctors is difficult

The process of trying to resolve questions about wrong doses or potential interactions is a source of tremendous frustration for pharmacists. In my experience, what usually happens is something like this. The pharmacist calls the doctor's office and says something like, "I have a prescription here that Dr. Smith wrote today for [Drug X] for Mary Jones. Our computer has flagged a "most significant interaction" between [Drug X and Drug Y]. Could you check with Dr. Smith to make sure we should go ahead and fill the prescription?"

What I'm really saying is that I'm not eager to fill the prescription since our computer flags the interaction as "most significant." I'm trying to put the ball completely in the doctor's court (and give the doctor full notice) so if the patient suffers harm, the doctor is to blame. Of course, it's not that simple because pharmacists have a right and duty to refuse to fill any prescription that the pharmacist feels is not in the patient's best interest. Pharmacists can be liable if the patient suffers harm from the interaction even though the doctor confirmed in a phone call that we should go ahead and fill the prescription as written.

The nurse/receptionist who takes the pharmacist's phone call does one of the following things.

Phone Scenario #1 (Least likely): The doctor is not busy and is standing nearby so the nurse/receptionist immediately says to the doctor, "CVS is calling about a prescription for Mary Jones. The pharmacist says there's a drug interaction."

Then the doctor either tells the nurse/receptionist to tell the pharmacist to go ahead and fill the prescription as written or the doctor tells the nurse/receptionist to tell the pharmacist to change the offending drug (to drug Z) to avoid the potential interaction.

Some doctors do indeed get on the phone and read the pharmacist the riot act for calling about what the doctor considers to be an insignificant interaction. That has happened to me a few times. It has the effect of dampening pharmacists' enthusiasm for calling that doctor in the future about potential interactions (and, indeed, for calling doctors about anything).

When I worked at one drugstore in North Carolina, a local doctor phoned one day and said that we were calling his office too often about potential interactions. That particular store is very busy with many different pharmacists rotating in and out on different days. These relief pharmacists understandably haven't worked in that store long enough to have learned the personal preferences of local doctors. These relief pharmacists have no idea that this particular doctor doesn't like to be phoned about potential interactions. I mentioned this to another pharmacist who worked there occasionally. This pharmacist suggested to me in disgust that the doctor needed to mail us a letter relieving us of any liability in the event that one of his patients suffered harm resulting from an interaction between drugs he prescribed. Obviously we never requested such a letter from that doctor. And obviously that would not relieve the pharmacist of responsibility for filling a prescription for drugs that interact adversely.

In my opinion, modern medicine is primarily about power, ego, status, and wealth. Health is further down the line. I suspect that it looks bad in the nurse/receptionist's eyes when a pharmacist phones and says that the doctor made an error in dosage or with regard to a potential interaction. So the doctor occasionally feels he needs to protect his ego and reputation in front of the nurse/receptionist by calling the pharmacist and reading him the riot act.

Phone Scenario #2 (Much more likely): The nurse/receptionist tells the pharmacist, "I'll check with Dr. Smith and get back to you." I would say that, on average, it may take forty-five minutes for us to get a call back from the nurse/receptionist. Most likely fifteen minutes to an hour, but it can easily be two or three hours before the pharmacist gets a return call from the nurse/receptionist. Many nurse/receptionists do not call back until the end of the day (5 PM or 6 PM). Some doctors do not address pharmacy calls until they have seen ALL their patients. (Likewise, when patients themselves call their doctors about some question, many doctors do not call the patient back until after the doctor has seen all his patients for that day.)

It is unrealistic for a patient to assume that the pharmacist can immediately resolve a dose or interaction question with a quick phone call to the doctor's office. Nurse/receptionists usually wait for an opportunity to ask the doctor about the dose or interaction. A few nurse/receptionists immediately call the doctor on the office phone system and the doctor gives an instantaneous answer. But that's doesn't seem to be particularly common in my experience.

If a customer brings a prescription to the drugstore after the doctor's regular office hours or on a weekend or holiday, getting in touch with the doctor is even more difficult. Yes most doctors pay an answering service for these situations. But, too often, when we do call the answering service, the doctor who calls us back is actually the on-call partner who knows nothing of the situation but, thankfully, he is usually willing to make the necessary changes in the prescriptions if warranted.

So patients should never expect that dose or interaction or illegible handwriting questions can be resolved quickly. Having a patient wait at the pharmacy for the matter to be resolved with the doctor is something that most pharmacists have learned is not a good idea.

Of course, many customers get very upset at having to wait. In addition, telling the customer what we're doing can be tricky. It doesn't instill much confidence in patients when we tell them "Your doctor just prescribed a dose that's far too high for a child" or "Your doctor prescribed a drug for you that may interact with another drug you're taking." If we say this to the customer, we are essentially saying that their doctor doesn't know what proper dosages are for the drugs he prescribes or their doctor doesn't know about interactions among the drugs he prescribes. So the pharmacist might say, "I need to phone your doctor to clear up something." Then the customer is in a complete fog as to what's going on. Many pharmacists are indeed quite forthright and do indeed tell the customer that the doctor prescribed a questionable dose or a drug that may interact with other drugs the patient is taking. Some pharmacists are indeed very direct in explaining what's going on. Other pharmacists try hard to protect the reputation of local doctors from whom we get lots of prescriptions. (Doctors can easily steer patients to competitors.) Some pharmacists don't care whether the explanation to the customer makes the doctor look bad.

There is tremendous variation in the threshold that different pharmacists use when deciding when to phone the doctor about a questionable dose or potential interaction. Many young pharmacists just out of pharmacy school call doctors' offices very often, whereas many veteran pharmacists call doctors only in cases of the most blatant or serious dosage or interaction questions. Young pharmacists working in busy chain drugstores soon learn that they don't have time to call doctors' offices as often as they were instructed to do in pharmacy school. In the real world, chain pharmacy is about quantity, not quality.

Physicians almost never call the pharmacist back promptly. Doctors seem to give priority to the patients being seen rather than drop everything and address the pharmacist's concerns. I think this contrasts with what doctors do when other doctors are on the phone. Short anecdote: When my father was visiting several doctors before being diagnosed with lymphoma, I accompanied him on several of these visits. One time my father mentioned to one of these doctors that he had recently been to another local doctor for an evaluation. Immediately, the doctor phoned that other doctor and got thru to him right away. My impression is that doctors give much greater priority when other doctors phone, in contrast to when pharmacists phone.

Sometimes we never hear back from the doctor's office. Sometimes the doctor is out of town, or on vacation, or not on call that weekend, etc. Not hearing back from doctors' offices is not unusual. Pharmacists often have to make an additional call to doctors' offices to remind the nurse/receptionists that we never received an answer to the dosage or interaction question. Consequently, many customers go home in limbo, without the prescription. We tell the customer we can't fill the prescription until the nurse/receptionist or the doctor calls us back. Some customers get angry. Other customers are accustomed to these difficulties in dealing with very busy doctors or their disorganized/incompetent staffs.

In general, I would say that doctors view pharmacists' calls as nuisance calls. The hierarchy in modern medicine is very rigid. Doctors are at the top of the pyramid and pharmacists learn very quickly we are not viewed by doctors as professional equals. Way too many doctors view themselves as gods. How dare the pharmacist phone and claim that there is a potential drug interaction or wrong dose!!!!! Very few doctors seem to view the pharmacist's call as one health professional (the pharmacist) consulting with another health professional (the doctor) on equal terms for the best interests of the patient.

Over my career of 25 years, I spoke with hundreds (perhaps thousands) of doctors. My view (and, I suspect, that of many pharmacists) is that issues of power and hierarchy are, at the very least, as important to doctors as is the health of their patients.

My pharmacy school was in the same medical center complex as the medical school. Pharmacy students see what types of students go into medicine. The competitiveness that is required to gain admission to medical school is often precisely the opposite personality trait that is needed to be a truly compassionate physician. It is my opinion that many pharmacists, as a result of years of talking to doctors on the phone, have a skeptical view of the humanitarianism of many doctors.

Let me emphasize that some pharmacists do indeed call doctors too much. Some pharmacists call about interactions that are unlikely to cause a significant problem. But, of course, an interaction can be much more serious in one person than another. Pharmacy computers seem to be programmed to flag every potential problem, rather than only the most serious problems. Some pharmacy computers grade the seriousness of the interaction as "Level 1," "Level

2," or "Level 3." Many times I have seen pharmacists call doctors about interactions that I would not have called about. So, from the perspective of doctors, it is fair to say that some pharmacists are making calls of marginal significance. Some pharmacists seem to like to parade their drug knowledge in front of doctors, as if the pharmacist is saying "Gotcha!"

I would say that half of the students in my pharmacy school class were serious students and serious people. The other half seemed to be interested in learning the least they could to graduate. I guess my point is that I don't really have much respect for perhaps half the pharmacists I know and I suspect that many doctors have come to the same conclusion as a result of some of the phone calls they (doctors) get from pharmacists.

A disturbing incident when my mother was in a hospice in Florida

Here's a disturbing incident that occurred when my mother was in a hospice in Florida. It illustrates many things about our health care system, including the fact that it can often be difficult to get prompt answers from doctors, even in emergencies.

I was fortunate to be able to be with my mother for the last several days before she died from colon cancer that spread to her liver. At our nearby community hospital, she was given a continuous drip of morphine for her intense pain. Her oncologist had given orders that the nurse on duty could supplement that morphine drip with a direct injection from a syringe as needed in the event of any breakthrough pain (i.e., anytime my mother experienced especially severe pain that exceeded the ability of the continuous drip of morphine).

For example, I vividly remember one occasion when my mother began moaning terribly in pain. I ran out to find her nurse who happened to be with a patient in a room a couple of doors down. I told the nurse that my mother was moaning in pain. The nurse immediately accompanied me to my mother's room and administered maybe half of a syringe containing morphine. This seemed to help my mother quite quickly.

After a few days in the community hospital, my mother was transferred to the local hospice. I rode in the medical transport vehicle with my mother from the hospital to the hospice, a distance of about ten miles. While sitting in my mother's hospice room, I noticed that something wasn't right. Where is the morphine? In the hospital, a bag or bottle of morphine was her constant companion, hung near the head of her bed.

I went to the nurse's station and asked my mother's hospice nurse (a very professional and caring person), "Where is the morphine?" Suddenly, one of the other workers at the nurses' station piped up and said, "We have a call out to her oncologist."

So I went back to the room and waited. And waited. And waited. No morphine. I knew that my mother would soon be in excruciating pain without the morphine. She still had some morphine in her system from the hospital but I knew her pain would return when the effects of the hospital morphine wore off. So I went back to the nurses' station and asked about the status of the morphine. That same worker (I don't think she was a nurse) told me again, rudely, "We have a call out to her oncologist." I asked her (almost pleading for anything at this point), "Can't you just call the hospital where we just came from and get a confirmation of the morphine order she had there?" This MEAN WOMAN again rudely told me that they were awaiting a return call from my mother's oncologist.

I was getting very nervous because my mother had been without the morphine drip for over an hour (possibly approaching two hours) and I was afraid that at any moment she would be in excruciating pain. So I told this MEAN WOMAN who was speaking to me as if I had no understanding of the medical system, "I'm a pharmacist. I know you have to stay on 'em [doctors] when they don't return calls." This MEAN WOMAN at the nurses' station suddenly shut up.

Even though I try very hard to avoid confrontations with people, this MEAN WOMAN could see I was very tired of her attitude. My mother's nurse was standing nearby and heard my entire conversation with this MEAN WOMAN at the nurse's station. But the nurse did not say anything.

Several minutes later when my mother's oncologist finally called the hospice, the nice nurse came in my mother's room with the morphine. She told me "You were absolutely right" [to confront that MEAN WOMAN at the nurse's station]. I had the impression that the nice nurse had had other bad experiences with that MEAN WOMAN. The nice nurse told me that my mother's oncologist requested that she relay to me his very sincere apologies for failing to arrange the morphine order prior to my mother's arrival at the hospice.

A few weeks later, I received what looked like a standard questionnaire from the hospice, asking me to answer a few multiple choice questions as a way to assess my experience during my mother's brief stay at that hospice. There was also a space to add any additional comments. I had wanted so badly to tell the hospice administrator personally about this entire incident, but I was afraid that the administrator would think it was the nice nurse who was the person who rude to me, rather than the MEAN WOMAN at the nurses' station. So I didn't make any comments.

My mother died less than 36 hours after arriving at the hospice. I stayed with her the entire time, sleeping on a cot that was in the room. I think each nurse's shift lasted 12 hours. My mother had a different nurse assigned to her for each of the three shifts. The first nurse was absolutely spectacular. The overnight nurse was horrendous. And the nurse the next morning was average. But I'll never forget that MEAN WOMAN at the nurses' station who was handling the call to my mother's oncologist for the morphine order. During this time of profound sadness as I stayed with my mother before she died at the hospice, the situation was made worse by that MEAN WOMAN at the nurses' station who was a first class asshole.

I think this incident illustrates the following: (1) Patients in hospitals and hospices need a friend or family member present (preferably around the clock) to try to assure that the patient is getting reasonable attention. (2) Don't assume that your doctor will arrange pain relief medication orders ahead of time when a patient is transferred from a hospital to a hospice. (3) Don't assume that the physician can be contacted immediately in the case of an emergency. (4) Don't assume that all hospice workers will be helpful.

Both of my parents died from cancer and they both had different oncologists. (My father died from lymphoma). My father's oncologist was arrogant, aloof, and, in my opinion, a real jerk. In contrast, I really liked my mother's oncologist. He was much younger than my father's oncologist and a really down-to-earth person who didn't seem to have a big ego.

The day that my mother was transferred from the hospital to the hospice, my mother's oncologist told me (at the hospital) that he made rounds through the hospice in the mornings so I would probably see him there if I were in the room with my mother. It turns out that I was indeed there the next day and the oncologist never showed up. I don't know what the reason was but I suspect it may have been because he was so embarrassed for having failed to authorize the morphine prior to my mother's arrival at the hospice.

My mother's oncologist seemed to have a British sense of humor even though I could not detect a British accent. When the nice nurse informed me that he sincerely apologized on the phone for not having made arrangements for the morphine prior to my mother's arrival at the hospice, the nurse said that he said he was "aghast" to be informed that my mother was at the hospice without morphine. That sounded precisely like a word he would have used.

I never saw that oncologist after this event so I was never able to discuss it with him. I could certainly have visited his office and told him about my displeasure, but I realize that things like this happen all the time in our health care system where patients routinely fall through the cracks. He was a decent enough person up to this event so I saw no reason to stop in to see him.

Chapter 6

Doctors from a pharmacist's perspective

When doctors prescribe the wrong dose

1. Compazine error. One Saturday I received a prescription for a child aged 2 years 9 months. The prescription was for Compazine 12.5 mg suppositories, a drug used to treat severe nausea and vomiting. The doctor's directions were "Insert 1 suppository rectally every 6 to 8 hours." If these suppositories were inserted every 6 hours (four times a day), the child would receive 50 mg of Compazine per day. However, the recommended dose for severe nausea and vomiting for a child weighing 30 to 39 pounds (my estimate of the weight of a child at this age) is "not to exceed 10 mg per day." (2003 *PDR*, p. 1491) If the child were given 4 suppositories per day, he could well have gotten five times the recommended dose.

The *PDR* (2003 ed., p. 1491) lists the following symptoms of overdosage, among others: "Symptoms of central nervous system depression to the point of somnolence or coma. Agitation and restlessness may also occur. Other possible manifestations include convulsions, EKG changes and cardiac arrhythmias...."

It so happened that I did not catch the doctor's error until after the child's father already picked up the finished prescription. We were very busy at that time and I was working as fast as my hands would allow me. About a half hour later, I got an uneasy feeling that the doctor had overdosed the child. So I looked up the recommended dose and discovered that the doctor had indeed made a big error.

The prescription had been written at the local hospital emergency room so I called there hoping the doctor was still on duty. Luckily, he was. I said to him, "I just filled a prescription for Compazine suppositories for [child's name]. You probably know more about pediatric dosing than I do, but isn't the dose you prescribed a little high?" I said "a little high" in an attempt to be nice. Actually, it was dangerously high. He said, "Okay, let's make it twice a day." I said, "That's still a daily dose of 25 mg which is still more than double the recommended dose for a child who weighs 30 to 39 pounds." Incredibly, he asked, "What's the recommended dose?"

I told him that the *PDR* says the recommended dose for nausea and vomiting in a child 30 to 39 pounds is "not more than 10 mg per day." He seemed to be quite concerned at this point. Then I told him that I had already dispensed the prescription and that the child's father had already left the store. Then he made a statement that irritated me. He said, "You went ahead and dispensed the prescription?" I said "It wasn't 'til after the child's father left that I got worried." I had the impression he was trying to shift some of the blame to me even though he was the one who had written the prescription. He was, however, essentially quite decent during our exchange. But he seemed to become even more worried. I told him, "I've got the father's home phone number and I'll give him a call if you like." He said, "Please do."

Luckily, the child's mother answered the phone when I called and luckily she hadn't given the child a suppository yet. I told her that the doctor and I decided that the child would be better off with a lower dose. I did not tell her that the doctor had made a potentially serious mistake and that I had failed to catch it before dispensing the drug. The mother didn't seem to be upset. She said that she would have her husband return the suppositories as I requested.

I called the doctor back and said that I had reached the child's mother and that she hadn't given the child a suppository yet. The doctor was audibly relieved. He then told me to change the prescription to 2.5 mg every 6 to 8 hours (a total daily dose one-fifth of his original order). Then he said "I really appreciate what you did a whole lot."

My comment: The doctor sounded very young and very hurried. I'm probably not as young but equally hurried. When customers demand that prescriptions be filled with lightning speed, errors like this are inevitable.

2. Albuterol error. One day I received a prescription from another doctor for Albuterol inhalation solution for asthma. This medication is put in a special breathing machine. It comes two ways: as a concentrated solution and as a pre-diluted solution. The user or caregiver is to mix, usually, half a cc of the Albuterol with 2.5 cc of a diluting solution before administration. This prescription was for a child.

When I received this prescription, it had a few numbers on it that made no sense. The child's mother told me that she was in a hurry. But I still had to call the doctor who wrote the prescription to clear up the confusion. The child's mother only seemed to be interested in getting the medication. She did not seem to understand or appreciate my efforts to clear up this doctor's confusing prescription.

The customer had just received the prescription from the local hospital emergency room. I called the doctor there and asked him what, in particular, two numbers were supposed to indicate. He told me that he had never prescribed that particular product before so he was not very familiar with it. He said that he had prescribed it as a result of the child's mother's request. He apologized for the resulting confusion. He said that he had started to prescribe the concentrated solution but the child's mother had asked for the dilute solution because she had used the dilute solution before. He said that he had never prescribed the pre-diluted solution before and asked me to describe the form in which it was available.

The doctor was very nice and apologetic. Yet the fact remains that he prescribed a product with which he was not familiar. This hospital emergency room is usually quite busy so I am not surprised that he did not have time to investigate the product before he prescribed it. I sympathize with him as regards his workload.

Yet the fact remains that this child could have ended up receiving six times the intended dose if this prescription had not been clarified. The child's mother did not seem to appreciate my efforts. She just seemed to resent that she had to wait while I cleared up the confusion.

I was recently told of another incident at another drugstore involving these same two products. A pharmacist who had been licensed less than four months told another child's mother that the concentrated solution could be given without being diluted. Somehow the child's mother found out that this was incorrect and returned to the pharmacy crying over the potential harm that could have resulted. Another pharmacist was on duty at that time and apologized for the error.

3. Tussionex error. Another doctor prescribed the cough syrup Tussionex for a 14-year-old girl, with the directions: "Take 1 to 2 teaspoonsful every 8 hours." The official prescribing information for Tussionex reads as follows (2003 *PDR*, p. 1174): "Adults: 1 teaspoonful every 12 hours; do not exceed 2 teaspoonsful in 24 hours. Children 6-12: one-half teaspoonful every 12 hours; **do not exceed 1 teaspoonful in 24 hours.**" The bold-faced print appears in the *PDR*.

This was a refill bottle that another pharmacist had originally filled. The customer's request for the refill took place on a weekend. The directions were so evidently an excessive dose that I retyped the directions on the label with the manufacturer's recommended dose. In my experience, Tussionex is one of the drugs most frequently prescribed with the wrong directions. Most doctors forget—or never knew—that Tussionex is unusual in that it is long-acting and it is used in small doses.

I didn't even notify the doctor's office that I changed the directions. It was so clearly an error that it was pointless to notify the doctor and risk appearing to "rub it in" that he made an error.

What usually happens is that we call the doctor's office and tell the person who answers the phone (usually the receptionist) that there appears to be an error in the doctor's directions. Then the receptionist tells the doctor or a nurse. I suspect that it is embarrassing for the doctor to be told by his receptionist or nurse that the drugstore is calling with what appears to be an error. Then (assuming it is indeed an error), one of two things can happen:

1. The doctor is honest with himself and agrees with the pharmacist that an error has been made. The doctor tells his nurse or receptionist to tell the pharmacist to correct the directions.

2. The doctor's ego and his desire to appear faultless in front of his staff cause him to tell his nurse or receptionist to relay to the pharmacist that the doctor wants it kept as he wrote it on the prescription. The doctor knows that he is clearly in error but refuses to acknowledge that fact.

In this case with the Tussionex, I felt there was no reason to notify the doctor's office, even if this incident had occurred during the doctor's normal business hours. (As I said, this was a weekend.) We get lots of prescriptions from this doctor, so why risk upsetting him? I know that he has a very busy practice and that mistakes like this are inevitable. Having spoken with him many times over the years as he relays prescriptions to us, he seems to be the type of doctor who would prefer that we just make the correction in the dose without making a big fuss about it.

The difficult part was telling the child's father that the directions we had typed on the label originally were what the doctor had written but that it was best to use a lower dose. I implied that the doctor knew better but must have been in a hurry. Whether or not the doctor actually knows the maximum recommended dose for Tussionex is something I don't know.

As I said, the doctor wrote on the prescription, "Take 1 to 2 teaspoonsful every 8 hours." Every eight hours means three times per day. So the doctor's directions could have led the child to take up to six teaspoonsful per day. This is three times the recommended adult dose. Sometimes doctors prescribe a somewhat higher dose when the patient is large. However, this 14-year-old girl appeared to be of average weight for her age. It is even stretching it somewhat to put her in the adult category because, at 14, she's only two years past the child category according to the manufacturer's recommended dose. So it is not stretching things a lot to say that six teaspoonsful per day could be six times the recommended dose. I asked the girl how often she was taking it and she said she was taking one teaspoonful in the morning and two teaspoonsful at night (three teaspoonsful per day).

So I acted as if the doctor knew the correct dose but just must have been in a hurry when he wrote the directions. Whether or not this is the case I'll never know, but at least it got me out of a fix. I didn't want to refill the Tussionex with the original directions that the previous pharmacist had typed on the label. I was legally liable for dispensing a drug with incorrect directions. My employer was also liable. I just acted as if it was no big deal and re-typed the directions on the label with the manufacturer's recommended directions. I implied that the doctor knew the correct dose but must have been in a hurry. I was protecting myself and my employer against a lawsuit. The doctor had clearly made an error.

When doctors don't welcome pharmacists' calls about drug interactions

In my experience, most doctors don't seem too happy to hear that a pharmacist is calling to point out a drug interaction. They too often interpret this as a turf battle or an implication that they are not sufficiently knowledgeable about interactions among the drugs they prescribe.

Pharmacists are overwhelmed with prescriptions, yet some doctors think we have nothing better to do than call about interactions. One doctor told my partner we were calling his office too often. I told this to another pharmacist who suggested we request written permission from the doctor never to call him again about drug interactions. But I doubt that would relieve us of liability in the event of a lawsuit.

One Saturday I called a doctor about his prescribing erythromycin for a customer who was on carbamazepine from a different doctor. This is a "Level 1," or "most significant," interaction. When the doctor finally called back, he said rudely, "I'm making a long distance phone call for this? The interaction is extremely mild!" He finally said (as if only to please me), "All right! Change the erythromycin to

Duricef!" I told the patient her doctor had changed her antibiotic, but not about the potentially serious nature of the interaction or how angry the doctor was that I called him.

Here is what the *United States Pharmacopoeia* says about the interaction between erythromycin and carbamazepine (*USP-DI*, 1997, p. 1351): "Erythromycins may inhibit carbamazepine metabolism, resulting in increased anticonvulsant plasma concentrations and toxicity; it is recommended that erythromycin be used with caution if at all in patients receiving carbamazepine."

On a different occasion, I called another doctor's office about another Level 1 interaction. I wanted to make sure I should dispense the drugs as written. When the receptionist called me back, she said, "I checked with the doctor, AND HE SAID IT'S OKAY!" Her attitude implied that I was an idiot for calling. I assume that is because the doctor was irritated that a pharmacist had called about yet another drug interaction and took out his anger on her.

Pharmacists are put in the impossible position of having to decide which patients will experience clinically significant effects from drug interactions. In any large statistical sample, some people will end up with adverse consequences from a drug interaction. Others will not.

I believe the doctor should be the one to weigh the statistical probability, not the pharmacist. The doctor should have ultimate responsibility for screening for drug interactions. He/she should have a duty to review all current meds a patient is taking (including the ones prescribed by other doctors) before prescribing another drug. Liability for detecting drug interactions resulting from doctors' carelessness should not fall on the shoulders of pharmacists. (Of course, if we had adequate staff in the pharmacy, I would more willingly accept part of the burden of screening for drug interactions.)

In understaffed pharmacies, we simply don't have enough time to call doctors as often as we should. Customers are in a hurry, and they don't seem to recognize the significance of our phone calls. Yet these same customers will not hesitate to sue us if they suffer harm from an interaction. When we do call, the doctor's response to the interaction often seems arbitrary or based on inadequate knowledge. Or the doctor simply uses the occasion to display his ego.

Because of doctors' attitudes, we may tell customers something like this: "Our computer flagged a potential interaction between your medications. I called your doctor and he feels there will be no problem." Essentially, we're telling customers that we, as pharmacists, are concerned about an interaction but their doctor is not, so if they develop a problem, BLAME THE DOCTOR!

Patients would probably be surprised to learn that considerations such as a doctor's ego factor into whether their pharmacist calls about a potential drug interaction. Customers likely assume that health professionals are collegial and that everyone works together for the benefit of patients. In reality, some doctors' attitudes and egos are a serious impediment to ensuring safety in the dispensing of medications.

I'm sure a few pharmacists enjoy parading their drug knowledge in front of doctors. And I'm sure many pharmacists call doctors about potential interactions that indeed have a low probability of causing a problem. But the longer a pharmacist has worked in a busy store, the quicker he realizes there simply is not enough time to devote to potential drug interactions.

Pharmacists: Do you have adequate time to call doctors about drug interactions? Are you worried that your pharmacy technicians are overriding significant drug interactions?

When doctors don't keep up with the latest drug warnings

In his excellent book on the FDA, Philip J. Hilts discusses how doctors often ignore FDA warnings in the official prescribing information, known as the label. Hilts quotes one FDA staffer, "Doctors aren't often paying attention. We may put crucial information in a label and have it end up as a dead letter." Hilts says, "Studies confirm it: the labels are largely unheeded and often completely unread." (Philip J. Hilts, *Protecting America's Health: The FDA, Business, and One Hundred Years of Regulation,* New York: Knopf, 2003, pp. 234-5)

I wrote the following in May 1995: A local doctor continues to prescribe the pain killer Toradol for an excessive duration of time.

He often prescribes it to be taken for ten days with four refills. This is a potentially 50-day supply. However, the medical literature says that Toradol should not be taken for more than five days because of the possibility of serious gastrointestinal bleeding and other problems.

The recommendation for short duration therapy with Toradol was a big story in 1995. How could this doctor have missed it?

One day I said to my partner, "There's a local doctor who's using a drug for much longer than is recommended." To my great surprise, my partner immediately said, "Yeah. It's Dr. Smith and it's Toradol." I was surprised that my partner had the same concern that I had.

I told my partner that one of us needed to call this doctor and wake him up because he's jeopardizing the health of his patients and exposing us and Revco to liability. Every time we enter "days supply" into the computer when filling one of his prescriptions for Toradol, the computer flags this as an excessive duration of therapy.

But Dr. Smith is such a know-it-all that we both decided that neither of us wanted to call him. We get a lot of prescriptions from Dr. Smith, so we fear that he'll direct his patients elsewhere if we tell him he's greatly exceeding the recommended total duration of therapy for Toradol. Hopefully some other drugstore in town will make him aware of this fact.

June 1995: The daughter of the customer my partner and I were concerned about brought in another prescription for Toradol. Against my better judgment, I went ahead and dispensed thirty more tablets. Later on that afternoon, I called the customer herself and asked her how long she had been on the Toradol. I could have looked it up in our computer records, but I wanted her to actually tell me how long she had been on the Toradol. She told me that she had been taking Toradol for a little over a year for her headaches.

The revised prescribing information (December 1994) for Toradol specifically states that patients should not take this drug for more than five days and that it should not be used for chronic conditions. There have been many reports of serious gastrointestinal bleeding and even death from this drug. It turns out that this customer has had ulcers in the past even though she told me she doesn't currently have an ulcer. (How can she be so sure that some ulceration is not occurring without her realizing it?) Toradol should be used even more cautiously in patients with a history of ulcers.

Sidney Wolfe, M.D., and his Public Citizen Health Research Group, advised against use of this drug as early as August 1993. ("Health Letter," August 1993, p. 5:)

A widely-used painkiller, especially used in patients after surgery, has been temporarily suspended from sales in Germany and the German government gave Syntex, the drug's U. S.-based manufacturer, three weeks to provide evidence that it should not be permanently removed from the market. The drug, which is in the same family of non-steroidal anti-inflammatory drugs (NSAIDs) as Feldene, Naprosyn and aspirin has been associated with a large number of cases of serious gastrointestinal bleeding, including dozens of deaths as well as life-threatening allergic reactions similar to Zomax, another NSAID which is no longer on the market.

...For now, we urge patients not to use ketorolac [generic name for Toradol].

The official prescribing information sounds equally scary. From the package insert, revised December 1994:

Toradol, a nonsteroidal anti-inflammatory drug (NSAID), is indicated for the short-term (up to 5 days) management of moderately severe, acute pain, that requires analgesia at the opioid level. It is NOT indicated for minor or chronic painful conditions. Toradol is a potent NSAID analgesic, and its administration carries many risks. The resulting NSAID related adverse events can be serious in certain patients for whom Toradol is indicated, especially when the drug is used inappropriately. ...

Toradol can cause peptic ulcers, gastrointestinal bleeding, and/or perforation. Therefore, Toradol is contraindicated in patients with active peptic ulcer disease, in patients with recent gastrointestinal bleeding or perforation, and in patients with a history of peptic ulcer disease or gastrointestinal bleeding. ...

The combined use of [intravenous, intramuscular, and oral forms of Toradol] is not to exceed 5 days. ...

Serious gastrointestinal toxicity, such as bleeding, ulceration, and perforation, can occur at any time, with or without warning symptoms, in pa-

tients treated with Toradol. Studies to date with NSAIDs have not identified any subset of patients not at risk of developing peptic ulceration and
bleeding. ...

The incidence and severity of gastrointestinal complications increases
with increasing dose of, and duration of treatment with, Toradol. ...

Toradol is a potent NSAID and may cause serious side effects such as
gastrointestinal bleeding or kidney failure, which may result in hospitalization and even fatal outcome.

Physicians, when prescribing Toradol should inform their patients of
the potential risks of Toradol treatment. ...

Remember that the total duration of Toradol therapy is not to exceed
5 (five) days.

I told our customer that the recommendation for a decreased duration in the use of Toradol was very recent. I told her that I was going to call her doctor to see whether he had heard about it. The fact
is that her doctor had plenty of time to hear about it but I needed a
way to make it sound like her doctor was a good doctor, even
though there are many people in this community who hold a very
low opinion of this doctor.

That evening, I called my partner at home and said that we
needed to do something about this situation NOW!!! He agreed,
particularly after I read him the warnings from the official prescribing
information and after I read him from Sidney Wolfe's "Health Letter."

My partner has worked at this store for nearly fifteen years. I
work in this particular store only on a part-time basis, yet I happened
to fill a few prescriptions for Toradol for this customer. We agreed
that it was best that he call the doctor and act like this was very new
information that the doctor possibly had not heard about, even
though, as I said, it's been in the medical literature for several
months.

My partner has spoken on the phone with this doctor countless
times in these nearly fifteen years, usually for routine questions like
permission to refill various drugs for our customers, and, significantly,
for help in deciphering his handwriting. This doctor has some of the

worst handwriting I've seen in the twenty years since I graduated from pharmacy school.

We concluded that if we were to make this doctor mad (a not unlikely possibility), my partner should be the one to handle the situation since my partner was the one who needed to maintain on-going relationships with the doctors in this town.

My partner called this doctor on a Monday morning. It turns out that the doctor didn't get mad but his reaction to the situation was quite inadequate and quite disappointing. For the recommendation that Toradol not be taken for more than five days, the doctor said that he had told the patient to always skip a day after five days (what a joke!) and that he had told her not to take more than twelve tablets a week, even though he allowed her to take it every week for over a year.

Then the doctor made an absolutely incredible statement. He said that it was his experience that warnings in the prescribing literature come and go and that it was his experience that one's own judgment should guide the physician's prescribing practices.

I guess this doctor has no use for the FDA. Why worry about official FDA warnings? Since he had not personally run into problems with his patients on Toradol, that fact apparently superseded data gathered from around the country and around the world.

In discussing this situation with me, my partner said that we should document all our concerns and conversations (with the patient and doctor) on the prescription and in the computer. I told my partner that I still was not satisfied. I said that we are still liable for dispensing a drug that we have reason to believe is not in the patient's best interest. As pharmacists seek a greater role in drug therapy decisions, lawyers are not exempting pharmacists from lawsuits when something goes wrong. In the past, it was usually only the doctor and the drug manufacturer that were found liable.

I told my partner that I plan to refuse to dispense any more Toradol to this customer and that he should do the same. I also said that I pray that she doesn't have any gastrointestinal bleeding in the meantime. I told him that we should possibly contact the Revco legal department for further guidance.

This customer gets all her prescriptions at Revco, so it would probably cause a problem in our relationship with this doctor if we told the customer that we would fill all her other prescriptions but refuse to dispense any more Toradol.

I transferred to a different city shortly after this episode, so, unfortunately, I never found out whether this customer continued to take excessive quantities of Toradol.

Doctors and placebos

In the early 1990s I worked at several drugstores in North Carolina, including one in a town called Henderson. Henderson is a forty minute drive on the Interstate from Durham, the city in which Duke University is located. Drugstores in a wide radius from Durham receive lots of prescriptions from the Duke University Medical Center. One day a customer handed me a prescription for her son from a Duke doctor. The customer decided to hang around in the drugstore and wait for the prescription to be filled—rather than return later to pick it up.

When I began filling the prescription a few minutes later, I noticed that the Duke doc had prescribed a drug with which I was not familiar. The Duke doc had prescribed Obecalp. I called the customer over and told her that I would have to phone her doctor at Duke because I wasn't familiar with Obecalp and I couldn't find it listed in any of our order books. The customer said that would be fine. She remained nearby as I called the Duke doc. Luckily, I got through to the Duke doc quickly. I said, "I have a prescription here for Obecalp for [patient's name], but I can't find it listed anywhere." He said, "Oh. That's placebo spelled backwards."

The doctor proceeded to explain the situation to me. He was considering prescribing Ritalin for this child (for attention deficit-hyperactivity disorder, I presume). He wanted to see whether the mother could actually tell a difference in her child's behavior on days that he took Ritalin and on days that he took the placebo. The plan was to alternate the Ritalin and the Obecalp (placebo) in some way—I can't recall the precise plan. Perhaps the placebo was to be taken every other day, or every other week, or every other month.

I told the Duke doc that, even though I was well aware of the placebo effect, I could not recall ever having actually dispensed placebo pills (commonly known as sugar pills or inert pills). He said, "Why don't you just dispense, say, a low dose of Vitamin C tablets if you don't have any placebo pills." (Placebo pills—containing no active ingredients—are indeed available from our suppliers under "Placebo," not "Obecalp.)

This doctor was extremely nice during the entire conversation, but I was left worrying that I had blown the cover on his experiment. The child's mother was standing nearby during this entire conversation and she must have heard almost everything I said to her child's doctor. I think I went ahead and dispensed Vitamin C tablets, as the doctor suggested, rather than actual placebo pills since we didn't have any placebo pills on hand. I did not tell the Duke doc that I may have ruined his experiment since the child's mother was standing nearby and had overheard most of my conversation. The mother now seemed to be highly curious about what was going on.

I greatly admire this Duke doc for considering the possibility that the child may not need the Ritalin. And I greatly admire his attempt to see whether the child's mother could tell any difference in her child's behavior on the days he took the Ritalin versus the days he took the placebo (actually Vitamin C tablets in this case). But I just wish the doctor had handled the situation a little differently by, perhaps, calling me before the child's mother arrived with the prescription for Obecalp. He could have called beforehand to explain to me what he was planning to do with this unconventional prescription for Obecalp.

Of course, I was equally guilty for handling this situation poorly, since the child's mother had heard almost all of my conversation with the doctor before I concluded that the doctor probably didn't want her to know that the Obecalp pills are indeed placebo pills (i.e., a dummy or inactive pill). I don't know how much of this experiment the mother was aware of before she walked into the drugstore, but she certainly understood much more after my bumbled conversation with the doctor.

Too many doctors seem to prescribe Ritalin reflexively, so I admire the way this Duke doc was trying to determine whether the child really needed the drug. But the way he and I handled the situation was not good at all.

Here's an unrelated but (perhaps) funny anecdote about placebos. This is a letter-to-the editor published in *Drug Topics*, written by a New Jersey pharmacist. This pharmacist, in cooperation with a physician, dispensed placebo pills to one of that physician's patients. (Letters, "Score 1 for placebo ... make that 2," *Drug Topics*, December 2010, p. 10)

In 1957, I was a brand-new pharmacist in a New York hospital. An elderly female patient of the arthritis clinic adjacent to my pharmacy had no clinical disease in reality but constantly sought treatment. The rheumatologist, the director, and I conferred and decided to give her a 2-month supply of saccharin tablets with ad lib refills [refillable as needed] to be taken 1 tid [one tablet three times a day]."

This went well for several months, with the patient reporting good results, until she came to my window one day, shouting, and accused us of giving her substandard medication. The previous night she had tried to commit suicide by taking the entire supply — "And look at me: I'm standing right here in front of you, and I'm alive!"

We sent her for a psych consult. I didn't know whether to laugh or to cry. *—Irving Gerber, RPh,* Fair Lawn, N.J.

There has been a great deal of discussion about whether it is ethical to prescribe placebos to patients without those patients knowing it. How would you feel if your doctor—without informing you—decided to put you on a dummy or inert pill to see, for example, whether your symptoms of depression or anxiety responded as well to the placebo pill as to, say, Prozac or Xanax? Would you feel that your doctor thinks you're nuts?

PART III

PHARMACISTS, TECHS, SUPERVISORS, CUSTOMERS

Chapter 7

Pharmacists' attitudes and biases

If you really want to understand how Big Pharma has been so successful in convincing Americans about the safety and effectiveness of drugs, it is insightful to understand the attitudes and biases of pharmacists and their surprisingly low level of skepticism toward these products. The typical pharmacist in the typical drugstore is much more likely to have a mercantile mentality than the mentality of a skeptical scientist. Too many pharmacists are largely unaware of—and uninterested in—the many serious critics of the pharmaceutical industry. Some pharmacists are angered and defensive when critics question the safety and effectiveness of the drugs we dispense.

In my opinion, given the track record of Big Pharma in minimizing the adverse effects of drugs and in exaggerating the benefits, pharmacists should maintain an essentially skeptical attitude toward a large number of the products in the pharmacy. But, in my opinion, pharmacists are largely an unquestioning group of people who basically accept the information we receive from Big Pharma. It is for this reason that I view pharmacy as akin to a religion in that pharmacists are essentially unquestioning of the dogma. When I attend continuing education seminars with pharmacists, the culture at these seminars is curiously similar to the culture one finds in organized religion: a suspension of critical thinking.

Many pharmacy customers probably assume that Big Pharma is unable to snow the public because pharmacists and doctors would protest if Big Pharma deviated too far from reality. However, in my opinion, pharmacists and doctors are not even close to playing the watchdog role that the public assumes. The fact that doctors and pharmacists are well-compensated by our medical system guarantees that these professionals will largely passively accept The World According to Big Pharma.

The public sees pharmacists as objective drug experts who eagerly keep abreast of the latest developments in the world of drugs. Well-informed pharmacy customers who are skeptical of big corporations probably expect pharmacists to be unbiased scientists who see through the exaggerations and distortions and lies of the drug industry. But, in my opinion, pharmacists and doctors have been largely bamboozled by the same immense promotional apparatus that inundates the public with soothing advertisements for powerful drugs. Big Pharma has an awesome power to create widespread acceptance of the concept known as *better living through chemistry*. The sheer volume of drug advertisements in the print and electronic media has the effect of force-feeding Americans with the view that there is a pill for every ill. So it is not surprising that doctors, pharmacists, and consumers are disinclined to think outside the pill.

Pharmacists basically do not question Big Pharma's focus on molecules and cells and rarely object to our medical system's striking lack of emphasis on any type of prevention. Big Pharma claims to be highly interested in the field of prevention. But the only prevention that Big Pharma is interested in is "prevention in a pill." This perversion of the generally accepted definition of prevention advocates the widespread use of pills to prevent the progression of an existing disease into a more serious disease, e.g., using antihypertensive drugs to prevent hypertension from causing heart disease. This concept of medicalized prevention is widely at odds with the generally recognized view of prevention which is based on lifestyle modification, good nutrition, proper weight, avoiding tobacco and alcohol, etc.

Maintaining a skeptical or critical attitude toward drugs would place a heavy burden on the pharmacist's psyche. It is very difficult to come to work every day as a pharmacy heretic, with serious questions about many of the drugs we dispense. But Big Pharma's track record of manipulating the outcome of drug studies and downplaying adverse effects of drugs should make pharmacists wonder whether much of the clinical data generated by the drug companies—and submitted to the FDA—can be trusted. As Melody Petersen writes in *Our Daily Meds* (New York: Farrar, Straus & Giroux, 2008, p. 206):

> **Dr. John P. A. Ioannidis, an epidemiologist who holds positions at Tufts University and the University of Ioannina in Greece, said in 2005 that the conclusions of most published scientific studies are just plain wrong. In an essay, Dr. Ioannidis blamed the industrial quest for profit, the growing number of conflicts of interest among scientists, the small size of many clinical trials, as well as the manipulation of their design, for creating an era in medicine when most studies turn out to be fiction.**
>
> **"There is increasing concern that in modern research, false findings may be the majority or even the vast majority of published research claims," he wrote in the journal *PLoS Medicine*. "However, this should not be surprising. It can be proven that most claimed research findings are false."**

One of the biggest misconceptions among Americans involving drugs is that the FDA actually directly conducts drug studies. In reality, the pharmaceutical companies carry out the studies and submit their data to the FDA. The FDA then examines the data regarding safety and effectiveness. A very large number of pharmacists are not aware of this basic fact that the FDA only examines data submitted by the drug companies. Many critics say that the drug companies have a powerful incentive to manipulate the data which they submit to the FDA.

Whenever books are written exposing the lies of the drug industry, I do not see pharmacists eager to read these books. Even though these books represent a major attack on many of the products that pharmacists routinely dispense, the major pharmacy magazines rarely discuss these books because of a fear of angering Big Pharma. Pharmaceutical industry advertising is by far the biggest source of revenue for the leading pharmacy magazines (*Drug Topics*, *U.S. Pharmacist*, and *Pharmacy Times*). So it is not surprising that these magazines are fearful of being too critical of Big Pharma. In my opinion, the public would be shocked to see that the ever-expanding critique of the pharmaceutical industry has essentially been swept under the rug by the major pharmacy magazines.

Pharmacy magazines like *Drug Topics, Pharmacy Times, US Pharmacist,* and the now-defunct *American Druggist* have been the publications most widely read by pharmacists. From my perspective the content of these magazines has a major influence on how pharmacists view the profession of pharmacy and the pharmaceutical industry. Pharmacists need to realize that the editors-in-chief, senior editors, and assistant editors at these magazines may not necessarily agree with the largely uncritical perspective toward drugs that these magazines must maintain to be attractive for pharmaceutical industry advertising. For the period of several years when I was writing articles/editorials for a couple of these magazines, I came to know a few of the editors as a result of communications we had regarding my submissions. Here are two short anecdotes:

One day one of the editors commented to me something like "I don't like to take pills myself. Occasionally I'll take an aspirin but I'm not too thrilled about that." Yet her full time job consists of writing about a wide range of pharmacy topics: new drugs, the profession of pharmacy, the drug industry, pharmacy associations, pharmacy benefit managers, chain drugstores, pharmacy schools, trends in pharmacy, etc.

On another occasion, I spoke with a different editor at another national pharmacy magazine. She informed me that she was about to lose her job because the magazine was ceasing publication because it was unprofitable. I asked her whether she had plans for another job. She told me that she had been offered a job ghostwriting drug articles that would be published in drug and medical journals. She said that she would write the articles and then (usually) physicians would attach their names to the articles as if they had actually written the articles. She said she turned down the job because it went against her principles. I told her that I admired her for sticking to her principles. She told me that it was more a matter of her simply being *physically incapable* of forcing herself to do it because she was so strongly opposed to it. Basically, the drug companies would tell her what to write, she would then write the articles, and a physician's name (or physicians' names) would appear at the top of the articles as if they had written the articles themselves.

Another reason that the major pharmacy magazines try to maintain a very supportive attitude toward pharmaceuticals is that many pharmacists become angry at significant criticisms of the products we dispense. Many pharmacists have a Pollyanna view of pharmacy and are angered by the suggestion that the products we dispense can sometimes be hazardous.

Too many pharmacists have unquestioningly accepted the "pill for every ill" mentality in modern medicine today in which every customer's complaint is answered with a product rather than an insight into prevention. Every health complaint becomes simply a matter of finding the "right" product. Most pharmacists seem to believe that good health is primarily a consequence of drugs rather than primarily a consequence of a healthy lifestyle, a clean environment, good nutrition, etc. Pharmacists seem to believe that human health is directly proportional to the per capita consumption of pharmaceuticals and that prevention offers little hope in comparison to drugs. Pharmacists have essentially bought into Big Pharma's narrative that implies the human body is like an old car that is constantly breaking down. Pharmacists seem to have little appreciation for the wondrous complexity of the human body or for the fact that *Homo sapiens* can thrive under the conditions that have been present for thousands of years.

It should be obvious to most people that conditions in modern societies are widely divergent from the conditions that our genes are accustomed to. It should be equally obvious that an inevitable consequence of this divergence is the long list of what is referred to as "diseases of modern civilization." Big Pharma fears that if the public understands the concept of Western diseases, there will be much less enthusiasm for pill solutions to lifestyle diseases. Big Pharma prefers to blame genes, viruses, and aging as the primary causes of illness because such culprits cast an inevitability to disease and thereby divert attention from simple things that people can do themselves to maintain health independent of doctors and drugs.

In my opinion, pharmacists' objectivity is significantly influenced by the fact that the management of chain drugstores expects pharmacists to give largely soothing answers to customers' questions about side effects. It is simply much faster for pharmacists to downplay adverse reactions when we are asked about the safety of drugs. Positive answers are much faster than taking the time to support any critical views we might have.

There is, in fact, tremendous variation in the types of answers pharmacists give when customers ask us about the safety and effectiveness of a drug that their doctor has prescribed. Some pharmacists make a serious effort to answer questions about side effects realistically, while other pharmacists downplay the possibility and significance of side effects. With understaffing, too many pharmacists simply don't have time to give thoughtful answers to customers' questions, even if they would like to. Compounding the problem is the fact that a large number of pharmacists try very hard to avoid all contact with customers for a variety of reasons:

• Conversations with customers can be very time consuming when we have a pile of prescriptions waiting to be filled.
• Some pharmacists are basically introverts who are uncomfortable speaking with customers.
• Some pharmacists don't want to be bothered answering "stupid" questions from customers who don't know anything about drugs.

In my experience, pharmacists are surprisingly ambivalent about newly discovered hazards of prescription drugs. Pharmacists don't often discuss the wider implications when drugs are withdrawn from the market for safety reasons. Drug withdrawals rarely prompt pharmacists to examine issues like whether the FDA is a captive of Big Pharma the same way that the Securities and Exchange Commission has been a captive of Wall Street, or whether the long term effects of drugs are as poorly understood by the FDA as complex financial instruments like derivatives were poorly understood by regulators. According to *The New York Times*, (Cyrus Sanati, "Greenspan Says He Was Mystified by Subprime Market," February 12, 2009), "Alan Greenspan, the former chairman of the Federal Reserve, told CNBC in a documentary to be shown [Feb. 12, 2009] that he did not fully understand the scope of the subprime mortgage market until well into 2005 and could not make sense of the complex derivative products created out of mortgages."

In twenty-five years as a pharmacist, I've worked with dozens of pharmacists. In my experience, pharmacists rarely discuss (among themselves) things like the safety of drugs. Pharmacists' belief in the safety and effectiveness of the products we dispense is so rock-solid that the withdrawal of a drug is seen as an aberration in a fundamentally sound system. In my experience, pharmacists do not seem to be aware of (or interested in finding out about) the many readily available articles that discuss the incredible pressure on the FDA to approve drugs faster. Pharmacists don't seem to be interested in reading the many book-length exposés of the pharmaceutical industry.

Therefore, in my opinion, pharmacists do not have a context in which to understand the significance of drugs pulled from the market. The withdrawal of a drug should tell pharmacists that the FDA did a poor job when it approved the drug. I never met a retail pharmacist who commented on FDA's competence in assessing the safety and effectiveness of drugs. I never met a pharmacist who bemoaned the fact that the pharmaceutical industry puts pressure on Congress to force the FDA to approve drugs faster.

Most pharmacists seem to think that the FDA is a powerful and strict agency. When major drugs like Redux (for obesity), Rezulin (for type 2 diabetes), Vioxx (for arthritis), Baycol (for elevated cholesterol), or Propulsid (for heartburn) are withdrawn, it is basically a non-event for many pharmacists, and it doesn't even begin to cause them to question their confidence in the fundamental safety and effectiveness of many of the other products we dispense. The withdrawal of a drug from the market should be a powerful lesson to pharmacists about how industry pressure on Congress causes the FDA to approve drugs too quickly.

I've never worked in a hospital pharmacy so I don't know whether hospital pharmacists discuss the issue of drug safety. If you ask a pharmacist in a drugstore (a "retail pharmacist") about safety issues, it is my opinion that most of these pharmacists are unqualified to discuss the subject of drug safety intelligently because they're not really interested in the subject. Retail pharmacists seem to have mainly a mercantile mentality and seem to view pharmacy as primarily a business.

The incredible workload endured by many pharmacists employed by the big drugstore chains has forced us to adopt a business outlook rather than the outlook of a skeptical scientist. Furthermore, doctors don't want pharmacists questioning the safety of drugs. Our employers certainly don't want us to question the safety of drugs. The big drugstore chains definitely do not like pharmacists who spend time raising safety issues with our customers. Such pharmacists would be viewed as unfavorably by the corporation as slow pharmacists. The big drugstore chains have total disdain for pharmacists who are slow or who spend too much time speaking with customers.

Many times I have been tempted to ask pharmacists what they think about the latest high-profile drug that's on the evening news because of some newly discovered adverse reaction associated with that drug. But I've hesitated to do so. Pharmacists just don't seem to be interested. They would view me as a troublemaker, as someone who is anti-drug, as someone who questions the profession of pharmacy. It would go over as well as my criticizing their religion.

One day I did mention to one of my best friends, a pharmacist, that I was concerned that the drugs we dispense have not necessarily been carefully and objectively screened for safety and effectiveness before being approved. His attitude was quite shocking. He implied that, with a wife and kids, he needed the income from his job and he didn't like me discussing the subject. It was as if somehow I had the power to make the public more discriminating and skeptical about the products we dispense every day. It was as if my conversation was somehow jeopardizing his livelihood. I changed the subject because he clearly wasn't interested in what I had to say, and, in fact, he had a very cold reaction to the entire subject. I don't recall him reacting quite so coldly to any other subject we've discussed.

In my opinion, there are several books that are absolutely essential for an understanding of pharmacy, the pharmaceutical industry and modern medicine. Yet I've never heard a discussion among pharmacists of the following books:

1. **Overdosed America**: *The Broken Promise of American Medicine* by John Abramson, M.D.

2. **Prescription for Disaster**: *The Hidden Dangers in Your Medicine Cabinet* by Thomas J. Moore

3. **Bitter Pills**: *Inside the Hazardous World of Legal Drugs* by Stephen Fried

4. **The Truth About the Drug Companies**: *How They Deceive Us and What to Do About It* by Marcia Angell, M.D.

5. **Powerful Medicines**: *The Benefits, Risks, and Costs of Prescription Drugs* by Jerry Avorn, M.D.

6. **Natural Causes**: *Death, Lies, and Politics in America's Vitamin and Herbal Supplement Industry* by Dan Hurley

7. **Best Choices From The People's Pharmacy** by Joe and Teresa Graedon

8. **Generation Rx**: *How Prescription Drugs Are Altering American Lives, Minds, and Bodies* by Greg Critser

9. **Selling Sickness**: *How the World's Biggest Pharmaceutical Companies Are Turning Us All into Patients* by Ray Moynihan and Alan Cassels

10. **The $800 Million Pill**: *The Truth behind the Cost of New Drugs* by Merrill Goozner

11. **The Big Fix**: *How the Pharmaceutical Industry Rips Off American Consumers* by Katharine Greider

12. **Protecting America's Health**: *The FDA, Business, and One Hundred Years of Regulation* by Philip J. Hilts

13. **The Merck Druggernaut**: *The Inside Story of a Pharmaceutical Giant* by Fran Hawthorne

14. **Inside the FDA**: *The Business and Politics Behind the Drugs We Take and the Food We Eat* by Fran Hawthorne

15. **The Whistleblower**: *Confessions of a Healthcare Hitman* by Peter Rost, M.D.

16. **Big Pharma**: *Exposing the Global Healthcare Agenda* by Jacky Law

17. **On The Take**: *How Medicine's Complicity with Big Business Can Endanger Your Health* by Jerome Kassirer, M.D.

18. **Critical Condition**: *How Health Care in America Became Big Business—and Bad Medicine* by Donald L. Barlett and James B. Steele

19. **Let Them Eat Prozac**: *The Unhealthy Relationship Between the Pharmaceutical Industry and Depression* by David Healy

20. **Hard Sell**: *The Evolution of a Viagra Salesman* by Jamie Reidy

21. **Hope or Hype**: *The Obsession with Medical Advances and the High Cost of False Promises* by Richard A. Deyo, M.D., and Donald L. Patrick, Ph.D.

22. **Last Well Person**: *How to Stay Well Despite the Health-care System* by Nortin M. Hadler, M.D.

23. **Severed Trust**: *Why American Medicine Hasn't Been Fixed* by George Lundberg, M.D.

24. **Medical Nemesis**: *The Expropriation of Health* by Ivan Illich

25. **Worst Pills, Best Pills**: *A Consumer's Guide to Avoiding Drug-Induced Death or Illness* by Sidney Wolfe, M.D., and the Public Citizen Health Research Group

26. **Disease Mongers:** *How Doctors, Drug Companies, and Insurers Are Making You Feel Sick* by Lynn Payer

27. **Medicine and Culture:** *Varieties of Treatment in the United States, England, West Germany and France* by Lynn Payer

28. **The Rise and Fall of Modern Medicine** by James LeFanu, M.D.

29. **Examining Your Doctor**: *A Patient's Guide to Avoiding Harmful Medical Care* by Timothy B. McCall, M.D.

30. **Talking Back to Prozac:** *What Doctors Aren't Telling You About Today's Most Controversial Drug* by Peter Breggin, M.D.

31. **Our Daily Meds:** *How the Pharmaceutical Companies Transformed Themselves into Slick Marketing Machines and Hooked the Nation on Prescription Drugs* by Melody Petersen

32. **Confessions of a Medical Heretic** by Robert Mendelsohn, M.D.

33. **What Doctors Don't Tell You**: *The Truth About the Dangers of Modern Medicine* by Lynne McTaggart

34. **Top Screwups Doctors Make and How To Avoid Them** by Joe and Teresa Graedon

35. **Overtreated:** *Why Too Much Medicine Is Making Us Sicker and Poorer* by Shannon Brownlee

36. **Worried Sick:** *A Prescription for Health in an Overtreated America* by Nortin M. Hadler, M.D.

37. **Overdiagnosed:** *Making People Sick in the Pursuit of Health* by H. Gilbert Welch, M.D.

38. **How We Do Harm:** *A Doctor Breaks Ranks About Being Sick in America* by Otis Webb Brawley, M.D.

39. **The Healing of America:** *A Global Quest for Better, Cheaper, and Fairer Health Care* by T. R. Reid

How can pharmacists be qualified to comment on the drug industry and the safety of pharmaceuticals when pharmacists aren't interested in reading what critics of the industry have to say? I have never heard a discussion among pharmacists of the drug industry's most high-profile critic, Sidney Wolfe, M.D., and his Public Citizen Health Research Group. When the TV networks seek the consumer perspective on some pharmaceutical issue, they often interview Dr. Wolfe. The media also often turn to Jerry Avorn, M.D., of Harvard, or Marcia Angell, M.D., former editor-in-chief at the *New England Journal of Medicine.* How is it that pharmacists are largely uninterested in what these people have to say? I know very few pharmacists who even know who these people are.

Many pharmacists seem to view the products on our shelves as completely without controversy. For example, why is it that whenever drugs are removed from the market, I never hear pharmacists asking themselves why the FDA didn't uncover the hazards before approving the drugs? I never hear pharmacists asking questions like how well the FDA really understands the drugs it approves. I never hear pharmacists asking if the drug industry has too much power over the FDA. I never hear pharmacists discussing journal articles like the very disturbing one appearing in *JAMA* stating that twenty percent of new drugs will eventually either be banned or will be found to have serious or life-threatening side effects. (Lasser, et. al., "Timing of New Black Box Warnings and Withdrawals for Prescription Medication," *JAMA*, May 1, 2002)

Well-educated pharmacy customers perhaps believe that pharmacists hotly debate controversial issues surrounding drugs. Less-educated pharmacy customers probably do not even know that there are indeed lots of controversies about the products in the pharmacy. Most pharmacy customers seem to have a wide-eyed optimism toward pharmaceuticals as a direct consequence of massive exposure to drug advertising on television.

I've worked in dozens of different locations for three of the largest drugstore chains in this country in my 25-year career and I've had conversations with a huge number of pharmacists. Controversial issues regarding the drugs we dispense are almost never discussed. Therefore I think the typical consumer should not view his local pharmacist as an unbiased, intellectually curious person who can give an insightful opinion regarding the safety and effectiveness of medications.

To obtain continuing education credits required for the renewal of our license, pharmacists routinely attend dinner-lectures sponsored by drugs companies. My local pharmacy association usually succeeds in arranging for a drug company to sponsor such dinner-lectures every month at the nicest restaurant in our area. The drug companies' obvious (yet unspoken) intent is to create good will so that, for example, when hospitals are deciding which drugs to stock in the pharmacy, the hospital pharmacists who attend these dinner-lectures will be favorably disposed to recommending the drugs from the sponsor of the dinner-lecture.

Each dinner-lecture has a guest speaker chosen by the sponsoring drug company. At one such event I attended, our local pharmacy association president preceded his introduction of the speaker by appealing to the pharmacists in attendance to remember to mail in their pharmacy association dues. Even though most pharmacists have a fairly nice income, our president's plea was met with the usual groans that accompany any plea for money.

Surprisingly, the drug rep for Pfizer, the company sponsoring this particular dinner-lecture, chimed in and said that Pfizer routinely makes donations to groups like pharmacy associations. My reaction was that these drug companies have too much money and that they spread it around like fertilizer, hoping to cultivate the good will of pharmacists and doctors. At this particular dinner-lecture, Pfizer gave each pharmacist the choice of one of the two most expensive items on the restaurant menu. I remember one choice was prime rib.

I frequently wonder why I never hear pharmacists talk about the clever tactics used by the drug companies (like sponsoring these dinner-lectures) to buy our allegiance. Even more damning, I never hear pharmacists discussing the central fact that drug companies have convinced pharmacists that the pharmaceutical treatment of disease is preferable to prevention.

These dinner-lectures sponsored by the various drug companies are most noteworthy because of the huge conflict of interest. A typical topic might be one of the following: 1) "Treating menopausal symptoms," sponsored by the maker of the hormonal drug Premarin, 2) "Updates on treating depression," sponsored by the maker of the anti-depressant Paxil, 3) "Advances in the treatment of erectile dysfunction," sponsored by the maker of Viagra, Cialis or Levitra.

Another highly notable thing about these dinner-lectures is, in my opinion, the nearly complete lack of skepticism among most of the pharmacists in attendance. In private conversations among ourselves before the seminars begin, I never recall pharmacists commenting on the drug being highlighted in that seminar. I never recall hearing pharmacists ask: "Is this drug any more effective than other drugs already on the market? Is it safer? How much of this is pure hype?"

What topics do pharmacists discuss privately among themselves at these dinner-lectures or at pharmacy association meetings or in the drugstore? In my experience, rather than engage in wide-ranging discussions of more weighty issues like national health insurance or the pros and cons of the various products we dispense, most pharmacists discuss much more mundane things like: plans for the weekend or an upcoming vacation, football and basketball games at their college alma mater, hassles with insurance companies, widespread under-staffing in the chain drugstore industry, working conditions at the various chain drugstores (Rite Aid vs. CVS vs. Walgreen's, etc.), the fact that the non-pharmacist store manager doesn't have a clue about the how easily a pharmacist can be sued when we make a mistake, etc.

Several years ago, I went out to dinner with a pharmacist and his girlfriend. Hoping to stimulate an interesting conversation, I made the following (true) statement: "In the last fifteen years, the only drugs I've taken are a half-dozen Tylenol and one course of penicillin when I had a root canal." That statement prompted the following exchange:

Other pharmacist: That's why pharmacists don't take much themselves, because they know what it can do to them.

Girlfriend: Well, you tell me what I should take. Aren't you being [pause, searching for the right word]

Me: Hypocritical?

Girlfriend: Yes, feeling that way and not telling customers you feel that way?

Other pharmacist: Well, I take things like Robitussin when I need it.

The topic of the conversation changed because the other pharmacist became somewhat uncomfortable being called a hypocrite.

As a relief (floater) pharmacist for a significant part of the time since I graduated from pharmacy school in 1975, I've worked in many drugstores and have had the opportunity to meet many pharmacists. It strikes me that pharmacists in general don't seem to be overly enthusiastic about drugs. People probably assume that pharmacists take quite a few drugs themselves because they know what's available for various conditions. But this is certainly not the impression I've gotten from being around pharmacists. I think pharmacists in general are wary of taking drugs themselves. However, I don't see this wariness being conveyed at all to customers in response to customers' questions about a drug or drugs their doctor has prescribed.

One day in 2008 I drove a neighbor to her doctor's office in Lake Worth, Florida. While she and I were sitting in the waiting room, we overheard a conversation between two other patients in the waiting room. One of those patients said, "My husband was a pharmacist. He didn't like drugs." Obviously that statement overlooks the many drugs that are highly effective, essential, and even life-saving, such as insulin, antibiotics, and thyroid hormone. Nevertheless, it does reflect a sentiment I've encountered not uncommonly among pharmacists.

I don't know for sure whether pharmacists take more or fewer drugs than our customers. But I suspect pharmacists take fewer. It might be interesting for someone to conduct a study by asking pharmacists whether they believe they take more or fewer drugs than our customers.

A significant part of the pharmacist's time is spent listening to customers describe side effects and checking reference material to see whether the side effects being described could be from the drugs the customers are taking. Surely this must convince pharmacists that side effects are very common, with frequencies more prevalent than stated in the official prescribing information, and much more common than implied in drug advertisements on television.

The big drugstore chains have long lists of rules governing everything that the pharmacy staff is allowed to do (e.g., no food in the pharmacy refrigerator, no sitting on stools while entering prescriptions into the pharmacy computer, no radios allowed in the pharmacy, male pharmacists must wear a tie and white pharmacy jacket, etc.). So I suspect that most pharmacists understand quite clearly in this rigidly controlled workplace that management would not look favorably upon us conveying to customers our own personal doubts about many of the products we dispense. If you ask a pharmacist for a frank discussion about the potential risks associated with a drug you're taking, I think it is safe to say that you won't necessarily get a frank answer. I bet that you'll get a typical reassuring answer that the big drugstore chains and Big Pharma will be happy with.

That same pharmacist with whom I went out to dinner was at my apartment one day. He and I seldom talk about drugs and I have never told him about my concerns about drugs because I am always afraid that I might get a reputation among pharmacists as one who criticizes drugs. At one point as he headed to the bathroom, he said to me, "Give me something to read." On my table was the latest issue of *Newsweek* in which there was a two-page article on the controversy surrounding the potential hazards associated with Upjohn's sleeping pill Halcion (Geoffrey Cowley, "More Halcion Headaches," March 7, 1994, pp. 50-52). I suggested that he read this article. After exiting the bathroom, I asked him what he thought of the article. He said only, "I sure wouldn't recommend Halcion to a member of

my family." Our conversation immediately proceeded to other subjects because I am afraid to indulge other pharmacists in significant
discussions about the potential hazards associated with the drugs we
dispense. I fear being labeled by other pharmacists as too critical of
drugs. I can easily imagine a pharmacist telling my supervisor, "Dennis criticizes drugs." I doubt seriously that my employer would look
favorably upon a pharmacist with a reputation for believing that
many of our customers take drugs of questionable safety and/or effectiveness, or that Americans are overmedicated.

If I were to ask pharmacists "Is it possible that Americans are
overmedicated?", the replies would vary tremendously. I suspect I
would get the coldest response from pharmacists who own the store
in which they work. In my experience, these "independent" pharmacists have the most mercantile outlook of all pharmacists. If I asked
this question of chain pharmacists during a very busy workday, I suspect they would say "Hell, yes." If I asked this question of hospital
pharmacists, I suspect they would be less likely to agree that Americans are overmedicated since hospital pharmacists typically fill prescriptions for people who are sicker than pharmacists working in
drugstores.

The pharmacist who I mentioned in the last two anecdotes was
one of my best friends but I never felt comfortable telling him that I
think Americans are overmedicated or that too many of the drugs we
dispense are poorly screened by the FDA. He just would not have
welcomed that conversation. He was proud of being a pharmacist
and he was especially proud of the athletic teams at his alma mater,
the University of North Carolina. But I would not describe him as an
intellectually curious person. I was with him one day when he said
to his girlfriend that if they got married, they could have a son who
could be a football player and a daughter who could be a cheerleader.
I guess I would have preferred that he wanted to have children who
grew up to be professors of sociology or political science. But, to
me, his football player/cheerleader comment summed up his simplistic outlook on life.

I worked as a pharmacist in only two states—West Virginia and
North Carolina—and I got to know a lot of pharmacists in those
states. Perhaps the pharmacists in those two states are more conser-

vative than those in say, New York City or Boston. Perhaps more liberal pharmacists are more open to discussing controversies about pharmaceuticals.

Many pharmacists are understandably reluctant to express doubts about drugs to our customers because such doubts could cause our customers to unilaterally discontinue one or more prescribed medications. Obviously there's tremendous liability if one of our customers discontinues a medication and suffers negative consequences. Thus many pharmacists keep quiet out of fear of being sued if someone discontinues a drug and something bad happens. Fear of lawsuits keeps pharmacists from having frank discussions with our customers. It's much easier to give optimistic answers to all of our customers' questions.

The fact that my pharmacist friend would not recommend Halcion for anyone in his family is, to me, quite revealing. The way in which he expressed it is also quite revealing. He did not say, for example, "I would express caution or skepticism if a customer asked me what I think about Halcion." In my experience, most pharmacists feel safe only when sharing their true feelings with their own family. Pharmacists seem to be quite afraid to voice these same concerns when customers ask us about the safety of drugs. It is, in fact, not uncommon for customers to ask pharmacists some version of "Is this a safe drug?"

My point is the routine hypocrisy I see among many pharmacists. While filling prescriptions, I see many instances of pharmacists making little comments to co-workers about the potential hazards of the drugs being dispensed. But I seldom see any such sentiments expressed when customers ask us about drugs.

Robert Mendelsohn, M.D., titled one of his books *Confessions of a Medical Heretic* (Chicago: Contemporary Books, Inc., 1979) because of his view that modern medicine is a church to which most Americans have a deeply religious devotion. Most pharmacists, in my opinion, fear criticizing modern medicine in front of our customers the same way many people fear criticizing organized religion. Rather than risk being sued and rather than risk angering the doctor who prescribed the drug(s), pharmacists usually keep their personal opinions to themselves.

A few years ago, I had the occasion to work with a pharmacy school graduate during her internship (the period just before she was licensed). To my surprise, she routinely gave me her perspective on individual classes of drugs as we filled prescriptions together. Here are her comments:

On anti-cancer drugs: They're too barbaric. They're too toxic. Medicine at its crudest.

On drugs for anxiety and depression: I'd never take one of those myself. These people have some problem with their life that a drug won't solve.

On oral contraceptives: Too dangerous. I'd never take them myself. Just read the side effects in the *PDR*.

On drugs for hypertension: Way too many people are put on 'em for mild hypertension. They need to focus on losing weight instead.

On estrogens: Dangerous.

On cholesterol-lowering drugs: They change body chemistry so who knows what other problems they could be causing.

On antibiotics: Doctors prescribe 'em way too much so you've got all the problems with resistance.

I asked this soon-to-be-licensed pharmacist whether criticism of drugs was widespread these days in pharmacy school. She said that maybe ten percent of her class would actually discuss (among themselves) the potential hazards of the drugs they were learning about. The other ninety percent, she said, didn't question things.

She told me that her main personal medical problem has been with her sinuses. She said that she has taken most of the prescription and non-prescription products for sinus problems. She said that these products made her feel weird. For example, she said that she took the once popular antihistamine Seldane (now removed from the market because of its potential for serious drug interactions). She said she felt so strange while taking it that, for example, she had to scrutinize each word she spoke to be sure it was relevant to her point.

She also said that she can't foresee herself taking much medication in her life and she said that her husband, who has been a pharmacist for six years, "won't take anything himself, not even an aspirin." She said that she felt sure pharmacists in general take less medication than the general public because of their familiarity with the potential risks.

The husband of this recent graduate is known to be willing to work as a pharmacist for sixty or seventy hours per week, without complaint. She tells me he works overtime to be able to afford his habit of buying boats (the ones that are small enough to tow behind a pick-up truck). He feels guilty spending his regular pay for other than family expenses. Her husband willingly—even enthusiastically—puts in long hours dispensing drugs that he would not take himself.

She also told me that she figures that pharmacists get more feedback (than doctors) from patients about side effects because she suspects the patients are too intimidated to talk to their doctors about side effects. She says that complaints about side effects from drugs are viewed by doctors as complaints about their competence in prescribing drugs. Consequently, she said, patients keep quiet.

Skeptical comments like these are, in my experience, quite uncommon among pharmacists. Even though I always look forward to big picture assessments of drugs, I have rarely encountered such frank discussions with pharmacists during my 25-year career as a pharmacist.

In my opinion, a high degree of skepticism is fully warranted because pharmacists dispense the products of an industry that has consistently shown a preference for placing profits above science. It is very naive to think that the pharmaceutical industry (or any industry) would place the public interest above profits.

In my career I have never heard pharmacists at work discuss among themselves a drug and say something like "It's a great drug" or "It's a great breakthrough." At required continuing education seminars, pharmacists often hear the speaker make such statements. But pharmacists routinely tell customers that the medication they've been prescribed is great, very effective, very safe, etc. I've never heard pharmacists praising medications among themselves in private conversations. It always struck me as odd that pharmacists routinely reassure customers about drugs yet these same pharmacists seem to lose that enthusiasm for drugs in private conversations with other pharmacists.

Pharmacists' lack of enthusiasm for the products we sell seems to contrast with some other workers in our society. I have, for many years, observed employees in various stores to see whether they seem to genuinely enjoy discussing the products they sell. In my experience, computer salesmen and car salesmen seem to genuinely enjoy discussing the differences between the various models, the latest innovations, etc. It doesn't seem to be drudgery to them. Lots of employees in bookstores, record stores, and clothing stores go home and indulge in activities that are quite similar to their work. Booksellers often go home and read books; record store employees go home and listen to music; and clothes salesmen genuinely enjoy discussing clothes, wearing clothes, etc. Radio station disk jockeys probably go home and listen to music. Auto mechanics and auto parts employees deal with cars all day, yet, in my experience, they're likely to go home and enjoy working on their own car. Home Depot employees seem to genuinely enjoy discussing home repairs and improvements.

In my experience, a similar level of enthusiasm does not exist with pharmacists. I don't know any retail pharmacists who eagerly await the arrival of the latest issue of pharmacy magazines to read about the latest drugs. I just haven't seen a genuine passion, enthusiasm, and interest in drugs among pharmacists.

Despite the rosy picture of pharmacy painted by professors in pharmacy schools, leaders of pharmacy associations, editors of pharmacy magazines, and management at chain drugstores, the filling of prescriptions is not an inherently enjoyable activity. Many pharmacists consider it to be a monotonous, boring activity like the filling of burger orders at McDonald's. But what makes pharmacy even more onerous is the fact that the consequences of a mistake in the pharmacy are much more serious than leaving ketchup, mayonnaise, or pickle off a burger.

In my opinion, the pharmacist's duties with the big chains are as mundane, mind-numbing, and non-creative as telephone operators, airline ticket agents, bank tellers, and clerks at McDonald's. How can pharmacists find their job fulfilling when it consists of filling prescriptions as fast as our hands and feet will allow, almost from the minute our shift begins to the minute it ends? How can pharmacists have a passion for filling a never-ending wave of prescriptions, at lightning speed, in dangerously understaffed pharmacies?

Pharmacists working for the big drugstore chains view themselves as hourly wage laborers. Because of widespread understaffing and constant worry about the bottom line, pharmacists have little choice except to focus on products rather than on the people who use those products. Pharmacy magazines and pharmacy schools say that pharmacy is very satisfying because pharmacists are able to help educate people about medications. In the real world, there's very little time for good communication with customers. Customers are lucky if they get more than one sentence when they ask their pharmacist a question.

I've never worked in a hospital pharmacy so I am not knowledgeable on that subject or on hospital pharmacists. But I have the impression that hospital inpatient pharmacists are more fulfilled by their work than are pharmacists who work for the big chains. Certainly hospital pharmacists usually fill prescriptions for people who are sicker than the customers served by chain pharmacists. That means that the average prescription dispensed by hospital pharmacists is less likely to be unnecessary. For example, conservative estimates are that one-half of prescriptions for antibiotics written by doctors outside the hospital are unnecessary. (These antibiotics are often written for the common cold.) I doubt that hospital pharmacists see chronic overmedication like drugstore pharmacists do.

It is quite striking that pharmacists seem to have accepted the notion that an important part of our job is to reassure the public about the safety of medications. Customers read the list of fifty—or more—side effects in the *Physician's Desk Reference* and then call the pharmacist and say they're not sure they want to take the medication their doctor has prescribed. The pharmacist then downplays the caller's concern by saying something like, "All drugs have side effects. Your doctor wouldn't have prescribed that medication if he didn't think it would help you." In my experience, nearly one hundred percent of people who read about their drug in the *PDR* are less enthusiastic about taking the drug after reading about it.

Despite personal doubts about some of the drugs we dispense, many pharmacists have a visceral hatred toward consumer drug advocates like Sidney Wolfe, M.D. and his Public Citizen Health Research Group (*Worst Pills, Best Pills* is among their publications). Some pharmacists react as angrily to any public criticism of drugs as they react to any criticism of their religion.

One pharmacist wrote an angry letter to the editor at *Drug Topics* (March 17, 2003, pp. 12, 14) after that magazine ran a cover story discussing the possibility that the government may begin testing medications compounded by pharmacists because of possible quality problems (mainly potency and contamination). This pharmacist ended his letter: "My message to you is to defend our profession, unite the pharmacist, make pharmacists proud to be who they are. Your job is to show the positive aspects of our profession, not the negative."

Many pharmacists view drug criticism as a challenge to their self-worth as health professionals. It would be quite taxing on the psyche of pharmacists to dispense drugs every day while simultaneously harboring serious doubts about many of these drugs or about the lack of emphasis on prevention in our health care system. Sociologists have a term "cognitive dissonance" which is "a psychological conflict resulting from incongruous beliefs and attitudes held simultaneously." It would be difficult for pharmacists to sling out prescriptions at lightning speed every day while harboring significant questions about many of those drugs. I found it very difficult to go to work each day because I was very disillusioned that the focus of modern medicine is so narrowly focused on molecules and cells rather than on prevention.

In my experience, pharmacy is not a dynamic, intellectually stimulating profession in which dissenting opinions are welcome. A pharmacist who says that Americans are overmedicated or that our health care system focuses too heavily on drugs is likely to be viewed by many pharmacists as a troublemaker. A pharmacist expressing such views would be greeted as unfavorably by many pharmacists today as when Copernicus questioned the prevailing wisdom by stating that the Earth is not the center of the universe.

Most pharmacy customers probably think that issues of drug safety and effectiveness are adequately handled by the FDA. Our more sophisticated customers are less likely to blindly accept assurances from governmental agencies. I suspect that some of these more educated customers assume (or hope) that pharmacists are world-wise people who objectively and dispassionately look at the risks versus benefits of drugs, whether certain drugs are really needed (is it all marketing?), whether conditions can be prevented without drugs, etc. In twenty-five years as a pharmacist, I can only recall a few instances in which pharmacists actually made insightful comments about certain drugs. Here are a few more examples:

One pharmacist I worked with said that "Way too many kids are put on drugs like Ritalin for hyperactivity. What the kids really need is more discipline from their parents." Upon hearing that one of our customers was opposed to her son's day care center claiming her son needed to be on Ritalin, another pharmacist said to me, "If the mother doesn't agree with the day care center, she should find another day care center."

Pharmacists are often skeptical when we fill prescriptions for weight loss drugs for women who are only slightly overweight. During the heyday of the diet pills Pondimin, Redux, and phen-fen, many pharmacists were quite skeptical of the widespread use of these drugs. Pharmacists would routinely make private comments to pharmacy staff like "These women just want to lose a few pounds to look better in a swimsuit." These weight loss drugs were approved by the FDA to treat people with a serious weight problem but, as often happens with drugs in every category, far more people end up getting prescriptions. After filling a huge number of prescriptions for these diet pills, one of the pharmacy technicians who I had known for a long time decided to go to her family physician for her own prescription. Though she did lose a few pounds initially, use of the weight-loss drug did not result in her keeping the pounds off.

In addition to criticizing the overprescribing of drugs like Ritalin and weight-loss drugs, pharmacists are very often critical of doctors who seem to write prescriptions too easily for pain pills. Pharmacists often comment to our techs that many of our customers appear to be hooked on pain pills like Vicodin, Lorcet and Tylenol w/Codeine. Pharmacists also often feel that too many of our customers are hooked on anti-anxiety drugs like Xanax and Ativan. Occasionally pharmacists make comments to techs that many of our customers wouldn't need to be on drugs for hypertension if these customers would exercise, lose weight, and eat nutritious food.

Even though I am disappointed by the extent to which pharmacists hide their own personal concerns in discussions with our customers, I believe that a large number of pharmacists might privately agree with much of the following:

- The pharmaceutical industry is out of control.
- Drugs have too often been rushed to market without proper testing by the manufacturer or scrutiny by the FDA.
- The drug companies have undue influence with Congress and the FDA.
- The drug companies routinely exaggerate the benefits of their products to doctors and on television while downplaying their risks.
- Drug advertisements on TV cause people to request often unnecessary drugs from their doctor.
- The drug companies charge outrageous prices for drugs that are— too often—just cousins of drugs already on the market (i.e., "me-too" or "copy-cat" drugs).
- The drug companies hype each of these copy-cat drugs as if they were equal to the discovery of penicillin or insulin.
- Doctors have bought into this pharmaceutical culture because it has been financially lucrative.
- Academic researchers have done likewise.
- Americans would be far better off with fewer drugs on the market.
- Americans have been misled about the safety and effectiveness of pharmaceuticals.
- The pharmaceutical industry has pulled the wool over the eyes of Americans.
- Most of our customers simply want a quick fix rather than make significant changes in their lives which might allow them to take fewer drugs.

• The drug industry would clearly like to expand the market for each of their products beyond that which is clearly justified based on the risks and benefits of each drug.

• When problems surface with specific drugs, the manufacturer routinely downplays the significance of the hazards or, worse, engages in a cover-up.

• According to George Lundberg, M.D., formerly the editor at *The Journal of the American Medical Association*, "U. S. pharmaceutical companies remain a world model for creating devious methods to get physicians and patients to do what the companies want, whether or not it is in the best interest of the patient." (George Lundberg, M.D., *Severed Trust: Why American Medicine Hasn't Been Fixed*," New York: Basic Books, 2000, p. 145)

I suspect that many pharmacists agree with many of these observations but they're afraid to tell our customers. Sometimes I am optimistic that pharmacists are able to see how manipulative and dishonest Big Pharma is. At other times I am very pessimistic and think that pharmacists have swallowed Big Pharma's pill-for-every-ill outlook in totality.

As regards the pharmacist who commented to me: "Way too many kids are put on drugs like Ritalin for hyperactivity" and "What the kids really need is more discipline from their parents," in my opinion there's no way that this pharmacist could make that comment to a parent without angering that parent. Obviously it makes chain management angry when we upset our customers. This lack of freedom to suggest that some drugs are overprescribed makes my job very unfulfilling. As another example, pharmacists (who may be so inclined) are reluctant to tell obese customers with elevated blood pressure that the single best thing to lower their blood pressure is to lose weight.

Pharmacists are often very reluctant to give information to customers that goes contrary to those customers' outlooks. Most customers seem to favor the reductionistic view of modern medicine that focuses on *treatments* for diseases rather than actual *causes*. Telling obese people that they need to lose weight has a tendency to upset these people. This places the burden on them to change their eating habits. Instead, they seem to prefer the drug industry narrative regarding obesity, i.e., it is a complex physiological malfunction requiring pharmacological management. Many obese people don't like being told that they simply need to learn to eat less food. They prefer to view obesity as a disease of unknown cause that requires continuing medical research to uncover arcane molecular and genetic secrets.

Even though human ancestors have thrived on earth for hundreds of thousands of years, the pharmaceutical industry has convinced Americans that our ability to survive depends on continuing innovation in drug research. Unless Big Pharma is allowed to innovate and make big profits, our survival is imperiled. But the biggest myth of modern medicine is that the increasing lifespan in the last hundred years is primarily due to doctors and drugs. In fact, the increase in the average lifespan is due primarily to the wealth effect (as nations become wealthier, lifespans increase) and public health measures like better sanitation, better protection from the elements (better housing), better nutrition, the availability of clean water, etc. Modern medicine has played a role but that role is modest compared to social, cultural, economic, and political factors. See Thomas McKeown (*The Origins of Human Disease*, New York: Basil Blackwell, 1988, p. 89):

> **The transformation of health and rapid rise of population in the Western world during the last three centuries have a common explanation: they resulted from a decline of mortality from infectious diseases. The infections declined mainly for two reasons: increased resistance to the diseases due to improved nutrition, and reduced exposure to infection which followed the hygienic measures introduced progressively from the late nineteenth century. *The contribution of medical treatment and immunization to the decline of mortality was delayed until the twentieth century, and was small in relation to that of the other influences.* [my italics]**

The introduction of antibiotics played a much smaller role in the increase in lifespan in the last hundred years than is commonly believed. The death rates from infectious diseases had already fallen to low levels by the time that antibiotics were introduced. See Leonard

Sagan, M.D., (*The Health of Nations: True Causes of Sickness and Well-being*, New York: Basic Books, 1987, p. 64):

> The introduction of antibiotics into clinical medicine in the late 1940s and early 1950s was indeed a moment of great historical significance. There can be little doubt that, when properly used, antibiotics can shorten the course of some infectious diseases; they often did so during the early days of the antibiotic era. Yet it is not at all clear that these agents have contributed to the overall fall in mortality from infectious disease. Why is that?
>
> As noted earlier, death rates from the infectious diseases had already fallen to low levels by the time that antibiotics were introduced. …the decline in infectious disease mortality began long before the appearance of the first antibiotic, penicillin, and even long before the widespread use of the first chemotherapeutic agents, the sulfa drugs. By 1950, when effective antitubercular drugs first became widely available, the death rate from tuberculosis, the major infectious disease of young adults, had already fallen to a small fraction of what it had been in the nineteenth century.

Also see the following:
• J. B. McKinlay and S. M. McKinlay, "The Questionable Contribution of Medical Measures to the Decline of Mortality in the United States in the Twentieth Century," *Millbank Memorial Fund Quarterly* (Summer), 405-428, 1977
• Norman J. Temple and Denis P. Burkitt (eds.), *Western Diseases*, Totowa, New Jersey: Humana Press, 1994

Pharmacists understand quite well that our job is to be supportive of pharmaceuticals, not lifestyle changes, not dietary changes. Our assembly line healthcare system is based on the rapid processing of patients/customers. This industrial production model relies on the dispensing of commodities, rather than on the education of the population. For example, dispensing antidepressants to depressed people is much more efficient for doctors than examining in depth the patient's life circumstances which may be causing the depression.

A medical system based on prevention, education and insight is not conducive to productivity and financial reward.

The big chains are absolutely obsessed with productivity. Whenever I see or hear the word *productivity* from our bosses, I know that they're looking for more brilliant ways to squeeze more prescriptions out of us in less time and with less staff.

A skeptical pharmacist in a drugstore will inevitably become restive. It is very depressing to me that the only place where a critique of modern medicine seems to be genuinely appreciated is in some universities, mostly in the fields of medical sociology and medical anthropology—but certainly not, in my opinion, in the school of pharmacy.

Shortly after graduation from pharmacy school, I became disillusioned with the quality of contact that I had with customers. Most contact usually consisted of a customer coming up to me and asking:

- "What's good for a cold?"
- "What's good for a cough?"
- "My baby hasn't had a bowel movement in three days. He just can't go. What do I need to get?"
- "What's good for a sore throat?"
- "What's good for a sore back?"
- "I'm always out of energy. Could you suggest a vitamin?"
- "My wife's nerves are acting up. Do you have anything that might help her?"
- "I have trouble sleeping. Could you suggest something?"

The population has been well-indoctrinated by drug industry marketing to respond to every symptom with the question "What's good for...?" (as opposed to the more enlightened response: "How could I change my life or habits so that I might avoid these problems?").

When someone approached me to recommend a non-prescription product, I began saying to myself: *Please don't ask me what's good for a cold or cough or sore throat or hemorrhoids or nerves or sleep or a sore back or loss of energy or diarrhea or constipation. Please don't ask me to recommend a quick fix.* I have heard that doctors prefer educated patients because they ask intelligent questions. I assume most pharmacists feel the same way.

There is something monumentally degrading by the extent to which modern medicine has stripped a feeling of competence from the average person in this country as regards his ability to comprehend the basics of health. That is why Ivan Illich subtitled his landmark book, *Medical Nemesis,* "The Expropriation of Health." (New York: Pantheon, 1976)

There is something degrading, demeaning, and pitiful that an adult would come to me and say "My wife hasn't been able to go for three days." There is something terribly wrong that one of the most frequently asked questions of pharmacists is "What's good for nerves?" There is something terribly wrong that a customer would interpret her personal anxiety, tension, depression, marital stress, or job dissatisfaction as simply an indication that her nerves are "acting up." Such a customer may have been abused or unloved as a child. To me, it is incredibly sad that she interprets her resultant depression as simply "nerves acting up."

How can any pharmacist find this job fulfilling when we dispense superficial drug solutions for complex problems in the lives of our customers? Pharmacists are expected to be supportive of drug solutions for problems in life that range from the trivial to the profound. That's why I think modern medicine's most serious crime may be its role in stripping the population of an independent ability to be a competent human being.

Working with a pharmacist who shared my skepticism would have made my job a little more bearable

Most chain drugstores are open around eighty hours a week, split between two full-time pharmacists, both of whom work forty hours. Even though there is not a lot of overlap in these shifts, we get to know the other pharmacist (our "partner") pretty well, especially if we work in the same store for months or years. Say one pharmacist works from 9 AM to 3 PM and the other pharmacist works from 3

PM to 9 PM. The first pharmacist usually needs to spend a few minutes telling the second pharmacist about any situations that are in limbo or any problems that are hanging. So we get to know that other pharmacist fairly well if we've worked with him or her for a few months or more.

Having a partner who is friendly and a hard worker can make the world of chain pharmacy somewhat less burdensome. Having a partner who, at least to some extent, shares our skepticism is even better. In my 25 year career, I've worked at maybe a hundred different locations for three huge chains. Most pharmacists are used to filling in for sick days or vacation days at nearby stores. So I've gotten to know a large number of pharmacists. Of course, pharmacists' personalities span a wide spectrum from those who are very nice people to those who are complete jerks.

Since I am the type of pharmacist who is not enamored with the pill-for-every-ill outlook that is so prevalent today in our society, I naturally enjoyed working with pharmacists who seemed—at least to some extent—to be able to see how absurd things often are in the world of pharmacy, in the world of health care, and in the wider society. For a few months, I worked with one pharmacist who completely accepted her job at face value. She seemed to have no doubt that the pills on our shelves were all safe and effective, and she seemed to have no doubt in her belief that health is directly proportional to one's utilization of drugs and doctors. Her rock-solid belief in the unequivocal value of what she was doing used to grate on me. It was much like two people on opposite ends of the political spectrum. One day, in my *hope springs eternal* attempt to introduce a little humility into her personality and world view, I mentioned to her that I had been reading some books critical of the drug industry and modern medicine. I asked her whether she cared to read them. She said that it so happened she was accompanying her husband on a short business trip a few days hence, and that she would probably have time to read the books since she anticipated spending significant time in the hotel room while he was at business meetings. So I brought her Ivan Illich's *Medical Nemesis* and Robert Mendelsohn's *Confessions of a Medical Heretic*. A few days after she returned from the trip, I asked her if she had looked at the books. She answered that yes, she had, but her body language strongly suggested that she couldn't care less what Illich and Mendelsohn had to say. This was in the early 1980s when these two books had been out for only a few years.

Working full time for months in the same drugstore can be quite tiresome when one's partner has a world outlook completely different from our own. Clearly I was on the far end of the spectrum as regards disillusionment with the pill-for-every-ill obsession in our health care system. Granted, many pharmacists will readily admit (to other pharmacists) that Americans are grossly overmedicated. But these same pharmacists don't seem to want to dwell on that topic. They seem to be willing to agree with that observation, but then they seem to want to change the subject. I suspect it is uncomfortable for pharmacists to linger too long on the observation that we are active participants in a medical system that pushes pills rather than prevention. Indeed, I would say that pharmacists are enablers of the current system, in that our acquiescence with the pill-for-every-ill outlook legitimizes the system in the eyes of our customers. Our customers think that surely pharmacists would not support a system that goes against their beliefs. But I would say that that is precisely what many pharmacists are doing.

Occasionally I would meet pharmacists who would make little comments like "If people would just take better care of themselves, lose weight, eat better, etc., they wouldn't need so many pills." I would instantly feel a degree of sympatico with these pharmacists. I once worked with a pharmacist who made a generalization that I found quite shocking. She seemed to be surveying all the pills in the pharmacy one day when she said to me, "I can't take any of this stuff." I sensed that she was expressing serious and heartfelt skepticism about the safety and effectiveness of many of the pills on our shelves. I acted like I didn't understand what she was saying. I hoped she would expand on her comment in a pure way, uninfluenced by my personal views. So I asked her, "What do you mean?" She said something like "This stuff is too dangerous!" That is indeed, in my experience, a rare comment from a pharmacist. Many pharmacists may privately agree with that view, but, in my experience, few are eager to verbalize it to other pharmacists. And obviously we can't imagine making such a statement to our customers. Of course, I am sure that she would agree with the obvious fact that many drugs are absolutely essential and even life-saving.

I was filling in one day at a store in which I had never worked before. During a lull in the workday, I had a brief conversation with the non-pharmacist store manager. He told me that he was interested in the subject of health. As he surveyed all the pills on our shelves, he said, "The further we get from the trees, the more problems we have." He was basically saying that the further humans get from a connection with the natural world (fresh fruits and vegetables, clean air and water, etc.), the more health problems we develop. What a refreshing thing to hear in a setting far removed from nature: i.e., a typical modern drugstore!

In my experience, most pharmacists are uninterested in reading exposé's of Big Pharma. Most pharmacists don't seem to want to be bothered with books like John Abramson's *Overdosed America*, or Marcia Angell's *The Truth About the Drug Companies*, or Jerry Avorn's *Powerful Medicines*, or Stephen Fried's *Bitter Pills*, or Melody Peterson's *Our Daily Meds*. In my opinion, most pharmacists would view me as a traitor to pharmacy if I focused too heavily on a critique of the safety and effectiveness of the drugs we dispense. Since I did not want to get a reputation with pharmacists or my bosses as someone who questioned the pill-for-every-ill outlook, I usually kept my opinions to myself. With at best one or two exceptions, I did not meet pharmacists in my 25-year career with whom I felt comfortable discussing a critique of modern medicine, or with whom I felt truly comfortable sharing the many books that so strongly influenced my disgust with a health care system based on pills rather than prevention.

Chapter 8

Why some pharmacy technicians are a threat to the public safety

Pharmacy technicians are those people you see in the pharmacy who wear white coats but are not pharmacists. They do things like accept prescriptions from customers, count pills, answer phones, stock pharmacy shelves, and operate the pharmacy computer.

For example, if you are allergic to penicillin, the person entering this fact into your computer record may be no more than a high school student. This critical information allows the computer to flag any subsequent prescription for penicillin or penicillin-like drugs. If the person entering this information does so incorrectly, your notifying the pharmacy of your penicillin allergy has been a waste of time.

Pharmacies are turning over more duties to techs. Techs decipher your doctor's oftentimes poorly legible handwriting to determine which drug you doctor prescribed. Commonly, it is the technician—not the pharmacist—who inputs the drug name, strength, quantity, number of refills, and directions (once a day, twice a day, every 4 hours, etc.). Techs attach those colorful little stickers to your prescription bottle like: "Take with food" or "Avoid prolonged exposure to sunlight" or "Take this medication one hour before or two-three hours after a meal."

Techs are allowed to do almost everything that the pharmacist does, under the pharmacist's supervision. The pharmacist is always responsible for checking the tech's work. There are a few things that techs are not allowed to do. For example, techs are not allowed to release a prescription without a pharmacist's approval.

The chains love techs. Techs usually make around $10.00 to $15.00 per hour. Pharmacists make $90,000 to $110,000 or more per year. The chains say that with profit margins squeezed by managed care, pharmacy technicians are essential to ensure a profit in the pharmacy. The chains say that techs hold down the cost of your medication.

There are several hundred thousand pharmacy techs in the United States. An increasing number of techs are becoming certified, allowing them to place the initials CPhT (Certified Pharmacy Technician) after their name. In addition, many of the nation's pharmacy technicians are attending technical schools or getting associate's degrees. Many techs favor licensure or certification, seeing it as a way to increase their wages. Some employers oppose the licensing of techs, figuring it will increase their labor costs.

Facts from the Pharmacy Technician Certification Board website (https://www.ptcb.org/AM/Template.cfm?Section=Regulations&Template=/CM/HTMLDisplay.cfm&ContentID=4108, accessed Aug. 23, 2011):

• Since 1995, the Pharmacy Technician Certification Board has certified 413, 447 pharmacy technicians through the examination and transfer process.

• The following states require certification of pharmacy technicians: Arizona, Idaho, Illinois, Iowa, Louisiana, Maryland, Massachusetts, Montana, New Mexico, Oregon, South Carolina, Texas, Utah, Virginia, Washington State, Wyoming.

• The following states do not require registration, licensure, or certification of pharmacy technicians: Colorado, the District of Columbia, Georgia, Hawaii, Michigan, New York, Pennsylvania, and Wisconsin.

Is licensure or certification of techs the answer to safety concerns? Or is lack of adequate staffing in the pharmacy the real problem? Can licensed or certified techs make up for dangerous understaffing in the pharmacy? Many pharmacists say that understaffing is the most serious problem in the pharmacy, causing a dangerous dispensing environment.

Many chains define a tech as anyone who helps out in the pharmacy, regardless of her level of experience. As soon as she walks into the pharmacy from the street, some chains define her as a tech. This is absurd and dangerous.

Auburn University School of Pharmacy conducted a study of pharmacy errors, concluding that "51.5 million errors occur during the filling of 3 billion prescriptions each year." (Eliz. Flynn, et.al., "National Observational Study of Prescription Dispensing Accuracy and Safety in 50 Pharmacies," *Journal of the American Pharmacist's Assoc.*, March/April 2003, pp. 191-200) Can pharmacists be expected to catch all the mistakes made by techs in high pressure pharmacies in which hundreds of prescriptions are filled daily? I have worked in pharmacies that fill up to 50 prescriptions per hour during the busiest times of the day.

A pharmacist can safely check the work of how many technicians? Tech-to-pharmacist ratios are hotly debated. Some observers say that with more than two techs per pharmacist, the pharmacist is unable to safely check all the prescriptions techs churn out. Common sense says that the faster people work and the less training they have, the more likely it is that errors will occur. The question is whether your pharmacist can catch all the inevitable errors in this fast-food environment.

Do techs increase the likelihood of errors in the pharmacy? In some cases, they undoubtedly do. Having a good tech, however, is almost like having another pharmacist present. It all depends on the quality of the techs. I know many techs who make fewer errors than pharmacists. I know many techs who I trust more than pharmacists to accurately type your doctor's directions on your label. It's not that these techs know more than pharmacists. It's just that some techs are inherently more careful than many of the pharmacists I know. Techs and pharmacists span the entire spectrum as regards accuracy.

Some techs and pharmacists rarely make errors. Other techs and pharmacists are an accident waiting to happen. You have no way of knowing whether the pharmacists and techs at your pharmacy are in the former category or the latter.

I worked in one very busy store in which the best tech could churn out as many prescriptions as the three or four worst techs combined. I know many techs who can churn out far more prescriptions than pharmacists. Given the choice between working alongside a great tech or a slow pharmacist, I would choose to work with the great tech every time.

With so many look-alike or sound-alike drug names like Prilosec and Prozac or Xanax and Zantac, should you trust a person with little or no formal training in drugs to decipher your doctor's handwriting? Is the tech sophisticated enough to investigate a poorly legible prescription to determine that acid reflux is your problem, implying that your doctor wants you to have Prilosec; or that depression is your problem, implying that your doctor is prescribing Prozac? If pharmacists often have difficulty reading doctor's handwriting, does it make you comfortable to know that the person attempting to decipher your doctor's handwriting may have just begun working in the pharmacy?

Upon becoming a pharmacist, I was surprised that many of the big chains would allow high school students and inexperienced techs to have such a critical role in filling prescriptions. I was surprised that on-the-job training has been accepted practice with something as critical as prescription drugs. Prescriptions are often filled so quickly that they are just a blur as they pass by technicians and pharmacists. Pharmacists frequently say to themselves, "Mrs. Smith was in today but I don't even remember filling or checking her prescriptions."

Should technicians run the pharmacy computer?

The pharmacy computer is the heart of the pharmacy and the repository for all the data about your prescriptions. If data is entered into the computer incorrectly, the current prescription and each subsequent refill will reflect that erroneous information. Unless there is some obvious reason to go back and change the data that's entered, a serious error can be perpetuated for months or longer. That means the customer can receive the wrong drug, the wrong strength, the wrong directions, etc., for the current prescription and subsequent refills.

Pharmacy software providers pride themselves on the number of warning flags they can raise as pharmacists and techs enter prescriptions into the pharmacy computer. This gives technicians the impossible task of separating critical warnings from those that are unlikely to result in significant harm. Pharmacists, themselves, are frequently uncertain about which warnings justify taking action such as notifying the doctor who wrote the prescription(s). Most pharmacists agree that expecting pharmacy technicians to evaluate these oftentimes complex warnings is absurd. Yet most of the big drug chains expect pharmacy technicians to input most of America's prescriptions and to evaluate the huge numbers of warnings that pop up as technicians speed through a large number of computer screens in the filling of millions of prescriptions across America every day. Granted, pharmacy computers usually grade the severity of each warning. But many techs seem to have a very relaxed attitude toward these warnings, regardless of the severity level assigned by the computer software. It is true that their level of concern often reflects the attitude of the pharmacists with whom the techs work.

U. S. News & World Report conducted a large-scale undercover investigation of pharmacists' ability to catch drug interactions. ("Danger at the Drugstore," August 26, 1996, pp. 46-53) The investigation revealed that pharmacy staff did not do a good job of catching potential drug interactions. Even though this investigation was conducted in the 1990s, I would be willing to bet that similar results would be obtained today, since the problem of pharmacy understaffing is probably more acute today than it was in 1996. Understaffing translates into prescriptions filled at incredible speed. Does it make any sense to have technicians screen your record for drug interactions that even pharmacists overlook? Some computer programs do not even require that the tech call the pharmacist over to view the most serious interactions and enter his secret password or authorization before proceeding.

Statistically, overriding a drug interaction warning is unlikely to harm the customer since most of the warnings that pop up on the computer screen do not require a change in the drugs the doctor has prescribed. Yet the chains seem to be gambling on statistics. Drug interactions vary tremendously in their potential to cause harm. In my experience, most interactions that the pharmacy computer flags have been of theoretical concern and do not require notifying the doctor who prescribed the drugs. For several years, I have been collecting articles that describe lawsuits against pharmacists. I see that "overlooking a drug interaction" is not one of the more common reasons for a lawsuit against pharmacists. The most common reason that pharmacists are sued is for dispensing the wrong drug (for example, dispensing Coumadin instead of Cardura). Another common reason for being sued is typing wrong directions on a child's liquid prescription medication (for example, "Give 1.5 teaspoonsful" instead of "Give 1.5 milliliters."

Employers say that technicians free up the pharmacist from mundane tasks like counting pills and operating the pharmacy computer. Supposedly this allows the pharmacist time to advise customers about the proper use of medications. It is a fact that employers greatly prefer to hire techs when business increases, thus making the pharmacist responsible for checking, for example, the work of three techs rather than two. The addition of techs does not necessarily give the pharmacist more time to advise customers, because chain staffing is usually kept at the bare bones level to increase profitability.

Pharmacy technicians are the workhorses of pharmacy. Busy drugstores often have one or two pharmacists supervise techs who prepare several hundred prescriptions per day. The onerous workload of this nation's increasing prescription volume is being placed on pharmacy techs. It's a high-pressure assembly line with the pharmacist responsible for verifying the end product.

I once had a conversation with the head of a state board of pharmacy. He compared the modern drugstore to one famous episode of *I Love Lucy* in which Lucille Ball places pies in boxes at the end of an assembly line. As the speed of the assembly line increases, more and more pies fall to the floor. The head of this state board of pharmacy told me that he worries that we may be heading in a similar direction in pharmacy.

Here's another food production analogy: The filling of prescriptions in America is much like the making of sausage: You don't want to watch the process. With some understanding of what's involved in the filling of prescriptions, if you were to step behind the pharmacy counter in a busy drugstore for a few hours and watch how prescriptions are processed, you might never again assume that:
• the right pills are in your bottle,
• the directions on the label are correct,
• your medications have been properly screened for drug interactions, or
• your pharmacist has had enough time to carefully check each prescription technicians have filled.
You might also see that time constraints sometimes force pharmacists and technicians to take educated guesses about doctors' poorly legible handwriting or questionable doses, and to sometimes override potentially risky drug interactions.

When pharmacists fill in at other stores for pharmacists who are sick or on vacation, we are at the mercy of those stores to have competent techs on duty. Most pharmacists are very familiar with the extremely unpleasant experience of working in an unfamiliar pharmacy with techs who make lots of errors, or working with no tech at all. Some pharmacists insist on proper tech staffing before agreeing to work in an unfamiliar pharmacy. Sometimes this gives the pharmacist a reputation for being uncooperative, too demanding, not a team player, etc.

As pharmacy customers become more impatient and expect instant service, many of the large chains have responded with drive-thru windows. This reinforces in the minds of our customers the perception that prescriptions are a commodity like hamburgers. It is very dangerous to add oftentimes untrained technicians to an already hyper-stressed environment. Do you want—in some cases—a high school student preparing your medication order as if she were preparing a burger order? Do high school students have the maturity required for the pharmacy? Are ongoing conversations about their boyfriends and social activities conducive to the accurate filling of prescriptions? Are you comfortable with people of widely varying experience levels having an increasing role with today's potent prescription drugs?

The practice of having techs run the pharmacy computer seems to be a corporate decision at most of the big chain drugstores. Yet some pharmacists refuse to let techs run the computer. These pharmacists feel that running the pharmacy computer is the most critical job in the drugstore and that only the pharmacist should be trusted to read all the warnings that pop up on the screen as we enter prescriptions. So the question is: *Should techs indeed be allowed to run the pharmacy computer even though doing so is routine in most pharmacies today?*

In my opinion, the corporate attitude of the big chain drugstores toward the doctorate in pharmacy degree (Pharm.D.) illustrates the same corporate attitude that endorses techs running the pharmacy computer. It is clear to me that the bean counters at the big chains believe Pharm.D.'s are overeducated for work in drugstores. The best indication of this is that many of the big chains want technicians to run the pharmacy computer, not the pharmacist. The most often stated reason is that this allows the pharmacist to be free to answer customers' questions, speak on the phone with doctors' offices, check prescriptions that have been completed by technicians, make recommendations to customers for non-prescription products for coughs and colds, etc.

Apparently many of the big chains do not attach much significance to the endless number of warnings (Drug Utilization Review or DUR alerts) that pop up on the computer screen. If you have any doubts whether the big chains think Pharm.D's are overeducated for retail pharmacy, consider the fact that the big chains don't think it is necessary for a pharmacist (B.S. *or* Pharm.D.) to review the warnings, contraindications, precautions, high/low dose alerts, drug interactions, etc.

Pharmacists: Can you name a task in the pharmacy that requires more education than responding to drug therapy questions or evaluating DUR alerts? Supposedly technicians are not allowed to screen for drug therapy problems but isn't that exactly what they're doing when they routinely zip past a blizzard of DUR alerts of varying levels of importance?

The pharmacy computer software generates a remarkable number of these DUR alerts. Pharmacists assumed that the evaluation of these DUR alerts is precisely the reason we were required to graduate from pharmacy school. Some of these warnings are highly complex and they leave the pharmacist scratching his head and wondering what is indeed the practical significance of these warnings. Some pharmacists choose to ignore the vast majority of warnings as simply "noise." Other pharmacists consult reference books in the pharmacy in order to understand more fully the implications of the DUR alerts.

The big chains design their computer systems as they see fit, with "filling and billing" functions given top priority. The fact that most of the big chains encourage the pharmacy technicians to run the pharmacy computer demonstrates to me that the big chains view the pharmacy computer as mainly a data-entry tool for the processing of prescriptions, rather than a medical tool for assuring that all prescriptions are screened for possible drug therapy problems.

Are pharmacists and techs like airline ticket agents? Airline ticket agents spend a large part of their day on the computer: checking fares, flights, the availability of seats, and entering the customer's name, address and phone number, etc. But airline ticket agents don't also need to examine the plane's maintenance records to determine the safety of the planes on which the customers fly. In contrast, the pharmacy staff must screen each prescription to be sure that there are no pertinent warnings, contraindications, drug interactions, etc. that can affect the customer's safety.

What conclusion can one reach other than that the big pharmacy chains do not place a lot of importance on the warnings? If the big chains took seriously the endless number of warnings, only pharmacists would be allowed to run the pharmacy computer. The big chains seem to view the operation of the pharmacy computer as simply a clerical job, not a job that requires substantial knowledge of drug therapy.

I bet that most pharmacists have often wondered what warnings the technicians are ignoring. In my experience, only a small percent of the warnings require changing anything about the prescriptions, so, statistically, the pharmacy staff finds little danger in having a relaxed attitude toward the endless number of warnings that pop up. But surely we are overriding a few very important warnings. In that huge sea of warnings generated by the pharmacy computer software, surely we are overlooking a few very important ones.

If the big chains are sued, they can claim that the pharmacist was negligent in overlooking the warnings that do indeed pop up on our computer screen. Thus the big chains can blame the pharmacist, rather than admit that staffing levels determined by the corporation don't allow the pharmacist enough "warm bodies" in the pharmacy to assure that all prescriptions are filled with maximum care.

I occasionally worked in one store with a tech who would call me over—in what seemed to be a random fashion—to look at various warning messages. She seemed to be proud of herself for being conscientious enough to call me over. Yet she seemed to have no idea which warnings were the most serious and which were unlikely to result in significant harm. I suspect that she, like many techs, overrode the vast majority of warnings, but, feeling guilty, wanted to assuage her guilt by randomly calling me over. She was more likely to call me over during times of the day when the pharmacy was less busy. She seemed to be much less likely to call me over when everyone in the pharmacy was stressed to the max as a result of our running far behind in the filling of prescriptions.

I am at least partly guilty in this situation. I should have stressed to her the importance of closely monitoring the grading system that the computer software uses to warn us about the severity level of each warning. But there just never seemed to be enough time. I felt that, since I was only filling in at that store occasionally, it was the duty of the regular pharmacists to teach her.

Because of all the things that can go wrong when techs run the pharmacy computer, some pharmacists insist on running the pharmacy computer themselves. However, in very busy pharmacies with several computer terminals, it is almost impossible to prohibit the technicians from running the pharmacy computer. High prescription volume often requires substantial use of the pharmacy computers by technicians.

Should a pharmacist's secret password or authorization be required to override computer warnings?

I used to work for a large national chain that required the pharmacist to review drug interactions by typing his secret password in the computer before proceeding. The computer screen would lock until a valid pharmacist's password was entered. This meant that the technician had to interrupt the pharmacist from whatever he was doing (like answering a customer's question or talking on the phone with a doctor's office). The technician would say something like "I need you to look at this drug interaction." The pharmacist had to walk over to the computer, examine the potential drug interaction, and then enter his secret password if the pharmacist determined that the drug interaction was unlikely to result in significant harm.

When our chain was sold to another large chain, all pharmacists at our chain began using the computer program used by the chain that bought our chain. Our new employer's pharmacy computer system does not require the pharmacist's secret password to proceed. Many pharmacists told me that they are scared to death that a technician will proceed past critical drug interaction warnings without notifying the pharmacist. Pharmacists worry about the real potential that a customer can be harmed, resulting in a lawsuit.

Our new employer held a meeting for the fifty or so pharmacists in our district. The purpose of the meeting was to familiarize us with the new computer system. There was a loud groan among many pharmacists in attendance when we were informed that the computer system we would be adopting (with transition to the new employer) did not require the pharmacist's secret password to proceed. The trainer told us, "It's a training issue!! Train your technicians to call you over whenever a drug interaction pops up on the computer screen!!" Pharmacists in attendance mostly said, "Yeah, right!!"

With dangerously inadequate staffing in too many pharmacies, pharmacists don't welcome frequent interruptions from technicians (or customers, for that matter). In many such cases, technicians become reluctant to interrupt the pharmacist and simply proceed past drug interaction warnings with the new computer system that doesn't require the pharmacist's secret password to proceed. Since, in my experience, most drug interactions are indeed overridden by the pharmacists themselves, technicians see that the course of least resistance is to override the interaction without interrupting the pharmacist.

Overriding potential drug interactions doesn't often result in harm to the customer, since most of the drug interaction warnings that pop up on our computer screen seem to be more of a theoretical concern than a real world concern. But the fact remains that this attitude toward drug interactions by techs and pharmacists occasionally results in overriding potentially serious interactions. Can anyone seriously deny that?

The big chains seem to feel that slowing down the prescription filling process by having pharmacists and technicians obsess over each potential drug interaction is not worth the time. It is as if the big chains prefer to pay customers who suffer harm from drug interactions rather than slow down the prescription filling process across the entire chain. The big chains seem to base their operations on how often they get sued for something, rather than basing it on assuring that prescriptions are filled with extreme care. Filling prescriptions with extreme care does not seem to be profitable under managed care. It is more profitable to herd customers and then pay that small fraction of customers who are inevitably harmed.

Many pharmacists were very unhappy with the fact that our new employer's computer system does not require the pharmacist's secret password to proceed past potential drug interactions. But the common attitude among the pharmacists I know seems to be: *This is just one more example of the ease with which the big chains place our license (and the corporation itself) at risk in order to fill prescriptions quickly.* One of the biggest surprises for me in pharmacy has been the ease with which big chains seem to expose themselves to tremendous liability (for both their pharmacists and the corporation itself). Many pharmacists feel that the big chains will continue in this reckless manner until the cost of settlements from lawsuits exceeds the cost of adequate staffing in the pharmacy.

Let me be perfectly clear that I do not mean to denigrate technicians. Some technicians are absolutely fantastic. There are many technicians with whom I would rather work than pharmacists. I know many technicians who are more accurate and faster than pharmacists. My concern is simply whether technicians are capable of determining the significance of oftentimes highly complex warnings when pharmacists themselves are often uncertain of their practical significance.

There is as much variation in the quality of technicians as there is in the quality of pharmacists. The public thinks that surely one pharmacist is as good as the next. Not so. Same with techs. Great techs are an absolute delight to work with. I've seen pharmacy managers who schedule the best techs to work the pharmacy manager's shift and leave the worst techs to work with the other pharmacists.

Some chains seem to feel that once we've got a warm body in the pharmacy, that's the equivalent of having a seasoned tech. When we have an opening for a tech, many pharmacists hire the first person who walks in the door and asks for a job. Pharmacists should, in my opinion, go back through their employment applications on file to find the most promising candidate. Hiring a good tech is one of the most important of the pharmacist's duties. Many pharmacists put a tremendous amount of thought into whom they hire as a tech. Other pharmacists hire the first person who asks for a job.

Hiring a tech is more difficult than I first assumed. I used to think that I was a good judge of people, that I could size them up after a short conversation and predict how well they would do as a tech. In one store, the store manager transferred one of his clerks to the pharmacy when we needed a tech. At the time, I assumed the store manager was dumping his worst clerk on us, and I guess I shouldn't be surprised that a store manager would not want to part with one of his top employees. I worked with her for a few weeks and was very disappointed in her performance. I had heard her tell another tech, "The more you learn, the more they'll expect you to do." So I assumed she was pretty much hopeless. Apparently something caused her to change her attitude, because she gradually became a super tech. To my amazement, she turned out to be one of the best techs I ever worked with. She was quiet but turned out to be fast as lightening.

Even though predicting who will be a good tech is very difficult, I wish more pharmacists would put a much greater effort into screening whom they hire. When I fill in at other stores, I find techs who are absolutely terrific, and others who are horrendous, a threat to the public safety. It seems that young pharmacists are more likely to hire the first person who asks for a job as a tech. Perhaps more experienced pharmacists realize how important it is to hire promising applicants.

Techs can definitely make the difference between a day that's tolerable and a day that's an absolute nightmare. I worked in one busy pharmacy in which we had three or four techs on duty at one time (plus two pharmacists), and a total of seven or eight techs on the payroll. I am not exaggerating in saying that the output of the top two techs was equal to the combined output of the other five or six techs.

I enjoy working with fast, accurate, and friendly techs and hate working with techs who are slow and immature. I'd rather work with a fast tech who makes a few errors than a slow tech who is extremely accurate. In the real world, many pharmacists would consider the slow tech to be a greater danger to the public. That is because the chaos caused by being covered with prescriptions is much worse than the usually straight-forward task of catching and correcting tech errors. I'd rather work with a tech who is extremely fast but makes a few mistakes during her shift, than I would to work with a tech who makes no errors but is painfully slow. Slow techs cause confusion in the pharmacy because prescriptions back up, customers start complaining, and tempers flare. Some techs can absolutely make the computer keyboard sing. Other techs seem to stare at the computer screen endlessly when they are stumped—rather than ask a pharmacist or another tech for assistance. Perhaps the tech doesn't want anyone to know that she doesn't understand something in the computer.

Error-prone techs are a particular hazard when working with floater pharmacists or pharmacists who fill in for sick days or vacation days. Many floater or fill-in pharmacists assume the techs they work with are accurate. That is a dangerous assumption. It is wise to be extra-vigilant when working with techs we are not familiar with.

Technicians often fight among themselves over whose turn it is to answer the phone or wait on a customer at the drive thru window. Understandably, techs don't like interrupting their work on the pharmacy computer to ring up a customer or accept a prescription from a customer who has just approached the pharmacy. I occasionally worked in a pharmacy in which the drive thru window is an incredibly long distance from the dispensing area. One day a pharmacist commented that the architect who designed the layout for that pharmacy should be hung from one of the rafters in the ceiling. Techs routinely became upset with each other over whose turn it was to walk the long distance to wait on a customer at that drive-thru.

Working with a tech who's a mature and interesting person can sometimes make my day almost tolerable. Pharmacy can be an intellectually deadening job even though pharmacists can't allow our brain to become less than fully alert in viewing drug interactions, contraindications, drug allergies, and in making sure the right pills are in the right bottle. In my opinion, the activity of filling prescriptions is inherently unfulfilling (profoundly so) because it is like a hamburger assembly line. (I have lots of adjectives to describe my dislike for my job: piece work, production work, intellectually unsatisfying, vacuous, monotonous, repetitive, robotic, physically exhausting grunt work in a factory.) Working with a fast tech who's also an interesting person can sometimes turn a nightmarish day into one that's tolerable. If she's cute, that's an added bonus.

I try hard to be a likeable person. Despite my best efforts, some techs and I just don't hit it off, probably due to us having totally different personalities.

Should maximum tech-to-pharmacist ratios be mandated?

Some state boards of pharmacy have maximum "tech-to-pharmacist ratios." In states that have such a regulation, what this means, for example, is that no more than two (or sometimes three) techs can be on duty for each pharmacist on duty. I've never heard of a maximum ratio of four techs to one pharmacist. State boards of pharmacy pass regulations mandating such maximum ratios in an attempt to force employers to hire a second pharmacist, i.e., when the prescription volume exceeds the capabilities of a single pharmacist to adequately check every prescription filled by that pharmacist and the techs. It is obviously cheaper for the corporation to keep hiring techs as prescription volume increases, rather than pay the salaries of two pharmacists working simultaneously.

Unfortunately, I've only seen such "tech-to-pharmacist ratios" actually enforced after the-fact. In other words, when the board of pharmacy investigates a particular pharmacy or pharmacist for an infraction of some type (a pharmacy mistake reported by a customer, a pharmacist found to be distributing drugs to dealers, a pharmacist found to be abusing drugs or alcohol, etc.), the investigator may notice that the tech-to-pharmacist ratio in that pharmacy is being exceeded. That infraction will be added to the other infraction(s) in the board of pharmacy citation.

In my opinion, if the state boards of pharmacy imposed severe penalties for exceeding these maximum tech-to-pharmacist ratios, it might have some effect. However, in the cases I've read about, the penalties for exceeding the maximum ratio amount to a slap on the wrist. As I state in my chapter on boards of pharmacy, I feel this is because the state boards of pharmacy are afraid of the immense legal and political clout of the big chains. And the state boards don't want to appear to be anti business in the eyes of state legislatures that are strongly pro-business.

I would, in fact, love to work in a pharmacy that had an excess number of techs. Yes, after perhaps three techs per pharmacist, the techs can churn out more prescriptions than one pharmacist can safely check. But I don't recall ever having the luxury of working with too many techs. The usual problem is having too few techs on duty.

During my entire 25 year career, I've only worked in one store which had two pharmacists on duty simultaneously. That pharmacy averaged over 300 prescriptions per day, a nightmare for a single pharmacist. But even at this store, there were days when one pharmacist was forced to work as the only pharmacist on duty, usually due to the illness or vacation of another pharmacist and due to the fact that no other pharmacists in the district were available to work that day.

I think the state boards are naïve if they think that their loose, after-the-fact enforcement of tech-to-pharmacist ratios will force the big chains to have, say, two pharmacists on duty at the same time. The big chains only have two pharmacists on duty at the same time when the volume for one pharmacist becomes extremely burdensome. Most chains have strict internal guidelines on the level of prescription volume required before two pharmacists are allowed to work at the same time. These guidelines are usually far above what pharmacists feel is realistic or safe.

Should techs be allowed to give advice to customers?

Some technicians have a habit of advising customers or answering customers' questions in a manner that exceeds the tech's level of knowledge. Sometimes this occurs because the tech is overzealous or over-confident, but sometimes the problem is that the tech knows that the pharmacist she's working with doesn't like to be bothered or interrupted with questions. Some pharmacists are simply arrogant and technicians understandably avoid speaking with these pharmacists. Working with pharmacists who don't like to be disturbed, the tech is placed in the uncomfortable position of feeling compelled to try to give advice to customers or answer customers' questions when the tech knows that the pharmacist is the person who should be answering those questions from customers.

Here is an example from the Institute of Safe Medication Practices (www.ismp.org) in which a technician gave a wrong syringe and wrong instructions to a customer. There is, of course, no way of knowing whether the pharmacist didn't have the time or desire to advise the customer. Some pharmacists love to talk with customers. Other pharmacists try hard to avoid speaking with customers because of shyness or because they're so far behind with a huge backlog of prescriptions.

Whenever you get a prescription filled or refilled, be sure that the pharmacist talks with you about your medications. This means more than just telling you the name of the medication. If the medication needs to be measured, ask the pharmacist to show you how to measure it. A mother gave her 7-week-old baby 5 mL of Tagamet (cimetidine) instead of 0.5 mL for acid reflux because a pharmacy technician gave her the wrong syringe. The technician told the mother that the "5" on the syringe meant 0.5 mL. After four doses, the baby was very drowsy, vomited and had loose stools. The mother took the baby to the emergency room for observation, but, fortunately, the baby did not have to be treated. When prescriptions are dispensed, no one but a pharmacist should be giving you advice about the medication. If a pharmacist does not offer to counsel you, insist on it.

A similar incident occurred involving the dispensing of the acid reducer Axid to an infant. In this case the medicine dropper was incorrectly marked by a technician. This incident, which occurred in 2008, resulted in a disciplinary action by the North Carolina Board of Pharmacy against pharmacist A. P.
(http://www.ncbop.org/Disciplinary%20Actions%20%20-PHAR-MACISTS/PickensAsa05790.pdf#search="error")

On August 25, 2008, [Pharmacist A. P.] dispensed a prescription for Axid to an infant patient with a medicine dropper that was incorrectly marked, so that the patient received approximately four and one-half times the prescribed dose of the medication. A technician had hand-marked the medicine dropper, and requested that [Pharmacist A. P.] confirm the marking. Without visually inspecting the medicine dropper, [Pharmacist A. P.] approved the marking. [Pharmacist A. P.] accordingly failed to physically review the dispensed product and the medicine dropper before they were delivered to the patient. Furthermore, when [Pharmacist A. P.] dispensed the drug, he failed to counsel the patient, instead improperly allowing the technician to counsel the patient.

The drug was administered to the patient, and the patient twice ingested the drug at the incorrect dose. As a result, the patient suffered from diarrhea for over a week while the large dose passed through her system.

What happens when you don't "Shake Well"?

Here's an example of a problem that can occur because of poorly trained or inadequately supervised technicians. I fear that this problem is more common than most pharmacists realize. First, some background on the critical difference between liquid medications that are solutions and those that are suspensions.

Most of the drugs in the pharmacy are tablets and capsules but a large number are liquids. Liquids are used primarily for children since children often have a hard time swallowing tablets or capsules. An exception to this generalization is that products for cough are usually in the liquid form for both children and adults.

Many of the products in the pharmacy need to be shaken by pharmacy staff before being dispensed to the customer. Then the customer (or parent) must shake the product again at home before it is swallowed. Drug products available in the liquid form are usually in one of two categories: solutions and suspensions. A solution is a product that does not normally need to be shaken. A non-pharmacy example of a solution is any of the soft drinks you buy in a supermarket such as Coke, Pepsi, Mountain Dew, Dr. Pepper, etc. These products obviously aren't supposed to be shaken before you drink 'em.

On the other hand, think of a suspension as a product like a salad dressing. When a salad dressing has been sitting on a shelf for a period of time, we see that a significant portion of the contents has settled to the bottom of the bottle. For example, we shake Italian dressing before pouring it over our salad. Very few people who know anything about salad dressings would ever consider pouring it over their salad without first shaking the bottle. A very similar situation exists in the pharmacy, i.e., there are several products that are analogous to salad dressings. These products must be shaken well before being dispensed. The trouble is that many pharmacy technicians are not fully aware of the importance of shaking these products when pouring them from our stock containers when filling a prescription. I have seen many instances in which techs shake the bottles in the most cursory and superficial fashion. Would you be contented with shaking your salad dressing, perhaps, once up and once down?

I've seen techs do that with pharmacy products that need to be shaken before being transferred to the customer's bottle.

Among the products that sit on the pharmacy shelves as suspensions (and thus need to be shaken before being dispensed to the customer) are Septra (trimethoprim/sulfamethoxazole) suspension and Tegretol (carbamazepine) suspension. These prescription products must be shaken before they are dispensed to the public because a heavy concentration of active ingredient settles to the bottom of these bottles while sitting on our shelves. These products must also be shaken well at home before *each* dose is taken.

Many technicians do not fully comprehend the importance of shaking these suspensions in our (typically) 16-ounce stock bottles before pouring out a smaller quantity to fill a waiting prescription. If the bottle is not shaken well, most of the active ingredient may be sitting at the bottom of the bottle so the first prescriptions filled from our stock bottle would tend to be subpotent, whereas the last prescriptions would tend to be superpotent. Notice that the little sticker we apply to your Rx bottle says "SHAKE WELL." It does not say "SHAKE LIGHTLY."

Many children's' antibiotics arrive at the pharmacy in the form of a dry powder, to which pharmacists or technicians add a specified quantity of water before dispensing the product. It is important that parents shake these products thoroughly before each dose is given to a child. Otherwise, most of the active ingredient is sitting at the bottom of the container.

Here is a real world example of the consequences of the pharmacy staff not adequately shaking a child's anti-seizure medication before dispensing it. (Kate Kelly, Pharm. D., "Shake Well Before Dispensing," *Pharmacy Times*, October 2005 http://www.pharmacytimes.com/article.cfm?ID=2652)

Obviously, it is important to ensure that the active ingredient(s) in a suspension is (are) properly dispersed throughout the vehicle before administration. "Shake well before use" is a common reminder (in the form of directions typed on the pharmacy label, an auxiliary label, or verbal instructions) given by pharmacists to patients who receive oral suspensions. Yet, how often is this important reminder forgotten by pharmacy staff

members when preparing a smaller quantity of a suspension from a large stock bottle? What happens if the stock bottle is not shaken or is inadequately shaken?

One mother knows all too well. In a report to the Institute for Safe Medication Practices, she explained that her son had been diagnosed with epilepsy, and his seizures were well controlled with carbamazepine (Tegretol) oral suspension. His prescription called for 8 oz of carbamazepine to be dispensed with each refill. Because the medication is available in a 16-oz stock bottle, smaller bottles were prepared for each refill.

Several days after starting a new bottle, the son had a recurrence of seizures that lasted about a week. During this time, his mother noticed that the suspension had a different appearance from the previous prescription. She mentioned this difference to the prescribing physician, who recommended getting a new refill. She was subsequently more aware of the appearance of the suspension whenever she had the medication refilled. Whenever the suspension looked different from what was expected, she would ask the pharmacist for a replacement, dispensed from an unopened manufacturer's bottle and shaken in her presence.

After a few of these occurrences, however, she insisted that the pediatrician write prescriptions instructing pharmacists to dispense the medication only in the 16-oz unopened manufacturer's stock bottle. She saved several of the more suspicious-looking suspensions dispensed in 8-oz bottles and sent them to the manufacturer. Assays performed by the manufacturer's Quality Control Division revealed that three of the bottles contained suspensions that were significantly less concentrated than the expected 100-mg/5-mL concentration, and one bottle of suspension was three times more concentrated than was expected!

The problem appears to have stemmed from pharmacy staff members not shaking or inadequately shaking the stock bottle of carbamazepine suspension before preparing the smaller bottle. If an unopened stock bottle of a suspension was inadequately shaken before preparing a smaller bottle, the suspension that was poured out could potentially be less concentrated than expected. The remainder of the stock suspension would then be more highly concentrated. Both situations could potentially lead to significant variability in doses, which could affect disease control (i.e., recurrence of seizures resulting from the less-concentrated carbamazepine suspension dispensed). This variability is particularly significant for drugs with a narrow therapeutic index. Even if the suspension is adequately shaken prior to dispensing, if patients do not shake the medication properly, similar variability in doses can occur.

In order to prevent such problems, pharmacy staff members should be sure to adequately shake all suspensions. Education may be required for pharmacy technicians and students, who may not be aware of the difference between a solution and a suspension. Visually check that the suspension is uniformly dispersed before it is transferred from its original container. Pharmacists involved in the final check of a suspension should verify with the individual who prepared it that this important step was performed before allowing the suspension to be dispensed.

Consider making auxiliary labels as reminders for pharmacy staff members that read "Shake well before dispensing," and add them to appropriate pharmacy stock bottles. In addition, attention could be drawn to suspensions by highlighting or circling the word "suspension" on product labels. Make sure that patients receiving suspension preparations are counseled so that they fully understand the need to shake the medication well before each use. The "Shake Well" auxiliary label, which commonly accompanies the pharmacy label on suspension preparations being dispensed, could easily be overlooked. It should not be used as the only means of communicating this important information, but rather it should serve as a reminder for patients.

Technician errors span the spectrum from those that are trivial to those that are potentially catastrophic. Here are some tech errors that I recall catching over a period of a few months:

Two drugs with similar generic names
(hydralazine confused with hydroxyzine)

This example illustrates the dilemma with techs. In one store in which I worked, one evening a customer came in with a swollen face. She approached me and asked, "Has my doctor called in a prescription for this?" She then pointed to her swollen face and said that that happens to her occasionally because she reacts to some (as yet undetermined) substance. I was startled by the swelling but she assured me that she had had it more than once before and that medication helps to clear it up. I went to the bin where we keep prescriptions that are ready to be picked up. I noticed that the computer label on the bag indicated that the contents was hydralazine, a blood pressure medication. I said to the customer, "What we have ready for you is a blood pressure medication." She was startled and said that that made no sense. I asked, "Have you not been on this drug before?" She said, "I don't even have hypertension."

I had that sinking feeling in my stomach as I sensed that all-too-common scenario: another prescription error. I went over to our pile of new prescriptions that had been filled that day and retrieved her doctor's phoned-in prescription. To my dismay, the prescription called for hydroxyzine (a drug that treats allergies or allergic reactions), rather than the blood pressure drug hydalazine. Without explaining to the customer that we had made an error, I changed the prescription to the proper medication. I did my best to act as if nothing had happened, even though she left with a very quizzical expression on her face, wondering what had indeed happened.

I was working the evening shift that day. It turns out that the pharmacist who had filled that prescription in the morning had not caught the tech's error. How do I know a tech had made the error? Let me explain: There were two techs working during the day, but only one remained with me to work the slower evening shift. After the customer left, I asked the remaining tech if she had any idea how this could have happened. As it turns out, the tech who was there with me has a lot less experience than the other tech. The evening tech told me, "I asked Mary if this was the right drug. She said it was." Mary is the more-experienced tech, by far.

So it turns out that the less experienced tech asked the more-experienced tech to verify the drug the doctor wanted. The less experienced tech picked the wrong drug. The more experienced tech did not catch the error when asked for verification by the less-experienced tech. And the pharmacist, who has ultimate responsibility for detecting errors, also did not catch the error. Two techs and a pharmacist missed this error. I remember the other pharmacist commenting to me, as she left for the day, "It's been a very busy day to-day."

Here is an example of an actual lawsuit in which Walgreen's was sued after mix-up involving these same two drugs (hydroxyzine and hydralazine) contributed to a patient's death. Any involvement by pharmacy technicians is not described. (Kansas City Injury Lawyer Blog: "Pharmacy Sued Over Fatal Drug Error," March 19, 2012, by The Horn Law Firm, Doug Horn, Lead Attorney http://www.kansascityinjurylawyerblog.com/2012/03/pharmacy-sued-over-fatal-drug.html)

The family of an elderly Kentucky woman has filed suit against Walgreens pharmacy after an alleged mix-up of her prescription medication led to her death. Mary Moore, a Louisville resident, had just left the hospital after receiving treatment for high blood pressure, kidney failure, and congestive heart failure on November 10, 2010. Her doctor had written her a prescription for the high blood pressure medication hydralazine. The pharmacy allegedly gave her the antihistamine hydroxyzine by mistake.

Because of the medication error, Moore's high blood pressure went entirely untreated for about two weeks. The pharmacy reportedly noticed the error and provided Moore with the correct medication, but by then "it was too late," according to the lawsuit. Moore could not tolerate the dosage of the blood pressure medication. Her blood pressure reportedly continued to increase, putting additional strain on her heart. This caused "decompensation" of both her congestive heart failure and her kidney disease. She was hospitalized again, and died on December 6, 2010.

Hydralazine, according to the National Institutes of Health, is a muscle relaxant used to treat high blood pressure. It allows blood to flow more easily by relaxing the muscles in the blood vessels. Hydroxyzine is an antihistamine used to treat allergic reactions such as itching, and to control symptoms of motion sickness. It can also treat anxiety and alcohol withdrawal symptoms. The NIH specifically cautions people over the age of 65 to not use hydroxyzine, as other medications that treat the same conditions are considered safer for older patients.

Moore's family filed a lawsuit in Jefferson Circuit Court in Louisville on February 15, 2012 against Walgreens and the pharmacist in charge at that particular location. The lawsuit claims negligence and wrongful death, as

well as strict liability, negligent failure to warn, and breach of warranty. The pharmacy's error in dispensing the wrong medication, according to the lawsuit, was a "substantial factor" in Moore's injuries, in enhancing her existing injuries, and in causing her death. The suit also alleges that, by not counseling Moore about the drug at the time she filled the prescription, the pharmacy violated state law. Had the pharmacist spoken to Moore at that time, the pharmacist likely would have noticed that the medication was incorrect, the lawsuit says.

PCE 500 and Entex PSE

A tech filled two prescriptions as follows. One was for the antibiotic PCE 500 mg (erythromycin), taken twice a day. The other was for Entex PSE, a drug used for colds, also taken twice a day. The tech filled both prescriptions correctly in every detail except one. She put the PCE 500 in the Entex PSE bottle. And she put the Entex PSE in the PCE 500 bottle. So the medications that the patient would have received were correct but they were in the wrong bottles. In this case, it would likely have resulted in no harm since both tablets are taken twice a day. Under other circumstances in which the label directions were different, the results could have been disastrous. Even in this case, if the patient had decided to take the decongestant only as needed and the antibiotic for the full course, he would likely have ended up taking the antibiotic for a few days and the decongestant for the full course, i.e., exactly opposite of what's usually recommended.

Ibuprofen 600 and Ibuprofen 800

There are lots of garden variety errors that occur in pharmacies. For example, a technician recently put Ibuprofen 600 mg (a drug that treats pain, inflammation, and fever) in a bottle that was supposed to be Ibuprofen 800 mg. This error was discovered before the customer received the wrong strength. This is a minor error but it is still an error.

Coumadin 4 mg confused with Cardura 4 mg

One technician put Coumadin 4 mg in a refill bottle that was supposed to be Cardura 4 mg. I told her that Coumadin is probably the most dangerous drug in the pharmacy and that I just prevented her from killing someone. I made a joke out of it because I didn't want her to lose confidence in her abilities or dislike working with me. Yet she needed to know that she made a potentially very serious mistake. Coumadin is a blood thinner. It is very similar to the substance that is used in d-Con rat killer. Rats eat the d-Con and then hemorrhage internally. Cardura is used for blood pressure. I was not kidding when I told her that Coumadin is the most dangerous drug in the pharmacy. In lawsuits against pharmacists and pharmacies, Coumadin is one of the drugs most frequently involved. This was, indeed, a potentially very dangerous mistake.

Expiration dates and refrigeration

Technicians frequently put wrong expiration dates on children's antibiotics. Most children's antibiotics arrive in the pharmacy as a dry powder. The pharmacist or technician adds water to the powder immediately before dispensing. Once the water is added, the antibiotic is good only for ten or fourteen days, depending on the particular antibiotic. The majority of these antibiotics (amoxicillin and Keflex, for example) are good for fourteen days. So, techs get in the habit of putting a fourteen day expiration date on the label of all these antibiotics, even the ones that are good only for ten days. Most of these antibiotics are supposed to be kept in the refrigerator during these ten or fourteen days. However, there are a few that are supposed to be kept at room temperature. As is the case with expiration dates, the techs often seem to be so accustomed to attaching labels instructing the patient to refrigerate these liquids that they do so even for the ones that are not supposed to be refrigerated.

After I discovered a mistake that one tech made and pointed it out to her, she said to me that she needed to slow down. I said, "No. You need to continue at the same speed. If you slow down, we'll get completely covered with prescriptions. It's my job to catch your mistakes."

Some more examples of tech errors:
• A tech filled a prescription for Levlen birth control pills with TriLevlen.
• A tech filled a prescription for Septra DS (a drug used frequently to treat urinary tract infection in women) with ten tablets rather than twenty specified by the doctor.
• A tech typed a label for Motrin suspension (a drug used for pain and fever in kids), "Take three-fourths teaspoonful" rather than what the doctor specified, "Take one and three-fourths teaspoonsful."
• A tech typed the directions for Naprelan (an analgesic and anti-inflammatory drug) as "Take 1 daily" rather than what the doctor specified, "Take 2 daily."
• A tech put a "Keep in refrigerator" sticker on two bottles containing tablets. These tablets are not supposed to be refrigerated. This clerk does everything with lightning speed and never looks back to see if she has made an error.
• A tech filled a prescription with Rondec DM Drops rather than plain Rondec Drops specified by the doctor. These are medications for colds in infants. One contains dextromethorphan (DM), a cough suppressant. The other does not.
• A tech filled a prescription with Cefzil rather than what the doctor specified, Ceftin. These are both antibiotics. I caught myself making the same mistake on a separate occasion.
• A tech gave a customer the correct pills in his two refill containers but switched the contents of both containers. In one container labeled glyburide (a drug used to treat type II diabetes), she placed methotrexate (a powerful drug used to treat cancer, rheumatoid arthritis, and psoriasis). In the container labeled methotrexate, she placed the glyburide.

This last example is a potentially very dangerous mistake. Of course, there's a good chance that if this customer had been on these drugs for awhile, he would have caught such an error and no harm would have occurred. Customers catch a lot of our errors. So an error that we make doesn't necessarily mean that harm will occur, even with potentially dangerous drugs. An ever-vigilant patient is a requirement in today's "speed is all that matters" environment.

These are, as I said, just a few of the errors that I recall catching in the last few months. If I were to list all the errors that I've caught techs making in the twenty-five years since I graduated from pharmacy school, the list would fill a book. Catching errors of varying levels of seriousness is a routine part of the pharmacist's job. The errors I've seen and caught are no different (in terms of seriousness) than those seen by every pharmacist in America.

Chapter 9

Do store managers have any clue about pharmacists?

I think that many of the big chains need to go back to the drawing board and figure out a better management structure for their stores. In almost every store I've worked in, there is a constant battle between the pharmacists and the non-pharmacist store manager. In the best-run stores, the pharmacists and the non-pharmacist store manager get along well and enjoy working with each other. But, in my experience, that is the exception.

The fundamental nature of the conflict between managers and pharmacists hasn't changed since I graduated in 1975. This conflict is truly Topic A in many of the stores in which I've worked. Many pharmacists talk about this situation constantly and passionately. Too often, the relationship between the pharmacists and the non-pharmacist store manager is like a bad marriage where both partners desperately need a divorce. We see each other so much that we get under each other's skin.

Pharmacists resent the fact that someone with so little appreciation for the problems in the pharmacy has so much power in the store. Pharmacists feel that our years of schooling entitle us to more respect than we receive from the non-pharmacy management. Pharmacists resent that someone who often has little or no college education is (or acts like he is) our boss. Many pharmacists feel that district managers too often hire low caliber management trainees.

Whether the non-pharmacist store manager does indeed have authority over the pharmacy is a question that's often avoided by chain management. Pharmacy supervisors tell pharmacists that the non-pharmacist store manager isn't really our boss. But the non-pharmacy supervisors seem to tell the non-pharmacist store manager the opposite.

In many stores, the pharmacy accounts for over half of the total sales. Pharmacists at these stores feel they should be given more respect for this fact. In contrast, the non-pharmacist store manager prefers to look at the situation in terms of square footage. The non-pharmacist store manager takes pride in the fact that he commands much more square footage than the pharmacists.

Pharmacists understandably don't want any more responsibility than we already have. Pharmacists don't have time to be in charge of the entire store. The solution that most pharmacists would like is for the non-pharmacy supervisors to tell the manager to keep out of the pharmacy's business. Many companies have a separate chain of command for the pharmacy but this doesn't prevent the non-pharmacy supervisors from getting involved in pharmacy affairs. In my ideal world, the non-pharmacy people would have absolutely no authority over the pharmacy and this fact would be made clear to all store employees.

The non-pharmacist store manager thinks we should be able to sling out prescriptions as quickly as McDonald's slings out burgers. I don't know any non-pharmacist store managers who seem to genuinely comprehend that each prescription we fill is a potential lawsuit—an event that can have devastating consequences for our customers and ourselves. Pharmacists view the non-pharmacist store manager's single-minded emphasis on speed as cavalier and ignorant of the realities of a litigious society.

As long as the non-pharmacist store manager views prescription drugs as a commodity similar to hamburgers, he will never truly understand pharmacists' concerns. Perhaps it is unrealistic to think that the non-pharmacist store manager would understand what worries pharmacists since our customers don't seem to understand either. The only thing that customers seem to care about is how long they will have to wait for their prescriptions to be filled. Customers seem to have absolutely no idea how easy it is to make an error in the pharmacy. Many customers are even surprised (or shocked) to learn that drugstores do indeed make errors.

Even many pharmacy technicians don't seem to truly understand how high the stakes are in the pharmacy. Some techs ask the pharmacist to take a quick look at a prescription because a customer is in a hurry. These techs don't seem to understand that if it's OK to look at one prescription quickly, then it's OK to look at every prescription quickly.

An outside observer would probably think that all store employees routinely take up for each other in our daily battles with rude and arrogant customers. But, too often, the tension between pharmacists and non-pharmacist store managers leads to back-stabbing incidents. I got into a dispute with a rude customer one day. The non-pharmacist store manager, who knew nothing about the situation, stepped in, taking the customer's side. The customer mailed in a complaint card to corporate headquarters, at the manager's suggestion. When a customer complains to the non-pharmacist store manager about something in the pharmacy, the manager often seems to enjoy giving customers complaint cards that are mailed to corporate headquarters.

The non-pharmacist store manager has a leisurely lunch and dinner each day in his office and can't understand why pharmacists don't have time for the same. Nor does he understand why we don't have time to go to the bathroom or sit down for a break. Too often, he seems to be jealous of our wages. He acts as though he's the boss of our pharmacy technicians.

The non-pharmacist store manager takes every opportunity to criticize pharmacists (behind our back) and he tells his supervisors that he would have a good store if he had better pharmacists. The pharmacy is always the source of all the problems in the store in the eyes of the non-pharmacist store manager.

When a floater pharmacist fills in for us, the non-pharmacist store manager has only one assessment of the floater the next day: "He (or she) was too slow!!" The non-pharmacist store manager does not seem to understand that pharmacists are slower in unfamiliar pharmacies. The non-pharmacist store manager's favorite subject is the speed of pharmacists. He tells our supervisor we're slow. "Slow" becomes our middle name.

The company encourages the non-pharmacist store manager to help out in the pharmacy and allow other non-pharmacy employees to do likewise during extremely busy times. In the best stores, non-pharmacy staff help out in the pharmacy frequently. I agree with the non-pharmacist store manager that this puts an extra burden on him because he doesn't get enough staffing to complete his own work on the sales floor so allowing the non-pharmacy staff to help out in the pharmacy puts him even further behind. Understandably he resents it when the pharmacist wants to pull a clerk off the sales floor to help out in the pharmacy.

The professional model stressed in pharmacy school (a professional pharmacist with highly trained colleagues and co-workers) is at wide variance from daily reality in the drugstore. Personality conflicts simmer for months—until, by chance, the pharmacist or non-pharmacist store manager transfers to a different store. Too often, even with new pharmacists or non-pharmacist store managers, the patterns of tension and resentment soon re-emerge. I don't deny that the pharmacist is sometimes to blame. Some pharmacists are indeed very immature.

The hyperstressful working conditions bring out the worst in all of us. Best friends become bitter enemies. Employees blame each other for being too slow, for spending too much time talking to customers, for taking too much time filling each prescription. In the extreme stress of understaffed drugstores, employees blame each other rather than pull together as a team.

The following e-mail was forwarded to me in 2006. It is written by a former K-Mart pharmacist who describes a very unpleasant interaction with the non-pharmacist store manager at K-Mart.

Here is how I handled my problem with the chains. It was unprofessional but it did make me feel better.

I used to work for K-Mart and life there was miserable. High volume, high pressure. I grew to hate it. I had a store manager who was a jerk. No other word for it. He was tough to work for. It was a chain pharmacy and I was chained to the counter.

Every day at noon, he (store manager) would pull my clerk to cover a register up front while one of the cashiers up there was on lunch hour break. My tech/clerk would come back at 1 PM only to go on her lunch. I had no lunch break. He would leave me all alone in the pharmacy putting extra pressure on me. One day I complained about the lack of help, the disservice to customers and the problems involved. He said "Get used to it."

My other pharmacist was on vacation so I was doing 12 hour days. One day, since it was a high volume store and it was busy, I told every customer during the morning that the computer was down and things would be all okay at 2 PM and that their Rx would be ready at 2 PM. I took in plenty of Rx's. I had them lined up and down the counter. I told customers who called in that their Rx's would be ready at 2 PM. During my two hour "lunch break" I did nothing. Absolutely nothing. I stopped, I ate, I had a cup of coffee, I read a magazine. I ignored the phone—all three lines. There were about 50 people waiting in the store.

At 1:55 PM I closed the pharmacy, locked the door, went to the main office and put the key in the wrong safe knowing it would be found only hours later. There were plenty of customers waiting for the 2 PM pick up. I told them the pharmacy was closed, their Rx's were not ready and to complain to the store manager about the lack of service. I waited while the customers lined up at the service desk and yelled at the store manager, and yell they did. Loud and clear. The customers were upset and vented complaints at the manager. I felt sorry for the customers but not the manager. He was under pressure and the customers threatened to call K-Mart (Troy, Michigan) headquarters. This would bring hell down on the manager.

I then told the store manager, "I quit." He got very upset and was visibly angry. Explosive would be more appropriate. He said, "What about all the unhappy, yelling customers waiting for their Rx's?" I said "That is your problem. Get used to it." I left and never went back to work for any chain ever again.

Life is good! I work where I am appreciated, from owner above and customers below. **—[Pharmacist B. K.]**

Here are two e-mails I received from pharmacists as a result of my editorial in *Drug Topics* titled "Pharmacists versus non-R.Ph. store managers." (Sept. 15, 2003, pp. 18, 21)

Subj: Drug Topics Viewpoint article
Date: 9/23/03
From: [Pharmacist G. P.]
To: dmiller1952@aol.com

Dennis,

I truly enjoyed your article on pharmacists vs. store managers. I am one of the few lucky ones. I work for a supermarket chain, and my store manager does not interfere with pharmacy, but rather supports and assists me to the best of his ability. Yet I hear the horror stories from my colleagues. Your points are very true. Community pharmacy has quite a ways to go. We are trained professionals in health care, yet many times we are simply viewed as another department, pill pushers, and treated with little respect. I recently had a customer call corporate because I asked him to wait 15 minutes and he insisted that I was "touching the pills". Just to retaliate.

I graduated from pharmacy school in 1999 at age 46 (my second career) and enjoy my job immensely. Yet my biggest gripe is how patients view us versus their physicians. On a day-to-day basis, I receive incorrect prescriptions from doctors, e.g. Levaquin 500 qid [four times a day] rather than qd [daily]; a refill with a higher strength than the one patient was originally on; Augmentin for children with a PCN [penicillin] allergy; Zocor 20 mg tid [three times a day]. The list goes on and on. Yet the patients are quick to "forgive," if you will, their physicians for the mistakes. Yet, they become furious when we make a mistake in filling; no mercy; it is as if they hold us to a higher standard, or yet, they forgive their physicians because they are "so busy." Well, so are we. They will wait 2 hours for the physician but expect us to fill their script in 10 minutes!!!

I work in community pharmacy by choice. I enjoy the interaction and 90% of my customers are appreciative and understanding. Yet that 10% have no respect for our profession and they would never speak to their physician the way they speak to us.

Getting back to your topic, one of my pet peeves is when a customer wants to register a complaint with the "store manager." I quickly approach them and explain that I am the pharmacy manager, but no, they want to speak to the store manager (who obviously has no concept as to what we do).

I feel that we as pharmacists must work diligently to promote our profession as one that is to be respected; in fact, we should be treated in the same category as physicians. Sometimes when I am counseling a patient, I will be interrupted by a patient who asks me to hurry up their script. It is downright insulting. Being of Hispanic descent, I marvel at the way Hispanics respect their pharmacists—a different respect, just like those from European culture.

Good luck to you.

[Pharmacist G. P.]

Subj: Pharmacist vs. non-R.Ph. store manager (Feedback)
Date: 10/9/03
From: [Pharmacist Z. M.]
To: dmiller1952@aol.com

Hello Mr. Miller,

I enjoyed reading your article in *Drug Topics* in the September 15th 2003 issue and it was like you were reading my mind. I don't know of any other health professional who is treated in the same manner that pharmacists are treated. It's like they think that we are machines and not human beings. We are not allowed to get sick, have family emergencies, take vacations, or leave the pharmacy on time. The same managers who want you to hurry up and fill prescriptions are the same individuals who want to leave at posted store hours although we have a backlog of customers waiting on their prescriptions and they would not approve the necessary help to service these customers. And, of course, they were supposed to help out in the pharmacy but they hate coming to the pharmacy to help out so they hide or wait thirty minutes to show up.

I feel the major problem that we have in our profession is that we don't have strong lobbying associations. Everyone looks at us as well-paid servants and part of the problem is that we don't speak up enough. Our profession needs more unity. The boards of pharmacy in each state only look out for the best interests of the consumers and they are a watch dog for them. But, as for us, we have no such organization. I really don't know how we are able to do our jobs as well as we do with store managers and the state boards breathing down our backs. We need to form a reliable organization that is going to look out for us. I don't know how much more our profession can handle with the managed care companies forcing their clients to utilize mail order and the poor reimbursement which insurance companies give us. It makes you wonder what I was thinking when I chose this as a profession. And pharmacy school does not even give you a clue of what to expect in the real world. All they tell you is that you are a professional and you must conduct yourself accordingly. But they never tell you that you will be the only person who understands that you are a professional. This is why we don't understand how someone who may not even have finished high school—let alone completed one year of college—can be our supervisor.

We need a change. I don't know how or when it's going to happen but if something doesn't happen soon, the baby boomers won't have anyone to fill their meds. I can't tell you how many pharmacists I know of trying to pursue a new career because they are so burned out and broken-hearted by the current plight of our profession.

Sincerely yours,
[Pharmacist Z. M.]

Chapter 10

District supervisors: *gung ho* for the corporation

District pharmacy supervisors are usually pharmacists who are in charge of somewhere around 10 to 20 pharmacies and 20 to 40 pharmacists, assuming an average of two pharmacists per pharmacy. District supervisors don't usually fill prescriptions themselves except in cases of a severe shortage of pharmacists. They usually travel between stores in carrying out their management duties, which include hiring pharmacists. Pharmacists might see their district supervisor once every two or three weeks. The district supervisor might stay in the store for an average of an hour or two with each visit. I've had more than a dozen district supervisors in my career.

Some of my district supervisors stress that no food is allowed in the refrigerator. Apparently, food in the refrigerator is unprofessional, causes a cluttered appearance, and poses a problem of cross-contamination with the drugs. (A moldy sandwich might contaminate the drugs in the refrigerator.) The prohibition against food in the refrigerator has always struck me as heartless. Would the supervisor be so cavalier if his own lunch or dinner were prohibited from being kept in the refrigerator? Food is one of the last pleasurable things at work for a pharmacist who's absolutely exhausted. If there were another refrigerator in the store (like in the break room), I wouldn't have a problem with the prohibition against food in the pharmacy refrigerator. As regards the possibility of moldy sandwiches contaminating drugs, the supervisors should simply stress that we need to be extra careful to make sure that the refrigerator is routinely checked for old food. Eating is a requirement for *Homo sapiens.* Somehow, many supervisors seem to view food as a luxury, not a necessity.

Some chains require pharmacists to wear a tie. I have always found a tie (and tight collar) to be uncomfortable, but many district supervisors get agitated when pharmacists don't wear ties. Is this gender discrimination against men? I am not aware of any dress code for female pharmacists.

One day my district supervisor told me, "You think too much about what you're doing." I was shocked by his comment because I felt I did a pretty good job of hiding my personal feelings about my job. Perhaps my body language revealed more about me than I assumed. Certainly my boss had no understanding of my profound disillusionment with my chosen profession. Nevertheless, I extrapolated his comment to its logical conclusion: I need to work my shift each day on automatic pilot rather than ruminate endlessly about the logic of basing a health care system on pills rather than on prevention.

One of my district supervisors was always disappointed to see that we were sitting on a stool when he visited our store--even for a short break. He actually made a big speech one day (on voice mail) about stools. He said that they should be kept off to the side somewhere and used at a minimum. We are forbidden to use stools when entering data into the computer because this creates the impression that we are lazy. Incredibly, the district supervisor hinted that stools would be banned from the pharmacy if he found them to be used excessively.

In pharmacy school, there is no dress code, class attendance is optional, and the professors let students be individuals. Chain pharmacy is nearly the opposite. Pharmacists must wear the company smock and name tag. When I graduated, tennis shoes were prohibited. This rule seems to have been relaxed, possibly because management finally (amazingly!) realized that pharmacists are more productive when they wear comfortable shoes.

District supervisors are adamant that we do everything to avoid confrontations with customers. What this means is that we cannot say even one word to incredibly rude and arrogant customers. We are required to swallow any personal attacks against us without any anger. For example, one of my district supervisors put out a voice mail: "Swallow your pride. Swallow your gum. But don't have a confrontation with the customer!" In my experience, when a pharmacist gets into an argument with a customer, and his or her supervisor finds out about it, chances are the supervisor will support the customer's side. That's because supervisors want to end the argument at the store level rather than have the angry customer contact people higher up the corporate ladder. Pharmacists shouldn't be surprised if their supervisor appears to inexplicably support the customer's side, even when that customer richly deserves to be forcibly removed from the store.

One day I overheard my district supervisor's phone conversation with another pharmacist. Apparently the pharmacist on the other end of the phone had gotten into a big argument with a customer. My district supervisor told the pharmacist on the phone, "Don't argue with him. Take his money." The implication was: *You can't get the customer's respect so get his money!* Presumably, making a sale and making someone poorer by the cost of his prescription should be satisfaction enough.

I once had a supervisor who directed all pharmacists, techs, and clerks in his district to answer the phone "Thank you for calling Revco. This is (employee's name). How can I help you?" During one period when this supervisor was tightly enforcing this policy, he listened closely to see how employees answered the phone when he called. The net result was that store employees became afraid to answer the phone, afraid that it was him calling. So all customers who phoned the store experienced long wait times before any employee in the store found the courage to answer the phone.

A prominent characteristic of chain pharmacy is the rigid hierarchy that closely resembles military hierarchy. I once had a district supervisor mention to me that one of the pharmacists in his district was guilty of "insubordination" for going over the supervisor's head and speaking directly with the division manager. The chain hierarchy usually consists of (starting from the bottom): staff pharmacist, chief pharmacist, district supervisor, division manager, regional vice-president, president.

Many pharmacists fear visits by their district supervisor, feeling that he comes to criticize us, not to help us. One of my former partners decided to make a career change by getting a Ph. D. in public health. I ran into her one day and asked her why she decided to leave pharmacy. She said, "The district supervisors would only tell you when you did something wrong. They would never tell you when you did something well."

We fear our bosses because they have the power to fire us if we don't fill prescriptions fast enough. The blood pressure of pharmacists often goes up when our supervisor visits our store. Our bosses' main concern is whether prescription volume (number of prescriptions filled per week) is up compared to the same period the previous year.

District supervisors routinely speak disparagingly of pharmacists in their districts who are slow. In twenty-five years as a pharmacist, I can recall only one instance in which a pharmacist was terminated because of an excessive number of dispensing errors. I am not saying that completely reckless pharmacists are retained forever. In my experience, inadequate speed and rudeness toward customers are much more likely to give pharmacists a bad name with district supervisors than dispensing errors.

The most serious confrontation I have ever seen between another pharmacist and a district supervisor involved the pharmacist's supposed inadequate speed in filling prescriptions. I happened to be in the pharmacy as my shift had just ended. I was tying up some loose ends. Even though I ended my shift fully caught up, a lot of customers came in at the same time with new prescriptions and my partner was covered up with prescriptions when our district supervisor walked in. The district supervisor almost immediately began criticizing my partner for being so far behind. My partner was very agitated by our supervisor's single-minded focus on speed, given the fact that corporate policy set staffing levels ridiculously low.

Our district supervisors often speak about other pharmacists in the district. It is highly unusual for a supervisor to say something like "Bill is very knowledgeable about drugs." It is much more likely for a supervisor to say something like "Bob can really crank 'em out!" (i.e., fill prescriptions quickly). Supervisors praise fast pharmacists to let it be known that speed is a very important criterion in our job evaluation.

District supervisors say that more errors are made when things are slow than when we're very busy. We complain to our district supervisor that the overwhelming workload increases the opportunity for misfills. Our district supervisor recites his favorite self-serving mantra: "More errors occur when things are slow because you're not focused." I'd like to ask him, "Does that mean we should regularly exceed the speed limit on the highway because speeding causes us to be more focused on our driving?"

It may just be the district supervisors I know, but when they're forced to work in a pharmacy themselves because of a severe shortage of pharmacists, they seem to make an inordinate number of errors in filling prescriptions. District supervisors place a high value on speed and it shows when they fill prescriptions. They are correct in believing that they are nearly immune to criticism from the company for dispensing errors (after all, they *are* the company). But they are certainly not immune to a lawsuit filed by a customer.

In my experience, it is not the best pharmacy students who become district supervisors. In my experience, the district supervisor personality is more extroverted, outgoing, and more likely to have been a party animal in school than a serious student. In pharmacy school, the serious students did not respect the party animals, but in the real world, the party animals are now our bosses. In my experience, the party animal personality is less concerned with accuracy than the serious student personality. In pharmacy school, the party animals seemed to be in college mainly to have a good time.

How well do our district supervisors really know the pharmacists under their control? I've seen many pharmacists put on a good act when our district supervisor is present. As soon as the district supervisor leaves, that pharmacist resumes his or her rudeness toward customers and techs. Sometimes the supervisors gradually learn what the pharmacist is really like. But I've seen many instances in which supervisors never figure out what the pharmacist's true personality is and how that pharmacist is, in reality, very bad for business.

I once worked with a pharmacist who was extremely professional and quite knowledgeable about drugs. She was very thorough and precise with paperwork. She took great care in learning the proper procedures for submitting claims to various insurance companies. Pharmacists would often call her for advice in solving some paperwork question or some quirk in insurance procedures. Yet this pharmacist had a very negative attitude toward customers. When the large chain we were working for bought a small local chain, my district supervisor asked her to transfer for a few weeks to one very high volume store that was just purchased. My district supervisor viewed her as one of his best pharmacists and he felt she would be of great assistance in transitioning that high volume store since this pharmacist was an expert in the policy and procedures for our chain. One day I visited her at that pharmacy. I asked her how things were going. I was not surprised when she said that the prescription volume was overwhelming. She commented to me that things would improve "when we get the volume down to a manageable level." In other words, she was saying that that store *has too many customers!* This statement would have been viewed as absolute blasphemy in the eyes of our district supervisor. My supervisor had no idea that that pharmacist's solution for the overwhelming workload in that pharmacy was to *shed customers.* Chain supervisors have one overarching obsession, i.e., that Rx volume grows, not shrinks.

I once had a district supervisor (in charge of, say, fifteen stores) tell me about an incident in which a local pharmacist had gone over the head of this district supervisor and complained about something to the division manager (in charge of, say, a hundred stores). My district supervisor was very unhappy with this pharmacist and referred to it as "insubordination." In pharmacy school, I never thought I'd hear the term "insubordination" coming from one of my bosses in the world of community pharmacy. If I were a pharmacist in the military, I could understand it. As a chain pharmacist, it was surprising.

The hierarchy in chain drugstores is, indeed, as rigid as that in the military. It looks something like this: staff pharmacist, pharmacist-in-charge (PIC), district supervisor, division manager, regional vice president, director of operations, and president. With thousands of stores, the big chains have a clearly defined chain of command. My district supervisor didn't look kindly on the pharmacist who did not seem to understand the power hierarchy.

Store level employees often referred to these people above the store level as "the suits." That's because they visited us in the stores wearing a suit or sports jacket, in contrast to store employees who wore smocks or pharmacy jackets. The suits enjoyed displaying their power over store-level employees by constant use of the telephone when visiting stores under their command. This was meant to show store level employees that "the suits" were important people.

A pharmacist once told me a story about division manager (in charge of perhaps one hundred stores) or regional vice president (in charge of perhaps five hundred stores) who visited one of the local stores and awarded a pharmacist, on the spot, somewhere around three thousand dollars for suggesting something that almost anyone could have suggested. Have you ever been in a grocery store and noticed those little advertisements that are about the size of a license plate attached to your shopping cart with a little plastic frame that is similar in shape to a license plate frame? This incident occurred a couple of decades ago and apparently this "suit" had not been in too many grocery stores. It is true that the use of such advertisements on shopping carts was not yet commonplace, but it was not rare. So this suit, in what I would describe as a display of power, awarded this pharmacist around three thousand dollars for suggesting that our drugstore chain begin using similar advertising attached to all of our shopping carts. I don't recall discussing this incident with anyone besides the pharmacist with whom I worked at that time. Both he and I agreed that the cash award seemed excessive, bordering on reckless. But that's the way power often shows itself.

The number of stores under the command of the various bosses was not set in stone. I think I recall my district supervisor having as few as a dozen stores, and as many as two dozen when he had to take temporary control over the adjacent district when that supervisor was transferred or quit. During this period when my district supervisor had two dozen stores, he mentioned to me that all he had time to do was "go around and put out fires." In other words he didn't have time to work with individual managers in any significant way. All he had time to do was things like intervene in a store in which the pharmacist-in-charge and the non-pharmacist store manager were close to killing each other (not a rare situation by the way).

Chapter 11

Things customers do that really irritate pharmacists

My pet peeves with pharmacy customers

1. Most customers don't seem to realize that pharmacists can and do make mistakes. Some customers are so confident in their pharmacist's abilities that they don't even question when the color or shape of their pills suddenly looks completely different. These customers have been led to believe that a change in the appearance of the pills always means they received a generic. A change in the appearance of your pills most often means that the pharmacist gave you a generic. But sometimes a change in appearance means the pharmacist has made a mistake. There are some customers who have very little trust in pharmacists. These customers immediately go home and count their pills to verify that we gave them the correct quantity. Not a bad idea.

2. Most customers evaluate pharmacists based solely on how fast we fill prescriptions. Customers do not realize that some pharmacists are much more thorough in calling doctors about illegible handwriting, questionable doses, and drug interactions. Customers do not realize that some pharmacists make many more errors than others. Customers do not realize that "speed" is not the most important criterion in judging a pharmacist.

3. Many customers think that clearing their throat or clanking their keys on the counter or staring at us will cause us to fill their prescriptions faster. They ask "Why does it take more than a few minutes to put a few pills in a bottle?" or "Why does it take so long to fill my birth control pills? The pills are already in the pack." or "Why does it take so long to fill a prescription for a skin cream? The cream is already in the tube." Customers do not realize that, even though there may be only one or two other people nearby, we have a backlog of maybe fifty prescriptions, including those for customers shopping elsewhere in the store. Customers seem to think that the pharmacist should be able to fill prescriptions as quickly as McDonald's fills burger orders. They have no idea that rushing their pharmacist increases the likelihood of an error.

4. Many customers expect vitamins to cure any and every problem. Customers ask us to recommend a vitamin for "nerves" or "lack of energy." Customers seem to interpret their anxiety, depression or angst as a sign that their nerves are "acting up." Customers don't seem to realize that vitamins are not the best way to address "lack of energy." Customers don't seem to be interested in advice that they should consider getting more sleep at night, eating more nutritious foods, or finding a job that isn't so exhausting, etc.

5. Many customers, when trying to decide which non-prescription drug is right for them, pick up a half-dozen products from our shelves (like Dimetapp, Coricidin, Contac, Sudafed, etc.). But these customers are absolutely unable to replace the products in the proper spot on the shelf. These customers seem to think that products for colds, coughs, sore throat, heartburn, constipation, diarrhea, gas, fever, etc. are randomly arranged on drugstore shelves. These customers do not realize how much time is consumed by store clerks in returning products to their precise location.

6. Many customers phone in the wrong prescription number and arrive at the pharmacy wondering why their prescription is not ready. I once had a customer who phoned in a prescription for his wife. When he arrived at the pharmacy and picked up the Rx, he told me that I had given him the wrong pills. It turns out that he had mistakenly picked up the wrong bottle. He thus gave me the wrong Rx number on the phone. He did not recognize the pills I filled as one

of the other medications his wife was taking. He made a big scene out of it, speaking loudly enough for several other customers to hear. He kept saying, "That's all right. Pharmacists make mistakes. Pharmacists are human." He seemed to take pleasure in accusing me of making an error, as in *Pharmacists think they're so important. I'll take him down a few notches.* I was never able to convince him that he had simply phoned in the Rx number for another of his wife's medications. I filled the Rx for the drug he meant to call in. Several other customers were looking at me the entire time, wondering whether they could trust me to fill their prescriptions. Yes, I've made mistakes in my career but this was not one of them.

7. Many customers get really mad at the pharmacist when we tell them that their insurance plan does not cover the drug their doctor has prescribed. The customers often seem to think that the pharmacist is intentionally trying to make life difficult. I once witnessed another pharmacist engaged in a heated exchange with a customer over the customer's obvious disbelief that the drug was not covered. Finally, the pharmacist used an explanation which I have since adopted myself: *This is between you and your insurance company!* This explanation is, in effect, saying, "Look buddy. I don't want to get in a big fight with you. You need to contact your insurance company." I have yet to see a customer who had answer for that.

8. Many customers have been thoroughly conditioned by Madison Avenue to want a pill for every ill. They seem to think that, for each medical condition, surely there must be a safe and effective drug. I wish customers would, instead, seek an understanding of their body and ask themselves what steps they might take to prevent diseases before they occur.

9. A few customers describe their symptoms (e.g., jock itch) to the pharmacist and then ask the pharmacist for a recommendation for a non-prescription product. Shortly thereafter, the customer leaves the store without purchasing that product (e.g., Lotrimin), or any other product, but the customer returns later and steals that product.

10. Many customers treat us like we're a clerk at McDonald's. I suspect that pharmacy drive-thru windows imply to customers that prescription drugs are similar to hamburgers. So pharmacists

shouldn't be surprised when pharmacy customers behave the same as McDonald's customers.

11. Many customers seem to interpret their doctor's illegible handwriting as a sign of intellectual brilliance. Their reaction is "Wow! My doctor is so brilliant that even the pharmacist can't read his handwriting!" Customers should be offended that their doctor doesn't make the effort to write clearly so that there is no chance the pharmacist will misread the Rx.

12. Many customers get mad when we tell them there are no re-fills remaining on their prescriptions. The customers yell, "No!! My doctor said I could have unlimited refills!!" The customers do not understand that state law requires the pharmacist to check with the doctor after a certain period of time, depending on the type of medi-cation.

13. Many customers seem to think they're the first to mention that "child-proof" caps are actually "adult proof." They jokingly say, "I have to get the kids to take the lids off for me!" These customers laugh approvingly at their powers of perception, not knowing that we've heard that observation a thousand times.

14. Many customers ask me to recommend a laxative. I often ask myself: *I became a pharmacist so I could spend my time recom-mending laxatives?* Customers don't seem to be eager to learn that laxatives are usually unnecessary, that fiber can decrease constipation, and that overuse of laxatives can cause the bowels to depend on these drugs.

15. Many customers don't seem to realize that if they would just lose some weight, they might not need so many pills for hyperten-sion or type 2 diabetes. Customers want to be able to eat all they desire and then swallow a diet pill that allows them to look great in a swimsuit.

16. Many customers blame the pharmacist when the customer's insurance co-pay increases. Customers should realize that the co-pay is not determined by the pharmacist. The co-pay is transmitted to the pharmacist immediately upon the pharmacist billing the prescrip-tions on-line.

17. Many customers wait until the pharmacist has completed fill-ing that customer's prescriptions before telling the pharmacist that

they have insurance coverage. This necessitates the laborious task of running each prescription back through our computer.

18. Many customers seem to think that generic drugs have something to do with genes since they call them "genetic" drugs. Many customers are unconvinced of the equivalence of generic drugs. They say, "No! I want the real thing!"

19. Many customers inexplicably think they need to speak with the pharmacist even when phoning in Rx numbers for prescriptions that need to be refilled. Pharmacists prefer that customers give these numbers to a tech or clerk.

20. Many customers phone in several prescription numbers and then arrive at the drive-thru window ten minutes later and can't understand why the prescriptions aren't ready. They should have asked us on the phone (or we should have told them) how long it would take. Drive-thru windows certainly create the expectation of instantaneous service at pharmacies. Many pharmacists feel that the drive-thru window is the worst thing that ever happened in our profession and that it is symptomatic of everything that is wrong with our health care system today, i.e., speed is the top priority. Quantity is valued more highly than quality.

21. Pharmacy customers rarely know when they have been well served. Customers rarely understand the significance of a pharmacist who catches a potentially serious drug interaction or a dose that's too high or a contraindication. Customers only care about how quickly their prescriptions are filled.

22. Many customers hand us several prescriptions, wait until after we've filled those prescriptions, and then inform us that they just want half the quantity the doctor specified on each prescription. Consequently we have to re-do each prescription.

23. Many customers are very interested in learning about their medications but are not interested in waiting in line while other customers ahead of them get that same type of information.

24. Many customers think that it is entirely reasonable to go their doctor for an antibiotic for the common cold. They do not understand that antibiotics are ineffective against viruses.

25. Many customers don't seem to be embarrassed easily. They routinely approach the pharmacy and ask what we recommend for gas—with several other customers hearing the conversation.

26. Many customers at the drive-thru window honk their horns, expecting prescriptions to be filled as quickly as McDonald's fills burger orders.

27. Many customers equate power with effectiveness. They frequently ask us "What's the strongest thing you have to knock out this cough?"

28. Many customers leave their doctor's office with a prescription but without a clear understanding of what the drug is used for.

29. Many customers discard our drug information leaflets without reading a single word.

Here is a rather common scenario. A customer phones the drugstore from home or comes into the drugstore and says that he needs to get his prescription(s) refilled right away because he's on his way to catch a plane and he forgot to have them refilled beforehand. Most pharmacists hate situations like this. We're running an hour or so behind and this customer expects us to put his prescriptions ahead of everyone else's. Other customers who have been waiting patiently in the store are equally turned off by these customers. I once saw a coffee mug in a pharmacy imprinted with a message pharmacists love: *Poor planning on your part does not necessarily constitute an emergency on my part.* In other words, just because you didn't remember to have your prescriptions refilled in a timely manner prior to your trip doesn't necessarily mean I'm going to drop everything to refill your prescriptions ahead of everyone else. Of course, our corporate bosses require that we keep messages like this out of sight of our customers. The corporate bosses don't like to see any negativity in the drugstore. Our bosses prefer the model of the pharmacist as affable automaton who absorbs an endless number of indignities without complaint.

Here's another common scenario: All four phone lines are for the sole pharmacist on duty. Customers are honking their horns at the drive thru-window. They're clanking their keys on the counter, clearing their throats, and asking how much longer it will be. ("Why does it take more than a couple of minutes to put a few pills in a bot-tle?")   They're bombarding me with questions like the following (many of which should clearly be directed at the non-pharmacy per-sonnel but the pharmacist and techs are more visible):

• What aisle is the motor oil on?
• Do you have any Coke or Pepsi products on sale this week?
• What are the possible side effects with the medication?
• What kind of dressing should I put on this cut?
• Where are your hearing aid batteries?
• Can you recommend a laxative for my three-year-old?
• What do you recommend for gas?
• What's good for lice?
• Where are your pregnancy tests? Which one is the most accurate?
• What do you recommend for poison ivy?
• What do you recommend for sunburn?
• What's the difference between all the products for yeast infection [Monistat, Femstat, Vagistat, GyneLotrimin, etc.]?
• Why hasn't my insurance company reimbursed me for the drugs I got two months ago?
• What do you think of DHEA (melatonin, zinc, chromium, etc.)?
• My doctor says I need to start taking calcium. Which brand do you recommend?
• Do you have any more diapers in the stockroom? You're out of the ones I usually buy.
• Why is my prescription so expensive?
• Why doesn't Medicaid cover my prescription?
• Can I use your phone to call a cab?
• Can you recommend a good multivitamin?
• I don't seem to have any energy. Can you recommend a vitamin for energy?
• What do you think of amino acid supplements for weight lifters?
• What's good for sleep?
• I'm in a hurry. Can you fill this prescription right away?
• Your Coke machine outside stole my money and didn't give me a drink. Who do I need to see?

• How come the generic is less than half the price of the real thing? Is it just as good?
• Can you leave those child-resistant safety caps off my prescriptions? I have to get the kids to take them off for me. [Customer laughs as if he is the first person to make this observation.]
• Is there anything cheaper over-the-counter that would be just as good as what my doctor prescribed?
• Can I just get half the prescription? I'll come back and get the rest on Friday when I get paid.
• Do you have a restroom I can use?
• My doctor was supposed to phone in my prescription. Is it ready?
• What's the best vitamin for a six-year-old who just won't eat?
• My doctor says I need to start taking iron. Which one do you recommend?

When customers describe their symptoms to me and ask me to recommend a non-prescription product, I have found that these customers don't usually like it when I give them an assortment of alternatives. Customers seem to think that each symptom has a precise solution, just like each math problem has a precise solution. Customers want a definitive answer like *two plus two equals four.* Customers interpret a variety of solutions as tantamount to my not really knowing what product is best for their symptoms. Customers like pharmacists who immediately and confidently recommend one specific product. Customers view this pharmacist as more intelligent than the pharmacist who provides a number of alternatives. Customers do not realize that many pharmacists are just "throwing a solution" at the customer so he or she will go away.

For example, a customer may ask, "What do you recommend for colds?" The pharmacist then answers quickly: "I recommend Sudafed. It's on aisle two." Many of these short-answer pharmacists view all customer questions as annoyances. Of course, some pharmacists hurriedly throw a drug name at customers because we are overwhelmed with a huge pile of prescriptions and we truly don't have time to give your question the time it deserves. For example, before recommending a product for colds, the pharmacist should ask whether you have any conditions that may make specific products unadvisable, such as high blood pressure or enlarged prostate.

Say a customer describes symptoms that sound like heartburn. There are a wide variety of ways this can be treated with non-prescription drugs. At the most basic level, the pharmacist could recommend the safest products, i.e., antacids like Tums, Rolaids, Maalox, or Mylanta. At the next level, the pharmacist might recommend stronger non-prescription products which may have more side effects, i.e., H2 antagonists like Tagamet HB, Pepcid AC, or Zantac 75. The next level above the H2 antagonists is the non-prescription proton pump inhibitors like Prilosec OTC, Prevacid 24HR, Zegerid OTC, and the house brand omeprazole. Proton pump inhibitors are the strongest of these three categories and carry the highest potential for side effects, including a distressing rebound hypersecretion of acid upon discontinuation of these drugs.

Alternatively, the pharmacist might describe ways in which heartburn can be prevented: by not overeating; by not lying down too soon after eating; by maintaining proper body weight; by raising the head of the bed six inches; by avoiding coffee, alcohol, fats, chocolate, and smoking; etc. A thorough pharmacist should also mention that the symptoms of heartburn can be mistaken for other conditions (e.g., angina).

In my experience, most pharmacy customers don't like such detailed answers. They want the pharmacist to confidently name one product only. I have had many instances in which I tried to give customers several alternatives only to have them reply forcefully and in a somewhat irritated tone: *SO WHAT DO I NEED!!??*

Normally, the best advice from pharmacists would be to give all the preventive measures a serious try. Only if all these preventive measures fail should the customer try a drug. But very few pharmacy customers want to give serious consideration to non-drug preventive measures. The fact that these customers are in the drugstore means they're leaning heavily toward a quick-fix solution. In my experience these customers will be disappointed in a pharmacist who does not have a similar outlook, i.e., a pill for every symptom.

Pharmacy customers make unusual requests

Here are a few brief anecdotes illustrating that pharmacy customers sometimes make unusual requests.

One day a customer approached the pharmacy with some produce he had just purchased at the supermarket next door. He said he suspected that the scales at the supermarket were inaccurate so he asked me to weigh the produce for him. He said he heard that pharmacy scales are very precise. I told him that our pharmacy scale could weigh—at most—a few ounces. There was no way I could weigh his produce which required a scale capable of measuring pounds.

On another day, a customer stood a few feet in front of the pharmacy counter and proceeded to take off the top of his electric shaver. He then blew really hard to clean the shaver. Tiny hair particles spread around the adjacent area. He then handed me the top of the shaver and asked me whether we carried the appropriate replacement blades/heads. How could he not realize how unsanitary it was to clean his electric shaver in the store by blowing?

One day a customer asked me if we had a laxative for one of his farm animals (a horse, I think). I didn't have the courage to ask him how he determined that this farm animal was constipated. I told him that I didn't know whether the laxatives we sold were safe for animals. I also told him that I didn't know what dose he would need to give to the animal.

One day a lady asked me whether the print on the tablets her doctor prescribed posed any harm. Did the ink used to print the drug name and identification number on the tablets pose any harm to her system when she swallowed the tablets? I assured her that the ink was harmless even though I had no direct knowledge to make that statement.

One day a man mentioned to me that he knew that Benadryl could cause drowsiness. He asked me what dose of Benadryl would be needed to put his mother's cat to sleep permanently. He told me that the cat was old and sick. I told him the truth: I had no idea what dose would be needed to kill the cat. I didn't tell him that I wondered whether what he planned to do was legal.

Did this customer purposely contaminate a medication so that he could sue us?

Here is an unusual story about an unusual pharmacy customer. I had just graduated from pharmacy school and I began work for a major chain in a small town in West Virginia. My boss told me that one of the pharmacy customers was in the process of suing the chain because a mold had grown in his pint bottle of potassium chloride liquid. Everyone seemed to know everyone else in this town. This customer had contacted a small law firm with only two attorneys. It turns out that both attorneys routinely came into our drugstore and routinely spoke with one of the pharmacy techs. My district supervisor brought me up to date on the lawsuit. He told me that the customer was going to bring me the bottle of potassium chloride liquid that contained the mold. I was to pack it carefully in a box and mail it to the manufacturer with a letter requesting that they inform us what foreign substance was in the bottle. A few weeks later, I received a letter from the manufacturer stating that, yes, there was mold in the bottle.

This was all very bizarre because no professor in pharmacy school had ever told us to watch out for the possibility that liquid medications from major manufacturers were prone to contamination with mold. Like I said, I had been out of pharmacy school for only a few months so I wasn't confident how I should handle the situation. Why had I never heard of mold growing in liquid medications? One day one of the two techs mentioned to me something like, "You know, Dennis, Mr. Smith is kinda strange. He's a retired chemist." So I began thinking: *What's really going on here?*

It turns out that the bottle that Mr. Smith had given me to send to the manufacturer was not the bottle in which we had originally dispensed the medication. I finally concluded that Mr. Smith had purposely succeeded in growing mold in that nearly empty bottle of liquid potassium chloride in an attempt to sue the drugstore chain. My district supervisor appeared to be accepting the customer's story at face value, not suspecting anything out of the ordinary. My district supervisor appeared to believe that the manufacturer had failed to adequately prevent mold growth in this product. So I told my district supervisor, "This whole thing is very strange. Mr. Smith apparently transferred the potassium chloride to a different bottle and, as a retired chemist, succeeded in growing mold in that bottle." I called one of the lawyers representing Mr. Smith and said something quite similar to what I had told my district supervisor. I said something like "Surely we're not responsible when a customer transfers a medication to a different container. He's a retired chemist and he appears to have undertaken a project of growing mold in this bottle in an effort to sue us." The lawyer listened carefully and, for some reason, the lawsuit against my employer did not proceed any further. I'm guessing that the lawyer had similar questions about the mental stability of Mr. Smith, but I don't know that for sure. Anyway, that lawyer and his partner continued to shop in that drugstore as did Mr. Smith. They all acted like nothing had happened.

I didn't hear anything more about Mr. Smith until a few months later when he returned the unused portion of a package of non-prescription sleeping pills and asked for a refund. I recall he said something like "It didn't work." Or "It didn't put me to sleep." He was conceivably telling the truth that the sleeping pill didn't put him to sleep. But most customers do not return products to the drugstore and ask for a refund, claiming that the product doesn't work (even though that is a potentially realistic scenario). What if every customer asked for refunds on non-prescription medications that didn't work for them (like products for colds, coughs, acne, warts, backache, etc.)? I can't recall whether we gave him a refund for the non-prescription sleeping pills. I assume we did if for no other reason than to keep him happy.

Chapter 12

Drug abusers, crooked employees, burglars, shoplifters

Screening of pharmacists and technicians for drug abuse, drug dealing, shoplifting, etc.

During the first half of my career, pharmacists and technicians were required to take a polygraph (lie detector test). I took a polygraph twice in my career: before being hired by Rite Aid and before being hired by Revco. On both occasions the polygraph examiner asked many variations of "Have you ever stolen anything at work?" One examiner prefaced this by explaining that he was not concerned with, for example, employees discovering (at home) store ink pens in their shirt pockets or smocks.

The polygraph was, needless to say, a very demeaning experience. In the second half of my career, the polygraph was dropped for pharmacists but prospective technicians and clerks were required to take a written test to determine their honesty. I recall that we went through a period of a year or so when the majority of the clerks and techs who took the written test were deemed a risk and therefore not recommended for hire by the company that developed the test.

I vaguely recall that one question on the written test was something like this: "Since everyone steals little things like candy bars every now and then, do you admit that you've stolen inexpensive things like that from stores you've worked in?" This question was obviously loaded in suggesting that everyone steals. It turns out that, in fact, not everyone steals. If a prospective clerk or tech answered that question in the affirmative, he or she would not be recommended for hire by the developer of the test.

One day I did something that was against company policy. We needed a technician for the pharmacy and it so happens that one applicant for that position was previously a sales clerk at that store. I thought I knew her well enough to predict that she would make a good pharmacy tech. I coached her before taking the test by saying, "The written test considers stealing anything—regardless of its value— to be wrong and reason to recommend against hiring. It considers stealing one cent to be just as bad as stealing something worth a hundred dollars. Don't be trapped into admitting that everyone steals small things occasionally." It turns out that she passed the test but, unfortunately, she was a lazy technician. I never in my career mastered the ability to accurately predict—from a job interview—how an applicant would actually perform on the job. Some applicants who I felt would be great often turned out to be a disappointment. On the other hand, I've seen many applicants hired by other pharmacists and managers who turned out to be good employees, even though I would not have predicted that from my initial impression of those applicants.

During the first half of my career when pharmacists were required to take the polygraph, I knew many pharmacists who were adamantly opposed to it. Most said it treated pharmacists as common criminals. There's no doubt that it was a very demeaning experience that I dreaded but I will grudgingly agree that the chains need some way to weed out pharmacists and techs who abuse or steal drugs.

I don't know whether smoking marijuana leads to using "hard" drugs, but I do know that many of my pharmacy school classmates were frequent users of marijuana. I've often wondered whether some of them succumbed during their careers to the temptation of having so many drugs at their fingertips. Clearly drug abuse is a significant problem among pharmacists. State boards of pharmacy routinely discipline pharmacists after uncovering evidence that those pharmacists are drug abusers or drug dealers. The disciplinary actions are often publicized in board of pharmacy newsletters sent to pharmacists.

Robberies, shoplifting, employee theft

I filled in regularly at one store which had a pharmacist who I thought was a great guy, very friendly, easy-going. The store manager at that store gradually began to notice that the number of "over-rings" on the pharmacy cash register was greater on days that pharmacist worked. I can't remember the details but I know that pharmacist was fired for bogus overrings. He apparently pocketed cash equivalent to the amount of each phony overring.

My district supervisor once hired a pharmacist who, according to the grapevine, was fired from her previous employer after she was found to be stealing Viagra and mailing it to her relatives in her home country. Polygraphs were not being administered when my district supervisor hired her.

Here's the problem, in my opinion: The big chains burn out pharmacists and then claim there's a shortage of pharmacists in America. As a consequence of such a high turnover in pharmacists, the big chains sometimes hire pharmacists who would not have been considered years ago. In the first half of my career, it was not unusual to find a pharmacist who had been with the same chain for ten years. Toward the last half of my career, a pharmacist who had been with the same chain for five years was considered a veteran.

Shoplifting is a tremendous problem in all types of stores across America, including drugstores. I was at a meeting of Revco pharmacists one day when a high-ranking Revco official stated that internal pilferage (i.e., by store employees) is greater than shoplifting from customers. I find that hard to believe but I assume he knew what he was talking about.

Another term for pilferage is "shrink." Chain drugstores bring in inventory crews maybe twice a year. After inventorying every item in the store and examining store sales, the store manager is presented with a "shrink" report. I recall that store managers were said to be doing an acceptable job when "shrink" was kept below three percent, i.e., when pilferage is kept below three percent of gross store sales. When pilferage was determined to be excessive, management would be instructed to take various preventive measures such as hiding security cameras behind lighting panels in the ceiling over cash registers (to see if any store employees were pocketing cash after bogus transactions).

I worked in only one drugstore that had a security guard. This was at the Revco in Heritage Square in Durham, North Carolina. Revco contracted with a security firm in Durham to supply our store with a security guard. That security guard worked 40 hours per week even though the store was open 80 hours per week. So, even at this store, there was no security guard present half the time the store was open. As best as I can recall, Revco decided to discontinue the practice of having a security guard in that store after this security guard was caught (by the store manager) stealing cartons of cigarettes. This store was in a high-crime area so the need for the security guard was obvious. There was a dollar store located directly adjacent to this Revco. The security guard at the dollar store would frequently come into our store on his breaks because he liked talking to our female clerks who ran the cash registers. I remember one day this security guard—during a break from the dollar store next door—actually caught someone in our store shoplifting a huge supply of deodorant products (a popular target for shoplifting, I later learned). I recall this guard from the dollar store next door telling me something like *Man, you need a security guard back in this store!* (after ours had been fired for stealing cigarettes). I agreed but unfortunately I was never in a position to approve the hiring of a security guard. Perhaps the reason for discontinuing the security guard contract in that store had something to do with the fact that Revco was apparently given a rent subsidy by some local or federal governmental entity in return for locating this store in a high-crime area. I had an occasion to speak with one of the management people at the security company that supplied us with the guard. This management person told me, "If it was up to me, I wouldn't put 'em in retail." His overtly racist statement implied that black security guards should be used only in situations like football games, basketball games, and concerts, as opposed to retail stores where there's lots of stuff to steal.

This store was very close to the interstate highway that runs through town. The back of the store is easily visible from that highway. One day I asked my district supervisor why all the stores—except ours—visible from the highway had a sign on the back door, making it easier for delivery trucks to determine which door belonged to which store. My boss told me that that was a conscious decision. He didn't want people driving down the interstate thinking, "Wow! Look how easy it would be to rob that pharmacy and then have an easy get-away on the interstate highway!"

I filled in at Revco in Hillsborough, North Carolina, for a pharmacist who was robbed at gunpoint by a person demanding drugs. That pharmacist was taken hostage for a few hours but somehow managed to escape. The incident caused the pharmacist to abandon retail pharmacy completely. After a week or two recovering from this traumatic event, he began a new career as a hospital pharmacist at Duke University Medical Center, safely away from anyone who might be intent on robbing a drugstore.

When I worked at one of the Rite Aid stores in West Virginia, the pharmacist who had worked in that particular store before me was licensed to carry a gun. Apparently he had been threatened by someone. My boss at that time told me that he (the boss) wasn't too happy that this pharmacist had a gun under his pharmacy smock every day at work. Due to confidentiality, I never found out the precise reason for that pharmacist leaving Rite Aid. I think it involved more than the gun.

When I worked at Revco in Oxford, North Carolina, one evening I happened to notice a man standing somewhat off to the side of the pharmacy looking closely at the prescription department shelves behind me. It is not unusual for customers to look at me or at our prescription department shelves while waiting for their prescriptions to be filled. But most of these customers seem to have a glazed look in their eyes, almost as if they were half-asleep and bored yet impatient while waiting for their prescriptions to be filled. This man was looking very closely at our prescription department shelves and I had an eerie feeling that something was wrong. Indeed, something was very wrong: The pharmacy was robbed late that night, long after all store employees had left. A big heavy rock was thrown through the exit door, shattering the glass. The store alarm indeed automatically notified the Oxford police, who arrived shortly. But the burglar (and, I assume, accomplices) had managed to get away after stealing a few bottles of controlled substances and our entire rotating Timex display which contained perhaps fifty watches. Apparently that suspicious-looking person from the night before was scanning our shelves in an attempt to locate the drugs he was interested in. I assume he knew that once the store alarm was set off, he needed to be out of that store in, say, less than a minute. My partner had been phoned in the middle of the night by the Oxford police. I was scheduled to work that morning. Upon arriving at the store shortly before opening time, I saw a big sheet of plywood covering the exit door. As the police investigated the burglary, my partner had placed that plywood over the exit door until morning when he phoned a glass company to repair the door. My partner told me he had been there ever since the police called him. My partner was checking our inventory to try to determine which drugs had been stolen. I did not tell my partner—or anyone else—about the incident that had occurred the night before, i.e., that I had observed a suspicious person looking intently at our prescription department shelves. I would have been blamed by my partner, by Revco district supervisors, and, I assume, by the Oxford police, for not taking more direct action by notifying the police of my suspicions. This incident occurred over fifteen years ago and I no longer work for Revco (now CVS), so I don't care if anyone knows now. The police told my partner that they had indeed arrived at the drugstore so soon after the alarm sounded at the police station that they (the police) were thinking the burglar or burglars were still in the store. They were not. After this incident, my district supervisor alerted all his stores to bolt the Timex display to the counter.

For a period of several months, I worked at a Revco in Durham at Wellons Village Shopping Center. We had several cashiers at that store who worked part-time while attending high school. One day, one of these young cashiers told me that she saw a young man steal a pair of sunglasses. The cashier implied to me that I needed to confront that young man before he left the store. Even though I was very busy in the pharmacy, I felt that I needed to approach that customer to show this cashier that the company took shoplifting seriously. I approached the customer but he protested to me that he had purchased the sunglasses elsewhere. Of course, I had no definitive proof that he was lying so I didn't pursue the matter. When he got home, he evidently told his parents what happened. I got a phone call from his father who proceeded to read me the riot act for accusing his son of shoplifting. From that incident, I learned to be more careful and selective in deciding when to believe a cashier who claims to see a customer stealing something.

Shoplifting at that store was especially bad. For a period of a few weeks or months, the store manager initiated a practice of locking all entrance and exit doors whenever she spotted a shoplifter in the act. She then phoned the police. By locking all the doors, the shoplifter could not leave the store. The store manager did this a few times but apparently she was told to discontinue locking the doors. Preventing the escape of shoplifters by locking doors endangers other customers trying get away from what could be a potentially dangerous situation, i.e., the shoplifter could pull a gun while being detained by the store manager.

One summer at this store I worked with a pharmacy student who had graduated pharmacy school but had not yet taken his licensing exam. One day this pharmacy "intern" lit out of the store in a flash, in pursuit of a shoplifter. It turns out that this intern was an athletic and somewhat macho kind of guy. He told me that he caught the shoplifter a short distance away from the store but decided against calling the police.

At this store we had a few part-time cashiers from North Carolina Central University, a predominantly black school. One day I received a call from one of these cashiers, named Vernon. Vernon was one of the nicest people I have ever known. He said that he wouldn't be able to come to work because he was being held at the Durham police station. He said that apparently his car was similar in appearance to one that Durham police believed was involved in a robbery. Vernon was exceedingly upset because he said he had been stopped by the police, with guns drawn, and told to lie on the ground. Vernon implied that, as a black man in a Southern town, he was at a terrible disadvantage. Vernon asked me whether I could help him some way. I was absolutely covered with a huge backlog of prescriptions, but I wanted desperately to leave the store to try to vouch for the character of Vernon, who I genuinely felt was the last person in the world who would be involved in a robbery. As much as I wanted to go to the police station, I felt my district supervisor would not see things as I did. Therefore, I decided to ask this same pharmacy intern to go to the police station. It turns out that somehow the police determined that Vernon was innocent so he was released just as our pharmacy intern arrived at the police station. Vernon told me that the experience of having guns pointed at him while he was on the ground was something he felt he would never forget. Vernon asked me whether I had any suggestions for what he could do to show his displeasure with the way he was handled by the police. Even though I do not doubt that the police did indeed think Vernon was potentially involved, I understood how upset he was. This incident left me with perhaps a modest insight into what can happen to a black college student, away from home, in a Southern town. I told Vernon, "North Carolina Central has a law school. Maybe you could go there and ask them if there is anything you could do." As best as I can recall, Vernon did speak with someone at the law school and I think he was told that there wasn't much he could do since the police did apparently genuinely think Vernon was a suspect. But I think Vernon was somewhat relieved to be able to discuss the incident with someone at the law school.

One afternoon when I was working at the Revco in Oxford, North Carolina, one of the (middle-aged) cashiers told me that she personally witnessed a customer putting a bag of candy in her handbag. This cashier implied that I was a wimp if I didn't confront the customer. So, even though I was busy with a pile of prescriptions in the pharmacy, I reluctantly approached the customer and asked her to open her handbag. The customer refused. There was a young girl with this customer, presumably her daughter. I would guess the young girl was around six years old. The woman handed the handbag to the young girl and told her to run home. Of course, this was an unacceptable turn of events because if I were to call the police, I would have absolutely no evidence. So I tried to grab the handbag from the woman and the young girl but I decided, *What the hell, this isn't worth it!* The child looked like she was ready to start crying and I feared that she would run out of the store and be hit by a car while running home and I would be held liable. So I let the customer leave with the young girl but I told her never to come in the store again. I remember worrying whether there were specific laws detailing the circumstances under which management is permitted to hold a customer in the store. I was afraid I was potentially in legal jeopardy for not following some guideline. Of course, Revco wanted store employees to do what we could to cut down on customer shoplifting, but I don't recall Revco ever giving us instructions on the specific circumstances that allowed us to detain shoplifters until the police arrived. On the one hand, I was worried about a lawsuit if I overlooked some technicality. On the other hand, I was thinking, "This is the South. They don't coddle criminals in this town." I never saw that woman in the store again but I did run into her one day at the post office. Upon seeing her in the post office, I recall thinking what an absurd world this is. The previous encounter was hyperstressful in the drugstore whereas the current encounter consisted of brief eye contact while standing in line waiting to mail a package.

Here's a short anecdote about the clerk who notified me that she saw this customer steal the bag of candy. As I said, this clerk implied to me that I was a wimp if I did not confront the customer. On another occasion a few months later, the tables were turned on this clerk. One day a policeman pulled up to our store with a suspect he had just apprehended. When this suspect was apprehended, he (the suspect) had in his possession a product that had a Revco price sticker on it. (This was before bar code scanners made price stickers unnecessary.) The policeman told me that the suspect claimed he had just purchased the product at our store. The policeman suspected that the product had been shoplifted. The policeman asked me if it would be okay to ask the sole clerk on the cash register whether she recalled ringing up a sale for that man. I said that was fine so the policeman asked that clerk if she would agree to look at the man in the back of the patrol car to see whether she recalled seeing him and ringing up the product. This same clerk had, a few months earlier, implied that I was a wimp if I did not confront the customer she claimed to have seen stealing a bag of candy. This was now an opportunity for this clerk to make a stand against shoplifting. But the clerk told the policeman, "No. I don't want to get involved." So the policeman drove away, unable to verify whether the suspect had indeed stolen the product from our store. I'm sure this clerk had forgotten the event several months earlier when she implied I was a wimp if I did not confront another shoplifter. I do not blame this clerk for refusing to help the policeman make a case against the suspect. This clerk probably feared retribution from the suspect. I'm only pointing out this clerk's hypocrisy.

I worked for Rite Aid in Hurricane, West Virginia for part of 1976 and 1977. One day the non-pharmacist store manager got a call from the Hurricane police department. An informant apparently had tipped them off that a burglar was planning to enter our store overnight via the roof air shaft, apparently to steal drugs from the pharmacy. The police told the non-pharmacist store manager that a few undercover policemen wearing plain clothes would enter the store intermittently throughout the evening in a very non-conspicuous manner, in case our store was being watched by the burglar. Sure enough, throughout the evening, a total of three or four people wearing unremarkable clothes entered the store and proceeded to the stockroom. Apparently the police had determined that the burglar's entry via the roof air shaft meant that the burglar would most likely set foot in the store first in the stockroom. Since the only restrooms in the store were in the stockroom, store employees (including myself) who went to the restrooms that evening witnessed the police preparations as they built barricades in the stockroom in anticipation of the overnight break-in. Interestingly, the barricades consisted entirely of big boxes of merchandise from our stockroom shelves. And even more interestingly, the biggest boxes contained baby diapers. I wondered how the police expected boxes containing baby diapers to stop bullets fired by the burglar. Later I concluded the boxes were mainly for hiding, not to stop bullets. Store employees viewed the entire situation as quite exciting and entertaining. There was almost a party atmosphere among store employees since excitement such as this is rare for a drugstore. Company regulations do not allow non-employees (including police) in the store without a store employee present (usually a manager, assistant manager, or pharmacist). Since he had to be present with the police in the store, the non-pharmacist store manager went home to get a portable television. He planned to watch television overnight in his office to avoid boredom. (I assume the Hurricane police were told by this manager that he would have to stay in the store, and apparently the police agreed.) If the burglar had been walking around in the store in an effort to determine whether everything looked okay for break-in overnight, surely the burglar would have sensed the party atmosphere among store employees and surely he would have sensed that something unusual was going on. Having three or four policemen with rifles in our stockroom was very exciting for store employees. Unfortunately, the store manager did not have the presence of mind to tell all the store employees to act as if nothing unusual was happening. Indeed, the store manager himself seemed to be caught up in the excitement. I am somewhat surprised that the police did not realize that the behavior of store employees risked making the burglar suspicious, if he happened to be walking around in the store as if he were a regular customer. At some time past the 9 PM store closing, only the store manager and the plain-clothed policemen remained in the store. The next day, all the store employees—including myself—were eager to hear what happened overnight. When I arrived at work the next morning, I was informed that, after several hours spent in the stockroom, the police decided to leave the store, apparently concluding for some reason that no break-in was likely that night.

Customers who are drug abusers

Many customers tell the pharmacist that they deserve an early refill on their Vicodin or other similar pain pill containing the narcotic hydrocodone. These customers sometimes claim they were standing by their medicine cabinet and "accidentally dropped the pills in the toilet." Customers who are hooked on pain pills think up an endless number of clever stories in an attempt to convince the pharmacist to refill their narcotic pain pills earlier than would be expected from the doctor's directions. Say a doctor prescribes a twenty-day supply of narcotic pain pills and indicates that the prescription can be refilled once if needed. When the customer comes back to the pharmacy after, say, ten days, and requests a refill, our computer flags this as early and therefore suspicious. Pharmacists are not supposed to agree to early refills if we suspect that the customer is abusing the drug by taking it far more often than the doctor's directions indicate.

I suspect that nearly every pharmacy in America is plagued by customers making up ingenious stories to justify early refills on narcotic pain pills and anti-anxiety pills like Xanax and Ativan. Pharmacists talk among ourselves about this problem all the time. You would probably be surprised by the number of pharmacy customers in this country who are either hooked on prescription drugs or are headed in that direction. Many pharmacists privately refer to these customers as "druggies," a moniker that reflects the endless stories that our customers invent in an attempt to snow the pharmacist into allowing early refills.

Another headache for pharmacists is forged prescriptions. Maybe once or twice a year, I receive what is clearly a forgery. I suspect this occurs so often because doctors sometimes leave their prescription pads in an exam room and then the patient (a drug abuser or dealer) steals the prescription pad and begins forging prescriptions on that doctor's prescription pad. Pharmacists can usually recognize the handwriting of local doctors. Consequently, when we receive a prescription with unfamiliar handwriting or with something else that looks suspicious like…

• an unusually large quantity of narcotic pain pills
• an unusually large number of refills
• refills on Schedule II drugs which—by law—can't be refilled

…we usually phone the office of the doctor who wrote the prescription. The doctor either confirms our suspicion that we have a forged prescription in our hand, or, occasionally, the doctor says we are mistaken and it is indeed a legitimate prescription.

Some pharmacists alert the police when we receive a forged prescription. Other pharmacists don't want to get involved. Some pharmacists feel that it is not our job to be policemen, so these pharmacists just hand the prescription back to the customer and say "We don't stock this drug." I've seen a few macho male pharmacists hand the prescription back and make some comment like "You ought to be glad I'm not calling the police." The customer/abuser/dealer then high-tails it out of the drugstore.

I once received a call from someone who said he was a detective on the local police force. He sounded quite polished and said that the police department had a few incidents recently in which pharmacies had been robbed overnight and the narcotic Percocet was stolen. This so-called detective then asked me whether we stocked Percocet in containers of 100 tablets or in containers of 1000 tablets. This sounded like a highly unusual question so I told this so-called detective, "No, we don't dispense enough Percocet to stock it in the 1000-tablet container." I suspect the caller was actually a fairly sophisticated drug abuser or dealer who was planning to rob us some night if I had been naïve enough to tell him that we indeed stocked Percocet in the 1000-tablet container. I considered calling the police department after this incident but I was very busy and it all seemed so bizarre that I didn't notify anyone. My hope was that, by informing the caller we stocked Percocet only in the small container, he would be prompted to look for another drugstore to rob. Unquestionably, I should have followed up with the police. But I was covered up with prescriptions and I simply didn't have the time to get involved. Many pharmacists feel that drug abusers and dealers are so numerous that we, as pharmacists, are never going to solve this problem that is so deeply rooted in our society. Why should we as pharmacists endanger our lives by helping to nail such dangerous criminals?

I once worked in a town of around ten thousand people. One day someone called me and identified himself as Dr. Kaplowitz. He proceeded to act as though he was phoning in a prescription for one of his patients. I hadn't worked in that town very long but I seemed to recall having spoken with Dr. Kaplowitz on the phone once or twice before. I seemed to recall Dr. Kaplowitz being quite self-confident, quite forceful, bordering on arrogant. This person who claimed to be Dr. Kaplowitz was none of the above. He said something like "I'm thinking about prescribing Vicodin for Jane Smith or maybe Lorcet. What do you think?" Such uncertainty is—or should be—a definite tip-off to pharmacists. I've never in my career had a physician call me who was so unsure of himself. An hour or two later, "Jane Smith" called and asked me whether the prescription phoned in by Dr. Kaplowitz was ready. I told her simply, "No. Dr. Kaplowitz did not call." I should have called the real Dr. Kaplowitz and told him that someone was pretending to be him, but it was a very busy day and I felt that surely no pharmacist in America would be fooled by such an amateurish imposter.

Many drug abusers approach the pharmacist and imitate a cough, hoping we'll sell them a cough syrup containing the narcotic codeine. Codeine can be habit forming so government regulations place this drug in a special class called "exempt narcotics." Pharmacists are allowed to sell these codeine-containing cough syrups to customers without a doctor's prescription. What usually happens is this: A customer describes his or her cough symptoms to the pharmacist or actually imitates a cough. If the pharmacist thinks the customer is telling the truth (admittedly a subjective assessment on our part), i.e., the customer does indeed appear to have a real cough, the pharmacist can sell one of these codeine-containing cough syrups. My guess is that every pharmacist in America has seen many people who are hooked on these products. Or these customers simply like the feeling that these products provide.

Many customers approach the pharmacist and state that they need to purchase needles for their diabetic grandmother's insulin injections. Here again, if the pharmacist believes the customer is telling the truth, the pharmacist can sell the needles. Drug addicts very frequently use the "for my grandmother" story to obtain needles to inject themselves with illicit drugs—not insulin. When pharmacists are suspicious of the customers' demeanor or appearance, we decline to sell the needles. We often lie by saying, "We're out of needles."

Pharmacists hear endless stories from customers seeking needles, codeine-containing cough syrups, and early refills on their narcotic pain pills. This procession of phony stories from customers convinces pharmacists that drug abuse is a tremendously huge problem in America. Many pharmacists become jaded toward almost anyone who has prescriptions filled for drugs like Vicodin and Percocet. Many pharmacists seem to assume that nearly everyone who is on these drugs must be a drug abuser or drug dealer who has been successful in snowing their doctor into writing such prescriptions. When pharmacists see customers with prescriptions for narcotic pain pills, some pharmacists assume these people have been "doctor shopping," i.e., going around to various physicians in the area looking for one who will write narcotic prescriptions. But pharmacists should keep in mind that there are many people who have a legitimate need for these drugs. My mother died from colon cancer that spread to her liver. During the final two months of her life, she unquestionably needed the Percocet that was prescribed by her oncologist. She was the last person in the world who would want to take Percocet unnecessarily. I was fortunate that I was able to stay with her for the final few weeks of her life. I recall taking one of her prescriptions for Percocet to a nearby pharmacy. It was at night and the pharmacist on duty was alone in the pharmacy. When I handed the Percocet prescription directly to the pharmacist, I detected that skeptical look in his eye assuming my mother must be a drug abuser. I wanted to say to him, "You asshole. She's dying from cancer."

PART IV

CHAIN DRUGSTORES

Chapter 13

The chain drugstore culture

In my 25-year career as a pharmacist, I've worked for three major drug chains, including the Rite Aid chain from 1975 to 1978. The focus on sales volume was always intense with each of the drug chains I've worked for. But the focus on sales volume at Rite Aid was extremely intense. I remember that the number one question my Rite Aid supervisors asked me (on the phone and in person) was some variation of this: "How is prescription volume looking this week?"

Back in the 1970s most of the sales figures that pharmacists and store managers sent to corporate headquarters were handwritten. Today, sales figures are transmitted to the corporate office electronically. I remember that on our weekly handwritten sales recap that we sent to our Rite Aid district office, the most prominent figures we submitted were the number of prescriptions we filled during the current week and also the number of prescriptions we filled during the same week the previous year. The previous year's numbers were obtained from a notebook we maintained containing weekly sales figures. The form, completed at the end of each week (i.e., Saturday), looked something like this:

• Number of prescriptions filled this week
• Number of prescriptions filled same week last year
• Dollar value of prescriptions filled this week
• Dollar value of prescriptions filled same week last year

Comparing the current week to the same week during the previous year was an important yardstick used by our Rite Aid bosses to determine whether our store was on an uphill trajectory or a downhill trajectory. Pharmacists working in stores on a downhill trajectory needed to have a logical explanation for the decline (e.g., a competitor recently opened a drugstore down the street), or else endure being blamed for killing the store. Pharmacists can directly affect the success of pharmacies by obvious things like being too slow in filling prescriptions, being out-of-stock of too many drugs, or being rude to customers.

I had several different district supervisors during my three years at Rite Aid. All of them seemed to have been programmed to ask that same question: "How are prescription numbers looking this week?" The obsession with sales figures led to efforts to inflate these numbers by whatever means necessary, legal or borderline legal.

For example, pharmacists were encouraged to give an additional refill or two on prescriptions. Say a doctor specified five refills on the prescription he wrote. For "maintenance" drugs (those that treat chronic conditions like hypertension, arthritis, depression, type 2 diabetes, etc.), Rite Aid's corporate attitude seemed to be that one or two additional refills wouldn't hurt anyone. Let me emphasize that we were not encouraged to exceed the specified number of refills for controlled substances or antibiotics. Exceeding the specified number of refills with controlled substances would have been (and still is) a serious violation of the law.

With maintenance meds, the corporate attitude seemed to be "John Smith isn't going to be cured of his hypertension any time soon so an additional refill or two is no big deal." Of course, the pharmacist was encouraged to phone the doctor for authorization for additional refills when the customer ran out of refills. But pharmacists working in seriously understaffed stores frequently take the course of least resistance: giving an additional refill or two without calling the doctor for authorization. It's much easier for the pharmacist to go ahead and refill "maintenance meds" an additional time or two than always call the doctor.

There are many pharmacists who would never consider exceeding the number of refills specified by the doctor. Other pharmacists have a much more relaxed attitude toward exceeding the specified number of refills (on medications that customers will likely use for a long time). Rite Aid encouraged a more relaxed attitude toward refills compared to the other two drug chains I've worked for. This was Rite Aid back in the 1970s. I am not qualified to say whether a similar attitude exists today at Rite Aid pharmacies.

The obsessive focus on prescription volume led to an interesting situation. For example, whenever a customer asked the pharmacist to recommend a multivitamin, our supervisors recommended that we walk to the sales floor, recommend a product, then carry that product (One-A-Day, Theragran, Myadec, etc.) back to the pharmacy and make a prescription out of it. We were to ask the customer for the name of his doctor and then act like we had just received a prescription from that doctor for the multivitamin we were recommending. We would type a label instructing the customer to, for example, "Take one tablet daily." We would then slap that label on the product. Magically, we could then record this as an additional prescription.

Say we filled 150 prescriptions daily on average. Say we made five separate recommendations each day for multivitamins. These additional five recommendations would allow us to report an additional five prescriptions filled each day, or thirty-five per week. So, say we filled a thousand prescriptions in a certain week. This tactic would allow us to report to our district headquarters that we actually filled 1,035 that week. The inflated figure was obviously phony but it played well in the numbers game that obsessed our supervisors. This practice let us know that prescription volume should be the number one priority for chain pharmacists. Pharmacists understood quite clearly that the numbers we reported each week were how our bosses judged us. Most pharmacists got the message and wanted to report numbers that pleased our bosses.

Tightly controlled workplace

The chain pharmacy workplace certainly has many more rules regulating personal behavior than does pharmacy school. Workplace regulations I have personally seen enforced during my career:

• No personal reading material allowed in the pharmacy (like *People* magazine, a favorite among female pharmacists).
• No radios allowed in the pharmacy.
• No chairs allowed in the pharmacy.
• Pharmacists and techs must not sit on stools while entering prescriptions into pharmacy computer. Sitting on stools creates the impression of laziness.
• Pharmacists must answer the phone within three rings and routinely return to any callers on hold to tell them the status of their call.
• Bottles on shelves must be straight as "little toy soldiers."
• No notes (like the phone number to the local sub shop) taped to walls, including walls outside the view of customers. Notes on the pharmacy walls create a cluttered appearance. If you want notes, get a notebook.
• Male pharmacists must wear a tie, a name tag, and white jacket.

Countless times I've watched pharmacists forcefully and confidently advising customers about the importance of taking prescribed medications religiously for elevated blood pressure and elevated cholesterol, while I've rarely seen pharmacists forcefully and confidently advising customers about the importance of maintaining ideal weight, eating nutritious foods, and otherwise having a healthy lifestyle, all of which might lessen the need for such drugs. Of course, pharmacists rarely have time for in depth conversations ("consultations") with our customers. Even though it's never verbalized, it is clear to most pharmacists that our employer doesn't want us advising customers about non-drug approaches to illnesses. Non-drug approaches circumvent the drugstore.

In my opinion, there is no greater contradiction in pharmacy than the perspective of the big chains (that pharmacy is mainly a distributive enterprise) and the perspective of pharmacy schools (that pharmacy is a cognitive enterprise). The culture in chain pharmacy is nearly opposite that in pharmacy school. From my perspective, pharmacy professors do not adequately prepare students for the transition from pharmacy school to the real world. Professors do not alert students about the culture shock we experience when we find ourselves ringing up diapers, deodorant, and suntan lotion at the pharmacy cash register along with prescriptions.

Fortunately, some pharmacists are able to take the more demeaning aspects of our job in stride. One recent pharmacy graduate commented to me, "I'll happily ring up groceries all day for what I'm being paid."

I have heard many pharmacy students say that their professors ridicule retail pharmacy (as opposed to hospital pharmacy) for being intellectually unsatisfying, not what pharmacy is really about, physically exhausting grunt-work in a factory. I've never worked in a hospital pharmacy so I am unqualified to say whether hospital pharmacy is more satisfying.

I wish someone would do a study comparing academic performance in pharmacy school versus satisfaction with chain pharmacy. My theory is that the higher the pharmacy student's grade point average, the less he or she is satisfied with chain pharmacy. Perhaps the intellectually curious students find the chain pharmacy environment to be deeply unfulfilling, vacuous, assembly-line piece-work/production-work. Perhaps the best students in pharmacy school are profoundly uneasy in the retail environment in which speed in filling prescriptions is valued much more highly than drug knowledge. Perhaps the pharmacists who were slackers in pharmacy school are more satisfied with monotonous, repetitive, robotic chain pharmacy.

Our chain pharmacy bosses certainly do not value highly those pharmacists who want to spend a lot of time examining potential drug interactions, phoning doctors about potential problems, advising customers, etc. The corporate bosses feel that pharmacists who want to spend their time discussing drugs should leave the retail environment, become a member of the pharmacy school faculty, and teach full time.

Professors in pharmacy school tell us that pharmacists will be paid for our drug knowledge. The drugstore chains have an entirely different outlook: We are paid for our labor. Supervisors with the drug chains relate to pharmacists below them completely in terms of sales—not health. Having a supervisor engage us in a conversation about some drug treatment would be unimaginable. Supervisors talk to us about three things: sales, sales, and sales. The most important question to supervisors is: Are the pharmacy sales figures up compared to the same period last year?

A district supervisor for a competing drug chain took me out to lunch one day in an effort to fill a slot in one of his stores. During our surprisingly frank discussion (perhaps this was his way of letting me know what kind of pharmacists he likes), he told me that most pharmacists just out of school have some unrealistic expectations of what it's like working in a drugstore forty hours a week. He told me that most of them leave the ivory towers of the universities with a "know-it-all" cockiness and that they take too long to learn (some never learn) that their job is just like "flipping hamburgers at McDonald's" all day long. He said that few graduates understand that, in the real world, they're being paid for their labor. He said they don't know that pharmacy (as practiced by the big chains) is one of the few professions where licensees are paid mainly for their labor. Whereas doctors, lawyers, professors, etc., are paid for using their heads, chain pharmacists are mainly paid for using their hands and feet. He said that the average chain pharmacist in this country fills somewhere between 100 and 200 prescriptions in an eight- or twelve-hour day and that this puts chain pharmacists in the category of piece-workers. He acknowledged that this is demeaning and that he was not pleased that our profession had degenerated to this. But he said he was tired of hiring pharmacists who didn't seem to be able to accept reality and perform accordingly.

This economic perspective in the drugstore quickly replaces the drug therapy perspective we had in pharmacy school. In fact, the economic perspective pretty much colors our attitudes and outlook in the drugstore. In cities where our chain has more than one outlet, pharmacists frequently spend a lot of time on the phone with pharmacists at the other outlets. We call these local pharmacists often to see if they have various drugs on hand that we're out of. Occasionally, when we can steal a minute or two, we talk about whatever is on our minds. In my experience, the most frequent topic between pharmacists is "How's business?"

The competitive drive being what it is, the pharmacist at the higher-volume store very often lords this fact over the pharmacist at the lower volume store. The importance of sales has been so thoroughly hammered into our heads that we use it as a yardstick to gauge our success as pharmacists. Superior prescription volume is a reason to feel superior to a another pharmacist. Superior knowledge about medicine or health or prevention is rarely the basis for such egotism. Success is, unfortunately, not measured in terms of the quality of the answers that the pharmacist gives to customers' questions. I've never seen a pharmacist criticized by a supervisor for giving poor or mediocre advice to a customer. On the other hand, supervisors are very often critical of pharmacists who are slow in the dispensing of prescriptions.

The unit malfunctioned

One day my partner and I were in the pharmacy and a customer walked up to us and said, "These don't look like my usual pills." We examined the contents of her bottle and, sure enough, the "floater" pharmacist who had worked the day before had given her the wrong pills. This floater had worked the last day of my partner's vacation. This floater had mistakenly dispensed Premarin 2.5 mg instead of Provera 2.5 mg. This was not a major error since these are both female hormones, yet it was indeed an error. After he gave the customer her correct pills, my partner said to me, "The unit malfunctioned yesterday." My partner has grown attached to the word "unit" as a way of expressing how our employer has turned pharmacists into robots. I usually use the word "automaton," but my partner thinks the word "unit" more closely captures the absurdity of our work environment. My partner uses the word "unit" to compare pharmacists to mechanical devices in the pharmacy like fax machines, cash registers, and laser printers. Commenting further on this floater's error, my partner said, "That's what Revco [our employer, a big drug chain that was sold to CVS] wants. They want us to *run 'em thru* [fill prescriptions at lightning speed]." My partner did not apologize to the customer for the floater's mistake. He just thanked the customer for coming back. My partner is tired of apologizing for errors that he feels are inevitable in the chain's "speed is all that matters" culture. He's tired of incurring the wrath of customers for errors made by other pharmacists in an impossible system.

Speaking with customers is discouraged even though management claims otherwise

My employer says that we should talk to customers, but most pharmacists are highly skeptical that the corporation really means it. I have heard numerous supervisors ridicule various pharmacists for spending too much time talking to customers. Talking with customers sure slows things down. For example, a customer might say she's experiencing a certain symptom and then want to know whether it could be a side effect of the drug she's taking. This would require me to pull out the professional insert or consult the *Physicians' Desk Reference* or *Facts & Comparisons* to search carefully to see whether that symptom is listed as a possible side effect of the drug.

Older pharmacists have told me that when they graduated from pharmacy school, they were forbidden to discuss medications with customers. They were supposed to refer the customers with their questions back to the doctor who prescribed the medication. These pharmacists weren't even allowed to put the name of the drug on your prescription label. Even though that was not good for teaching customers about their medications, it certainly made life simpler for those pharmacists. Not having to answer customers' questions sure would make my job easier and I would have less legal liability.

Mystery shoppers

My employer periodically sends around "mystery shoppers" for secret undercover evaluations of store employees and store management. The mystery shopper does not identify himself or herself. He or she checks things like: whether another cashier is called when there are over three people in line at the cash registers, whether all employees are professional and courteous to customers, and whether employees greet customers and make eye contact. The mystery shopper also checks the amount of time it takes the pharmacy staff to fill prescriptions—as if we were not already working as fast as we can, in fact, already at unsafe speeds. In most of the stores, we usually have to fight our urge to go to the bathroom or eat. We fight like hell just to keep up with the prescription flow. Yet management acts as though we're leisurely viewing *Playboy* magazine all day long.

Pushing non-prescription drugs

An important part of the pharmacist's job is to help move the non-prescription drugs in the store. This isn't too difficult. Customers have been well-programmed from radio, television, and magazine advertisements to interpret every discomfort as the need for a product from the pharmacy. As Ivan Illich (author of *Medical Nemesis: The Expropriation of Health,* New York: Pantheon, 1976) would say, the customers have been trained to *need on command.*

Selling non-prescription drugs is one of the parts of my job that I hate the most because I need to leave the prescription department to show the customer the product I recommend. In the prescription department, at least there is the mystique from not seeing or knowing precisely what the pharmacist is doing. But on the sales floor I feel surely the customers see me purely as a merchant trying to move products. I usually recommend the most popular product for each particular ailment. For example: Dimetapp for colds, Robitussin for coughs, Sucrets for sore throat, Preparation H for hemorrhoids, Mylanta for excess acid, Centrum for a vitamin, Advil for mild pain,

Neosporin for minor cuts or abrasions, Donnagel for diarrhea, Metamucil for constipation, Cort-Aid for poison ivy.

I recommend only well-know products because, if the customer doesn't find any benefit from that product, I have a big company like Proctor & Gamble or Bristol-Myers Squibb behind me. This way the customer can't say, "The pharmacist recommended some dumb product that didn't do me any good." By recommending a well-known brand name, I have the entire hype department of a multi-national drug company supporting me. This way the customer would be challenging the mountain of hype from that company. The customer can't claim I recommended some unheard of product.

My instructors from pharmacy school would surely feel I am disregarding their fancy justifications for the various products. And they would be right. I feel it is amazing how thoroughly the drug companies have done their job of selling Americans on the pill-for-every-ill concept. It is apparent to me that many people believe whatever marketing pitch they hear on television. I feel sorry for many customers because of their simplistic understanding of health, yet, at the same time, I am amazed they are so confident that their single-minded pursuit of quick-fix solutions is logical.

Occasionally when someone describes some innocuous symptoms and then asks me what we have for it, I say, "I don't know of anything that would be good for that." Invariably the response is, "Well, thanks anyway" and the customer has this expression on his face: *This Is A Dumb Pharmacist.* So I have come to the conclusion that I'd better make a recommendation when asked.

Quick-fix medicine is not fulfilling

Pharmacy professors tell students that pharmacy is very fulfilling because pharmacists help people with health problems. In my opinion, helping people find a quick-fix solution is not fulfilling. Dispensing products as fast as my hands and feet will allow is not fulfilling. Giving advice can be more fulfilling but, too often, we don't have enough time to give advice. Most customers aren't interested in gaining the insight that might allow them to prevent their problem whether it be depression, insomnia, vaginal yeast infection, jock itch, type 2 diabetes, elevated cholesterol, elevated blood pressure, constipation, diarrhea, heartburn, headache, etc.

How can pharmacists find it fulfilling when our days are spent dispensing Botox for facial wrinkles, Paxil for shyness, Vaniqa for female facial hair, Ritalin for hyperactivity, Anafranil for excess hand-washing, DDAVP for bedwetting, Sarafem for premenstrual dysphoric disorder, Xanax for panic attack, Imitrex for migraine, Sonata for insomnia, Rogaine for baldness, TriCyclen for female acne, Renova for wrinkles, Nexium for acid, Imodium for diarrhea, and Meridia for obesity? Most of these conditions are preventable or treatable without drugs or they're conditions for which Big Pharma has succeeded in making the public feel inadequate (e.g., baldness, female facial hair, wrinkles, impotence, shyness).

We're just a number

A medical sociologist once told me "The socialization process in medical school is stronger than a prison." In my opinion, pharmacists go through a similarly powerful socialization process with the big pharmacy chains. Socialization into the corporate culture involves a loss of individuality. Several pharmacists have told me that they feel more like a number than a person as we fill prescriptions at some mega-chain that has absolutely no concern for us as a human being.

Most people are surprised to learn just how big the mega-chains are. Here's a ranking of the chains by number of pharmacies in 2005 (Sandra Levy, "Chain industry is alive and well: NACDS profile," *Drug Topics*, Nov. 20, 2006, p. 48):

1. CVS—5,370 pharmacies
2. Walgreens—4,953 pharmacies
3. Rite Aid—3,323 pharmacies
4. Wal-Mart—3,289 pharmacies
5. Albertson's—1,945 pharmacies

Having so many stores means that corporate is obsessed with standardization, predictability, uniformity, and control. It means that each outlet of Chain X should be indistinguishable from the others, that pharmacists should be interchangeable in the various locations, and that the shopping experience at each store should be identical. Efficiency dictates that interactions between customers and employees be limited. The fast food model requires socialization into the overarching corporate ethos and a homogenization of pharmacists that leaves little room for those who yearn to find their own path. Students in pharmacy school who hope for creativity in their career will almost certainly be sorely disappointed with the rigid and regimented chain culture. The chain drugstore requires achieving control through automation or de-skilling of the workplace because people are inherently unpredictable and inefficient. The big chains want to routinize and mechanize the workplace as much as possible so that unskilled workers can replace skilled workers.

The big chains view pharmacy as a business, not a profession. The chains aggressively fight unions. Pharmacists working for the big chains occasionally go on strike, illustrating that labor/management issues are just as important in chain drugstores as they are at General Motors, Ford, and Chrysler. Pharmacy unions fight for better pay for pharmacists, but the unions also fight for things that many workers in our society take for granted, like meal breaks and bathroom breaks. In drugstores that have only one pharmacist on duty at a time, having that pharmacist leave for a few minutes to eat lunch or go to the bathroom causes an impatient public to complain about poor service. The chains see pharmacists as wage laborers who provide a product, rather than professionals who provide a service (screening for drug interactions, checking dosages, advising customers about proper use of medications, etc.).

A never-ending loop of happy drug messages on the store audio system

Chain pharmacists have surprisingly little control over the environment in which we work. For example, many of the big chains produce their own advertising messages at the corporate level which are then piped into each store. This bathes customers and store employees in a never-ending loop of pill-for-every-ill messages…all day, every day. To me, the effect is much more irritating than background music like Muzak. That's because these in-store messages usually have some annoyingly cheerful announcer pretending he's Ron Radio. I often wonder whether our corporate bosses ever considered the effect that constant repetition of these messages has on store employees. The corporate bosses seem to feel that store employees are no more adversely affected by this verbal pollution of our workplace than the products sitting on our shelves. A bottle of Robitussin cough syrup and a tube of Preparation H are unaffected by this noise pollution but I don't think the same can be said for human beings. I often feel like a lab rat being tested to see how many advertising messages I can withstand without developing some drugstore equivalent of *going postal*.

It seems to me that this constant assault by advertising messages has a numbing and dehumanizing effect on store employees. It is as if the corporate bosses have no respect for store employees as human beings. I often wonder whether our customers are similarly annoyed by these messages. Surely this continuous repetition of messages about drugs convinces customers (and, yes, pharmacists) that pills are the answer to every health problem. To the best of my recollection, none of these messages have dealt with the importance of proper diet, proper weight, exercise, etc., because such approaches circumvent the drugstore.

Should drugstores sell candy, cigarettes, and alcoholic beverages?

Three of the leading substances causing disease in America (sugar, tobacco, and alcohol) are readily available in drugstores. When your drugstore chain advertises that it cares about your health, ask yourself how that is possible if that chain sells cigarettes, alcoholic beverages (beer and wine), and candy. Sugar, alcohol, and tobacco are either addicting or cause craving. Obesity, dental cavities, alcoholism, and lung cancer can be the end result of the excessive use of products easily obtainable in most drugstores.

Drugstores sell alcoholic beverages while the pharmacist fills prescriptions for Antabuse, a drug that helps alcoholics quit. Drugstores sell cigarettes while the pharmacist fills prescriptions for people with lung cancer. Is it not hypocritical for drugstores to sell cigarettes and also sell nicotine gum and patches to help you quit smoking?

Americans associate holidays with candy. The drugstore aisles overflow with candy each Halloween, Easter, Mother's Day, Valentine's Day, and Christmas. As everyone knows, candy causes dental caries and contributes to obesity, which in turn contributes to type-2 diabetes and hypertension. Is it hypocritical that we sell candy in the front of the store and fill prescriptions (Xenical and Meridia) for obesity in the pharmacy? We also fill countless prescriptions for acetaminophen w/codeine and penicillin VK as a result of the dental caries caused by candy.

Is it strange that many public schools are prohibiting soft drink and candy vending machines while pharmacies sell lots of soft drinks and candy? Is it time to jettison the idea that people should bring a box of candy when they visit friends or relatives who have recently been discharged from the hospital? Is it time to re-examine our cultural practice of celebrating special occasions by buying a box of candy at the drugstore for one's spouse, girlfriend, or mother?

Would somebody please clean the men's restroom?

Would you eat in a restaurant with filthy restrooms? People assume that if the restaurant restrooms are filthy, chances are that the kitchen is unsanitary and the staff is ambivalent about cleanliness. Many customers react the same way to restrooms in drugstores. I've often wondered how customers react when they see the filthy restrooms at some of the drugstores I've worked in.

The cleanliness of the restrooms tells a lot about the way in which the drugstore is run. In many stores, the restrooms are always clean. In other stores, the restrooms are usually filthy, unless it happens to be just a day or two after the weekly or twice-a-month contract floor cleaners did their work. These floor cleaners clean the restrooms as part of the floor cleaning contract.

At many stores in which there is an ongoing conflict between the pharmacists and the store manager, the cleaning of restrooms becomes an issue of power and status. The store manager feels that he has more power than the pharmacists since the store manager controls more square footage than pharmacists. At stores in which there is not, say, a male part-time high school student who can be assigned the job of cleaning the restrooms, this task can fall on the shoulders of the only other non-pharmacist male in the store, i.e., the store manager. The store manager doesn't want to clean the restrooms himself because he fears he would suffer a diminution in status in the eyes of the pharmacists. So if there is no other male in the store other than the store manager, the restrooms are often left filthy until the scheduled arrival of the contracted floor cleaners.

I've worked in stores in which the store manager kept the restrooms locked, forcing customers and employees to ask for the key for entry. This allowed him to screen the people who could use the restrooms. The store manager didn't want to make it too easy for customers to enter the restrooms.

Some store employees tell customers "We don't have public restrooms." I recall seeing a memo from corporate stating something like, "Keep in mind that many of your customers have medical conditions which may require them to have access to restrooms. Therefore, restrooms should be made available to customers." Of course, this memo didn't address the fact that many customers leave a filthy mess in the restroom that store employees must clean up. It's easy for corporate to tell us to keep the restrooms available to the public. That's because the corporate hotshots don't have to clean the restrooms themselves. I'd love to see the corporate suits cleaning restrooms.

I worked in one store in which the store manager did not keep toilet paper in the restrooms. (Employees and customers had to request it beforehand.) I asked him about this once and he said that he was tired of finding whole rolls of toilet paper dumped in the toilet. I never understood why customers would be so angry or crude as to dump a full roll of toilet paper. Were they protesting the way they were treated by store employees? Were they angry at our prices? Were they upset having to wait for their prescriptions to be filled?

At most stores in which I've worked, the women's restroom is cleaner than the men's restroom. Perhaps male anatomy (standing versus sitting) makes it inevitable that the men's restroom will be less clean than the women's restroom. It is possible that women have been socialized into keeping clean restrooms whereas men view the cleaning of restrooms as beneath them, a feminine activity. Some men seem to view filthy restrooms as a macho thing. These men seem to feel that concern about restroom cleanliness is for women only.

I worked in one store in which the sales floor area was always well-maintained and the products on the shelves were always straightened ("front faced"). But the men's restroom was always filthy. That was in a store with a lazy male manager but a very hardworking female who essentially functioned as the floor manager. She kept the store shelves well stocked and clean and she made sure that the women's restroom was always in good shape. Under-standably she didn't touch the men's restroom. Surely it is not fair to ask female employees to clean the men's restroom.

Like many pharmacists, I've often needed to stay after store clos-ing to get caught up before going home. This means I have often been in the store by myself. I confess that, under these circum-stances, I've often utilized the women's restroom because the men's restroom is simply too gross and I'm too lazy or too tired or too fed up with the store manager to clean the men's restroom myself.

The only period during which I've routinely cleaned the men's restroom myself was back in the days when the pharmacist was the store manager. I happened to be the manager of a new store in Bur-lington, North Carolina. With the exception of the other pharmacist, I was the only male in the store. Knowing the other pharmacist as I did, I'm sure there's no way that he would have cleaned the restroom himself. Most male pharmacists would rather kill themselves than clean a drugstore restroom.

Chain drugstores are intellectually deadening

Customers probably think that chain drugstores are centers of lively and passionate discussion about the safety and effectiveness of prescription and non-prescription drugs. Is there indeed a frank discussion among chain pharmacists about the pros and cons of various drugs?

In my experience, the chain drugstore environment is almost exclusively focused on production, i.e., numbers of prescriptions and numbers of dollars. It is quite unusual for pharmacists to engage in significant discussions among themselves about drugs. Many pharmacists entering the real world after pharmacy school are shocked to see that the focus of their job in the chain drugstore is almost the exact opposite of the focus in pharmacy school. In pharmacy school, the study of drugs was our primary focus. At the chain drugstore, filling prescriptions as fast as we can is our primary focus.

In my 25 years as a chain pharmacist, I rarely saw pharmacists at work engaging in the types of drug therapy discussions with other pharmacists that would make our pharmacy school professors proud. Conversations among pharmacists usually focused on everything *except* pharmacology: plans for the weekend, plans for an upcoming vacation, family matters, difficult bosses and co-workers, understaffing, attitudes of local doctors, the pros and cons of working for CVS versus Walgreens versus Wal-Mart versus Rite Aid, the fact that the non-pharmacist store manager too often doesn't have a clue about the stresses pharmacists feel as a result of understaffing, and last—but certainly not least—attractive female customers.

It is clear to pharmacists soon after graduation from pharmacy school that drug chain supervisors do not think highly of pharmacists who are overly fixated on the "drug therapy" side of pharmacy. In fact, engaging our district pharmacy supervisor in a discussion about some drug therapy is very difficult for me to imagine. District pharmacy supervisors (who are, by the way, usually pharmacists themselves) are clearly primarily interested making sure that Rx volume in each of his stores is on the upswing.

It is also my experience that chain pharmacists rarely discuss among themselves significant events like the FDA adding critical black box warnings to the official prescribing information, or the FDA taking the drastic step of removing drugs from the market.

For thirty years, I've been hearing that the pharmacy school model of the pharmacist as drug expert will become the dominant model. However, the big chains are unyielding in their disdain for this "clinical" orientation of newly-graduated pharmacists. The big chains want pharmacists who can fill prescriptions at lightning speed. The big chains certainly don't want pharmacists who spend too much time discussing drugs with customers, calling doctors about potential drug interactions, or otherwise functioning as the public expects. The big chains view prescriptions like any other commodity in the marketplace. Shortly after graduation from pharmacy school, young pharmacists working for many of the big chains become shocked, saddened, and disillusioned when they fully comprehend the fact that they are no more than highly paid piece-workers on a production line based on McDonald's, complete with a two-lane drive thru.

When I was in high school and college, I thought I'd like to work for a big corporation. I was completely invested in the idea that corporations are efficient, exciting, and meritocratic. I felt sure that working for a corporation would be an interesting experience. When I graduated and began working for the big drug chains, I found a reality that was far different from what I had expected. I discovered that efficiency in the chain drugstore industry means mind-numbing and exhausting repetition: filling an endless river of prescriptions as fast as my hands and feet would allow. Efficiency in the chain drugstore means a never-ending quest by the corporation to figure out more ingenious ways to squeeze more production out of pharmacists and technicians.

Instead of being intellectually challenging, I found the big drugstore chains to be intellectually deadening. In my opinion, the big chains would be more accurately described as anti-intellectual:

• The big chains are completely uninterested in issues like whether Big Pharma exerts too much pressure on the FDA.
• The big drug chains aren't interested in safety issues surrounding drugs.

• The big chains aren't interested in examining, monitoring, or reporting the short term or long term adverse effects of drugs.

• The big chains aren't interested in discussing whether Americans are overmedicated. In fact, the big chains clearly *want* Americans to be overmedicated.

• The big chains aren't interested in the profound social implications of the mass prescribing of antidepressants to adults and, increasingly, to children.

• The big chains aren't interested in the tremendous overprescribing of antibiotics for the treatment of the common cold. The big chains aren't interested in the severe problems that the overprescribing of antibiotics causes in the development of drug resistance.

• The big chains aren't interested in the field of prevention—because prevention usually means finding alternatives to drugs.

• The big chains aren't interested in examining the striking age-adjusted variations in the incidence of diseases around the world and learning what this tells us about the powerful potential of prevention.

• The big chains aren't interested in pollution, in the ubiquity of toxic substances (including carcinogens) in our environment, in pesticide residues on fruits and vegetables, in cancer clusters around factories that discharge hazardous materials into the air and water.

• Clearly the big drugstore chains are more interested in the treatment of cancer than in its prevention.

• The big chains are opposed to any type of prevention that circumvents the drugstore.

• The big chains aren't interested in discussions about whether drugs are overprescribed.

• The big chains aren't interested in discussions about whether drug advertisements on television prompt consumers to ask doctors for drugs that may be unnecessary.

• The big chains aren't interested in the controversy surrounding the widespread prescribing of drugs like Ritalin for children who do poorly in school because they don't pay attention ("attention deficit") or won't sit still ("hyperactivity").

• The big chains aren't interested in the consequences of the over-prescribing of post-menopausal estrogens, including increases in stroke, heart disease, and breast cancer.

• The big chains aren't interested in whether Big Pharma exaggerates the benefits of drugs and minimizes the risks.

• The big chains aren't interested in examining the extent to which the placebo effect accounts for so much of the benefit that patients receive from pharmaceuticals.

• The big chains aren't interested in examining whether our health care system should be based on prevention rather than pills.

• The big chains aren't interested in a social critique of pharmaceuticals.

• The big chains aren't interested in the many booklength exposés of the pharmaceutical industry.

So why would any intellectually curious pharmacist want to work for the big drugstore chains? How could the complete mercantile focus in the drugstore appeal to any pharmacist who is interested in examining drugs in a broader social, cultural and even political context? How can a pharmacist who is a strong advocate of prevention be happy amidst the commodity fetishism that describes our daily existence in the drugstore? The big chains want pharmacists who fill prescriptions fast and who do not have doubts about the pill-for-every-ill focus of modern medicine.

Thousands of times in my career I have made recommendations for non-prescription products in response to customers' requests, even though I'd never use those products myself. Thousand of times I've made recommendations for products for colds, cough, insomnia, constipation, diarrhea, etc., even though I'd never take those products myself. Countless times I recommended Centrum when customers asked me to recommend a vitamin even though I don't take vitamins myself. In my opinion, one's focus should be on eating a nutritious diet rather than on attempting to fine-tune one's vitamin intake based on the latest magazine article or TV story that extols the virtues of vitamins. For whatever symptoms a customer describes to me, there's absolutely no chance that I would make a recommendation for a non-drug approach if my district supervisor is standing anywhere near me.

Soon after graduation from pharmacy school, I concluded that customers want definitive answers when they ask the pharmacist:

"What's good for…" (cold, cough, sore throat, backache, muscle aches, hemorrhoids, constipation, heartburn, dry eyes, minor cuts/abrasions, acne, diarrhea, insomnia, lack of energy, etc.). Customers do not like it when pharmacists answer these questions by suggesting lifestyle changes, dietary modifications, weight loss, adequate sleep, exercise, etc. Customers like pharmacists who forcefully and confidently answer, "You need X" (Sudafed, Robitussin, Myoflex, Preparation H, Pepcid AC, Sleep-Eze, Sucrets, Kaopectate, Metamucil, etc.).

Why I resist wearing a white coat

In pharmacy school, students were required (or highly encouraged) to wear our white coat during lab exercises. As best as I can recall, this was because, in some lab exercises, we handled chemicals that were potentially hazardous and thus the white coat could protect our skin and clothes. But the primary reason that we wore a white coat in our labs seemed to be because our professors viewed lab exercises as simulating real world pharmacy and the professors wanted us to get used to a "professional" appearance. Perhaps one third of the students in my class wore their lab coat all the time (i.e., in lecture halls *and* in the labs). These students seemed to be proud wearing their white coat. I resisted wearing my white coat because I never accepted the pill-for-every-ill outlook in pharmacy school and at CVS, Rite Aid, and Revco.

In the drugstore, wearing the white coat sent a subtle message to our bosses that we were loyal team players. Not wearing a white coat implied that a pharmacist was somehow rebellious and marched to the beat of his own drummer. I never felt comfortable wearing a white coat because it made me feel that I had sold out to the entire belief system of quick-fix medicine: suppressing symptoms with drugs, minimizing potential hazards of drugs, ignoring the powerful potential of prevention, placing the treatment of disease with drugs ahead of the prevention of that disease, accepting the hierarchical power structure which gave (oftentimes immature) supervisors power over pharmacists.

As someone who maintains a skeptical view toward the commodification of health, I am uncomfortable wearing the uniform that implies I am a team player in that enterprise, that I have accepted the goals and outlook of that enterprise, that I am part of a conspiracy to convince our customers that pills are better than prevention, that my primary allegiance is to the belief system I was taught in pharmacy school, that I accept The World According to Big Pharma. To me, wearing a white coat or uniform implies embracing the collective outlook of a group, being proud to be a member of that group, accepting the ideals and beliefs of that group. The word "uniform" comes from "one" plus "form." The chains would love for all pharmacists to look alike with a crisp white uniform and think alike—affable airheads who don't mind filling prescriptions at unsafe speeds at the pharmacy version of McDonald's.

My white coat increased the distance between me and customers. A white coat is somehow like a barrier. It says to customers, "I am the pharmacist. I am the drug expert. You are ignorant of drugs."

Here's an anecdote about white coats: The big chains had many rules for everything we did in the pharmacy (such as: no food in the pharmacy refrigerator, no radios or personal reading material in the pharmacy, no sitting on stools while using the pharmacy computer, products on our shelves should be "straight as little toy soldiers," phone-answering dialog should be "Thank you for calling Revco. This is [pharmacist's first name]. Can I help you?") But the corporate demand that really got under my skin was the requirement to wear a white coat.

District supervisors visit the pharmacy for perhaps an hour every two weeks. Too many district supervisors don't have a clue how pharmacists act toward customers when they (the district supervisors) are not in our store (i.e., the vast majority of the time). I have known many pharmacists who are very rude to customers and store employees. I have often thought that the first thing these district supervisors need to do is confront that pharmacist about his or her attitude toward customers or other employees. Every pharmacist knows that many pharmacists become a different person when our district supervisor is in the store, but that pharmacist immediately reverts to being a jerk toward customers and other employees as soon as that district supervisor walks out the door. District supervisors only know what they see, and those pharmacists become little angels when our district supervisor is present.

Rather than address such major problems like the rudeness of certain pharmacists, our district supervisor sees only what's in front of him: a pharmacist is not wearing a white coat. The district supervisor walks into the pharmacy and the first thing he notices is whether the pharmacist is wearing a white coat. A district supervisor once told me, "You need to wear your white coat." I answered him by saying, "The air conditioner in this store does not work very well." This was a correct statement but his reply was simple, "Well, you still need to wear it." Clearly, adherence to corporate policy is more important than the personal comfort of pharmacists.

The chains' *Alice in Wonderland* view of pharmacy mistakes

Alice in Wonderland is a well-known work of literary nonsense in what is called the "fantasy genre." In the world of pharmacy, a prominent example of the fantasy genre is the rationalizations given by chain spokesmen to reporters inquiring about pharmacy mistakes. Case in point: *USA Today* did a 3-day series (Feb. 11-13, 2008) on pharmacy mistakes. *The USA Today* series essentially placed the blame for pharmacy mistakes on the common practice of understaffing at the big chains. The big chains came out looking like they place high-speed production above accuracy.

Following a serious pharmacy mistake, spokesmen for the big chains are often interviewed by newspaper and TV reporters in the city in which the error occurred. Over the years, I've noticed that these chain spokesmen routinely make the following points, none of which—in my opinion—reflect the real world. These statements to the media are highly regrettable because, in minimizing the reality of serious mistakes, they perpetuate the current system of fast food pharmacy that guarantees errors. These explanations for pharmacy mistakes have an *Alice in Wonderland* quality about them because, quite often, the opposite is true. It is as if the chain spokesmen are living in some parallel universe.

Let's examine each of the chains' fantastical rationalizations individually. In soothing and reassuring tones, chain spokesmen say:

1. "Millions of dollars invested in technology will drastically reduce pharmacy errors." In reality, the chains want a technological solution to a human problem. A major cause of pharmacy errors is under-staffing but the big chains want the public to believe that errors are a technical problem with a technical solution, rather than a human problem that requires adequate staffing. Aside from the fact that some pharmacists are simply careless and would make mistakes re-gardless of the Rx volume, the primary problem in the pharmacy is the lack of an adequate number of properly trained techs and/or the need for more than one pharmacist on duty at a time. I know phar-macists who privately welcome the huge jury verdicts against chains in dispensing error cases. These pharmacists hope that the huge set-tlements will embarrass the chains into providing adequate staffing.

The big chains tell us that technology will make our lives easier. But the truth is that the big chains cut staffing commensurate with any efficiency gained by technology. The big chains dangle the carrot in front of us that technology will allow a more relaxed pace in the pharmacy. In reality, any gains in productivity brought about by technology will be met with an equivalent decrease in staffing. In-deed, the primary reason for adding technology in the pharmacy is to cut staffing.

2. "Every pharmacist will tell you that one error is too many." This is one of the chain spokesmen's favorite red herrings. It is a clever way of implying that the chains are approaching the elimination of phar-macy errors, that the number of errors is minuscule. If the chains feel that one error is too many, how would they characterize the millions of errors that are estimated to occur each year across this country? In fact, chain pharmacy is nowhere near eliminating errors. Rather than decreasing, it's just as likely that the frequency of errors is actually in-creasing each year as the big chains focus on production rather than safety.

3. "There are no quotas. Scripts per hour are only guidelines which can be modified as needed in the store." That's the most absurd statement I've ever heard in my life. Chain pharmacists have absolutely no power to increase R.Ph. staffing levels and thus lessen the burden of overwhelming and dangerous workloads.

4. "More errors occur when things are slow in the pharmacy because pharmacists are not focused." This is the chains' favorite mantra. It is like saying speeding on an icy highway is good because the inherent danger forces us to be more careful.

5. "No pharmacist is pressured to fill prescriptions faster than he or she feels comfortable." Yeah, Right! What about those computer systems that track the number of prescriptions not completed within 15 minutes of having been entered into the pharmacy computer? This data is compiled by corporate and often results in admonishments from our bosses to complete prescriptions more quickly.

6. "Safety is our number one priority." Nope. Speed is the chains' number one priority. Indeed the entire chain drugstore concept is based on speed and volume, just like at McDonald's.

7. "There is no correlation between high prescription volume and errors." The chains say that pharmacy mistakes occur in low volume stores and in high volume stores. The chains conclude, therefore, that there is no relation between volume and pharmacy mistakes. That is as illogical as saying that highway accidents occur at every speed, therefore there is no correlation between speed and auto accidents. It is like saying there should be no speed limits on highways because auto accidents occur at slow speeds as well as fast speeds. The reality is that speed kills on the highway and that speed in the pharmacy endangers the public safety.

Privately, chain management knows there's a correlation between volume and errors. But when reporters ask about such a relationship, chain management denies there is one. Using their tortured logic, we should be able to handle double, triple, or quadruple our current Rx volume without the hiring of additional techs or pharmacists.

If there were no correlation between volume and errors, why don't the chains expect each pharmacist to fill, say, three thousand prescriptions per shift rather than, say, three hundred? Clearly the chains do recognize that there are physical limits to human production. The chains claim that those limits are much higher than pharmacists believe.

Apparently speed causes errors in every human activity except the filling of prescriptions. I would like to ask chain executives to name any human cognitive activity in which speed does not increase errors. I can't think of a single one. Do you want your dentist rushing when he's making an impression of one of your teeth for the dental lab to prepare a crown? Do you want your heart surgeon rushing when he's giving you a triple bypass? Do you want your electrician rushing when he's re-wiring your circuit breaker panel? Do you want your automobile mechanic rushing when he's working on your brakes? Do you want your accountant rushing when he's doing your taxes? Do you want your pharmacist rushing when he's checking a counter full of prescriptions filled by rookie technicians?

Some of the contestants on the TV game show *Jeopardy* come up with some really stupid answers (or, more precisely, questions). Part of the reason is that those contestants are under heavy pressure because they're on television and there are two other contestants who are trying to buzz in first. Likewise, pharmacists are under tremendous pressure from customers and corporate management to fill prescriptions quickly. But somehow, according to chain management, being overwhelmed with prescriptions does not increase the occurrence of errors. Pharmacy is unique among human activities in that speed does not increase the occurrence of errors.

You've all heard that HASTE MAKES WASTE. Supposedly, this old dictum applies to every human activity except the filling of prescriptions. In the view of chain executives, HASTE MAKES MONEY.

When efficiency is all that matters

When I was in college, I used to think "efficiency" was an unequivocal good. I was attracted by the chain drugstore model because I bought into the concept that chain drugstores are efficient.

Even though I am often critical of chain drugstores today, I admit that they try hard to cut their unit cost for filling each prescription.

The chains enthusiastically embrace the latest technology to improve efficiency. When I first graduated, pharmacists had to write the Rx order each week by hand into a bulky order book. Later, the introduction of the Telxon allowed us to punch the product order number into this hand-held device. More recently, automatic replenishment freed pharmacists from the time-consuming and deadening task of eyeballing each product on our shelves on a weekly basis.

In the past, all the clerks in the drugstore punched time cards upon starting their shift, when leaving for lunch/dinner breaks or 15-minute breaks, when returning from those breaks, and when their shift was over. I vividly remember the extremely boring and laborious task of calculating each employee's time card into tenths of an hour each day. Now, each clerk simply punches his or her employee number into the high-tech cash register which doubles as a computer in automatically adding up each clerk's hours.

These advances in technology undoubtedly help the pharmacist. But technology can have a downside. Many pharmacy computers now have the ability to transmit data to our bosses about our speed and efficiency in filling prescriptions.

Many pharmacists feel that the chains care more about their technology than their employees. Pharmacists have been told routinely that improvements in technology will allow us more time to spend with customers. This has always been a bald-faced lie. The fundamental reason for the chains introducing the latest technology is to cut staffing. Staffing levels are cut commensurate with each technological advance.

Efficiency is what the chain drugstore is all about. The chain concept is meant to facilitate economies of scale. Mass purchasing of products allows lower unit costs. Chainwide computerization means that stores can be run more efficiently. In contrast, the basis for the independent drugstore is customer service. The chains want the public to think that we offer customer service that's as good as independents, but that is very often not the case. I've had bosses who ridicule pharmacists (behind those pharmacists' backs) for spending too much time talking with customers. The chains say they want us to speak with customers, but most pharmacists realize quickly that the chains don't really mean it. For example, the chains have always viewed patient counseling as a major drag on productivity that adds nothing to the bottom line.

The narrow focus on efficiency in chain drugstores comes at a huge cost to customers, to employees, and to society. Equating health with the efficient delivery of products comes at a tremendous cost that the big chains don't want to discuss. Search Google for "pharmacy mistakes" for one illustration of the many costs of placing speed and efficiency above everything else. Many pharmacists feel that the chains have made the cold calculation that it is more profitable to sling out prescriptions at lightning speed and pay any customers harmed by mistakes, rather than provide adequate staffing chainwide so that mistakes are a rarity rather than a predictable occurrence. I'd love to see a study that compares the per store error rate at chain drugstores versus independents.

When efficiency is all that matters in a business, the employees are viewed as machines rather than as human beings. Management at the big chains is endlessly disappointed that they are not able to remake the genomes of store employees so that those employees are robots. Pharmacists should realize that if the chains figure out a way to completely automate the pharmacy, we would be toast overnight.

When efficiency is all that matters, employees see that chain management views us only as a necessary evil to be barely tolerated until the chain can figure out a way to automate our jobs. Store employees resent not being treated as human beings, so they take out their resentment on our customers. If chain management doesn't care about us as human beings, why should we care about customers as human beings? Thus rudeness toward customers is not surprising in the chain drugstore model.

The narrow focus on efficiency in the drugstore has costs far beyond that of disillusioned store employees. Pharmacists know that we don't have time to do much more than throw a few words at our customers. Our customers end up not understanding their medications. Our society pays a heavy price for this assembly-line model that says that human health is directly proportional to the per capita consumption of pharmaceuticals. Our entire health care system is based on quantity rather than quality. In this model of health care, the concept of prevention becomes a quaint dream of the distant past. Americans remain ignorant of the non-pharmacological determinants of human health. This model based on efficiency promotes a quick-fix pill for every ill rather than a fundamental understanding of those lifestyle choices than can have a profound effect on one's health.

Very often, the pharmacy staff doesn't care enough to cultivate good relationships with local doctors and the receptionists who phone in prescriptions. I've seen floater pharmacists who are very rude to customers and doctors/receptionists because these floaters feel they'll just be working in that store for a day or two. So why care if customers, receptionists, and doctors are angered by the pharmacist's attitude? Many pharmacists feel that making customers angry is fine because we have too many customers to handle now with the ridiculous staffing levels.

The chains spend huge sums on marketing to attract customers into our stores. Too often, customers arrive to discover bright shiny new stores complete with two lane drive-thru windows and...Guess what?...deeply discontented employees. These employees, in effect, spend their time discarding those customers brought in by the chain's marketing. A pharmacist once commented to me that the best place to locate an independent is beside a chain because the chain will draw people to that location with advertising and then the independent can thrive off all the unhappy customers discarded by the unhappy workers at the big chains.

I've seen so many instances in which the chains had to pay pharmacists time-and-a-half overtime because the chains can't keep pharmacists. The chains are forced into bidding wars to attract pharmacists who, very often, don't want any part of the reckless game known as chain pharmacy. From my perspective, the chains end up paying much more in labor costs than if they had just treated their pharmacists well to start with.

I don't know if I'm unique but many times I would have happily forgone a pay raise in favor of an increase in tech staffing. I don't think that increased salaries for pharmacists can make up for miserable tech staffing levels. Many pharmacists have felt that there has never been a true national shortage of pharmacists, just a shortage of pharmacists willing to work in the chains' dangerously understaffed pharmacies. Do the chains not care that a large number of their pharmacists are questioning why they chose pharmacy as a career?

I have often wondered how this model of routinely burning out pharmacists and training new ones can be profitable. The chains would rather keep hiring young eager graduates who are willing to work at unsafe speeds, burning them out, and endlessly repeating this cycle. Apparently this is more profitable than keeping existing pharmacists happy. It doesn't take long for pharmacists to realize that the pace is not compatible with his or her mental or physical health. From the chains' perspective, I assume this high turnover in pharmacists dramatically cuts down on pension responsibilities.

When the chain I worked for was bought out by another large chain, most of the best pharmacists ended up going elsewhere. In my opinion, the new pharmacists who were hired to replace these veteran pharmacists were, very often, of a lower caliber (less professional, less customer-friendly) than the ones they replaced. As working conditions became more unbearable and the best pharmacists left, I found my bosses hiring pharmacists who never would have been hired in the past.

The chains' desire to make the pharmacist easily accessible to customers can have unintended consequences

There is considerable disagreement among the various drugstore chains regarding how accessible the pharmacist should be to the public. Some chains construct the pharmacy so that the pharmacist is easily accessible for questions, recommendations for non-prescription products, etc. Customers routinely ask the pharmacist questions like:

What do you recommend for a cold?
What's the strongest thing you have to knock out this cough?
I don't have any energy. Can you recommend a vitamin?
What aisle is the motor oil on?

Do you have a restroom I can use?
Do you have any diapers in the stockroom? You're out of the ones I usually get.

Other chains feel that having the pharmacist so easily accessible slows down prescription filling. I doubt that the chains would admit it publicly but I think they probably would privately agree that constant interruptions from customers increase the occurrence of pharmacy mistakes. I once read a commentary by a pharmacist who said that if the chains expect pharmacists to work in high volume stores, management needs to get the pharmacist away from the public, i.e., the pharmacy should be constructed so that the pharmacist can't be interrupted by customers every fifteen seconds.

With federal HIPAA regulations, there's a great deal of concern over privacy in health care today, but spending a few minutes hovering near the pharmacy can reveal a lot of private information. Many pharmacies have a glass partition of some type separating the pharmacist from the public. In most of these pharmacies, there is often a consultation area, sometimes off to a side. But if there are three or four people standing in line waiting to speak to the pharmacist in the consultation area, those people can sometimes get an earful of private information listening in on the conversation between the pharmacist and the person at the head of the line.

Here's a common scenario: In many drugstores, the vitamins are shelved directly in front of the pharmacy, not by coincidence but by design. This allows pharmacists to answer customers' questions about vitamins and to make specific recommendations. In those stores where there's no partition between the pharmacy staff and the public, you could—if you were so inclined—spend a few minutes hovering around the vitamin section (or whatever products happen to be in front of the pharmacy). You might hear a lot of information that is private. You could hear pharmacists calling doctors offices to clarify poorly legible prescriptions. You might hear a pharmacist on the phone to a doctor's office saying, "I have a prescription here for Bob Smith. It looks like Viagra [for erectile dysfunction] but I just wanted to make sure." Or you could hear a pharmacist asking, "I have a prescription here for Mary Jones. It looks like either Prozac [antidepressant] or Prilosec [acid reducer]." Or you could hear the pharmacist saying, "Can we refill John Smith's Detrol LA [for bladder control]?" Listening in on pharmacists' phone conversations with doctors' offices might reveal that one of your neighbors has a yeast infection or herpes or that he/she takes pills for anxiety, depression, insomnia, etc. Equally disturbing is the possibility that you might overhear conversations between two young technicians talking about their boyfriends while filling your prescriptions. You ask yourself, *Shouldn't they be concentrating on my prescriptions rather than talking about their boyfriends?*

I filled in occasionally at one chain drugstore in Henderson, North Carolina, in which the pharmacy was specifically designed so that the pharmacist would be very easily accessible to speak with customers. It was an unusual triangular-shaped design in which the pharmacy actually juts out toward the sales floor. Customers could stand four feet away from me the entire time I was working on their prescriptions and they could easily observe me counting their pills if they so desired. There was no partition of any type between me and the customers. On one particular day, the pharmacy was terribly understaffed. It was only me and one technician who I would describe as a real scatter-brain. We were running far behind and things were extremely stressful. At one point, this tech said to me in a normal speaking voice, "I don't know if I'm coming or going." Comments like this between pharmacy staff are not that unusual. But what was unusual about this was that, as best as I can recall, there were perhaps seven or eight customers within fifteen feet of us, and perhaps three or four of them were within five feet. Judging by the expression on the face of one nearby customer, I am absolutely certain that she heard this tech's comment. This customer appeared quite concerned to hear what this tech said to me. The customer had every right to be concerned because the stress level in the pharmacy was incredible, a perfect opportunity for a mistake. Of course, I tried to act like I hadn't heard anything unusual, but in reality I wanted to strangle that tech for speaking loud enough for (at least) one customer to hear.

Chapter 14

The McDonald's-ization of pharmacy

Speed may be the core concept that describes chain pharmacy today, just as speed is the core concept that describes fast food franchises like McDonald's, Burger King and Wendy's. Chain pharmacy is based on high volume. High volume and understaffing dictate that employees work at breakneck pace.

Countless times throughout my career, I've worked with pharmacists in their sixties or early seventies and I've felt sad that, after a long career, these pharmacists are still forced to run around the pharmacy like young graduates still in their physical prime. I'm sad when I see these older pharmacists racing back and forth between the pharmacy shelves, then back to the computer, then over to the cash register, then back to answer the phone, then over to the drive-thru window, then back to the register to counsel a customer, then up to the manager's office to get change for the register, then back to check an Rx filled by a tech, then over to a corner of the pharmacy to take a quick bite of a sandwich without customers watching. Many of these steps are repeated 100 to 200 times a day.

It is very sad to see a pharmacist at any age engaging in racetrack pharmacy, but it is extra sad to see pharmacists in their sixties or early seventies being forced to run around the pharmacy with the same speed and stamina as a pharmacist 40 years younger. I feel it is demeaning to these older pharmacists. Countless times I ask myself if that's what I want my life to look like when I'm that age.

Unlike many professions in which mastery of the pertinent skills makes one's job easier each year, the pharmacist's job actually becomes more grinding and exhausting as he gets older. That is because the pharmacist's job today primarily utilizes his hands and feet rather than his drug knowledge.

Recent graduates are very happy to be out of school and they're very happy to be earning a nice paycheck, so they're usually quite willing to put up with this pace. After a few years, many of them begin to question how much longer they can maintain that pace. That's why many pharmacists question whether there is indeed a shortage of pharmacists in America, or simply a shortage of pharmacists willing to work at full throttle all day, every day, under meat-grinder conditions. The big chains are notorious for squeezing blood out of young naive pharmacists, burning them out, and then crying about a shortage of pharmacists, for which the big chains have only themselves to blame.

I'd like to ask pharmacists: How long will you be able to maintain your current pace before you find yourself totally burned out? Or is it actually possible that you will find fulfillment in your career by aspiring to enter the ranks of the fastest pharmacists in America? Did you major in pharmacy so that you can prove to the world that you have what it takes to be a fast pharmacist? When you describe your job to your spouse or parents, do you say that speed is the most important factor in your job?

There are possibly three characteristics that are most commonly used to describe pharmacists:

1. The pharmacist has a good rapport with customers and co-workers.
2. The pharmacist is knowledgeable about drugs.
3. The pharmacist fills prescriptions quickly.

From my experience, of these three traits, the big chains unquestionably place the highest value on the third quality: *fills prescriptions quickly.*

In pharmacy school, I felt that my drug knowledge would surely be my biggest asset in my career. In the real world, I discovered that, far more important than my drug knowledge is the speed with which I fill prescriptions. Fast pharmacists are held in high esteem by co-workers, supervisors, and customers. Supervisors ridicule slow pharmacists behind their back. Pharmacists who spend too much time counseling customers, obsessing over drug interactions, and double-checking prescriptions are held in especially low esteem by management. Pharmacists are viewed by management like production workers at a General Motors assembly plant.

One pharmacist wrote a letter to *Drug Topics* describing how some chains monitor pharmacists' speed (Kern Stafford, "Racing the red light," *Drug Topics*, Sept. 1, 2003, p. 16):

...the pharmacist must check literally hundreds of prescriptions on each shift. To slow down will mean, in some chains, a red light showing on the computer screen signifying a pharmacist is behind in checking. This red light affects his bonus and invariably brings the area managers and district managers down on him. If a student really wants to go to pharmacy school for eight years, get that Pharm.D. degree, and then stand in one spot racing the red light with hundreds of prescriptions coming off the conveyor belt, good for him. The money is good, $85,000 and more in some places. But what about the health of the consumer, the drug interactions that are ignored, all in the name of speed?....

The big chains carry out "time and motion" studies to make the pharmacy run more efficiently. The big chains regret that they are not able to re-engineer the genome of pharmacists to make us faster, more accurate, and more efficient like a machine. The suits at the big chains lose sleep over the terrifying thought that a pharmacist somewhere in the chain is actually caught up. If a pharmacist is caught up, that is a sign tech staffing needs to be cut, yet again.

Pharmacists complain that the speed with which we're forced to fill prescriptions endangers the safety of our customers. Our supervisors tell us that more errors occur when the pharmacy is slow because our attention wanders. That is like saying speeding on an icy road is good because the inherent danger forces us to pay attention.

New technology is supposed to make the pharmacist's job easier but it seems that the pace in the pharmacy worsens every year. Pharmacy technology has indeed made the pharmacist's job easier in some ways. Counting machines (pill counters) make the counting of pills less onerous and time consuming. Pharmacy computers are great for "filling and billing" functions. Computerized automatic replenishment of drugs means the pharmacist doesn't have to spend an hour or two each week eyeballing every product on his shelves for the weekly warehouse order. Another innovation is the automatic calculation of the hours that techs and clerks work. Pharmacists no longer have to add up, with a calculator, the hours on each employee's time card at the end of the week. There are many examples of labor-saving and time-saving technology in the pharmacy. The logical question is "Why doesn't the introduction of new technology in the pharmacy make the pharmacy a more relaxed place?" The answer: With each new labor-saving technology, staffing is cut proportionately to the amount of labor that the innovation saves.

Compounding the problem of speed in the drugstore is the widespread expectation among customers for a quick fix for every ill. Customers are not interested in significant discussions about ways they can prevent their condition, nor do pharmacists have the time (or, in many cases, the desire) to engage in such conversations. With the commodification of health in this country, customers have come to believe that the solution to whatever ails them is simply a matter of finding the "right" product. If pharmacies are simply about the distribution of products, can we blame our customers for placing so much importance on the speed with which we provide those products? In this view of pharmacy, prescription drugs are a commodity just like toothpaste, shampoo, and deodorant. In reality, prescription drugs are powerful substances that can cause serious problems if not used carefully.

Drive-thru pharmacy

The profession has itself to blame, at least partly, for the culture of speed at the drugstore. With the widespread use of drive-thru

windows at pharmacies, we have convinced our customers that prescription drugs are like hamburgers, i.e., the final product should be
ready within a couple of minutes. Not surprisingly, the number one
question that customers ask us is "How long will it take?" Customers wonder why it should take more than a couple of minutes to fill a
prescription for birth control pills since the pills are already in the
packet, or a prescription for a skin condition since the cream is already in the tube.

Most chain pharmacists feel passionately about the subject of
pharmacy drive-thru windows. In my experience, nearly all chain
pharmacists hate the drive-thru since we don't have nearly enough
staffing to handle it. People drive up and ask the pharmacist to get
them a pack of cigarettes or a roll of film while we've got five to ten
people inside staring at us, waiting for us to fill their prescriptions. In
total disgust, one pharmacist said to me, "I'm going to start asking
them if they want fries, too!" When she was finally transferred to a
store without a drive-thru window, she said to me, "You wouldn't
believe how happy I was to lock that drive-thru window the night of
my last day at that store."

One day I asked a floater pharmacist whom I've known for several years whether he had ever worked in one of the newer stand-
alone stores. (A floater pharmacist is one who does not have an assigned store. He fills in wherever he's needed for vacations, sick
days, etc.) These stand-alone stores are not part of a strip shopping
center as are most of the stores in the chain I work for. He said that
he had no desire to do that because he doesn't like "working at Hardee's." (Hardee's is a fast-food chain specializing in roast beef sandwiches.) He said that all these new stand-alone stores have drive-thru
windows and that he absolutely hates drive-thru windows.

All the pharmacists I know who have worked at a store with a
drive-thru window feel that they're absurd because they increase the
already present danger of a mistake in a hyperstressful work environment. Most pharmacists also seem to feel that drive-thru windows are demeaning to pharmacy because the drive-thru windows
imply that prescriptions are analogous to fast food. The drive-thru
window reinforces customers' views that lightning-quick prescription
service is reasonable.

Pharmacists today are trying to convince the public that we do far more than simply dispense drugs. We are available to answer your questions and to advise you on the optimal use of your medications. Pharmacists are very worried about the rapid growth of mail order pharmacy facilities. Pharmacists fear that customers will be satisfied receiving medications from a mail order facility located in some distant part of the country. Pharmacists are afraid that mail order pharmacy will replace community pharmacy. Thus pharmacists are very concerned about job security and the profitability of the community pharmacy. The extreme popularity of drive-thru windows at drugstores tells our customers that prescription drugs are no different from any consumer product that can arrive in the mail, like books from Amazon.com. So far, pharmacists have not been very successful in convincing the public that there is value in face-to-face contact with pharmacists.

As we lean our head out the drive-thru window and shout a few words above the traffic noise ("Be sure to take this antibiotic until it's all gone," for example), the parallel to the McDonald's drive-thru window becomes inescapable. McDonald's dispenses fast food. Pharmacists today dispense fast prescriptions and "quick-fix" remedies. Discussions of things like what's actually causing someone's disorder are not even considered important. Our medical system no longer has time to examine causes. There's only time for the prescribing of pills. In my opinion, this can only be described as a cold and impersonal health care system.

It is no longer possible to become a pharmacist with a bachelor's degree in pharmacy (B. S. Pharm). All the pharmacy schools now require a doctorate (Pharm. D.) to become a pharmacist. This illustrates the absurdity in pharmacy today. The people who are graduating from pharmacy schools now are armed with more education than pharmacists in the past. But the movement in this country is away from face-to-face contact with pharmacists. Even though all the newly-graduating pharmacists now have doctorates, the big drugstore chains don't like the idea of pharmacists spending time talking to customers because it slows down production. And the big insurance companies are pushing people to have prescriptions filled at distant mail order facilities where the only contact with a pharmacist is via a toll-free phone number. The pharmacy schools are promoting the idea of the pharmacist as drug advisor. The marketplace, however, has not embraced this role for pharmacists. The marketplace is forcing pharmacy and pharmacists into the fast food model which views the pharmacist's advice as unnecessary or a luxury that the system can't afford.

Drive-thru windows may be great for burgers, banks, and dry cleaners, but they can be disastrous for prescriptions. After one mix-up at our pharmacy drive-thru, my partner said to me, "This really scares me. Customers need to realize that these aren't cheeseburgers that we're dispensing!"

The pharmacists I know agree that pharmacy drive-thrus are demeaning to pharmacy and represent a decline in professionalism. The drive-thru implies that prescriptions are analogous to fast food and that lightning-quick service is reasonable. Contrast the professionalism instilled in students while in pharmacy school with the real world of McPharmacy.

The public seems to feel that pharmacists do little more than dispense products. Pharmacists are trying to convince the public that we dispense critical drug information to go along with that product. The growing popularity of drive-thru windows creates the impression that it is indeed simply products that we dispense.

I don't know a single pharmacist who enjoys working in stores with drive-thru windows. I heard that one local pharmacist went to work for a competitor when he heard that his employer was replacing his store (in a strip mall) with a freestanding version with a drive-thru.

Customers have the perception that drive-thru windows can provide the pharmacy equivalent of McDonald's with scripts filled instantaneously, no waiting involved. Even repeat customers have a hard time understanding that prescriptions are different from burgers.

Some pharmacists refuse to allow customers to wait at the drive-thru. Yet some customers protest that they've got a sick child or elderly parent at home and that they need to return with the medication right away. Some pharmacists will go ahead and put these prescriptions ahead of others in line. Other pharmacists refuse to give special treatment to drive-thru customers.

Some of the drive-thru windows are bullet-resistant, creating a barricade-like setting complete with pneumatic tubes. The interaction with the pharmacist is as mechanical and sterile as a bank drive-thru. Is this the most conducive environment in which to educate customers about their medications, i.e., through microphones, speakers, with the engine roaring, and the car stereo blasting? You've never really experienced pharmacy until you've attempted to answer customers' questions at a drive-thru window without pneumatic tubes, where car exhaust fumes drift into the open pharmacy window.

Drive-thru windows may be good if we want to change the name of our store to something like Drugs-R-Us or Speedy-Rx or Drug-In-A-Box. And when customers ask for a two-month supply of their meds (rather than their usual one-month supply), maybe we should begin saying that the customer wants to SUPER SIZE his Rx order.

As if we didn't already have enough problems in the pharmacy, now we've got to endure the absurdity of people honking their horn at the drive-thru window, wondering why their prescriptions haven't been filled in two minutes. I once witnessed the second-in-line customer at our drive-thru honking his horn at the customer in front of him for being at the window too long. Or was he honking his horn at us (the pharmacy staff) for failing to move traffic through the window as quickly as McDonald's?

In one store, I was told that a customer at the drive-thru got the wrong medications as follows. The tech went to the window and asked for the patient's name. The tech misunderstood the patient's name and picked up the Rx bag for a customer with a similar-sounding name. The tech then read the name on the Rx bag to the customer at the drive-thru. Apparently the noise of the engine interfered with clear communication. The customer nodded in agreement when the tech read the name on the Rx bag. The customer went to the local emergency room when he discovered the error (after he had taken some of the wrong medication). There was no harm to the customer but I am told that he did indeed sue. I did not hear the final outcome of the lawsuit. Probably my employer quietly agreed to a small settlement. In my opinion, this type of error would be less likely to occur if the customer had picked up the medication inside the store rather than at the drive-thru window. I make the following observation only half-jokingly: It seems that the customer was guilty of *contributory negligence.* The customer contributed to the error by choosing to pick up his medications at the drive-thru window. Pharmacy customers need to realize that communication at the drive-thru window can be difficult and that drive-thru windows increase the chances of an error at the drugstore.

On days that we're severely understaffed, the pharmacist on duty may decide to close the drive-thru window for a few hours. In my experience, this always irritates the non-pharmacist store manager because he (the non-pharmacist store manager), like our customers, thinks drugstores dispense burgers. I've seen many non-pharmacist store managers who sit comfortably in their office (resting, eating, talking on the phone, etc.) for periods of time that pharmacists can only dream of. Yet these same non-pharmacist store managers call our district manager when the pharmacist closes the drive-thru window in response to dangerous understaffing.

I worked in one store in which the drive-thru window is located an insanely long distance from the rest of the pharmacy. One pharmacist there said that the architect who designed the layout of that store deserves to be hanged from a rafter in the ceiling. The technicians at this store were engaged in an ongoing grudge match with each other. Each tech criticized the other techs for not taking their fair share of the long walks to assist customers waiting at the drive-thru window.

There was one pharmacist at this store who was an absolute stickler for following rules. But he followed only those rules he agreed with. He was, of course, well aware of the pharmacy board's counseling requirement but he felt that the insanely long walk to the drive-thru window released him from his duty to counsel customers at the drive-thru.

The boards of pharmacy are good at mandating lots of things that pharmacists view as non-critical. For example, the boards enforce regulations specifying that we have on hand certain reference books or compounding equipment that we never use. But where are the boards when we need them to do something useful like outlawing drive-thru windows as a threat to the public safety?

Pharmacists who have been out of school for only a few months very often begin comparing our jobs to McDonald's or Burger King. It doesn't take long for these young graduates to become disillusioned. In my experience, the McDonald's analogy is possibly the single most frequently used description of our workplace by pharmacists on the front lines of chain pharmacy. The only difference of opinion among pharmacists as regards the fast food analogy seems to be which specific burger outlet pharmacists cite in comparison. For example, one pharmacist posted a message on the Internet discussion group sci.med.pharmacy: "The drive-thru has really cheapened the image of the pharmacist as a professional. Drive-thru windows have given people the impression that going to the drugstore is like going to Burger King or the bank."

A few years back, Merriam-Webster added the term "McJob" to one of its dictionary revisions. I recall reading a news story that noted McDonald's wasn't too happy with this addition. Many pharmacists refer to our workplace as McPharmacy. One pharmacist sent me an e-mail in response to one of my *Drug Topics* editorials. He wrote simply: "Pharmacist for 38 years: 13 in hospital pharmacy, 14 as store owner, 11 in chain pharmacy. Our profession in the chain pharmacy setting has deteriorated to what I refer to as 'McPharmacy.' Need I write more?"

A third-year pharmacy student wrote to me:

It's so funny that you are comparing pharmacy to fast food. Maybe I'm a little out of the loop here, and maybe this comparison has been made by others but I haven't heard it yet. I thought I was the only one who saw such a similarity between the two. Last week, I went inside the local In & Out. It was the first time I had been in a fast food joint in a long time. While I was waiting for my order, I watched the workers do their thing and I started to get a bit of anxiety, as it seemed all too familiar, despite the fact that I had never ever worked fast-food before. And then of course it hit me. It reminds me of work at the pharmacy. The fast pace, the long lines, the hierarchy, the audience watching and waiting for their order, the drive through!!! I went home and told my mom that I'm nothing but a glorified fast food clerk. Sometimes I'm even the cook (we do compounding at our pharmacy and the standards we use really suck, just like at a fast food place). You are so right about the fast food model and I'm so glad someone with your experience and background sees it that way too. I thought I was going nuts. I feel better now.

Even though the comparison to McDonald's is made constantly in the retail setting, some of our colleagues are angered by this analogy. This analogy often seems to be strongly frowned upon by pharmacists who don't actually toil on the front lines. Among some pharmacists in supervisory, administrative, or executive positions, discussions of working conditions are avoided the way some parents avoid discussing sex with their kids: pretend it doesn't exist. The pharmacy schools, pharmacy boards, and pharmacy associations often consider the McDonald's analogy to be too negative, too cynical, too divisive. Some pharmacists say that the term "McPharmacy" disrespects and trivializes pharmacy. The schools, boards, and associations avoid discussing working conditions because if these groups acknowledged the problem, they would be viewed as wimps for not trying to do something to remedy the situation. These pharmacists with jobs other than dispensing often have a vested interest in downplaying complaints about working conditions voiced by pharmacists on the front lines. These pharmacists do whatever they can to protect their current position so that they can stay away from the hyperstressful environment in drugstores where pharmacists fill prescriptions as fast as their hands and feet will allow. The pharmacists with jobs other than dispensing often seem to have a callous attitude toward their disillusioned colleagues in drugstores, feeling that being positive is more important than being frank: "Stop whining!" "Find another job!" "Don't renew your license!" "Leave the profession!"

Drug Topics occasionally publishes letters from disgruntled pharmacists. The magazine also publishes letters from pharmacists who write something like, "I'm tired of reading letters in *Drug Topics* written by pharmacists who are unhappy! These pharmacists need to do more than complain! They need to find a job with a different employer or leave the profession."

Should pharmacists on the front lines of pharmacy be castigated for using the McDonald's analogy? Should our colleagues who are offended by this analogy bully pharmacy magazine editors into avoiding references to fast food? In my opinion, the pharmacists who would like to prohibit use of the McDonald's analogy prefer a Pollyanna view of pharmacy. They seem to prefer to gloss over the fact that many of our colleagues are genuinely disillusioned with the big drugstore chains. The critics of the fast food analogy strike me as callously unconcerned about their colleagues who, in many cases, are wondering why they ever chose pharmacy.

Despite salaries of close to $100,000 per year directly out of pharmacy school, many young pharmacists are seriously questioning their career choice soon after graduation. Do the pharmacists who are happy with their jobs have a right to silence their disillusioned colleagues? One pharmacist wrote to me, "I cried twice last week. My job is eating me alive." Is it callous for us to suggest that this pharmacist simply discard her years of schooling and leave the profession?

The fast food model makes the practice of pharmacy nothing like the profession pharmacists hoped they were entering. Pharmacists are trained in pharmacy school to be drug experts but the big chains don't want any part of that. Working for the big chains is a production job, just like so many others in the manufacturing sector of our society. Pharmacists are valued for the speed with which we fill prescriptions. In contrast, many pharmacists would like to be evaluated by the quality of advice we give to customers, and how well we are able to help customers achieve a successful outcome with their medications.

The big chains, in adopting the fast food model, want to decrease counseling and decrease circumstances in which a pharmacist's judgment is necessary. Many pharmacists working for the big chains know that their bosses have utter disdain for pharmacists who spend too much time counseling customers.

McDonald's serves fast food. In my opinion, compared to mom's home cookin', McDonald's food isn't really that tasty. It has what can perhaps be referred to as a mass-produced quality and taste. But I suppose McDonald's food can indeed be loosely defined as "food." Similarly, drugstores sling out prescriptions at an incredible pace. Yes, we get the right drug to the right customer most of the time. But few pharmacists would say that we have the time to perform our job in a superior manner. We don't have enough time to counsel our customers adequately or to give adequate attention to potential drug interactions. Sometimes we're forced to take educated guesses when confronted with doctors' poor handwriting or questionable doses.

I'm getting tired of hearing the big chains complain about a pharmacist shortage. I think it is more accurate to say that there is a shortage of pharmacists willing to work in a sweatshop environment that values speed and production only. Quantity is valued much more highly than quality. Churning out prescriptions is valued much more highly than educating our customers about proper use of their medications.

Among the pharmacists I know, most of them remain only a few years, at most, with one chain and then switch to another chain in hopes that surely conditions can't be this bad throughout the industry. Many pharmacists can name several of their colleagues who have left the profession, gone part-time, or happily placed their dispensing career on hold to raise a family.

Many pharmacists resent the fact that the fast food industry doesn't seem to have a problem in providing adequate staffing for the dispensing of hamburgers, while many of the big drugstore chains are clearly unable or unwilling to provide adequate staffing for the dispensing of a far more critical product: prescription drugs.

The message sent to the public by drive thru windows is directly opposite the message that most pharmacists hope to send to the public. The public logically asks, "If drugstores aren't associated with speed, why do they have drive thru windows?" Our message should be that pharmacy is about advice on using medications for maximum benefit. The drive thru window convinces the public that pharmacy is simply about products, not advice. Pharmacists have inadvertently given the public the impression that pharmacy is simply about the speedy dispensing of products, that the pharmacist's relationship with customers is mainly mercantile, not cognitive.

In my experience, in contrast to chain pharmacists, independent pharmacists seem to love the drive thru window. Independent pharmacists would probably characterize the drive thru as being about convenience, not speed. The difference is that independent pharmacy owners can increase staffing sufficiently to handle the drive thru, whereas chain pharmacists don't even have enough staffing for stores without a drive thru. Staffing levels at chain drugstores are tightly controlled by the corporate office based on numbers of prescriptions filled. For example, chain pharmacists can usually determine technician scheduling, but not the number of technicians we can hire or the 'budget hours' for technicians.

Perhaps we can trace many of the current problems in pharmacy to the time when the fast food model was first applied to the drugstore.

In response to one of my editorials in *Drug Topics* in which I complained about the speed with which pharmacists are forced to fill prescriptions, the wife of a pharmacist wrote to me saying her husband is a "fast fill pharmacist." (I assume he must be an independent pharmacist. I don't know many spouses of chain pharmacists who would find fault with my criticism of understaffing in chains.) How can the label "fast fill pharmacist" be a description pharmacists aspire to? Does being a "fast fill pharmacist" lead to a fulfilling career? Did we enter pharmacy because we all yearn to "fill 'em faster"? Should pharmacists be proud that "speed" is one of the most important criteria used in judging us?

Pharmacy customers have two primary concerns: How much will it cost and how long will it take. Yet for each prescription that pharmacists fill, we have to check at least five absolutely critical things:

1. the right drug is being dispensed
2. the directions are correct
3. the dosage is reasonable
4. there are no drug interactions
5. the prescription is being filled under the correct customer's name.

If a pharmacist fills 200 prescriptions on his shift, he has to check at least one thousand things (200 X 5 = 1,000), an error in any of which can be disastrous.

It is true that McDonald's clerks, like pharmacists, need to be careful in filling orders, but clearly the consequences of a misfill at the drugstore are potentially a lot more serious than misfilling an order at McDonald's. If McDonald's gives someone a Big Mac instead of a cheeseburger, the customer is unlikely to sue or go to the hospital. At McDonald's, the worst thing that will probably happen is that the customer will be very rude to the clerk who made the mistake. At the drugstore, the worst thing that can happen is that our mistake kills the customer.

McDonald's is sued for ridiculous reasons like failing to warn a customer that the coffee is hot. (That was an actual lawsuit several years ago.) Pharmacists are sued for failing to warn customers about uncommon side effects of drugs, like the anti-depressant trazodone causing priapism—an unusually prolonged erection. (*Drug Topics*, May 6, 2002, p. 42).

McDonald's clerks don't have to learn strange lingo like *hs* (at bedtime), *qid* (four times a day), *pc* (after meals), *ac* (before meals), and *qd* (daily) as pharmacy technicians do. McDonald's clerks don't have the learn a huge list of long generic names in order to fill customers' orders. McDonald's employees usually find hamburgers, fish sandwiches, and Apple Turnovers nicely arranged on stainless steel shelves near the cash registers. In contrast, pharmacy technicians need to learn a long list of generic names so that they will know that cyclobenzaprine is shelved beside Flexeril, prochlorperazine is beside Compazine, doxazosin is beside Cardura, methocarbamol is beside Robaxin, etc. McDonald's has only a few dozen items on the menu, whereas the average pharmacy may have a couple thousand items in its inventory.

So, for our customers who think that drugstores are just like McDonald's (i.e., orders should be ready in less than two minutes), here is my list of reasons why your local drugstore is *not* McDonald's:

• McDonald's doesn't have to screen each order to make sure there are no duplicate therapies, inappropriate dosages, or drugs interactions.
• McDonald's does not accept insurance cards. McDonald's doesn't have to call insurance companies about rejected insurance claims.

• McDonald's doesn't have to explain to customers the fine details of insurance companies' complex tiered co-pay schedules.

• McDonald's doesn't have to deal with arrogant doctors (and their staff) or their illegible handwriting and incorrect dosages.

• McDonald's doesn't have to call doctors' offices for refill authorizations.

• McDonald's doesn't have to call answering services to track down doctors after office hours.

• McDonald's doesn't have to keep records indicating that they were only able to partially fill an order and, consequently, owe a customer, for example, 14 additional Prevacid 20mg.

• McDonald's doesn't counsel customers.

• McDonald's doesn't have orders coming in via phone, fax, and the Internet.

• McDonald's doesn't have to tell customers what foods or drinks to avoid.

• McDonald's doesn't have to tell customers what to do if a dose is missed.

• McDonald's doesn't have to tell customers about side effects, contraindications, precautions, warnings, and potential drug interactions. McDonald's doesn't have to ask customers if they are allergic to penicillin. McDonald's doesn't have to warn pregnant women about the use of certain products.

• McDonald's doesn't have to show customers how to measure 0.5 ml on a dropper or the proper technique for instilling eye drops.

• Whereas McDonald's can just scoop a bunch of french fries into a cardboard container, pharmacists and techs need to count pills precisely. Each french fry is worth one or two cents; in contrast, pharmacists often handle pills than cost several dollars each.

Both drugstores and fast food outlets have to contend with drive-thru windows and impatient customers. Unless the pharmacy has the latest pneumatic tubes, pharmacists (like McDonald's clerks) have the pleasure of inhaling car exhaust fumes as we lean our head out the window to hand our customers their orders. Drugstores and fast food outlets both have high school girls who work part-time and who are more interested in jabbering about their boyfriends than filling orders correctly.

Sheryl Szeinbach and colleagues at The Ohio State University College of Pharmacy co-authored a study examining whether pharmacy drive-thrus contribute to errors. They concluded that this is indeed the case. (Emily Caldwell, *OSU Research News*, "Pharmacists Believe Drive-Through Windows Contribute to Delays, Errors." http://www.pharmacy.ohio-state.edu/news/med_errors.cfm):

Consumers who pick up their prescription medications at a pharmacy drive-through window might be jeopardizing their own safety in the name of convenience.

A new study indicates that pharmacists who work at locations with drive-through windows believe the extra distractions associated with window service contribute to processing delays, reduced efficiency and even dispensing errors.

The surveyed pharmacists reported that the design and layout of their workplace has an impact on dispensing accuracy, especially the presence of drive-through window pick-up services.

The study suggests pharmacy design should emphasize minimal workflow interruptions but it also offers a caution to consumers to check their prescription medications, especially those obtained from a pharmacy's drive-through window, said Sheryl Szeinbach, the study's lead author and a professor of pharmacy practice and administration at Ohio State University.

"Maybe we ought to stop and consider: 'Am I likely to get the same level of service from the drive-through as I am actually interacting face-to-face with a health-care professional?'" Szeinbach said.

With the number of prescriptions dispensed annually in the United States nearing the 4 billion mark, Szeinbach said the public is best served by pharmacists with the fewest possible distractions. Even with stringent internal quality controls, pharmacists nationally make an estimated 5.7 errors per 10,000 prescriptions processed, according to the study, which translates to more than 2.2 million dispensing errors each year.

Responding pharmacists attributed about 80 percent of dispensing errors to cognitive problems that Szeinbach said could be associated with various disruptions that interfere with their work.

The survey results were published in a recent issue of the *International Journal for Quality in Health Care*.

Szeinbach and colleagues surveyed 429 U.S. pharmacists working at pharmacies located within mass merchant retailers, traditional chain drugstores or independently owned shops. The questionnaire sought pharmacists' perceptions of how their practice was affected by the pharmacy layout and design, the presence of a drive-through window and the availability of an automated dispensing system. Specifically, they were asked whether those factors had a positive or negative influence on errors in dispensing, communication between staff and pharmacists, prescription processing time, efficiency and physical mobility in the practice setting.

Participating pharmacists were asked to respond to questions using a scale from 1 to 5, with 1 indicating pharmacists strongly disagreed with suggestions that their practice was affected by these factors and 5 meaning they strongly agree.

While the responding pharmacists agreed that the layout and design of their workplace could contribute to errors and reduce efficiency, the presence of a drive-through window elicited a much more definitive response, Szeinbach said.

"The drive-through window, overall, poses a huge problem with respect to causing dispensing errors, contributing to communication errors, delaying processing and forcing staff to take more steps," Szeinbach said. "Think about it – that window has to be in an area that's convenient for the patient driving up to the window, yet may not – and obviously is not – convenient to the pharmacist and the staff. The link between drive-through and dispensing errors alone should be a concern to the public."

She said the findings suggest that consumers should always check the prescription medications they pick up at a pharmacy to confirm they received the right medicine.

According to the survey, pharmacists perceive that the drive-through window has the biggest impact on causing pharmacists and their staff to take extra steps (average agreement response of 3.7 on a 5-point scale); reducing efficiency (average response of 3.8); and causing delays in prescription processing (average response of 3.7). The respondents also attributed dispensing errors (average response of 3.2) and communication errors (average response of 3.3) to the presence of a drive-through window.

Szeinbach suggested the addition of a drive-through to a pharmacy has the potential to place unreasonable multitasking demands on professionals whose job includes counseling patients about medication use, not simply dispensing the drugs.

"A pharmacist or staff member could be responsible for four or five tasks, and serving people at the drive-through window is just one of them," she said. "Some people seeking the convenience of the drive-through window don't care about getting information. They just want the medication, and they want it as fast as possible. They should probably think about that and at least look at the medication and make sure it's OK. And if they have questions, it may behoove them to come into the pharmacy."

She noted that an additional study comparing actual error rates at pharmacies with and without drive-through windows is needed to verify her results.

"There's a potential bias that could exist against drive-through windows," she said. "But since the responding pharmacists pointed out the drawbacks of both drive-through windows and the entire layout and design, and their responses are fairly consistent, it leads me to believe their perceptions are probably accurate."

Szeinbach co-authored the study with Enrique Seoane-Vazquez and graduate students Ashish Parekh and Michelle Herderick, all of Ohio State's College of Pharmacy.

The chain drugstore environment is certainly not conducive to viewpoints that question pharmaceuticals. The typical chain drugstore is highly regimented and requires strict adherence to corporate rules. The modern drug chain is tightly controlled to the point of being nearly coercive. It is in such an environment that non-conformist ideas are highly frowned upon. Our job is to fill prescriptions as quickly as we can and not to question whether non-drug approaches may be more logical.

I can understand that corporations need conformity, efficiency, discipline, and a willingness by employees to work hard. I'm all in favor of efficiency and hard work and discipline. I realize that corporations need conformity if they are to avoid total chaos. But chain drugstores are run on the McDonald's, Burger King, and Wendy's models. Time and motion studies are done to maximize productivity. All this may serve to make the drug chain more competitive and allow us to sell drugs at a lower price (independent drugstores do, however, often beat the chains' prices). But the consequence of rigid conformity in procedures is a rigid conformity in ideas.

As the huge insurance companies dictate the nature of our medical system, pharmacists are forced to process more customers in less time. This results in a resentment by pharmacists toward the system. Customers are viewed as the problem. More customers means more workload, yet staffing always lags far behind workload.

The system is absolutely draining pharmacists of compassion. If we're running behind all day, each customer who approaches the pharmacy is only making the situation worse. Many pharmacists hope that business will not increase (blasphemous thoughts to the corporation) because an increase means that we will have to do more work with little or no increase in staffing.

As you approach the pharmacy, many pharmacists think: *Here comes another customer to get me even further behind.* Customers become the enemy because they rush us when we're already stressed to the breaking point. Even though there may be only few customers waiting near the pharmacy counter at a given time, this doesn't mean that the pharmacist isn't running an hour or two behind with a backlog of prescriptions that customers will be returning to pick up.

I once saw a sign in a restaurant that reminded me of my job: "Waitresses are like swans—calm and collected on the surface but paddling like hell underneath." We pharmacists paddle like hell to keep up with the prescription flow. The system is absolutely turning pharmacists into automatons. Pharmacy has become an endurance contest to see whether we can make it through the day without getting drowned by the prescription flow and without losing control of our emotions.

Pharmacist Bob Crocker from Farmville, North Carolina, ran for a seat on the North Carolina Board of Pharmacy in June of 1995. I received a postcard from him in the mail seeking support for his candidacy. He made several observations about pharmacists' working conditions. His observations about working conditions are as relevant today as they were in 1995.

Fellow Retail Pharmacist

I called a fellow pharmacist a few weeks ago and asked if he could meet me for lunch. He informed me he didn't get a scheduled lunch break and didn't have enough help to leave the pharmacy for even a few minutes. I thought to myself "even galley slaves get a lunch break." I don't know if this situation is the "exception" or the "norm" – but it should be the EXCEPTION!

I have heard from numerous sources that the [North Carolina Board of Pharmacy] has received several letters complaining of dangerous work conditions and asking for help in remedying the situation. To me it is unconscionable to set legal requirements for a professional and not provide him the ability to control his work environment to meet those requirements.

IT IS TIME FOR A CHANGE. Retail pharmacists need someone on the Board who knows what they face on a daily basis. I can be that person. I am a "working" retail pharmacist with both chain & independent experience.

Here's a typical letter to the editor that pharmacists find routinely in the pharmacy magazines. Sometimes pharmacists are brave enough to sign the letters even though we fear that our employer may see them in the magazines. Obviously the big chains would like to keep descriptions of pathetic and dangerous working conditions out of the pages of national pharmacy magazines. The following letter was published as "Name withheld by request." ("Burned-Out Pharmacist," *American Druggist*, May 1995, p. 8)

If honest want ads were run by discount store chains and chain drug stores, here is how they would read: Our pharmacists must be able to—
1. Work 10 hours a day without a break.

2. Answer the phone in three rings while ringing up sales, helping customers, and filling prescriptions.

3. Fill 150 to 250 prescriptions daily, one every three minutes.

4. Control bodily functions in order to limit bathroom breaks to one or two a day.

5. Deal with young, immature assistants who are jealous of your wages.

6. Take constant abuse from customers, store managers, and associates with a smile.

This mess has come about only in the last 10 years. Bottom lines and store traffic should not obliterate patient care. It's time to speak up for the profession. Everyone must protest these conditions. The companies cannot retaliate against us all.

Upon graduation from pharmacy school, young pharmacists very often suffer severe culture shock when they experience the real world of the chain drugstore. Professors in pharmacy schools prepare students to be highly-trained drug experts but the big chain drugstores don't want drug experts. The big chains want fast food experts. I think the pharmacy schools should practice "truth in advertising" by discussing with students what pharmacy is like in the real world. Over the years, I have heard several pharmacists suggest that a class-action lawsuit should be initiated against pharmacy schools for grossly misrepresenting the real world.

What kinds of pharmacists are most likely to have long-term survival in the chain environment? I have concluded that pharmacists with an "attitude" and a thick skin are the ones who are best able to tolerate their jobs. If you are too compassionate, you will soon be run over by rude and impatient customers. A warm and caring pharmacist in a busy chain drug store will soon be mowed down by a clientele that is too often arrogant, aggressive, and abusive.

The fast food model is the only one that works in a typical understaffed pharmacy. Pharmacists often refer to our job as "herding the masses." The education-prevention-caring-listening model simply doesn't work at McPharmacy. If we pharmacists spend too much time giving advice to customers, we're causing the herd to bottleneck. Rudeness increases the speed of herding customers. The friendlier I am to customers, the more they want to tell me their life story or at least their medical history. Countless times people tell me that their spouse is recovering from a heart attack or from bypass surgery or from cancer and all I have time to do is simulate a facial expression that I care. In reality, the speed of the prescription assembly line has drummed out most of my compassion. If I have customers making faces at me all day implying that I'm too slow, how much compassion do you think I have left to sympathize with their health problems? I think many of my colleagues would agree that chain pharmacy can destroy a pharmacist's empathy.

I once spoke with a pharmacist who had just graduated from pharmacy school and was licensed for only about a week. Not surprisingly, he was having trouble entering cardholder information into the pharmacy computer for customers with various prescription insurance plans. Many insurance companies have some unique little quirk with cardholder information that makes pharmacists' lives miscrable. This pharmacist told me that he had just made an observation about crowd control. He said that there can be several customers waiting calmly and patiently for their prescriptions. Then, all of a sudden, one customer makes some jackass comment about having to wait too long. Hearing this rude comment, all the other customers collectively become agitated and seem to adopt a herd mentality such as: "Yeah! You pharmacist son-of-a-bitch who is part of the price-gouging drug conspiracy in America. HOW MUCH LONGER IS IT GOING TO BE!!!???" He told me that one of his classmates had experienced the same feeling and that this classmate announced to those waiting at that store, "Now wait just a minute! This isn't Burger King! You'll get your prescription when it's ready!" Throughout this book, it may appear that I repeat the hamburger and fast-food metaphor excessively, but that is only because pharmacists routinely use it to describe our very stressful jobs.

I need to have an attitude if I want to be able to herd customers efficiently and if I want to avoid being run over by an impatient public. It is a fact that the friendlier I am with customers, the more likely that they are to want to talk. And the more likely they are to ask me a question for which I don't know the answer. So then I'd have to take more time to consult reference material. If I'm just barely cordial and very business-like, customers are less likely to set me back with long, involved questions.

Chapter 15

Are chain drugstores a threat to the public safety?

Do chain drugstores have a higher error rate per 1,000 prescriptions compared to locally-owned, independent, "mom and pop" drugstores?

Do the big chain drugstores have a higher error rate (per thousand prescriptions filled) in comparison to the error rate (per thousand prescriptions) at locally-owned, independent, "mom and pop" drugstores? I don't believe I've ever seen a study that attempted to answer this question directly. But a survey of Oregon pharmacists by the Oregon Board of Pharmacy in July 2011 strongly suggests that working conditions at chain drugstores are inferior to working conditions at locally-owned independent drugstores. Most pharmacists feel that there is a direct relationship between working conditions and pharmacy mistakes. The survey found that only 25.9 percent of *chain store* pharmacists agreed working conditions promoted safe and effective patient care—compared to 76 percent of pharmacists at *independent* pharmacies. (Oregon Board of Pharmacy, "Working Conditions Survey," July 2011
http://www.oregon.gov/pharmacy/Imports/OBOP-Pharmacy_Working_Conditions_Survey_Results11.11.pdf?ga=t)

If it is true that chain drugstores have a higher error rate per thousand prescriptions in comparison to locally-owned independent drugstores, what could explain this? Here is my theory.

If I were a pharmacist who owned the drugstore in which I worked, I would be extremely afraid of making an error in filling prescriptions because I would worry that a serious error in a small community could damage my reputation in that community and severely hurt my business. Do chain pharmacists care any less about making mistakes than pharmacists who own the drugstore in which they work? In my opinion, it depends on several factors.

I've worked for three large chains in my 25-year career. I worked for a small independent for only a few months during a summer in which I was in pharmacy school. All three of the chains I worked for had at least a thousand drugstores, divided into local districts usually consisting of fifteen to twenty drugstores. At each chain, I had a "district manager" who was in charge of these fifteen to twenty stores.

With a large turnover in chain pharmacists during most of my career, my district supervisor (or his secretary) would fill openings with any of the thirty to forty pharmacists in the local district. Thus, for example, it was quite common for the district secretary to call me and ask if I would be willing to work at a nearby store on my day off. "Nearby" could mean anything from a store that was two or three miles away to one that was thirty miles away. Most of the stores within the district were within an hour's drive of each other.

During these times of pharmacist shortages or pharmacists' vacations or sick days, a large number of pharmacists could end up filling in at given stores. It would not be uncommon, for example, to have a different pharmacist on duty at a particular store each day of the week. For example, Pharmacist A worked there on Monday, Pharmacist B worked there on Tuesday, Pharmacist C worked there on Wednesday, Pharmacist D worked there on Thursday, etc. No continuity at all.

What are the consequences of having so many pharmacists filling in at a store, as opposed to having one or two pharmacists who have worked at that store regularly for many years? The most likely consequences are 1) chaos, 2) bad morale, 3) rudeness toward customers,

4) rudeness toward the doctors and nurses who phone in prescriptions, 5) "lost" prescriptions (for example, a customer dropped off a prescription on Tuesday and returned on Wednesday only to find that the pharmacy staff can find no trace of that prescription—it happens more often than you think!).

"Fill-in" or "floater" pharmacists often have a bad attitude because they hate to arrive at a drugstore and find poorly-trained techs or no techs at all. This can be a prescription for disaster, i.e., the combination of poorly-trained techs (or no techs), high prescription volume, and a pissed-off pharmacist filling in at an understaffed store with which he is unfamiliar.

My point is that small, locally-owned, independent drugstores often have a totally different culture from that at the chain drugstores. With the pharmacist/owner present most of the time, there is a stability at independent mom-and-pop drugstores that is very often lacking at chain drugstores. The pharmacist/owner has the power to keep good technicians and he has the power to hire an adequate number of technicians.

In contrast, a chain pharmacist filling in at any of the fifteen to twenty stores in the local district is in an utterly different situation. That fill-in chain pharmacist has no control over the number of techs who happen to show up for work that day or the training level of those techs. That fill-in chain pharmacist has no incentive to nurture long-term relationships with local customers or with the doctors and nurse/receptionists who phone prescriptions to that drugstore.

Many fill-in chain pharmacists feel that they parachute into one drugstore in the district for one or two days and then they may never work in that drugstore again for many months, if at all. So why give a damn about that store? If these fill-in pharmacists arrive at that drugstore and find poorly trained techs (or no techs) and that fill-in pharmacist is "slammed" with a deluge of prescriptions, that fill-in pharmacist's attitude is very often, "Screw this company!" Such an attitude can lead to carelessness and mistakes.

Only pharmacists understand the sky-high stress levels, disgust, and sometimes rage that often results from working for a huge corporation that routinely places us in positions that jeopardize our license and make errors inevitable. Our attitude is often, "If this chain doesn't give me enough trained staffing for the safe filling of prescriptions, why should I give a damn about this chain and this store?"

The subject of "working conditions" is possibly the number one topic (hassles with customers' insurance may be number two) of pharmacists who write letters to the editor at pharmacy magazines like *Drug Topics*. The majority of these letters complain bitterly about our working conditions. But there are always a few pharmacists who write "I love my job" or "If you're unhappy, find another job." It is a fact that chain pharmacists are the largest single category of pharmacists, exceeding the numbers of pharmacists who work at independents or hospitals. So the alternatives for employment outside chain drugstores are not always great.

To be fair, there are very many chain pharmacists who are extremely concerned about mistakes, and who are extremely concerned about maintaining good relationships with customers, doctors, and nurses in the local community. Thus it is a generalization to say that pharmacists at chain drugstores have a higher error rate per store than pharmacists at small, locally-owned, independent drugstores.

Nevertheless, in my opinion, real-world conditions mean that the morale at the average independent drugstore is likely to be better than at the average chain drugstore, and that attitudes toward customers and doctors at independent drugstores are likely to be better than at the average chain drugstore. Chain pharmacists very often have a feeling of overwhelming powerlessness as we experience daily the reality of having no control over factors (like staffing levels) that can lead to serious errors. You do not want a pharmacist filling your prescriptions who feels utterly overwhelmed, panicked, and powerless. In addition, many pharmacists feel a sense of rage against the chain for such work environments.

Some chain pharmacists have worked at the same location for many years and they are very happy in their jobs. I don't personally know many of these happy pharmacists, but I see from pharmacy magazines and the pharmacy blogosphere that they do exist. Some of them are recent graduates who love their paycheck and have not yet realized (or have suppressed the fact) that their daily high-speed, high-stress, high-stakes reality is not conducive to their long-term career satisfaction and their physical and mental health.

Some pharmacists have suggested that young female pharmacists (who make up an increasing percentage of graduates from pharmacy schools) are more likely to accept bad work environments without complaint, in comparison to males, or in comparison to pharmacists who have worked for chains for more than a year or two.

The chain drugstore model seems to mean burning pharmacists out and then replacing them with recent graduates who are too naïve or docile to question things. After six or more years of college, it often takes a year or two for pharmacists to realize (or accept) that the real world is nothing like what they learned in pharmacy school. This leaves a huge number of pharmacists with a feeling of disgust toward their alma maters for misrepresenting the fact that the real world of chain drugstores is nothing like the model of pharmacist-as-drug-expert that they were taught in pharmacy school.

The Oregon Board of Pharmacy survey of pharmacists' working conditions (July 2011) was covered by both *The Oregonian* and by *Oregon Public Broadcasting*. Excerpts from both of those websites regarding this survey are below.

"Workloads, chain stores add to safety risks, Oregon pharmacist survey says"
The Oregonian, OregonLive.com
Feb. 12, 2012
Nick Budnick
http://blog.oregonlive.com/health_impact/print.html?entry=/2012/02/workloads_chain_stores_add_to.html)

A retired Paisley minister experiences sudden Parkinson's disease symptoms, so severe he believes death is imminent—only to learn it's due to the wrong medication.

A pharmacy technician in Hillsboro sells an Ativan prescription to the wrong man, who gets pulled over for driving erratically.

An Astoria woman suffers a cardiac arrest, and later learns her pharmacy for months had overdosed her with thyroid medication.

These are among the estimated hundreds of pharmacy errors reported in the last few years, either to state agencies or in lawsuits. And some pharmacists say errors are happening more than ever.

A recent survey by the Oregon Board of Pharmacy reported that more than 350 chain pharmacists—more than half of those responding—said their working conditions don't promote safe and effective patient care.

Many complained it is getting worse. "I feel that we are operating on the edge of disaster," wrote one. "It is a danger zone for us and our patients."

Last summer, the state board hosted an online survey for roughly 5,700 licensed pharmacists licensed in Oregon. The results were gratifying and disturbing, says board member Ann Zweber. She hadn't expected so many to respond—more than 1,300; unfortunately, many responded by reporting safety concerns.

"People had a lot to say," she says. "It concerns me greatly."

The survey results describe a profession in transition. Independent pharmacies, which once dominated Oregon, now number just 214 out of about 750 retail pharmacies, according to state records. As independents give way to large chains and mail-order operations, increased competition is inserting a bottom-line mentality into the way people get their pills.

Only 25.9 percent of chain store pharmacists agreed working conditions promoted safe and effective patient care—compared to 76 percent of pharmacists at independent pharmacies.

Not only that, more than 200 hundred chain pharmacists commented about workload and safety.

The survey data isn't perfect. It's anonymous and pharmacists were allowed to self-report their type of workplace. But the board believes the survey is credible, Zweber said.

Many complained of having to fill more prescriptions each day with fewer staff; of 12-hour shifts with scant breaks; and constant distractions, such as administering immunization shots to augment profits.

One reported quitting a chain job because of feeling "like I'm going to jeopardize the patients every time I stepped into that pharmacy." Another said because of lack of staff, "we have seen a huge increase in errors. We used to have a couple per month, now we have a couple per week and sometimes more than one in a day!"

Blake Rice, a pharmacist who used to sit on the state board, thinks many errors are caught internally by improved safety procedures. But he agrees chain stores don't protect the public, giving drugs "the same lack of oversight as the sale of bread and milk or canned beans."

There is no data to definitively show more pharmacy errors are occurring, or that they happen more often in chains. Pharmacies do not have to report errors to any public agency. The pharmacy board considers roughly 80 cases a year involving reporting errors. The Oregon Patient Safety Commission encourages voluntary reporting, but only 94 pharmacies have signed up.

The Institute for Safe Medication Practices solicits confidential reports of pharmacy errors from consumers and pharmacists. The group is seeing a steady increase in such reports nationwide, said Michael Cohen, a pharmacist who heads the group.

He said the group is sending its own survey. "It's hard for the pharmacists who work at these chains to complain too loudly to their manager or go public because they work there and they don't want to undergo any type of job issue," Cohen said.

Joseph Lassiter, a Pacific University pharmacy professor who sits on the Oregon Patient Safety Commission, said the Oregon survey results are disturbing. "This survey is a signal for us that there's something going on."

The board of pharmacy is considering rules to keep an eye on working conditions. The rules do not set strict workload levels, but allows the board to fine or suspend a pharmacy license over safety issues.

Patrick Bowman, owner of Tualatin Pharmacy, says he's not surprised at the survey. He founded his business 11 months ago after working in chains. "I don't have headaches anymore. I don't have trouble sleeping anymore," he said. "People come to me because they're not a number."

"Preventing Pharmacy Errors"
Oregon Public Broadcasting
AIR DATE: Wednesday, February 22nd 2012
http://www.opb.org/thinkoutloud/shows/preventing-pharmacy-cr-rors/

When you get a prescription filled, you assume that the pills in the bottle are the ones that your doctor prescribed. But if there's a mistake, the consequences could be serious. The Oregon Board of Pharmacy sent out a survey to about six thousand licensed pharmacists, trying to get a better idea about the state of the industry and pharmacists' working conditions. About 20 percent responded. The results of the non-scientific study were surprising. About 75 percent of pharmacists working for chain stores said they felt working conditions did not promote patient safety. About 25 percent of those working in independent pharmacies said the same. Board member Ann Zweber told the Oregonian that the results concerned her greatly.

GUESTS:
—Ann Zweber: Member of the Oregon Board of Pharmacy, instructor of pharmacy at Oregon State University, part-time pharmacist at Bi-Mart
—Joseph Lassiter: Pharmacy Professor at Pacific University, member of the Oregon Patient Safety Commission

---

Comments posted by Oregon pharmacists
on the Oregon Public Broadcasting website

I'm a practicing retail pharmacist who took part in this survey last year. I would have been surprised had the results of this survey NOT shown that most pharmacists feel as though their working conditions were not safe on the whole. We work very long hours (12-hour or more) and get very few breaks since most of us, if not all, are salaried and not expected to adhere to hourly labor laws. I am very disturbed when we find a mistake and we take it very seriously at my workplace. While we have put many procedures in place to prevent such mistakes and thus many procedures to deal with mistakes, they are inevitable, we are human. It seems as though the state of retail pharmacy has gotten to a point where people expect their prescriptions filled as fast as they expect a cheeseburger and french fries at a fast food chain. It is no wonder with drive-thrus in pharmacies and commercials promising 15-min wait times that people have developed ridiculous expectations of pharmacists. Also, it seems as though most pharmacies are always cutting how many hours we get for technicians and auxiliary help. We need more people in place to prevent more mistakes. **–Oregon pharmacist #1**

I'm a retail pharmacist in the Portland metro area who graduated within the past 5 years. I have been with my current company since I started school as an intern and then hired on as a pharmacist. In the years that I have been with the company, I have seen drastic decreases in the amount of technician hours a store is allowed with subsequent increases in job expectations. When I started I remember being thrilled with the profession and being able to talk to people and help them, and as much as corporate pharmacy would like you to believe that they are there to do this, we as pharmacists are stretched to the limit with our workloads. It absolutely kills me when someone comes in who really needs medical help, or needs advice on an OTC product, and I have to give them a very short/abrupt answer just so I can get back to spitting out prescriptions. As for errors in the pharmacy, they are on the rise. Pharmacists are forced to rush through verifying prescriptions. I consider myself very accurate at data verifying, but very rarely actually get the chance to think about the whole patient profile. I often catch myself thinking of things to look at after I hit enter, instead of having an extra two or three minutes to actually evaluate the patient profile. I also don't take breaks ever, and when I go to the bathroom (God forbid), I can almost count on being paged back to the pharmacy in ten seconds time. **–Oregon pharmacist #2**

I have professionally advised pharmacists caught in management squeezes in large chain store settings. Many times a pharmacist has to supervise pharmacy techs who actually answer to non-pharmacist managers in the larger retail setting of a supermarket or large chain pharmacy. Pharmacists actually have little supervisory clout within the organization and are subject to constant demands to speed up service and provide whatever the customers want. This results in mistakes, stressful personnel conflicts and a lack of accountability for the pharmacy function. I would not go to a large chain pharmacy because of the safety concerns in that environment. **–Roboturkey**

I thought I would be working till 65 and then part time after that since I enjoyed my job as a pharmacist. Things changed as the independent stores fell to the chains and their main focus is on SPEED! It has become McPharmacy, few patients want to listen to counseling, sit in their car at the drive up texting away. Speed is most important to the patient however many (most) of them refuse to provide the pharmacy with their current insurance information. More time is spent dinking around trying to find out who we are supposed to bill than actually filling the prescription. I miss the days when I actually had time to talk to the patients who seek advice, current time pressures do not allow in-depth discussions.

Long hours, no lunch, no breaks...many a day I worked 8 hours without a bathroom break. Technicians' hours have been slashed, so more and more the pharmacist is like a plate spinner, hoping to heaven that no plates drop and break. Corporate pharmacy would like nothing better than to have NO pharmacists on the payroll and as soon as they get a machine to replace us.

In the meantime they keep increasing the workload, adding vaccines, blood pressure checks, Medicare part D counseling, and cutting tech hours. Installing monitors on computers to track speed of rx filling.

I am a dinosaur from the days when pharmacists knew their patients and had time to talk to them and help with their healthcare decisions. Back in the old days when patients sometimes called you

"Doc" and not while they were on their cell phone. I used to enjoy going to work. When it got to the point of shifts ending in tears of frustration, I had to quit. **–Frustrated pharmacist**

I am a relatively new retail pharmacist (licensed less than three years) practicing in the Portland area. I completely agree with "PortlandPharmacist" but would like to emphasize the topic of "cutting hours" for ancillary staff as well as pharmacist hours and how it relates to safety in the pharmacy. Just a few years ago in a pharmacy that averaged around 1000 prescriptions per week, most pharmacies would have two pharmacists working together (overlapping with 2-3 technicians and a clerk) for at least 4-6 hours per day on busier days (Mon/Tues) and maybe 2-4 hours on less busy weekdays. It was possible to take a lunch, breaks and finish all of the prescriptions, daily filing, inventory control, ordering, re-stocking, cleaning etc.

Then, as the economy started taking a turn, and Wal-Mart's "$4.00 List" came out, our company decided that the current "labor model" wasn't working. They started basing the number of [staffing] hours they would give each pharmacy to operate with on the previous years' prescription volume, assuming no growth, and they decided to keep the pharmacies open later each night. Oh… and they implemented an "autofill" service that added to our prescription volume initially, but in many cases, we end up filling the same prescription 2-3 times because patients (still) don't pick up their prescriptions within the time allotted. So, they cut several hours out of every pharmacy's labor budget/schedule and eliminated several positions while asking us to work longer hours and duplicate work/fill additional prescriptions unnecessarily and significantly increase our vaccination services. This eliminated almost all pharmacist overlap and forced pharmacists to start working alone on weekends and evenings with no ancillary staff help and marginal help during the busier times during the week.

Pharmacists went from focusing on whether the prescriptions they were filling were clinically appropriate, correct, and that their patients were benefiting from their therapy with minimal or no side effects, providing thorough counseling (Medication Therapy Management-MTM) to just trying to get the right pills in the bottle before the end of their shift. Pharmacists are doing all of the ancillary work that used to be covered by technicians and clerks on top of all the added responsibilities of providing professional health services, immunizations, and final verification that all prescriptions in the pharmacy are correctly filled during their shift.

I saw a steady decline in morale and our work environment made many people see patients as the enemy because when they call or come to the counter they are interrupting our ability to get the work done. This is exactly the opposite reason why we became pharmacists. We wanted to promote patient safety and educate patients about the safe use of medications as well as prevent prescribing errors, but there isn't time for that in the average retail pharmacy anymore. We are overeducated pharmacy clerks (with doctorate degrees) answering the phone, running the cash register, ringing up donuts and dish soap while juggling 10 or more drug related issues per minute with our one technician yelling "Override!"

I have found and fixed many errors made by other pharmacists and admittedly I do not always report them because I don't have time. I have reported the serious errors and I have reported myself when I've made an error because I wanted to believe it would make a difference if the conditions of the pharmacy environment at the time of the mistake would be a reason for the company to give us our labor hours back. It doesn't matter and I have never been spoken to about any mistakes that I have made or reported.

I have worked several 12-13.5 hour shifts (not including travel time) with no pharmacist overlap where my ancillary staff is either untrained or not intelligent enough to occupy the position they are in. Training of pharmacy technicians and the hiring process for them are separate topics we could discuss as it pertains to patient safety. Most mistakes start with the technician typing a prescription incorrectly. This happens several times per day in most pharmacies unless you are working with an experienced, conscientious, fastidious technician. They are very rare and if you have one, it makes all the difference. The most egregious errors I have witnessed were made solely by pharmacists working alone or in understaffed busy pharmacies.

The errors occurred due to not looking at the pills in the bottle that they were labeling (that had been counted by a machine or technician) or by not actually reading the stock bottle that they were putting a label on, resulting in the patients receiving the wrong medication and having serious side effects. The side effects could have been life threatening and/or deadly.

Whether you are salaried or hourly, it is impossible for pharmacists to have a 30-minute uninterrupted lunch break if there is no pharmacist overlap. It is unlawful for any prescription to be sold if it is labeled as "New" (even if it is not new) without having a pharmacist consult with the patient. This happens on all highly controlled (C-2) medications and many refills that have been newly authorized by a physician ("reassigns" labeled as new). Whenever there is a question about an over-the-counter medication, the pharmacist has to be interrupted. If a patient has a question about a refill, the clerk or technician must interrupt the pharmacist to answer the question before the medication is sold. If a patient comes in and wants to get a flu, shingles, or travel vaccination, we are supposed to be readily available to provide this service, so once again, our break or lunch is cut short, postponed, or interrupted.

Many pharmacies are finding themselves getting one, two, even three days behind on filling prescriptions. It is disheartening when every person that comes to the pharmacy expecting their prescriptions to be ready finds they are not ready and the pharmacist has to stop what they are doing and fill that script on the spot. This constant interruption is a set-up for mistakes. Not to mention the pharmacy is understaffed on top of having the extra burden of being behind. It is a downward spiral only alleviated by the salaried managers staying late every night or coming in early to "clean-up." The managers in most cases are working 50-60 hours per week (but getting paid for 40) but would never in a million years complain to "corporate" for fear of appearing weak or incompetent. It is very sad. We used to get paid for every hour we had to stay over and we were allowed to work as long as it took to get the work done. Now that they have eliminated most of the "slow" or "weakest links" in the pool of pharmacists, with little or no regard for the quality or supply of technician help, we are all saying "Something's Gotta Give." Currently it is our health (the pharmacist's physical and mental health), our attention to "customer service," patient safety, and our career satisfaction. Does someone have to die before they realize the new labor model is not working?

All pharmacists that graduated after 2003 receive a doctorate degree. Most of us have 8 or more years of college education. We have a great responsibility to provide safe, professional healthcare services to the public. If we work for a corporation, we have little control over the tools we are given to provide the professional services we are licensed and highly educated for. We have unlicensed, unprofessional, middle management, high school dropouts micro-managing labor hours (likely because their bonuses are affected by it) and ultimately affecting safety outcomes for patients.

In school they say, "If you don't like retail then go do something else." Why does it have to be that way? Why not change retail pharmacy so it provides a professional environment for pharmacists to provide safe, professional healthcare services as well as have career satisfaction and feel like we don't have to kill ourselves attempting to make sure patients get the correct medications in a timely manner? Is it too much to ask that we close for an hour for lunch, and actually have a clean, quiet place to eat that lunch? Is it too much to ask that we not be shamed into standing for 12 hours for fear of appearing lazy or weak if we sit on a stool (if the pharmacy even has one)? I know of several pharmacists that have had deep vein thrombosis (blood clots in the legs), strokes, or are heavily medicated themselves on antidepressants, anti- anxiety, and pain meds. These issues are undoubtedly related to working conditions and stress levels. We joke around saying things like "corporate would prefer that we wear a catheter or a diaper so we don't have to leave for a bathroom break." It's just pitiful. We all have hope that somehow things will change because we enjoy the direct patient contact that retail provides and so we hang in there, but really, does someone have to die, patient or pharmacist, before retail pharmacy provides a safe, professional environment for everyone involved? **–Change Retail Now!**

I have been a pharmacist in a retail setting for 20 years. I agree with every word you've said. And I'll bet you work for Safeway, just as I do. I complain often to my district manager about our unsafe working conditions, as they relate to the health and safety of all of us working in retail pharmacies (I guess I can speak only for Safeway pharmacists) AND as they relate then to patient safety. I have been in contact with the Board of Pharmacy a couple of times in the past month begging them to DO SOMETHING about the very unsafe state of retail pharmacy in Oregon today. I, like you, know that the only thing that will prompt some legal/regulatory changes is for patient deaths to occur. I am furious and sad and just plain exhausted. I am a pharmacy manager and I can't wait to get out of this business. **-Zoemee2**

You guessed it. I do work for Safeway. It is very sad indeed. I hope the Board of Pharmacy will do something that corporate can't maneuver around with some clever policy change like our laughable meal and rest period policy. It looks great on paper but try actually implementing it in an understaffed pharmacy. It just doesn't happen. I'm hopeful that something good will come out of all the negative attention pharmacy is getting. If nothing changes, I will be looking at other options. **-Change Retail Now!**

Insurance-mandated mail order prescriptions play a major role in the erosion of patient care. As an independent pharmacist I find myself bailing out the mail order system when a prescription is not delivered on time. The cost of filling these prescriptions usually is far greater than the reimbursements. The mail order system saves the insurance provider money by shifting the cost of delivery errors to the local pharmacy. We recently filled a prescription that had a total reimbursement of 36 cents. This Rx took no less than 1 and 1/2 hours of phone time with the doctor, the insurance company, the mail order company. We often spend a great deal of time helping mail order subscribers pick out appropriate over the counter medicines. If we are lucky the patient brings in their list of current medicines, otherwise they have to go from memory of the medications and health conditions. Your corner pharmacist has always been trusted to give out free advice. I hope we can survive the mail order and loss leader chains. **–Thomas Field, RPh**

Chapter 16

Pharmacists' own words about working conditions

This chapter consists of three parts:
1. "Letters-to-the-editor" from various pharmacists published in major pharmacy magazines
2. Comments posted by pharmacists on two Internet pharmacy discussion groups (pharmacyweek.com and sci.med.pharmacy)
3. An editorial written by pharmacist Charles Duhon that was published in *Drug Topics*.

---

1. Letters-to-the-editor at various pharmacy magazines regarding pharmacists' working conditions

---

Letters-to-the-editor #1
[This pharmacist says he's "had enough" and "will no longer practice pharmacy."]

I am writing to you as a pharmacist who as of today will no longer practice pharmacy. My feelings and thoughts about the profession are so strong that I wanted to compile them in a letter that you might want to publish for other pharmacists and the industry, to possibly stimulate change.

It's change that has been needed for a long time. OBRA is a tremendous spark plug, but the real changes will occur in the coming months and years as pharmacists like me finally say, "I've had enough!"

There's a passiveness that has allowed pharmacists to put up with all the injustices dealt them in their practice settings. My experience has been in chain retail, where the abuses have always been at the ridiculous level. I perceived that the level of what was expected of me was so high in terms of quality, professional duties, and non-pharmacy job responsibilities that I could not personally meet it. This has led to a building frustration, a lack of job satisfaction, and a stress that has pushed me out of the practice. The battle of "pharmacy as *fast food*" versus "pharmacy as true profession" makes it impossible to fulfill what's expected of us by the public and the profession. The OBRA counseling requirements just may be "the straw that broke the camel's back"!

I'm a very strong advocate of quality communication and of teaching every customer (patient) anything that will improve his or her health. This desire for a decent quality practice of the profession has to go out the window when the scripts pile up and 90% of the incoming phone calls are for the single pharmacist on duty who has to ring the register, answer OTC questions, get change to the front register, [all] without a technician or anyone in the store who has been properly trained to dive in and get that level of "quality" back to where it should be!...

It has also been my experience, in 12 years of pharmacy practice, that pharmacists have always been grossly overworked—expected to be salesmen, bookkeepers, and "nice guys"...at all times, despite any and all stressful circumstances....

The pharmacist gets little appreciation, little sense of having actually helped anyone, the stress of knowing he cannot possibly do what's expected of him, and the frustration of knowing his existence and value to society in the first place are constantly questioned! In talking to my pharmacist partner, we decided that it was necessary to have an "attitude" just to get us through our workday, because our working situation was so stressfully bad. Where is pharmacy taking its pharmacists?

The "professional puppet"—the pharmacist—may rear back and fight when finally, after years and years of punishment, he wakes up and demands decent treatment....

[Right now] it's a spineless, voiceless, robotic type of pharmacist I observe around me. With this as a profile of the profession, I don't see any significant changes occurring anytime soon. What I probably will see are a lot of pharmacists going to stress-management programs and the profession being possibly "gobbled up" by other, stronger interests and powers. We'll see. But as for me. . . I'm outta there!

—Mark W. Tillack, R. Ph., Charlotte, N. C., "Enough's enough," Letters to the Editor, *Drug Topics* (Feb. 7, 1994, pp. 12, 14).

Letters-to-the-editor #2

[This pharmacist calls pharmacy "a horrible profession."]

I graduated from St. John's University College of Pharmacy, Jamaica, NY, in 1995 in hopes of having a fulfilling career as a pharmacist. I have yet to find such a position. I worked at a hospital where the conditions were terrible and then at a chain pharmacy on Long Island for three months. In search of better working conditions, I moved to Florida where I currently work at a chain drug store. I have to say, "I hate my job!" Pharmacy working conditions are the same everywhere: Horrible!

A typical day starts with scripts and problems left from the day before and people waiting for the store to open. My pharmacy has six phone lines, two fax lines, a drop off/pickup window and a drive-through. Usually there is one pharmacist to deal with all these possible incoming problems. Today my tech called in sick and I have a register person who has never worked in the pharmacy before. By the way, my tech didn't graduate high school, can hardly count to 100 without help and gets paid less than a register person at Burger King. So much for tech training.

After just five minutes at work I feel the pressure. All six phones are ringing and people at the drop-off window are already complaining. Someone is yelling in the drive-through to speak to the manager because he's been sitting in his car too long. My store manager is not a pharmacist. He is 23 years old and can fire me for poor customer service. I go home hating the world, my job and my life.

What a reward for five years of education! I have been told that I get paid too much money. Plus, if I make a mistake filling one of the 400 scripts in my typical day, with basically no help, I can get sued for everything and feel terrible that I hurt someone. But the pharmacy would remain open and someone else would take my place. Employers don't care. I have been told that if I don't like it, leave. How can we still call pharmacy a profession? ...

According to the Gallup poll we are the most respected profession, yet I have had people curse at me, spit on me and throw stuff at me, usually due to an insurance problem or having to wait for their prescription. I consider myself an excellent pharmacist with the knowledge to provide information to people, but in reality it doesn't happen.

I would like to stand up for my dignity and personal sanity. But if I do, I will lose my job. Pharmacy is a small world and your name will get around if you are seen as a troublemaker.

Pharmacy is a horrible profession and I see no end in sight. The associations have not done anything to help our cause nor do I expect they will in the near future. We need studies conducted in every state on how many pharmacists actually enjoy their jobs. Please help us by continuing to publish articles on the poor work environment. It gives us some hope that maybe in the distant future we will be able to do what we were taught to do: provide care and information to our patients in a caring environment. The public needs to be educated and maybe they would have some patience with us. All we want is to be able to do our jobs well and we can't do that without proper help. Thanks.

—A young, frustrated pharmacist licensed in New York and Florida
Letters, "Pharmacy: A 'Horrible' Profession," *American Druggist*, January 1999, p. 10.

Letters-to-the-editor #3
[This pharmacist asks, "Should I leave the profession?"]

As I read your editorial in the November issue, "Stand Up for Pharmacy," tears rolled down my face. I had just finished working a full weekend at my retail store, Saturday and Sunday, 12-hour shifts, alone.

I came home complaining to my husband how much I dislike my job now. I feel like a robot. Customers demand faster service while waiting times are increased due to insurance rejections, etc. I have never felt so stressed, not to mention the lack of breaks. I have three children ages five, two and six months and I need to keep my focus and maintain a positive attitude at home. It's becoming an impossible task but I can't afford to stop working.

I have been contemplating returning to graduate school to earn a Pharm. D. because I love the patient counseling aspect of pharmacy practice but I must find a way to leave the frustrations of the retail-bench setting. I wonder if the time and money spent on graduate school will be worth the sacrifice. Or should I leave the profession all together? My only hope is that pharmacists will stand up for our profession and changes will be made. I hope all the other states will conduct a survey like New York did, but more important, I pray that everyone involved will open their eyes and realize how devastating and disastrous things will become if nothing changes. I'm ready to take a stand. What can I do?

—Pharmacist in Massachusetts
Letters, "Where To Turn?", *American Druggist*, January 1999, pp. 10-11.

Letters-to-the-editor #4

[This pharmacist writes in response to an article in Drug Topics (March 18, 2002, p. 21) describing a pharmacy disaster in Southington, Connecticut in which a customer died as a result of a pharmacist mistakenly dispensing opium tincture instead of paregoric.]

I have quite a bit to say about your March 18 article "Lawsuit alleges fatal paregoric mix-up," but I'll try to keep it short. I used to be a pharmacist for CVS in Connecticut and would "float" through most of the stores in the area where the misfill occurred, including the Southington store. I also went to pharmacy school with the pharmacist whose name was on the prescription and worked with her several times at her store.

Your article left out many important facts. First of all, with the switch to Pharm. D. at the state's only pharmacy school, we were left with a crippling shortage of pharmacists at CVS. Many of the stores were closed several times a week for lack of a pharmacist. Imagine coming into a store that has a two-day backlog of prescriptions, not to mention angry, screaming customers. Also, in some stores with two pharmacists per shift due to heavy prescription volume, the second pharmacist was "pulled" to keep another store from closing. This happened in the store in question many times to my knowledge. Having one pharmacist to fill 500+ prescriptions in 12 hours (plus answer phones, tend the drive-in window, check Rxs, and monitor technicians) leaves little choice for us to "take our time when filling a prescription ... and not rush from one script to the next." This is, in my opinion, a very naive statement to make, especially coming from a lawyer who I'm sure knows nothing about working the bench.

Why are we, as pharmacists, not defending each other? Why are we agreeing to work in those potentially dangerous situations? The pharmacist in question may not remember me, but I certainly remember her. She is conscientious, intelligent, and hardworking in an impossible situation. This mistake could have happened to any one of us. The victim, and the pharmacist, are the result of a corporate push to open new stores on every corner with no thought of who will staff them. I have been in this same situation many times. I was labeled as a "troublemaker" by my district manager because I began to refuse to work in stores where I felt there was not enough help and too much room for error.

No job is worth making a mistake you can't undo. Please, I'm begging all pharmacists, let's stick together and start demanding better working conditions, for our sake, and our patients' sake.

—Heather Fontaine, R.Ph., Atlanta, GA, Letters: "Demand Better Conditions," *Drug Topics*, May 6, 2002, pp. 12, 14

Letters-to-the-editor #5

I cannot believe that working 12- and 13-hours days or 50- to 70-hour weeks is conducive to good, safe pharmacy practice. ...I have yet to work in an independent retail practice that has placed upon it the same extraordinary demands found in a busy chain store, both in terms of prescription volume and the need for personal counseling by the pharmacist.

I am appalled that any chain would allow a pharmacist to work 60, 70, even 80 hours a week, which happens regularly. Were I an attorney representing a client who suffered an injury related to a dispensing error, my first question to the pharmacist (and his employer) would be, "How many hours had you worked in the five days immediately preceding the error?"

It is my belief that pharmacist fatigue is a bigger contributor to dispensing errors than workload. Pilots and truck drivers are limited by law as to how many hours they may work without mandated idle time, thus helping to ensure the public safety; why do we expect more from ourselves?

—Mitch Fields, R.Ph., Royal Oak, Michigan, "Is this safe pharmacy?", *Drug Topics*, April 7, 1997, p. 12.

Letters-to-the-editor #6

It is incredible that pharmacy corporate officials, academics, and state boards do not simply observe the pharmacist during a normal workday and realize immediately the legion of reasons that contribute to dispensing errors. They are almost ridiculously obvious to even the most casual observer. Most of us are so stressed by many of the issues discussed in the poll that it is miraculous that there are not more errors.

When are retail pharmacy corporate officials, academics, and state boards going to come down to earth and address the real issues facing the practicing pharmacist? What person in the performance of such a critical service is regularly required to work 12-hour shifts without meal breaks and with limited comfort breaks, while attempting to be a switchboard operator, receptionist, insurance billing clerk, and cashier, as well as performing critical professional duties, all at breakneck speed?

It is time for retail corporate officials, academics, and state boards to get the stars out of their eyes and stop spewing their idealistic rhetoric long enough to look and listen. They must see the reality of how the pharmacist is actually required to perform, and hear what the pharmacist is trying to tell them regarding these conditions. Then and only then can the subject of dispensing errors begin to be positively addressed. The recent rash of bad press about pharmacists should be a loud wake-up call to more groups than pharmacists.

It is time that pharmacists stand up for themselves and say, "Enough!" Our patients deserve better, and our profession deserves better, and we as individual pharmacists deserve better.

Since my employer sees any views, comments, or ideas such as those expressed above as an "attitude problem" rather than legitimate feedback about an alarming situation, I hesitate to sign my name, but I hope that fact does not preclude the use of my letter.

—Name withheld by request, "Wake up to reality," *Pharmacy Today*, Jan. 15, 1997, p. 5.

Letters-to-the-editor #7

Why is it that pharmacists are expected to work 8-13 hours straight in one day without a break, lunch, or just some time to relax? There is a trend in this country that doctors have adopted by closing their office for lunch approximately one hour per day. In this time nothing takes place and all the phones are turned off. They still have patients! I don't know of one doctor who went out of business because he slowed down for one hour a day, and yet pharmacy management feels that this would cause such a hardship for the customers.

I have also heard the argument that it would not be cost-effective to give a pharmacist an uninterrupted lunch and break. I just wonder how cost-effective a multi-million-dollar lawsuit would be when a mistake that was made by an exhausted pharmacist was determined to be due to the unreasonable schedule that the pharmacist was forced to work.

This is not an isolated problem, it is widespread over the entire country. Wake up pharmacy leaders! People have not worked like this since the days of the sweatshop....

I don't care about all of this political stuff that is in *Pharmacy Times*. I don't care about insurance reimbursement. Let's concern ourselves about the unprofessional workload first and get pharmacists feeling professional again, then we can think about the other issues.

—Stephen D. Davis, R.Ph., "Unprofessional Workload," *Pharmacy Times*, March 1997, pp. 17-18.

Letters-to-the-editor #8

I have noticed that a number of Walgreen's stores are popping up with drive-through service. Now this may be great for the patient/customer, but I see it as another headache for the pharmacist who is already overworked with walk-ins and telephone orders. When will pharmacy stop being viewed and treated like McDonald's, and respected as a profession with a professional who is an expert on medications? ...

Pharmacists are professionals who know and understand medications. We should be there to counsel and advise patients on medical needs. We are not robots designed to churn out 350 scripts in a day, we are definitely not insurance agents who know about copays and deductibles, and finally we are human beings, not supermen from the planet Krypton. If pharmacy is going to continue to be like McDonald's, then let us have the support hours McDonald's has. After all, if a person accidentally gets a pickle when they didn't want it, is it going to kill them?

—Elas Dray, R.Ph., "Future of Pharmacy," *Pharmacy Times*, September 1996, p. 14.

Letters-to-the-editor #9

I am going to tell you what is wrong with retail pharmacy today. It has nothing to do with managed care, i.e., drug formularies, OBRA '90, declining margins on third party prescriptions. It's about greed, selfishness and non-loyalty to employees. ...

The simple truth is that retail chain pharmacy has nothing to do with patient care; the only thing the big boys give a hoot about is money, money and more money. The pharmacist's job is to fill customers' prescriptions at the speed of light (the faster you fill, the more money they make), explain their drugs only so the chain doesn't get fined for noncompliance with OBRA, and get them out as soon as you can.

–Lawrence Barusch, R.Ph., Clifton Park, New York, "Revco: A Friend for Life?" *American Druggist*, March 1997, p. 8.

Letters-to-the-editor #10

After reading many articles and editorials expressing pharmacists' plight for fewer interruptions, more technician help, much-needed and deserved lunch, dinner and bathroom breaks, and the need for a more "professional" environment, I've come to a conclusion.

On one particularly busy day, one of our regular customers could tell we were swamped and wanted to do something nice for us. She offered to bring us lunch. She asked, "Have you had your lunch break yet?" It was all we could do to not burst out laughing at such a silly question. I begrudgingly told her we did not get lunch breaks. Nor any kind of break for that matter, but I kept that to myself. The woman was extremely surprised and somewhat taken aback upon hearing my response. She couldn't believe that pharmacists don't get breaks, and, needless to say, she didn't bring us lunch.

Which brings me to my point. These articles and editorials that describe pharmacists' working conditions are only in pharmacy journals and are not likely to be read by average citizens. If our plight was more publicized, people might take notice. They may well be concerned that their prescriptions are being filled often by worn-out, food-deprived, urinary-challenged pharmacists who would function much better if they had better working conditions and got to sit down and detach the phone from their heads occasionally.

–Angela Stadler, R. Ph., Charlotte, North Carolina, "Give Us a Break," *American Druggist*, April 1997, p. 8.

Letters-to-the-editor #11

In pharmacy, most of us have at one time or another been the victim of a corporate policy that doesn't allow pharmacists to act professionally. No time for meals, no time to use the restrooms, no time to legally comply with OBRA regulations, no time to consult with patients, no time to adequately ensure that prescriptions are filled correctly. You know the story. We all know the story.

We can wait for the pharmacy boards to change the business by mandating tech-to-pharmacist ratios or pharmacist workload limits. But the dollar power of Big Business will stall any bills considered in the legislature. We can wait for Big Business to change the profession (through massive layoffs due to technology and outrageous use of technicians to perform pharmacist functions).

Or we can demand protection and change in our business by unionizing. Few pharmacists have considered unionizing but we need the strength that a union could provide.

Standing alone we have no bargaining power. We are at the mercy of our employers to adequately staff the pharmacies.

—Name withheld by request, "Time to Unionize," *American Druggist*, April 1997, p. 17.

Letters-to-the-editor #12

...In what other profession do you have to worry about finding time to take a bathroom break? In what other profession do you constantly feel guilty for trying to take 30 minutes to eat a meal, relax, and regroup to work the next few hours? Is it any wonder colleagues are leaving the profession and new pharmacists quickly become disillusioned with it?

These working conditions affect the safety of the public. It is only logical that a pharmacist working under these conditions day in and day out has a greater chance of making an error than someone who works under more humane conditions. Boards of pharmacy are charged with the protection of the public safety. Unfortunately, most boards have chosen to ignore working conditions in the mistaken belief that working conditions of pharmacists are a business issue rather than a public safety issue. Personally, I do believe boards should be setting some standards. ...

—Stanley L. Tetenman R.Ph., Auburn, Maine. "The Enemy Is Us," *Drug Topics,* April 16, 2001

Letters-to-the-editor #13

Regarding the article "Pharmacy boards of two minds about R.Ph. breaks," which appeared in *Drug Topics,* Feb. 19 issue, I lasted nine months as a retail pharmacist. The job, if done right, is grueling as well as emotionally and physically costly. I cannot believe that breaks are even an issue. What other profession or nonprofession works employees for 12 hours without scheduled breaks? I lost 15 pounds from a 100-pound frame in the nine months I worked in retail. My partner would get so nervous about coming to work that she would regularly vomit from the anxiety.

We are an educated group of professionals, and we are treated like slave labor. The current conditions are deplorable and need to change. I would never encourage a young person to pursue a career in pharmacy. Pharmacists have such a huge responsibility and workload but are not given the support they need to perform the job even marginally.

I have spent the last nine years as a hospital pharmacist and, because of the working conditions of that environment, would never even consider going back into retail.

—E. Stewart, R. Ph. (Etstewart5@aol.com)
"Retail work is grueling," *Drug Topics,* April 16, 2001

Letters-to-the-editor #14

...No one knows what we go through in a day but us. The closest people to understanding us are our techs, because it is they who see us being abused, disrespected, overworked, and walked on daily.

Just yesterday, during the worst part of the dinner rush, my two techs were stuck at the counter, leaving me to process, fill, check, and try to get the phone. Needless to say, I began ignoring the phone. As more and more lines were ringing, the assistant store manager started answering the phone and paging me to get the lines on hold. It took all of my willpower to keep my mouth shut and not blow up on him. You would think that someone who works in the same building as we do would have some idea what we go through. I guess that's too much to ask.

Hard as we try, we can't even fully make our families understand. I've told my wife, who is a teacher, everything imaginable about pharmacy. But she still is shocked when I tell her I don't have time to chat when she calls me in the middle of the day. "Why are you so hungry?" she'll ask. "Because I've worked all day and eaten only a Kudos bar and two packs of Smarties." They just don't get it. ...

—Jason Martinazzi
dr_of_rx@hotmail.com
"We're misunderstood," *Drug Topics*, Dec. 8, 2003, p. 22

Letters-to-the-editor #15

...The chain pharmacy retail sector lags considerably behind in examining profiles for drug interactions due to the fact that the pharmacist must check literally hundreds of prescriptions on each shift. To slow down will mean, in some chains, a red light showing on the computer screen signifying a pharmacist is behind in checking. This red light affects his bonus and invariably brings the area managers and district managers down on him. If a student really wants to go to pharmacy school for eight years, get that Pharm.D. degree, and then stand in one spot racing the red light with hundreds of prescriptions coming off the conveyor belt, good for him. The money is good, $85,000 and more in some places. But what about the health of the consumer, the drug interactions that are ignored, all in the name of speed.?....

—Kern Stafford, "Racing the red light," *Drug Topics*, Sept. 1, 2003, p. 16

Letters-to-the-editor #16

...I managed to stick out 4 years at CVS before the night of January 2, the Monday after New Year's and the busiest day of the year, when I worked a 14-hour shift with one 10-hour technician, filled

240 prescriptions, fell asleep driving home, and ended up crashing my car into the median. As soon as I woke up, I gave notice. Now I work at a grocery pharmacy for the same money, with much better hours and 10 times less stress.

CVS is an extreme case among retailers. Its new hires are almost always either recent grads or people who have bounced around the pharmacy world so often that they have nowhere left to go.

When are we pharmacists going to rise up and say that this treatment is completely unacceptable?

—Conchetta Lesser, PharmD, Phoenix, Ariz. "Wake-up call," *Drug Topics*, December 2011, pp. 8-9.

Letters-to-the-editor #17

...I spent my career at a drug company, retired 10 years ago, and returned to retail. The R.Ph. [registered pharmacist] works more than half the time without any [technician or clerk] help. I feel like a grocery clerk ringing up milk, soup, bread, etc., the way I did as a 16-year-old cashier in a supermarket. Some profession. We are nothing more than "high-priced clerks," who spend too much time with insurance problems, waiting on obnoxious, rude, impatient people who consider us as clerks; and work in high-pressure jobs that don't pay what we are worth. Pharmacy is no longer a profession. It's no wonder the young pharmacy students want no part of retail, as it is underpaid, understaffed, and overworked.

—Paul D. Rowe, "Associations are wanting," *Drug Topics*, April 19, 2004, p. 16

Letters-to-the-editor #18

Having read *Drug Topics* for years, I am increasingly glad I decided upon hospital pharmacy over the retail setting.

I have worked in the same hosoptial for 17 years, and I can honestly say I like my job. I have great co-workers, plenty of quality technician help, time for lunch and breaks, respect from management, involvement in many clinical activities, and I never have to deal with insurance problems—all in a safe and secure setting.

Almost every Letter to the Editor and many articles in *Drug Topics* are about how terrible retail pharmacy is, of which I am well aware.

Considering a pharmacist I know recently had to tackle and disarm a gunman (gunwoman actually), and that my other retail pharmacist friends hate their jobs, it would take a very significant pay increase or something like 10 weeks of vacation (which obviously will never happen) to ever persuade me to work in the retail setting.

—Jennifer Prazenica, R.Ph., Kittanning, Pennsylvania. "Job Satisfaction," *Drug Topics*, April 2012, p. 21

---

2. Comments posted by pharmacists on two Internet pharmacy discussion groups (pharmacyweek.com and sci.med.pharmacy) regarding pharmacists' working conditions

---

Pharmacy discussion group post #1

Internet discussion group: Pharmacyweek.com
Author: emmyjay (3/23/2006)
Subject: RE: retail setting vs. hospital setting

Oh my God, where do I start???? I would HIGHLY recommend that you spend some time in a retail pharmacy. See if a local big chain will let you job-shadow a few days (especially a Monday at the beginning of the month). You will soon see what a nightmare it is.

1. Rarely do you have enough competent tech help

2. When you come in first thing in the morning, your voice-mail is already full of refill requests, so you are running behind right off the bat

3. Customers are rude, demanding, nasty, impatient, and give you no respect

4. You are bombarded by phone calls from doctor's offices, patients, people who AREN'T your patient but want to get your opinion of what their regular RPh told them, people who get their drugs mail-order but still want you to spend time answering their questions, and people who just need someone to yak at

5. INSURANCE HASSLES!! Non-formulary drugs, drugs that need prior authorization, refill-too-soon rejects, requests for early fills, etc. Every phone call takes forever and you get that much more behind in your rx filling

6. Patients who expect you to know every insurance company, plan, copay, and deductible amount off the top of your head. "I don't have my card with me—just bill Blue Cross"...

7. People who come in at 5pm with no refills on their controlled substance rx but expect you to fill it anyway.

8. Drug-seekers and narc abusers who bullshit you with stupid stories (my dog ate my Vicodin) that insult your intelligence.

9. People who think just because there's nobody waiting at the counter, you're not busy. They don't see the 40 rxs lined up back behind the counter, not to mention the dozen on voice mail and the other dozen called in by the docs!

10. Medicaid patients who bitch about $1 copay, then go up front and buy cigarettes & beer.

11. People who pay no attention to the letters their insurance company sends them, then yell at you because you're charging them a $10 copay instead of $5.

12. Working at a furious pace for 8-12 hours with (maybe) 1 potty break, no meal break, and praying you don't make a mistake and hurt or kill somebody!

There is a reason they pay so much to retail pharmacists. Nobody wants to do it. They lure new grads with the big bucks, but most quit within a couple of years. It will wear you down and make you a nasty person. Don't take our word for it—go and witness it yourself. Talk to some pharmacists who work in retail and see what they have to say.

Hospital can be very hectic as well, depending upon the staffing situation, but it's nowhere near as bad as retail. In my area, hospital pays about $5/hr less than retail but my mental health is worth the pay difference!

http://www.pharmacyweek.com/job_seeker/discussions/thread.asp?board_id=2&conference_id=18&post_id=22699&thread_id=5500&paging_CurPage=2   (Accessed 4-26-06)

Pharmacy discussion group post #2
Internet discussion group: Pharmacyweek.com

Got out of retail long ago, but still remember the pain. My relatives don't understand when I try to explain what a hellhole retail is. They always say, "it doesn't look busy" just cuz there's nobody standing at the counter. They don't see the 40 rxs [prescriptions] in line & all 7 phone lines blinking, plus the computer screen saying "prior auth required" or "non-formulary", etc. AAARRRGGGHHH!

I wish Oprah or 20/20 would do a show about it. Film a busy retail store on a Monday at the beginning of the month that only has 1 RPh [pharmacist] and a couple of techs. SHOW people that all the insurance crap is NOT OUR FAULT!!! And that for every rx [prescription] that is brought to the counter, there are 5 more off the voice mail & from doctor's offices. And show people what NOT to do: don't make us call your doc for refills; don't park at the drive-thru; don't ask for 5 other things along with your rx at the drive-thru; pay attention to changes in your insurance; I could go on and on.

I don't know how you retail dogs stay sane and not kill anyone............
Emmajay 7-19-05

http://www.pharmacyweek.com/job_seeker/discussions/thread.asp?board_i d=2&conference_id=18&post_id=21376&thread_id=5126" \l "pid21376"

Pharmacy discussion group post #3
Internet discussion group: Pharmacyweek.com
Author: SlaveRPh (2/15/2005)
Subject: RE: New pharmacists getting a dose of reality

Well golly gee. Isn't this what I have been talking about for a long time? The big lie about pharmacy. You see most jobs are nothing more than assembly line functions. I'm surprised someone has not filed legal action against the schools for misrepresenting what pharmacy really has to offer. It's very sad that people who are so intelligent end up doing nothing with their knowledge. And its not going to change in the near future. Heck this clinical stuff was being pushed 30 years ago. It's gone nowhere. Why? Because it doesn't fit the system. I have found maybe 3 pharmacists over the last 40 years who were happy. They both owned their pharmacy. How could anyone with a 6 year degree be happy with the environment found in most pharmacy jobs? My god 6 years and you work at the local grocery store or mass merchandiser. Those are the places you think about when you think about a professional and rewarding career in pharmacy? And more time is spent fighting PBM's and the ignorant public just to fill a script than is ever spent on professional functions. I hope more articles like this [John Strahinich, "Bitter pill: New pharmacists getting a dose of reality," *Boston Herald*, February 13, 2005] get printed and all students read them. It's not too late to get out of pharmacy if you're a student. A doctor and you can't even get a potty break or lunch break. Absolutely ridiculous.

http://www.pharmacyweek.com/discussions/thread.asp?board_id=2&conference_id=18&post_id=20291&thread_id=4831&paging_CurPage=3#pid20291

Pharmacy discussion group post #4
Internet discussion group: sci.med.pharmacy
12-21-2003

...because physicians are spending less time with patients, the pharmacist is receiving more and more calls with medical questions. Why don't they call their doctors? I don't know why you were prescribed Neurontin. Shouldn't you know? I mean you went to the doctor for SOMETHING. I would be glad to discuss the various off label uses of Neurontin plus its plethora of side effects, but you are going to send the script off to mail order anyway!

This past week was hellish. I finally decided to tell everyone it would be a 2 hour wait (with the exception of mothers with children or adults with elderly parents). I couldn't help but notice that most customers don't extend the favor of calling refills in a day in advance, or keeping up with their own insurance plans. Why should I convenience someone who is making my job that much harder?

I WILL take bathroom breaks and eat lunch. Being busy does not equate to working faster. My mistakes can kill you or get me sued. If you want to be part of the problem, you are encouraged to go to another store. I tried consulting for several years but grew weary of the hotel stays. Tried hospital and am now waiting for an opening to go back.

skipperdogs.
skipperdogs@whatever.com

Pharmacy discussion group post #5
Internet discussion group: sci.med.pharmacy
12-21-2003

...I don't have any statistics, but from conversations with young pharmacists in my state, there is quite a large number that are disenfranchised with pharmacy, particularly retail and hospital. When asked my opinion on the future of our profession, the best I can offer is usually a shrug and "If only" RPhs took back the profession, were allowed to practice what they learn, and make a living by that practice. I find it increasingly difficult to recommend an intelligent young person choose pharmacy for a career....

Glenn Gilbreath Jr., Registered Pharmacist
Wizard57M@SurfBest.net

Pharmacy discussion group post #6
Internet discussion group: Sci.med.pharmacy
From: Ftino (FSCIORTINO@worldnet.att.net)
Subject: Re: pharmacist shortage
Date: 2003-10-17

There is no pharmacist shortage. There are a lot of "vacant job positions" because working conditions are terrible. Many pharmacists won't work more hours or have cut back hours because they hate the job. CVS lost over a dozen pharmacists in my area. Not because they died or retired but because they QUIT. Now they are "short". That's not a shortage.

Pharmacy discussion group post #7

Internet discussion group: Sci.med.pharmacy
From: skipperdogs (skipperdogs@whatever.com)
Subject: Re: Worked to Death
Date: 2003-04-22

I and my two technicians/cashiers did 119 scripts from 9 am to 12 noon today. That's 40 per hour. I had a customer "jesus christ"ing and "goddamn"ing at the register because he thought I was taking too long on his refill which he failed to call ahead with. I guess he wanted me to up it to 50 per hour. I am going to have to write a legal disclaimer for those types of customers to sign whereby I am not responsible for any errors/deaths resulting from their fast-food pharmacy excursion. No. I did not rush him through nor put him ahead of anyone else in line. I know full well he would be the first person to sue me if something was done incorrectly.

Pharmacy discussion group post #8

Internet discussion group: Sci.med.pharmacy
From: Dazed&Confused (nate@nowhere.net)
Subject: Oh, what to do... Any rural US pharmacists read this newsgroup?
Date: 2001-04-19

Hello all. ***WARNING—Whining Ahead***
I am just finishing my first year of a Pharm.D. program and am wandering what the &*## I'm doing here. I'm from a small town and plan on returning to a small town (pop. <10K) after graduation.
For some masochistic reason, I work as an intern for one of the major chains, and I absolutely hate it. I think I thought that if I could stand working there, I could work anywhere. Now I know I couldn't stand it if I were to have to work there full-time. It's one of the busiest (if not the busiest) of their stores in this town (pop ~600K), and

it's what I'd expect working at a McDonald's in hell at noon hour would be like. Not a day goes by that at least one of the female pharmacists or techs aren't in tears. (It may sound sexist, but its a fact.) I usually get by OK, as insults, etc. don't bother me much. I'm pretty thick-skinned at my ripe old age, but I have absolutely no skills in consoling people, and it does bother me to see my coworkers so upset all of the time (bit of a softie deep down I guess). That statement itself kinda scares me, as it sounds like it's an "us against them" situation, and that's not the way it should be. Getting jaded and cynical before my first year is even over is a bad sign. Granted, the vast majority of our customers are civil and understanding, but we're busy enough that the small percentage of true buttheads adds up to substantial numbers.

I guess I'm just looking for pity, or a shoulder to cry on, because I am so close to quitting. It's not something I want to do, as I'm kinda an old fart already, and I've had to bust my butt to get to where I am now, like working 7 days a week during most of my undergrad. But yet, the old proverb about throwing good money after bad keeps coming to mind.

So, if any small-town pharmacists happen to read this newsgroup, I'd love to hear some positive comments on your personal situation. (Are there any?) I plan on being a floater for a few years after graduation, eventually taking over a pharmacy of my own as someone retires. (Pipe dream?) If anyone has done something similar, I'd like to hear about that too.

Well, thanks for letting me babble on. —Nate

Pharmacy discussion group post #9
Internet discussion group: Sci.med.pharmacy
From: Name withheld (kmcl@zianet.com)
Subject: Wal-mart customers
Date: 2000/04/01

I just got home from another overwhelming day at Wal-Mart. I find it hard to continue day in, day out being insulted, harassed, pressured, accused of not doing theirs fast enough, etc., by customers. We often fill a little less than one prescription per minute. That's not fast enough for most customers, who arrive with 25 people ahead of them, and expect a 5 minute wait. Sure, they're in a hurry to go home to their soap operas, but we are hurrying as fast as we can up to 12 hours straight. If they want it fast, at least they could call it in a few hours in advance. I have been tempted to just lock the door and walk out. Does this ever end?

Pharmacy discussion group post #10
Internet discussion group: Sci.med.pharmacy
From: Liza57 (liza57@aol.com)
Subject: Re: Wal-mart customers
Date: 2000/04/05

Nope! It doesn't ever end—not in a retail pharmacy. But there are some things you can do for yourself. First, SLOW DOWN !!!! As was said before, you are setting yourself up for Rx errors that could cause a serious problem with your customer/patient and will ultimately affect you and the Board of Pharmacy when the mistake gets reported to the Board. No obnoxious customer should force you into feeling that you have to move faster to feel competent in your profession.

Second, realize that there is no way you can please every customer. Don't try to please everyone. Just do the best you can and when someone bitches about the how long it takes you to fill their prescription, ask them quietly and nicely whether they would care to have you fill it or would they care to take the Rx somewhere else and pay a higher price, which IS their prerogative. If they say yes, go back to work. If they say no...well...you certainly have enough to do already, right?

Third, take a really deep breath when you start to feel this frazzled. Step OUT of the pharmacy for a few minutes and take a few more deep breaths and keep repeating that you are doing your best and that faster doesn't mean better/safer for your customers and that NO ONE (customers included) should have this amount of power over you—to make you SO STRESSED OUT! I know this one takes practice. I've been doing this for 20 years and it still gets to me, too, but I'm getting better at it.

Pharmacy discussion group post #11

Internet discussion group: Sci.med.pharmacy
From: Liza57 (liza57@aol.com)
Subject: Re: public health issue.
Date: 2000/03/23
Re: What public health issue is most important to the profession of pharmacy? Why?

I believe the most important public health issue involving the profession of pharmacy involves prescription errors and the impact those errors have on the health of those involved in such incidents. I believe the error rate has risen due to a decline in the amount of ancillary help within the pharmacy thanks to low reimbursement rates from third party providers. I believe that corporations (both hospital and retail ~ independent or chain) were wrong to accept such low reimbursement in the first place and I don't feel that a pharmacist's ability to practice pharmacy in a competent manner should be jeopardized because of poor business choices. I also believe that it's time to step back and re-evaluate things like drive-through windows in pharmacies for convenience that can lead to yet more problems with drug therapy thanks to a lack of counseling. I think that this issue is by far the most critical issue facing pharmacy AND public health.

Pharmacy discussion group post #12

Internet discussion group: Sci.med.pharmacy
From: Paul (arghhspam@ctel.net)
Subject: Re: Pharmacy working conditions - New laws, N.C.
Date: 1998/12/25

I would probably bet that a break or two during the day would let all of us pharmacists live a little longer. Still, I don't know how I would ever be able to be caught up enough to take a 15-30 minute break. It might make it worse upon returning and attempting to catch up. My two techs have worked thru most of their lunch breaks (unpaid) for a long time just to try and keep up. What do you do about the truly sick patient or the one who has driven an hour (I live and work in the boonies) to get their meds? Do you make them wait? Would they get upset and go elsewhere? I don't know how you could make the system work. I think that all the pharmacies would have to close at the same time and for the same amount of time, just to be fair and consistent. In response to the original thread of this post, the profession is not fun, rewarding, stimulating or respected. It's just a job, as well as a few other adjectives that shall not be stated here, and I don't care where you work or who you work for, the grass isn't any greener. It's the same no matter where you are, it just plain stinks. On the bright side however, the money is pretty good and it does pay the bills. —Paul

---

3. Editorial written by Oklahoma pharmacist Charles L. Duhon

The following is an editorial written by Tulsa, Oklahoma, pharmacist Charles L. Duhon (Viewpoint: "Is pharmacy a profession or a trade?", *Drug Topics*, Oct. 23, 2006, p. 52):

I've been in the retail practice environment for more than 30 years and have realized that at the very heart of our profession lies a cancer that's been eating away at its core for decades. The cancer is called inadequate staffing, and it has caused myriad ills to befall the profession. I'm convinced that one of the primary contributors to the pharmacist shortage today is the disillusionment factor caused by stress brought on by inadequate staffing. I've known many R.Ph.s who early in their careers chose to pursue other career paths because of work environment issues. I've seen many female R.Ph.s, who are often secondary breadwinners, opt out of their profession because of intolerable stress levels due to inadequate staffing.

It should be obvious there is a problem when one of the most profitable drug chains in the nation, which offers high sign-on incentives and salaries cannot keep pharmacists. The chain is quick to blame the pharmacist shortage. What it, like most retail chains, fails to acknowledge is that the shortage has been created to a great extent by the working conditions behind the counter.

One national chain has added a new high-tech innovation to the practice of pharmacy. If you are filling scripts fast enough, a green light appears on the computer screen. If you fall behind, a red light appears. Records are kept and the red-light R.Ph.s are deemed incompetent because they are too slow. It is amazing to realize that, after six years of college taking such courses as biochemistry, pharmacognosy, physiology, and physics, your competency level is judged solely based on the number of Rxs you can fill per hour.

When are we going to realize that this is an albatross around the neck of our profession? The sheer fact that several state boards have attempted to address this issue gives it legitimacy. North Carolina and West Virginia are two that have passed legislation addressing this ongoing problem. In Oklahoma, I formed a committee to come up with a solution. We formulated a plan whereby any pharmacist who felt he did not have sufficient staffing could document it on a state-provided form. The board would investigate each incident, thus encouraging all employers to be competently staffed at all times. We formulated legislation that was passed, only to be blocked by the legal departments of a number of large chains.

I firmly believe that it is in the best interest of the state board and the people we serve each day, and more significantly in the best interest of the profession, that we be adequately staffed at all times. How can we project a professional image and be taken seriously by other healthcare providers as long as we keep trying to provide pharmaceutical care at the same time we are ringing up purchases, fighting with insurance carriers, entering data into the computer, and manning the drive-up window?

The pharmacy schools have been telling us for years that pharmacy should expand from providing products to providing services. But we will never get there until we are willing to recognize that we have a major problem with inadequate staffing and we are willing to come together as a profession to figure out how to fix it. We must be willing to surgically remove the tumor at all cost so that the patient might survive.

My tenure in this profession is almost over, and when I look back over the years I've invested in this great profession, I have mixed emotions. I know that I've helped many people physically, emotionally, spiritually, and sometimes financially. I know I made a difference when it came to helping people, but what have I done for the profession? In that regard I have failed miserably—primarily because I, like most other pharmacists, have allowed the cancer to grow and done very little to stop it.

I felt the pain 30 years ago when, right after graduating, I was sent to a high-volume store that filled more than 300 Rxs a day and had only one cashier. I saw the pain on the faces of my colleagues as they changed jobs over and over again trying to find a better work environment. I knew about the cancer and for years did little to correct it. If you ignore the pain long enough, the ailment that causes the pain will consume you. We've ignored the pain for too long, and the ailment has begun to consume us.

Ask yourself, "What have I done to change what is happening?" If your answer is "nothing," then you have only yourself to blame.

Chapter 17

Should pharmacists admit fault for errors caused by working conditions?

Many of our pharmacy leaders tell us that we should immediately fess up after a mistake. Let me make the case why I don't think the issue is quite that simple.

I happened to be visiting my mother and stepfather when my stepfather noticed that half the pills in one of his Rx bottles looked strange. It turns out that a national chain mistakenly dispensed Glucophage (for type 2 diabetes) to my stepfather instead of Toprol XL (for blood pressure). My stepfather has never had diabetes. I told my stepfather that I would like to accompany him when he asked the pharmacist what happened. During my stepfather's conversation with the pharmacist, I never identified myself as a pharmacist nor did I say a single word. I've witnessed similar scenarios too often in my career. The pharmacist who made the mistake was not on duty but the pharmacist-in-charge spoke carefully. He told my stepfather, "I'm sorry for the inconvenience." He did not say "I'm sorry for the error." I confess that I probably would have handled the situation similarly.

The issue of whether pharmacists should admit an error and apologize to the customer is one of considerable controversy to pharmacists in the trenches. Several years ago at a day-long meeting of about two dozen of the chain's pharmacists in my local district, our supervisor and his boss said that we should admit errors to customers and apologize. There was a great deal of discussion of this point. I have come to the conclusion that it was indeed a corporate decision that the pharmacist responsible for the error should apologize to the customer.

During our lunch break that day, the half-dozen pharmacists sitting around my table discussed this idea of admitting our error and apologizing to the customer. A couple of older pharmacists said they had never done it that way before and they didn't want to start now. The implied best way to handle errors was to try to obfuscate the whole thing by claiming, for example, that the drug is a generic. If the customer may be in danger, obviously we have to take more direct action. We always correct the error by saying something like "It's made by a different company but we'll give you the one you had before."

One of these older pharmacists said that most auto insurers recommend that policyholders not admit fault. I went home and checked my State Farm car insurance policy and, sure enough, on the back of my wallet card are these exact words: "Do not admit fault. Do not discuss the accident with anyone except State Farm or Police."

So why would my employer (one of the largest drug chains in the country) suggest that we admit fault to the customer and apologize? At our table, we concluded that the corporation was trying to protect itself by isolating us on a limb and then, if necessary, cutting off that limb. We figured that the chain would endeavor to get rid of us through various means or transfer us to a different town if the dispensing error were so serious that it received widespread publicity in our community. As a result, most of the pharmacists I know are not eager to admit fault and apologize to customers.

I wouldn't necessarily mind apologizing in the following manner: "On behalf of (Walgreens, CVS, Wal-Mart, Rite Aid, etc.), I apologize for the error." But this is precisely the opposite of what our employer wants. Our employer wants us to blame ourselves as individual pharmacists rather than blame the corporation for the understaffing that guarantees errors. The corporation wants to divert attention from its own negligence and responsibility to provide conditions in which accuracy is more than a matter of being lucky.

Why should all the blame be directed at the pharmacist when he is often simply the victim of a dangerously understaffed pharmacy? Are you to blame when the store you're working in (for example, for a pharmacist who is sick or on vacation) has poorly-trained techs, or no tech, or a tech who is off sick, or a tech who is on vacation? Are you to blame for the fact that your employer intentionally understaffs pharmacies to increase profitability? Are you a victim of the system just as much as the customer who received the wrong drug?

I simply have a hard time admitting fault for an error in which there are factors beyond my control. Little did I know in pharmacy school that the most difficult problem in my career would be having adequate staffing. It is shameful that pharmacists are not given enough staffing for the safe filling of prescriptions. Pharmacy school professors tell us we are professionals. In the real world, we quickly realize that we are piece-workers on a fast food assembly line.

If you are an independent owner and you dispensed the wrong medication, perhaps you have a greater responsibility to admit fault. After all, you have the power to determine staffing levels in the pharmacy. In contrast, employee pharmacists who work for the big chains are powerless to set tech staffing levels.

By admitting fault, will we increase the likelihood of the customer initiating a lawsuit? Are we essentially telling the customer that he has legitimate grounds for legal action? After one error that my partner made, he mentioned to me that he didn't know whether he should call the customer at home and apologize. My partner did decide to call the customer. My partner said the customer appreciated the apology. But it turns out that the customer sued my partner and our employer anyway. I never learned the outcome of the lawsuit. I felt it was too sensitive to discuss.

As regards the incident involving my stepfather, I was not angry at the pharmacist who was responsible. I know that the McDonald's model of pharmacy makes errors like this inevitable. Nevertheless, we all know pharmacists who are an accident waiting to happen. If the pharmacist responsible for the error in my stepfather's Rx was simply reckless and careless, a forgiving attitude would probably not be warranted.

In my opinion, there are two types of pharmacists: The first type tries very hard to prevent errors. These pharmacists lose sleep worrying about the possibility of errors. The second type of pharmacist slings out prescriptions all day long seemingly unaware of the tremendous liability riding on each prescription and without a clear understanding that the legal profession is salivating over the chance to take a big bite out of our posterior.

Who is to blame for pharmacy mistakes?

The issue of pharmacy mistakes is possibly the most serious issue facing our profession. Why have we been unable to solve this problem? I blame the following:

1. State boards of pharmacy—In my opinion, the state boards need to have the authority to levy hefty fines against those employers who don't provide adequate staffing for the safe filling of prescriptions. The fines need to be more than a slap on the wrist. As it is now, the big employers find it less expensive to pay customers harmed by pharmacy mistakes, rather than hire adequate staffing. The state boards need the muscle and willpower to aggressively go after the big employers, rather than slap them with a fine that means nothing to these multi-billion-dollar corporations. The fines need to be big enough so that the big employers conclude that understaffing and the inevitable pharmacy mistakes are simply not a profitable business model.

2. National Association of Boards of Pharmacy (NABP)—According to its website, NABP is "the impartial professional organization that supports the state boards of pharmacy in protecting public health." In my opinion, this places NABP in a unique position to make a difference with the issue of pharmacy mistakes. I would like to see NABP take its role seriously in protecting public health by making a forceful presentation to Congress that safe staffing in pharmacies must be assured. Surely NABP could do more in this regard than it is now, i.e., nothing.

3. American Pharmacists Association—Many pharmacists harbor a tremendous amount of contempt for APhA for not focusing on those working conditions (primarily staffing levels) that make errors inevitable. The American Medical Association seems to be far more effective in addressing working conditions for doctors than APhA is for pharmacists. Many pharmacists are incredulous that APhA appears to be too timid to fight for pharmacists' working conditions. Many pharmacists feel that APhA's timidity in addressing this issue is more than enough reason to refuse to join that organization.

4. State legislatures—The anti-regulatory ideology that predominates in America today (even after the near-collapse of our financial system) holds that the market should be left to its own devices to fix every problem, and that no governmental agency should intervene in the private sector. Accordingly, workplace issues such as understaffing are conveniently viewed by state legislatures as employer-employee issues rather than public safety issues. But state legislatures have a duty (like state boards) to protect the public safety. Fear of being labeled by state legislatures as anti-business causes leaders of pharmacy boards, NABP, and APhA to avoid focusing on understaffing. Unfortunately, state legislatures have tremendous power to overturn helpful workplace regulations that any pro-employee state board dares to pass. I would like to see some head of a state pharmacy board put his job on the line by standing up to the big chains even at the risk of being labeled by that state legislature as anti-business. We need courageous leaders who put this issue above their own job security. It seems that our leaders prefer to bask in the prestige that accompanies their positions, rather than use their visibility to make a real difference for pharmacists in the trenches.

5. Employers—I know many pharmacists who privately welcome the huge multi-million dollar jury awards against the big employers as a result of serious and/or fatal mistakes. Many pharmacists hope that these huge jury awards will embarrass and shame the big employers into providing adequate staffing so that pharmacy mistakes are a rarity. As it is, pharmacy mistakes are a predictable consequence of this business model based on slinging out prescriptions as fast as McDonald's slings out burgers. Many pharmacists are disgusted that McDonald's seems to be far more capable of providing adequate staffing for the preparation of hamburgers, whereas the huge drug-store chains seem to be incapable or unwilling to provide adequate staffing for the preparation of a far more critical product: prescription drugs.

6. Pharmacists—Every pharmacist knows that many of our colleagues are an accident waiting to happen. These pharmacists would make errors regardless of prescription volume and regardless of staffing levels. Some pharmacists seem to have no clue about how high the stakes are with each prescription we fill. They seem to be completely oblivious to the fact that lawyers are salivating over the possibility of taking a huge bite out of our posterior.

7. Pharmacy customers—Our customers deserve a big chunk of the blame for pharmacy errors because they—like our employers—seem to judge pharmacists solely by how fast we fill prescriptions. Unfortunately, drive-thru windows send an unmistakable message to customers that prescriptions are no different from burgers.

8. Cultural factors—Our quick-fix, pill for every ill culture has commodified health. When health is seen simply as the result of the consumption of commodities, it is not surprising that the rapid distribution of those commodities is seen as paramount. Mistakes are inevitable when pharmacy is seen primarily as a distributive activity rather than a cognitive activity.

A shorter version of this discussion was published as an editorial in *Drug Topics* ("Should you admit fault after a dispensing error?" June 16, 2008, p. 60). With each of my editorials in *Drug Topics*, I include my e-mail address in case pharmacists care to comment. Here are three of the e-mails I received following my editorial:

E-mail from pharmacist #1

Dennis,
    I just finished 7 straight days totaling 80 hours (6 X 12 hr. days and one 8 hour Sunday), working with one 24hr/week experienced tech, the other 5 techs are inexperienced, and they all do data entry. Not an envious situation. They learn from their mistakes as I point

them out and correct them. And brother are they ever doing a lot of learning.
[Anonymous pharmacist]

E-mail from pharmacist #2

Hi. Thanks for your excellent article on pharmacists and apologies. I could not agree with you more.

Several years ago, I was working for a grocery chain pharmacy. I had a technician who was incompetent, insubordinate, and mentally unstable. I had tried to fire this tech for over a year, but Safeway pharmacy management would not let me do this, despite the fact that I was the pharmacy manager and supposedly was responsible for staffing the pharmacy.

One day, a regular customer returned to the pharmacy with the complaint that she had received a prescription intended for another patient. She had taken two doses of the medication and had suffered no ill effects from it, but was understandably angry. We were still keeping manual signature logs at that time, and when I looked to see who had given the wrong Rx to this patient, it was that technician!

The patient had refused counseling, so I never saw what was actually given to her. The patient asked for a written apology from Safeway, and my store manager and pharmacy district manager tried to persuade me to write a personal letter of apology to her. I refused, as I saw a great deal of personal liability in doing this. Certainly, the technician was under my supervision at the time that this error occurred, but I had no realistic way of preventing it, short of watching over each prescription she passed to the customers, and this store was way too busy and understaffed to allow this. And if I had been allowed to terminate this employee as I had tried to several times before, this event would not have occurred.

The patient brought suit against Safeway, not me, and they ended up making a five-figure settlement to her. This event was not tied to me or my license in any way. I did feel horrible for the patient as she was a good customer, and also a good person. But I refused to make the pharmacy's staffing problem my own personal problem.

There was a huge teachable lesson for corporate pharmacy managers in all of this, but they never got the message, as the tech in question is still working for the chain. Fortunately, I am not, having left to pursue a very happy career in biopharmaceutical manufacturing operations for Amgen.

Have a good day!

[Pharmacist R. H.]

E-mail from pharmacist #3

Hi Dennis,

I read with interest your editorial in *Drug Topics* about pharmacists admitting to errors as they happen. I am a retail pharmacist and appreciate your opening dialogue on a topic that needs serious attention—the state of current pharmacy. You hint at many sad and dangerous trends in our business—understaffing, increasing errors, strained relationship between corporation and pharmacist, lawsuits, liability, and lying. Each of these can and should be discussed by all pharmacists. But I had read years ago that pharmacists tend to be an introverted group, so it's not surprising that we have been led like sheep to the "job" each day.

…Errors do happen, and part of our job is education. One of the myths out there is that pharmacies don't make mistakes. Think of how many times someone has come in and whispered "I am bringing my prescriptions over here because they made a mistake at CVS," or some other pharmacy. I always let them know at that moment that mistakes are made in EVERY pharmacy, as we are all staffed by human beings. I encourage them to call if ever anything looks different, and that in this day of hectic doctor visits and busy pharmacies you (the customer) need to look out for yourself and ask questions.

Several years ago our local paper (*Portland Press Herald*) had a lead story titled something like: "Pharmacy Errors—All Pharmacies Make Mistakes But Why does Rite Aid Get Sued More?" This was actually an eye-opening article. The writer had done his research and checked the number of errors/complaints that were brought to the attention of the Maine Board of Pharmacy, and sure enough the numbers were similar for most chains. But the number going to trial (at that time) was much higher for Rite Aid. The conclusion of the article was that how a patient is treated at the time of the incident is critical. If you are arrogant or callous in your approach, you are more likely to get sued. Since reading this article I have made it a point to develop good relationships with customers from the start. When the shit hits the fan, I want that angry customer to be a friend. If you have been an arrogant pharmacist (and there are plenty out there), then you are writing your own legal prescription. Keep that personal liability insurance handy.

...I will also say that I keep memos of correspondence between myself and the corporation when it comes to staffing. If I ended up in court I would present papers and emails to show that I tried to warn the corporation that we were dangerously understaffed. I won't go down alone; I'll drag as many of my supervisors into court as possible. Sad that this is how I look at my job, but this is my liability insurance.

Your article, hopefully, will be another push toward galvanizing pharmacists to be a more cohesive group. We are the only ones that can change this. Think about it—what if pharmacists walked off the job like the air traffic controllers did back in the 70's? Hopefully that would never happen but my point is that we need to ALL work toward change. The corporations have no interest in that.

Keep up the dialogue.

[Pharmacist B. Y.]

PART V

STATE BOARDS
OF PHARMACY

Chapter 18

State boards of pharmacy disciplinary actions

The purpose of the board of pharmacy in each state is to protect the public. The state boards do things like licensing pharmacists to ensure that those pharmacists are competent. The boards try to prevent pharmacists from breaking laws pertaining to drugs. The most common disciplinary actions taken by state boards of pharmacy are usually for one of the following three reasons: (1) the pharmacist abuses drugs and/or alcohol, (2) the pharmacist is involved in illegally selling or distributing drugs, or (3) the pharmacist makes an error in dispensing drugs (for example, giving a patient the wrong drug, wrong dose, wrong directions, etc.).

Most of my career as a pharmacist was spent in North Carolina. How common are pharmacy errors in North Carolina? In my opinion, they are probably just as common as in most other states, despite some well-intentioned workload regulations that were passed by the state board of pharmacy. During the years I worked in North Carolina, most of these workload regulations were ignored by employers unless or until, for example, the board got involved in investigating an error that was reported to the board of pharmacy. In my experience, only a tiny fraction of errors are ever reported to state boards of pharmacy, mainly because pharmacy customers do not know they have that option, or because they do not perceive the error as having been serious, or because they shrug it off by telling themselves, "Errors happen. Pharmacists are human."

The NewsChannel 36 investigative team at television station WCNC in Charlotte, North Carolina analyzed a spread sheet with five years worth of errors that were reported to the North Carolina board of pharmacy from 2006 through 2010. The WCNC-TV investigative team found that the most common error was the substitution of the wrong drug, which happened 226 times in that five year period, accounting for more than half the documented errors. Other errors included wrong dosage, wrong directions, wrong patient (one patient's drugs given to a different patient), and the wrong count or number of pills or tablets in the bottle. (Stuart Watson, NewsChannel 36, Charlotte, North Carolina, "Pharmacy board documents hundreds of pharmacist errors," Posted on WCNC.com on May 3, 2011. http://www.wcnc.com/news/iteam/NC-Pharmacy-board-documents-hundreds-of-pharmacist-errors-121189759.html#)

Errors reported to North Carolina Board of Pharmacy: 2006 -2010
(Analysis by WCNC-TV in Charlotte, North Carolina, May 3, 2011)
Wrong medication: 226
Wrong dose: 80
Wrong directions: 77
Wrong patient: 24
Wrong count: 12

Here is a sample of disciplinary actions taken by the North Carolina Board of Pharmacy for pharmacy mistakes that were reported to that board. Most of these mistakes involve the wrong drug being dispensed, or the right drug was dispensed but in the wrong dose, or the wrong directions were typed on the patient's label. These disciplinary actions are from the January 2002 and October 2001 issues of the *Newsletter* published by the North Carolina Board of Pharmacy (www.ncbop.org). Starting with the April 2002 issue, the North Carolina Board of Pharmacy stopped providing detailed descriptions in that *Newsletter* of disciplinary actions, so I am unable to provide more recent examples that are as detailed as those below. A notice in the April 2002 issue of the *Newsletter* states, "The format for "Disciplinary Actions" will change with this *Newsletter*. In this and all future *Newsletters*, there will be information listing a general summary of actions taken by the North Carolina Board of Pharmacy." From my perspective, there is no reason to assume that the incidence of pharmacy errors has decreased in the interim. (Please note: Brand name drugs are capitalized. Generic names are in lower case.)

DISCIPLINARY ACTIONS—JANUARY 2002

Clonidine dispensed instead of Premarin

[Pharmacist J. Z.] was the subject of a Prehearing Conference held April 9, 2001 with Mr. Watts regarding the **dispensing of clonidine on a prescription which called for Premarin 0.3 mg** and the patient ingesting one dosage unit of clonidine before discovering the error. Recommendation: Letter of Warning and directed to be more careful in the dispensing of drugs in the future and comply with statutes and regulations governing the practice of pharmacy and the distribution of drugs. Accepted by: [Pharmacist J. Z.] 6/28/01; the Board 7/17/01.

Tussionex dispensed instead of prednisolone

[Pharmacist V. F.] was the subject of a Prehearing Conference held May 21, 2001 with Mr. Overman regarding the **dispensing of Tussionex on an order for prednisolone.** The Tussionex was also labeled prednisolone. Recommendation: Caution and within 90 days of Board's acceptance of this order he shall submit a written proposal to the Board for the lawful and accurate dispensing of multi-orders of liquid prescription drugs to the same patient and that for 12 months from the date of the Board's acceptance of the order the respondent shall notify the Board's director of investigations of any error committed by him if the patient leaves the store with the prescription. Accepted by [Pharmacist V. F.] 6/23/01.

Amoxicillin dispensed instead of naproxen

[Pharmacist J. M.] was the subject of a Prehearing Conference held June 20, 2001 with Mr. Haywood regarding the **dispensing of amox-**

icillin on an order for naproxen with the patient ingesting the incorrect product for three days before the error was discovered. Recommendation: Warning to exercise greater care in his dispensing practices in the future; review his practice environment and make any changes necessary to prevent the occurrence of dispensing errors; not violate any law or regulation governing the practice of pharmacy. Accepted by [Pharmacist J. M.] 7/10/01.

Incorrect directions on Cefzil label

[Pharmacist A. C.] was the subject of a Prehearing Conference held April 26, 2001 with Mr. Rogers regarding the **dispensing of Cefzil to a patient with incorrect directions on the label** and also indicating no refills when refills were left on the prescription. Recommendation: Letter of Caution for his actions in this matter and cautioned to be more careful in the dispensing of drugs in the future and to comply with statutes and regulations governing the practice of pharmacy and the distribution of drugs. Accepted by [Pharmacist A. C.] 6/26/01.

Wrong strength of Tapazole dispensed

[Pharmacist S. S.] and The Medicine Shoppe were the subject of a Prehearing Conference held May 21, 2001 with Mr. Overman regarding the **dispensing of Tapazole 100 mg. on an order for Tapazole 5 mg.**; failure to conduct Drug Utilization Reviews on prescription drug orders; failure to make and keep an accurate record of prescription drugs compounded in the pharmacy; failure to make and keep records regarding patient's refusals to accept counseling on new drugs. Recommendation: For the actions in committing an error in the dispensing of a prescription drug the license is suspended for a period of 3 days, stayed 1 year with specific conditions. Accepted by [Pharmacist S. S.] 7/13/01; accepted by [Pharmacist S. S.] on behalf of The Medicine Shoppe 7/13/01.

DISCIPLINARY ACTIONS—OCTOBER 2001

Zoloft dispensed instead of metronidazole

[Pharmacist C. B.] **Dispensed Zoloft on a prescription for metronidazole**; no patient counseling offered; the patient ingested the wrong medication for a period of four days before the error was discovered. Official Board Warning.

Incorrect directions on Dilantin

[Pharmacist J. H.] Heard by Board Member Crocker. **Filled an order for Dilantin suspension with incorrect directions** for administration on the vial resulting in the patient being hospitalized for approximately eight days. Recommendation: License suspended seven days, stayed two years with active three-day suspension of the license and other conditions. Accepted by [Pharmacist J. H.] March 19, 2001; the Board April 17, 2001.

Incorrect directions on Histinex DM

[Pharmacist D. H.] Heard by Board Member Watts. **Dispensed Histinex DM Syrup to a patient with incorrect directions** on the vial. Recommendation: Letter of Concern. Accepted by: [Pharmacist D. H.] March 13, 2001; the Board April 17, 2001.

Synthroid dispensed instead of Maxzide

[Pharmacist R. R.] Heard by Board Member Nelson. **Dispensed Synthroid on a prescription for Maxzide** with the patient ingesting the wrong medication for approximately seven days before the error was discovered. Recommendation: License suspended five days, stayed three years with active suspension of one day and other conditions. Accepted by: [Pharmacist R. R.] April 10, 2001; the Board April 17, 2001.

Incorrect directions on Dilantin

Indian Trail Pharmacy. Heard by Board Member Overman. A pharmacist working at that facility **dispensed Dilantin liquid with incorrect directions** on the bottle with the patient receiving nine administrations of the product before the error was discovered. Recommendation: Permit suspended one day, stayed two years with conditions. Accepted by: [C. S.] on behalf of Indian Trail Pharmacy March 20, 2001; by the Board April 17, 2001.

Zyrtec and Lipitor dispensed in same vial

Eckerd Drugs, 945 N Harrison Ave, Cary. Heard by Board Member Crocker. Pharmacist **dispensed Zyrtec 10 mg with both Zyrtec and Lipitor 10 mg dispensed in same vial.** The error resulted from Zyrtec and Lipitor being placed in a "Baker Cell" without the knowledge of the pharmacist. The patient ingested at least four dosage units of Lipitor as a result of the error. Recommendation: Letter of Warning with the pharmacy to implement an effective Policy and Procedure for automatic devices used in the dispensing of prescription drugs. Accepted by: [J. C.] on behalf of Eckerd Drugs March 27, 2001; by the Board April 17, 2001.

Wrong strength of isosorbide dispensed

[Pharmacist R. B.] Heard by Board Member Haywood. **Dispensing isosorbide 60 mg on a prescription for isosorbide 30 mg.** The patient did not ingest any of the incorrect medication. Recommendation: Reprimand and violate no laws governing the practice of pharmacy or the distribution of drugs. Accepted by: [Pharmacist R. B.] April 17, 2001; the Board May 15, 2001.

Hydralazine dispensed instead of hydroxyzine

[Pharmacist K. S.] Heard by Board Member Nelson. **Dispensing of hydralazine on a prescription for hydroxyzine 25 mg** with the order being refilled several times from the original dispensing date, resulting in the patient ingesting the incorrect product. Recommendation: License suspended five days, stayed three years with active one-day suspension of the license and other conditions. Accepted by: [Pharmacist K. S.] May 2, 2001; the Board May 15, 2001.

Fiorinal dispensed instead of Florinef

[Pharmacist O. O.] Heard by Board Member Nelson regarding the **dispensing of Fiorinal on an order calling for Florinef** with the patient ingesting three dosage units before the error was discovered. Recommendation: License suspended five days, stayed three years with active one day suspension and other specific conditions. Accepted by: [Pharmacist O. O.] April 23, 2001; the Board May 15, 2001.

Vibramycin dispensed instead of vitamins

[Pharmacist L. R.] Heard by Board Member Watts. **Dispensing Vibramycin 100 mg on a prescription for vitamins** with the patient ingesting the incorrect medication for approximately 34 days before discovery of the error. Recommendation: Warning to exercise greater care in his dispensing practices in the future. Accepted by: [Pharmacist L. R.] May 10, 2001; the Board May 15, 2001.

Sulfasalazine dispensed instead of sulfadiazine

[Pharmacist H. M.] Heard by Board Member Rogers. **Dispensing sulfasalazine 500 mg to a patient on a prescription order for sulfadiazine 500 mg.** Recommendation: Letter of Warning for his actions in this matter. Accepted by: [Pharmacist H. M.] May 30, 2001; the Board June 26, 2001.

Prednisone dispensed instead of glipizide

[Pharmacist M. D.] Heard by Board Member Rogers. **Dispensing prednisone 5 mg to a patient who was to receive glipizide.** Recommendation: Letter of Warning for her actions in this matter. Accepted by [Pharmacist M. D.] May 30, 2001; the Board June 26, 2001.

Verapamil dispensed instead of Zantac

[Pharmacist T. L.] Heard by Board Member Watts. **Dispensing verapamil to a patient on a prescription calling for Zantac** with the patient ingesting two dosage units of the incorrect medication before the error was discovered. Recommendation: Letter of Warning for his actions in this matter. Accepted by: [Pharmacist T. L.] May 23, 2001; the Board June 26, 2001.

Pharmacist committed seven errors in six months

[Pharmacist W. F.] Heard by Board Member Watts. Embezzlement or otherwise diversion to his own use of approximately 900 dosage units of hydrocodone; during the first six months of the year 2000 **committing seven errors in the dispensing of prescription drugs to patients;** history of alcohol and controlled substance abuse for approximately 25 years. Recommendation: License suspended indefinitely, stayed five years with specific conditions. Accepted by: [Pharmacist W. F.] May 15, 2001; the Board June 26, 2001.

Propylthiouracil dispensed instead of Purinthol

[Pharmacist D. M.] Heard by Board Member Watts. **Dispensing propylthiouracil to a two-year-old patient on a prescription calling for Purinethol** with the patient ingesting the wrong medication from January 10 until June 20, 2000, when the error was discovered. Recommendation: License suspended 30 days, stayed three years with an active suspension of seven days to begin no later than June 30, 2001, and other conditions. Accepted by [Pharmacist D. M.] May 17, 2001; the Board June 26, 2001.

Morphine dispensed instead of Roxicodone

[Pharmacist A. A.] Heard by Board Member Watts. **Dispensing morphine 15 mg on a prescription calling for Roxicodone 5 mg** with the patient ingesting 81 morphine 15 mg dosage units before the error was discovered. Recommendation: Letter of Warning for her actions in this matter. Accepted by: [Pharmacist A. A.] May 17, 2001; the Board June 26, 2001.

Wrong dose of doxepin dispensed

[Pharmacist P. H.] Heard by Board Member Overman. **Dispensing of doxepin 10 mg to a patient on an order calling for doxepin 100 mg.** Recommendation: Warning to exercise greater care in his dispensing practices. Accepted by: [Pharmacist P. H.] June 15, 2001; the Board June 26, 2001.

Chapter 19

Why pharmacists are so disgusted with state boards of pharmacy

I have very mixed feelings about the state boards of pharmacy publishing (in their newsletters and/or websites) disciplinary actions taken against pharmacists. For those pharmacists who try very hard to avoid mistakes, but occasionally make them anyway, I have the greatest sympathy. If these pharmacists make an error because of inadequate staffing in the pharmacy, I consider it unfair to blame the pharmacist rather than the employer. Employers benefit from understaffing because it forces everyone to work harder, thereby increasing the productivity and profitability of the pharmacy. But understaffing also increases the chance of pharmacy mistakes.

There are a very large number of mitigating and aggravating factors that, in my opinion, should be considered before pharmacists are disciplined by state boards of pharmacy. Here are just a few:
• If a pharmacist makes a mistake because he was working overtime due to, for example, another pharmacist's vacation or illness, I find it hard to blame the pharmacist for being exhausted. However, if the pharmacist made the mistake because he asked to work those extra hours (and there were other pharmacists available), then blaming that pharmacist may be more reasonable if he claims the mistake was due to the fact that he was exhausted from the long hours on his feet.

• If a pharmacist makes a mistake because he was up all night with a sick child, then I have a hard time blaming the pharmacist.

• If a pharmacist makes a mistake because he was unfocused due to the fact that he just had an unavoidable fight with his spouse, children, or boss, I have a hard time blaming the pharmacist.

On the other hand,

• If a pharmacist makes a mistake because he was simply careless (for example, he was more interested in chatting with one of his young female techs or clerks) and there was adequate staffing in the pharmacy, it is probably more reasonable to blame the pharmacist.

Fear is a powerful motivator causing pharmacists to be careful. These fears include: 1) the fear of being sued and ending up in court, 2) the fear of harming one of our customers as a result of a mistake, 3) the fear of being disciplined by the state board of pharmacy, and 4) the fear of having our name listed in the board of pharmacy newsletter.

For those pharmacists who are extremely careful yet occasionally make errors, I feel it is unfair to publicize their names in the board of pharmacy newsletter. For those many pharmacists who are an accident waiting to happen, publicizing their names in the board newsletter may be one of the biggest things that can give these careless pharmacists a wake up call.

Potentially the most serious mistake I made in my 25-year career was when I did not catch a doctor's error on a prescription. In this case, a local doctor wrote a prescription for the sleeping pill Halcion with directions, "Take one tablet 3 times a day." Obviously sleeping pills are usually taken once a day (at bedtime). At that time, Halcion had just come on the market, and, as much as I hate to admit it, I dispensed this drug without knowing what it is used for (i.e., it is sleeping pill). The doctor had clearly made an error in the directions and I did not catch that error. I typed "Take one tablet 3 times a day" on the label just as the doctor specified. If the customer had reported this error to the state board of pharmacy, I would have been very upset but perhaps I would have deserved being disciplined for this error.

As best as I can recall this incident, there were not any exacerbating circumstances that I can blame for my role in this error. I did not make this error because of understaffing. It is true that I was some-times exhausted at this store. I was routinely working fifty hours a week because this was in a new store and my district supervisor hadn't yet found a second pharmacist to split the eighty hours the store was open each week. "Floater" pharmacists filled in whenever I asked for a day off. I can't remember whether I was fatigued that particular day.

Surely I should never have dispensed Halcion (or any other drug) without knowing what it is used for. But I did and I am lucky that no harm resulted. The customer apparently called his doctor and asked the doctor about the directions. The doctor phoned me and asked, "Why would you put three times a day on a sleeping pill?" I asked the doctor to hold on for a few seconds while I pulled the hard copy of the prescription from our files. What I discovered when I pulled the hard copy from our files was that the doctor had indeed mistakenly specified "three times a day" on his handwritten prescrip-tion. I told the doctor, "I have your prescription here in my hand. You wrote "tid" [the Latin abbreviation for three times a day]." I think I then offered to fax him the prescription so he could see that he had made a mistake. He did not ask to see a copy of the prescrip-tion so I assume he believed me that he had made the mistake. The doctor's main question was why I had not caught the error. So the doctor and I were basically even. The doctor had screwed up and I did not catch the mistake.

If this customer had indeed taken the pill three times a day and attempted to drive a car, the results could have been disastrous. I as-sume that the customer realized that the Halcion is indeed a sleeping pill, so I assume he knew enough to question why the label in-structed him to "Take one tablet 3 times a day." Many customers are on so many medications that they have a hard time keeping track of what each one is used for. And many pharmacy customers are illiterate or poorly literate or elderly and never question things. This customer had the misfortune of being the recipient of the most seri-ous mistake I made in my career, but I am lucky that he knew enough to question things.

Pharmacy customers need to realize that only a tiny percentage (maybe as few as one in a thousand) of mistakes made by pharmacists are reported to state boards of pharmacy. Why? Most customers do not know that they have this option. Many customers do not realize that pharmacy mistakes can vary in significance from those that are trivial to those that are deadly. Many customers have a hard time believing that pharmacists and techs do indeed make mistakes. Many customers are, thankfully, quite forgiving. When my stepfather was given a drug for Type 2 diabetes (he's never had Type 2 diabetes) by mistake instead of his blood pressure pills at a local WalMart pharmacy, my stepfather said to me "Accidents happen. If it happens again, I'll get mad." Even though I've seen or heard about many mistakes made by pharmacists in the stores I've worked in during my career, I can't specifically recall hearing that a single one of those mistakes was reported to the state board of pharmacy.

The purpose of the state board of pharmacy is to protect the public from harm as it relates to pharmacies. Since pharmacy mistakes can and do cause harm to the public, many pharmacists feel that state boards of pharmacy should be a powerful force in preventing these errors. Pharmacists feel that working conditions (including inadequate staffing) are a primary cause of pharmacy mistakes. Therefore pharmacists feel that boards of pharmacy should take a very aggressive role in prohibiting those working conditions that contribute to pharmacy mistakes. Many pharmacists feel that state boards of pharmacy have been afraid to blame the big drugstore chains for inadequate staffing. Many pharmacists feel that the state boards are afraid to challenge the immense legal and political clout of the big drugstore chains. In a phone conversation, the head of one state board of pharmacy told me that the worst part of his job was dealing with lawyers representing pharmacists and/or the big chains.

In my opinion, another factor that prevents state boards from blaming the big chains is that the boards don't want to be seen as having an anti-business outlook in the eyes of state legislatures if those legislatures indeed have a largely pro-business orientation. In the event of a pharmacy mistake, many pharmacists are disgusted and angered by the fact that many state boards focus aggressively on the weakest player (the individual pharmacist) but appear to be afraid to focus on the strongest player (the big drugstore chains). Pharmacists feel that the big drugstore chains routinely understaff pharmacies to increase profitability and that, therefore, mistakes are inevitable.

Many pharmacists hope that the reporting of mistakes to boards of pharmacy and local newspapers will result in efforts that require adequate staffing for pharmacies. It just doesn't seem to be happening. Unfortunately the public seems to have a hard time believing that the big chains are often reckless in how they staff pharmacies.

Issues of working conditions and public safety are not unique to pharmacists. Many nurses complain that unbearable workloads endanger hospital patients. Medical residents complain that their long work weeks cause fatigue which decreases their level of performance, putting patients at risk. Airline pilots say that pilot fatigue endangers passengers. Are all these examples strictly employer/employee issues between nurses, medical residents, and hospital administrators, or between airlines and pilots? Or are they public safety issues? Long-haul truck drivers who are exhausted from spending too many hours on the highway are clearly a hazard to the public safety.

At what point do employer/employee issues justifiably become public safety issues? Are nurses, pharmacists, medical residents, airline pilots, and long-haul truck drivers simply crybabies in search of cushy jobs? At what point does governmental regulation of the private sector for public safety reasons trump the rights of private corporations to control their workplace? How many deaths must occur before regulators are justified in intervening? Republicans typically favor less regulation of the workplace than Democrats.

The pharmacy boards act as though pharmacists' working conditions are a private matter between employers and employees. Pharmacy boards seem to feel that if pharmacists dislike their working conditions, they are free to change jobs. Indeed, some pharmacists write angry "letters to the editor" telling their disillusioned colleagues: "If you're unhappy, CHANGE JOBS!!"

Is it simply a matter of disgruntled pharmacists changing jobs? Each year the pharmacy workplace shows more resemblance to a factory assembly line. The mail order model of high volume dispensing seems to be the direction in which the profession is headed, to the dismay of many pharmacists. It may be that alternatives for disgruntled pharmacists are diminishing as more employers embrace the fast food model. Even though the schools of pharmacy continue to promote the model of the pharmacist as drug expert, the big chains have shown little enthusiasm for that concept. The schools of pharmacy convince students that they're professionals. So it comes as a powerful shock when these students graduate and begin working as licensed pharmacists and discover that the big chains are only interested in how many widgets (prescriptions) we can produce per hour. When the big chains talk about productivity, what they mean is getting pharmacists, techs, and clerks to do more work with less staffing.

One definition of a dysfunctional family is a family that avoids addressing the most pressing issues facing it. For example, a dysfunctional family avoids discussing a father who is an alcoholic or who abuses his children or beats his wife. In my opinion, pharmacy boards are significantly dysfunctional because they are afraid to openly confront the most crucial issue facing chain pharmacists: working conditions.

The boards of pharmacy say that they can't do anything about pharmacists' working conditions. The boards say that if pharmacists have complaints about working conditions, we need to form a guild or union. Are the pharmacy boards simply passing the buck? Is this a legitimate position for the boards to take? Or is it simply a cop-out? Should employee pharmacists let the boards off the hook so easily? Or should we organize and hold their feet to the fire and force them to address the immediate concerns of employee pharmacists?

In my opinion, the boards of pharmacy are afraid to challenge the immense power of the big chains. What happens when some pharmacy group stands up to the big chains? The big chains or their proxies may take you to court as the North Carolina Board of Pharmacy discovered several years ago when that Board tried to address pharmacists' working conditions.

Even though I admire the North Carolina Board's efforts to pass a regulation requiring a lunch break for pharmacists, I don't see how such a regulation would have a major impact on our workplace. No employer is so stupid as to say we can't take a lunch break. Many pharmacists choose to skip meals for the simple reason that we're so far behind in filling prescriptions that taking a break would put us even further behind.

I don't see how the National Association of Boards of Pharmacy (NABP) can continue to say that pharmacists' working conditions are outside their purview when they see that the North Carolina Board has taken courageous stands in an effort to address this issue.

Employee pharmacists need to collectively put pressure on the leaders of the state boards and NABP. We need to get the dead wood out of the pharmacy boards. The boards of pharmacy tell us that they don't have any power to improve working conditions and that they can only pass regulations that protect the public safety. But surely pharmacies that are dangerously understaffed are a threat to the public safety. Surely a pharmacist who hasn't eaten any food or taken a break in ten hours is a threat to the public safety.

In my opinion, the state boards of pharmacy, as official state regulatory bodies, need to capitalize on their ties to state legislatures in order to address pharmacists' working conditions. Employee pharmacists need to hold the state boards and NABP accountable in their responsibility to protect the public safety. We need to put pressure on the boards to address working conditions the same way that the boards put pressure on us to counsel customers even though, too often, pharmacists don't have enough staffing to allow proper counseling.

Pharmacists are tired of hearing that the state boards' hands are tied by the organizational structure of state governments. The state boards need to stop making excuses and learn to think outside the box. Let the state board members jawbone the state legislators at non-official gatherings if necessary, like at social functions, football games, etc. We need results—not excuses—from state boards.

The Auburn University School of Pharmacy study (Elizabeth Flynn, et. al., "National Observational Study of Prescription Dispensing Accuracy and Safety in 50 Pharmacies," *Journal of the American Pharmacists Association*, March/April 2003, pp. 191-200. (http://www.medscape.com/viewarticle/451962) concludes that "51.5 million errors occur during the filling of 3 billion prescriptions each year." Since most pharmacists feel strongly that there is a direct relationship between understaffing and errors, I think the boards are being less than honest when they claim that they have no role in the pharmacist's workplace. If the state boards and NABP are to properly carry out their role in protecting the public safety, they have a duty to speak out about pharmacists' working conditions.

The boards have credibility with state legislatures because the boards are not seen as promoting the economic interests of pharmacists. The boards need to use their position as watchdogs over public safety to get the attention of the state legislatures. If the main function of the boards of pharmacy is to protect the public safety, then, based on the occurrence of 51.5 million errors each year, the boards are doing a very poor job of protecting the public from this unacceptably high number pharmacy errors.

I have received a large number of e-mails from pharmacists who are fed up with state boards of pharmacy. These pharmacists feel that the state boards are negligent in their duty to protect the public safety by failing to address the threat posed by dangerous dispensing speeds. Pharmacists should realize that, collectively, we have tremendous power to influence the agenda of the state boards. If huge numbers of pharmacists complain to state legislators about the state boards, surely the boards will feel the heat.

We need true leaders at all the state boards, not people who pass the buck to protect their own position. (One state board director told me that "prestige" is a big reason why some people desire to be on state boards of pharmacy.) We need dynamic leadership and people who are willing to take courageous stands in the fight for employee pharmacists. Too many pharmacy boards are wimps on the issue of pharmacists' working conditions. Collectively, pharmacists need to become more forceful and sophisticated in shaping the agenda of pharmacy boards. A major shake-up is long overdue.

David Work, formerly the executive director of the North Carolina Board of Pharmacy, is an attorney and a pharmacist. He is one of the few people with a prominent role in pharmacy who has taken a courageous position in the fight for better working conditions for pharmacists. Pharmacists should encourage him to seek the helm at one of pharmacy's major national organizations or associations. In my opinion, he should be one of the most prominent voices for pharmacy and pharmacists.

Even though I would like to see state boards of pharmacy mandate adequate staffing in pharmacies, I admit that writing such a regulation would be difficult. For example, a regulation might state that, for example, a pharmacy filling 200 prescriptions per day must have "x" number of techs on duty, a pharmacy filling 300 hundred prescriptions per day must have "y" number of techs on duty, and a pharmacy filling 400 prescriptions per day must have "z" number of techs on duty. Wording a regulation in that way fails to take into consideration the quality of each technician. It is important to realize that techs vary in performance from those who are the greenest rookies to those who are absolutely fantastic. The best techs can work circles around the weakest techs. A pharmacy filling, say, 250 prescriptions on a particular day can be bearable with good techs, but it can be an absolute nightmare with weak techs. Mandating certification of techs is not, in my opinion, the answer. Certification of techs does not mean that those techs are fast or smart. I'd rather work with non-certified techs who are fast and smart, rather than work with certified techs who are slow and not very bright. At the very least I would like state boards of pharmacy to make an attempt to mandate adequate staffing, even though I acknowledge writing such a regulation would be difficult. In my dream world, a pharmacist would have the ability to walk out of a pharmacy that he felt was inadequately staffed and a threat to the public safety. In the real world, such a pharmacist would stand the very real risk of being fired.

Many pharmacists have a great deal of anger toward state boards of pharmacy for not standing up to the big chains and requiring conditions and staffing in drugstores so that errors are not inevitable. Pharmacists express these sentiments routinely in private conversations among ourselves and, often, in letters to the editor at pharmacy magazines. The following letter-to-the-editor published in *Drug Topics* is one of many examples (Ann Greene, R.Ph., "A Matter of Time," *Drug Topics*, October, 2010, p. 13). This letter was in response to an article in that magazine about Rajendra Bhat, a former Medco pharmacist who went on a hunger strike to protest production requirements at that huge pharmacy mail order facility. Although most pharmacists would probably agree that a hunger strike is an extreme reaction to workloads, these same pharmacists would probably emphasize that Mr. Bhat's main point is exceedingly important.

Re: "Desperate measures" [*Drug Topics* Viewpoint, Sept. 2010]:
I have been a retail pharmacist for 20 years and have seen the error rates progressively getting worse. I find it appalling that a state board could turn its back on not only the pharmacists but the patients as well. Rajendra Bhat should be commended for taking a stand while the rest of us cowardly pharmacists trudge on, knowing that patient lives are in danger.

The major chains care only about money; they add more responsibilities, such as immunizations, while providing no additional help. It is only a matter of time before a major tragedy occurs. Shame on Medco, shame on the board, and shame on the retailers who have the same quota systems in place.

--Ann Greene, R.Ph., Nottingham, Penn.

An Ohio grand jury indicted pharmacist Eric Cropp for manslaughter and reckless homicide in the death of a two-year-old child, which resulted from an improperly compounded IV solution. The medical error occurred in 2006 at Rainbow Babies & Children's Hospital where the child, Emily Jerry, was a patient undergoing chemotherapy. According to testimony presented before the Ohio board of pharmacy, the prescription for etoposide with a base solution of 0.9% sodium chloride was instead compounded by a technician with a base solution of 23.4% sodium chloride. Three days after receiving the medication, the child died. The grand jury declined to indict the technician, Katie Dudash. (Reid Paul, "Former pharmacist indicted for manslaughter after med error," *Drug Topics*, Sept. 17, 2007, p. 10. See also the Emily Jerry Foundation emilyjerryfoundation.org and http://emilyjerryfoundation.org/man-seeks-nationwide-law-after-toddlers-death/) This case settled for seven million dollars. Pharmacist Eric Cropp served time in prison for the pharmacy mistake.

Emily Jerry's father blames the Ohio State Pharmacy Board for the death of his daughter. I know this will sound extreme on my part, but I firmly believe that pharmacists across America should publicly ridicule state boards of pharmacy and the National Association of Boards of Pharmacy for being too timid to take meaningful action that actually decreases the occurrence of pharmacy mistakes. Here is the comment from Emily Jerry's father on the website (emilyjerryfoundation.org) he set up to promote the prevention of pharmacy errors. (http://emilyjerryfoundation.org/discovery-channel-to-air-%E2%80%9Csurfing-the-healthcare-tsunami-bring-your-best-board%E2%80%9D-on-april-28th%E2%80%9D-featuring-initial-interview-between-christopher-jerry-and-eric-cropp/

...I truly believe that the Ohio State Pharmacy Board, at that time, should have really been held culpable in Emily's death. The reason I say this is due to the simple fact that it was determined that a pharmacy technician had actually made the fatal error that had killed Emily. After the incident, the pharmacy technician had mentioned that she never really knew that highly concentrated sodium chloride (salt) could actually kill people. With that in mind, I have always asked myself why the Ohio State Pharmacy Board at that time had absolutely no training requirements, licensing requirements, or oversight of pharmacy technicians in the state of Ohio. To make matters worse, they had to know that pharmacy technicians were being used on a daily basis at all of Ohio's medical facilities to routinely compound IV medications going directly into patient's circulatory systems. With that being said, I believe the Ohio State Pharmacy Board was really not doing their primary job, which was to protect the residents of their state from unsafe pharmacy practices. Bottom line, as Emily's father, had I known that there would have been a very high likelihood, or probability, that a pharmacy technician who had little, to no, training would have been compounding my daughter's IV medications, I never would have allowed it to happen. I would have insisted that only a registered pharmacist, with years and years of training, prepare all of Emily's IV medications during the course of her treatment.

PART VI

PHARMACY SCHOOL

Chapter 20

How much chemistry is needed to work at a chain drugstore?

Back in the 1970s when I attended pharmacy school, a bachelor's degree (B.S. Pharm.) required five years. Today the bachelor's degree has been eliminated and all graduates must have a doctorate in pharmacy (Pharm. D.) which usually takes six years. I had two years of college curricula in what is called "pre-pharmacy" and three years in pharmacy school.

My most prominent memory of my five years in college is the heavy emphasis on chemistry. Who can forget all those courses in inorganic chemistry, organic chemistry, medicinal chemistry, and biochemistry? To this day, I can't understand why my formal education placed such a heavy emphasis on chemistry. Contrary to the perception of the general public, there is very little that I need to know about chemistry to function competently as a pharmacist with one of the big drugstore chains. Even though the public associates pharmacists with chemistry, that is an outdated view of pharmacists today, just as the "mortar & pestle" is an outdated symbol for pharmacy. The chemistry requirements in pharmacy school seem to be a holdover from the days when pharmacists were called "chemists."

My organic chemistry class consisted of pre-pharmacy and pre-medical students. One day in this class I remember the professor mentioning that he had been approached by some pre-med students about making the class more meaningful to aspiring health professionals. The professor commented that that was a reasonable request and that the issue would be examined. However, I didn't detect any increase in relevance after that point. I doubt that the subject of organic chemistry can be made very relevant to health professionals. Just as you can't change the stripes on a zebra, you can't change the nature of organic chemistry. I just don't think that organic chemistry is essential to being a pharmacist or doctor. At that time, I considered it somewhat idealistic that these pre-med students approached the professor with a request to make the class more relevant for future health professionals. Now I realize they were absolutely right.

There was a general perception among pre-pharmacy and pre-med students that the chemistry and physics classes were "hurdle" classes used by admissions committees to evaluate applicants. If a student did well in those classes, it was assumed that he could do well in pharmacy school or medical school. Like the heavy emphasis on chemistry that was required to become a pharmacist, I have never understood the physics requirement. Even back in the 1970s, it should have been perfectly clear that physics had very little to do with pharmacy. Today, many pharmacy schools require calculus for admission, but it was not required when I applied to pharmacy school. I had taken calculus because I was previously an engineering major. I can say with absolute certainty that I never used my knowledge of calculus in my 25-year career in chain drugstores.

In pharmacy school I had no idea that memorizing things like the structural formula of drugs would turn out to have no use in my career. Knowledge of structural formulas would have been beneficial if I had become a medicinal chemist. But I think the whole point of my medicinal chemistry class was understanding the relationship between the molecular structure of a drug and its biological activity. I think this was called the "structure-activity relationship," but I'm not sure. I no longer remember the structural formula of a single drug, nor have I needed to. I forgot that information soon after graduation. During my entire career as a chain pharmacist, there has never been a single instance in which I needed to know the structural formula of a drug.

Pharmacists: If you were to rank all of your required college courses in terms of relevance to your career, where would you place chemistry on that list? When is the last time you needed to look up a drug's structural formula? When is the last time that you looked up the structural formula for Prozac, Prevacid, Plavix, Pravachol, Procardia, or Protonix? When is the last time that a drug's structural formula had any bearing on any decision you made or on any prescrip tion you filled? When is the last time a doctor or customer asked you a question that required you to look at the structural formula of a drug? Do you know which drugs can stimulate an allergic reaction to sulfa from your recollection of structural formulas containing a sulfur atom?

I am not saying that we should not have a single course in chemistry. Complete ignorance of medicinal chemistry would not be wise. For example, pharmacists would not be able to have an informed opinion about the differences between "me-too" drugs without some understanding of the similarity in their structural formula. Pharmacists know that the differences between some drugs is simply a minor molecular modification that is sufficient to qualify for a separate patent.

My point is that chemistry should not be the primary focus of a pharmacist's education as it was when I was in pharmacy school. At most universities, chemistry is still a very significant part of the pre-pharmacy and pharmacy school curricula. I can still remember the endless amount of time I spent memorizing and writing structural formulas. Thirty-five years later I don't remember a single one! All that I remember is the core benzene ring which I wrote a thousand times.

Even though chemistry was the foundation of my pre-pharmacy and pharmacy school curricula, I am hard-pressed to recall a time I relied upon my chemistry knowledge in the drugstore. In the real world, pharmacists have infinitely greater need to know the drug interactions associated with Coumadin, in comparison to the structural formula for Coumadin. In fact, we have no need to know the structural formula for Coumadin or any other drug.

If chemistry is so important to being a pharmacist, why are there no continuing education courses offered today to pharmacists on the subject of chemistry? In my entire career as a pharmacist, I can't recall a single chemistry CE course at any of the live CE seminars or in any of the pharmacy magazines. I can't recall ever seeing any chemistry CE lessons in *Drug Topics, US Pharmacist,* or *Pharmacy Times.*

Retail pharmacists draw upon their knowledge of pharmacology routinely. For example, answering customers' questions requires a knowledge of pharmacology and drug therapies, not chemistry. Yet my college years consisted of more classes in chemistry than pharmacology. How is it logical to have so much chemistry in college if it's not used after graduation? Of course, chemistry is important for understanding things like incompatibilities when intravenous drugs are mixed in the same bottle, but I had far more chemistry than is needed to understand IV incompatibilities. As a chain pharmacist, I've never prepared an IV.

Pharmacy school curriculum needs to be more relevant. Certainly we need to understand economics to run a drugstore but does that mean we need a minor in economics? We need to know psychology to understand our customers and co-workers but does that mean we need a minor in psychology? We need to understand the cultural attitudes and misconceptions about disease causation that are common in various ethnic groups but does that mean we need a minor in medical anthropology? There are certainly times when my ignorance of Spanish inhibits my communication with Hispanic customers, but does that mean pharmacists need to become fluent in Spanish while in pharmacy school?

Certainly excellence in any, or all, of these subjects makes a better pharmacist and a more well-rounded human being. I am not making the case for ignorance or mediocrity. I am simply suggesting that all courses—including chemistry—should be given a focus in pharmacy school that is proportional to the needs of pharmacists in the real world. Having chemistry as the foundation of a pharmacist's education is, to me, absurd. In my opinion, pharmacology and therapeutics should be the central focus of the college curriculum.

Many pharmacists feel that pharmacy faculty are not living in the real world. Following my editorial in *Drug Topics* ("Reflections on pharmacy school after 30 years," Nov. 19, 2007, p. 36) questioning the emphasis in pharmacy schools on chemistry, I received an e-mail from a professor of medicinal chemistry in which he asserted that pharmacists need a level of understanding of chemistry that would cause most retail pharmacists to roll their eyes. For example, he stated "…understanding the drug omeprazole [Prilosec] requires that a practitioner understand acid/base chemistry, the acid catalyzed formation of a sulfenamide, and the nucleophilic attack that inactivates the Na/K-ATPase that fuels the proton pump." I can state categorically that pharmacists in the real world do not need to know that.

I received a lot of e-mail as a result of this editorial questioning the need for the fixation on chemistry in pharmacy school. Most of the e-mail I received from pharmacists who work in the trenches was highly favorable. I did, however, receive quite a few e-mails from pharmacy faculty who were livid that I had the audacity to suggest a much more limited role for chemistry in pharmacy school. An unintended—and, in my opinion, unfortunate consequence of this editorial involved the reaction from the American Association of Colleges of Pharmacy (AACP). [http://www.aacp.org/governance/SEC-TIONS/chemistry/Documents/Chem_StrategicPlanningCommitteeReport.pdf] At least in part as a result of my editorial, this association, which represents colleges of pharmacy across the country, passed a resolution stating that any pharmacy school that does not have medicinal chemistry as part of its curriculum would be "viewed as non-compliant with Standards 2007." The AACP noted that there were pharmacy schools that were dropping or had dropped chemistry, and that this was unacceptable. A document titled *Chemistry Section Strategic Planning Committee Response to Charges* includes the following: the "response of [Lucinda Maine, Ph.D., R.Ph., executive Vice President and CEO at AACP] to Dennis Miller's *Drug Topics* commentary (published in the April issue and attached) was appropriate." Another section of this document titled *Resolution from the Section of Teachers of Chemistry* states,

Be it further resolved that the AACP leadership communicate to the Accreditation Council for Pharmacy Education (ACPE) its expectation that any School or College of Pharmacy that fails to incorporate medicinal

chemistry or any other essential discipline into their required professional curriculum will be viewed as non-compliant with Standards 2007....

To the many professors of medicinal chemistry who sent me angry e-mails, I replied by asking them to provide a single example of how a chain pharmacist would need to use knowledge of chemistry in the drugstore. The silence was deafening. Only one professor attempted to provide such an example and it was the precise example I would have guessed he would provide. He said that knowledge of medicinal chemistry would help pharmacists recall which drugs can cause a sulfa allergic reaction based on the pharmacist's recalling which drugs contain a sulfur atom in their structural formula. From my perspective, it is much safer to use the pharmacy computer to flag drugs capable of causing a sulfur allergy, rather than rely on our memory of long-forgotten structural formulas. Only one professor could come up with this one example (sulfa allergy) which he stated proves that knowledge of chemistry is necessary in the drugstore. In my opinion, this speaks volumes to the weakness of the case for the intense focus on chemistry in the education of pharmacists. If I were to have stated in my editorial that pharmacists never use their knowledge of pharmacology in the drugstore, I would have been laughed out of the profession. It is easy to provide an endless number of examples in which pharmacists rely on our knowledge of pharmacology. Clearly the focus on chemistry in pharmacy school advances the occupational and intellectual interests of the chemistry faculty far more than it does the needs of pharmacists in the trenches.

Pharmacy faculty specialize in areas such as 1) "clinical" pharmacy (this discipline teaches pharmacy students and pharmacists how to help people optimize the use of drugs); 2) pharmacology (the study of the actions and effects of drugs); 3) pharmaceutics (this discipline focuses on the formulation of drugs into dosage forms such as capsules, tablets, liquids, injections, skin patches, creams, suppositories, etc.); 4) medicinal chemistry; 5) pharmacy law; 6) pharmacy administration; and 7) pharmacognosy (the study of drugs that are derived from plants or animals).

"Clinical" pharmacy is the discipline having the closest contact with the public. One professor of medicinal chemistry sent me an e-mail after my editorial in which he said that several of his "clinical" colleagues agreed with me that pharmacy students need far less emphasis on chemistry. He proceeded to excoriate me anyway implying that I wanted the clinical-types to take over the profession. Indeed, clinical pharmacy is the dominant specialty in pharmacy today and professors in other areas often fear that their specialty is taking a back seat to the clinical pharmacy faculty.

In my opinion, the focus on chemistry in the pharmacy school and pre-pharmacy curricula raises a fundamental question about the role of chemistry in human health. Is human health primarily dependent on the manipulation of molecules and cells with pharmaceuticals? Or is human health primarily determined by the proper nourishment of cells and tissues with nutritious foods, and by factors such as the maintenance of ideal body weight, exercise, a clean environment, the avoidance of tobacco and alcohol, etc.?

My basic disagreement with the focus on chemistry is that I don't view *Homo sapiens* as a collection of molecules and cells that are constantly prone to malfunction and constantly in need of pharmacological governance. To focus on chemistry in human health is to miss the big picture. My view is that the road to human health is primarily through prevention, not through chemistry. I disagree with the mechanistic, reductionistic approach that focuses on chemistry. I disagree with Big Pharma's basic orientation: better living through chemistry.

I am certainly not opposed to pharmacists having a well-rounded education. For example, if pharmacy schools want to graduate well-rounded students, I wish the curriculum would rise above its reductionistic fixation on molecules and cells. From my experience the public health perspective is sorely lacking in pharmacy schools. In my opinion, pharmacists desperately need to be taught about the social, cultural, economic, and political factors that have a major impact on health. I'd like to see courses in medical sociology, medical anthropology, social psychology, etc. In my opinion, the hegemony of the molecular focus in pharmacy school does not provide pharmacists with a well-rounded education.

Countless times I've read or heard statements such as "It's the lifestyles of Americans that's killing them." This, of course, refers to our obesity, hours in front of the television or computer, no exercise, poor diet, processed foods, alcohol, tobacco, pizza, desserts, candy, fast food, etc. There doesn't seem to be much serious disagreement in the mass media about the importance of lifestyles in preventing disease. So you would think that pharmacists would have courses in pharmacy school on sociology and psychology since society, culture, and personal behavior profoundly affect lifestyles.

It is quite rare that any of the major pharmacy magazines have articles discussing lifestyles, diet, exercise, etc., so I suspect that the absence of such articles implies to pharmacists that these subjects are unimportant. But pharmacists need to realize that the types of articles published in magazines are carefully chosen so that they will not upset the major advertisers in these magazines. In the case of pharmacy magazines, the biggest advertisers—by far—are the pharmaceutical companies. I have written seventeen editorials for *Drug Topics* and I concluded early in the process that any article I submitted that was too critical of Big Pharma would be quickly rejected.

Based on the articles in pharmacy magazines, pharmacists can easily conclude that the human body is a machine that is completely unaffected by social, cultural, psychological, economic, and environmental factors. Big Pharma only very grudgingly accepts that nutrition affects human health. In my opinion, Big Pharma's most shocking coup has been the complete removal of *Homo sapiens* from the natural world. Even though social and psychological factors can have profound effects on lifestyles (which, in turn, have profound effects on our health), sociology and psychology courses are uncommon and/or low profile in pharmacy school. The pharmacist's college years are dominated by a molecular and cellular focus on disease. I had so many chemistry classes in college that I felt I graduated with a degree in chemistry. The public often views pharmacists as akin to chemists, so it may seem unbelievable to the average pharmacy customer when I say that I can't recall a single instance in my 25-year career in which I actually called upon my knowledge of chemistry to fill a prescription or to answer a customer's or a doctor's question about drugs.

Since graduating from pharmacy school, I have found that studying human personality, culture, and society are far more insightful in understanding the root causes of the *diseases of modern civilization* than studying chemistry and pharmacology. In pharmacy school, students are taught surprisingly little about non-drug ways to prevent disease, but we are taught an incredible amount about the pharmacological management of disease. Pharmacists are taught that utilizing drugs to treat disease is far better than utilizing knowledge of culture and human behavior to prevent disease. The extent to which Big Pharma has been able to convince the public that health has more to do with pharmaceuticals than prevention is, to me, absolutely breathtaking. Big Pharma has been incredibly successful in molding public perception toward a mechanistic/reductionistic view of health, rather than toward what I consider to be a far more logical and common-sense view that places *Homo sapiens* squarely in the natural world. When people view their body as a machine, they are far more likely accept pharmaceutical solutions than when they view their body from an ecological perspective. The drug industry pushes pharmaceuticals but, equally importantly, Big Pharma pushes a narrow mechanistic view of the human body. Big Pharma has been outrageously successful in promoting synthetical chemicals (drugs) foreign to human evolution as the only solution to address what I consider to be, in essence, the maladaptation of *Homo sapiens* to conditions in modern societies. This approach has been immensely lucrative financially for drug companies, doctors, pharmacists, insurance companies, advertising agencies, etc.

I wish we had courses in pharmacy school in medical anthropology comparing disease incidences around the world. Required reading for pharmacists should include the National Cancer Institute's 205-page book *Cancer Rates and Risks* (NIH Publication No. 96-691, May 1996) which contains a large number of startling statistics on the huge variability in the incidence of cancer around the world, even when adjusting for the fact that average life span is higher is many Westernized countries. Wouldn't it be eye opening for pharmacists to discuss the possible reasons for the large variations around the world in the incidences of cancer? For example, the age-adjusted incidence of prostate cancer in black males in Atlanta is 127 (one hundred twenty-seven) times as great as the incidence of prostate cancer among males in Qidong, China (p. 25). The age-adjusted incidence of breast cancer in white females in the San Francisco Bay Area of California is 30 (thirty) times as great as the incidence of breast cancer in the African country The Gambia. (p. 27)

Pharmacists should also be required to read studies such as one by Weissman, et. al., in the *Journal of the American Medical Association* ("Cross-national epidemiology of major depression and bipolar disorder," *JAMA*, July 24, 1996, http://jama.ama-assn.org/cgi/content/abstract/276/4/293) which found high variability in rates around the world in the incidence of major depression. Population-based epidemiological studies using similar methods from ten countries (United States, Canada, Puerto Rico, France, West Germany, Italy, Lebanon, Taiwan, Korea, and New Zealand) found:

...The lifetime rates for major depression vary widely across countries, ranging from 1.5 cases per 100 adults in the sample in Taiwan to 19.0 cases per 100 adults in Beirut. ...In every country, the rates of major depression were higher for women than men. ...The differences in rates for major depression across countries suggest that cultural differences or different risk factors affect the expression of the disorder.

Pharmacy schools need to get over their outdated obsession with chemistry and, instead, introduce students to epidemiology and cross-cultural comparisons of disease incidences around the world. I doubt that most pharmacists are even aware of the sociological categorization of societies as industrialized vs. non-industrialized, urban vs. rural, and modern vs. traditional. For that matter, I doubt whether most pharmacists really understand the dichotomy holistic vs. reductionistic.

The chemistry-physics-biology focus in pharmacy schools and medical schools reinforces and legitimizes the narrow focus of the pharmaceutical industry. Big Pharma's approach to illness is extremely limited and one-dimensional: utilizing synthetic pharmaceuticals to overwhelm the delicate processes of nature. A focus on biology would be more logical if such a focus were on understanding biology in its broadest context, rather than Big Pharma's reductionist view of biology.

Since most people agree that the lifestyles of Americans are what's killing them, shouldn't health professionals be educated about our society? In my opinion, giving health professionals a solid understanding of sociology, political science, and anthropology would be far more advantageous in understanding the determinants of health than focusing on chemistry, physics, and reductionist biology.

In becoming a pharmacist, I had an incredible number of chemistry courses. While sitting in my chemistry classes and during my chemistry lab sessions, I never really understood the overwhelming fixation on chemistry. I assumed that an understanding of chemistry must be central to an understanding of human health. I have since come to realize that the focus on chemistry promoted the narrow view beneficial to Big Pharma. I have come to understand that the chemistry focus in pharmacy school reinforces a health care system that is primarily concerned with profits rather than human health. Understanding chemistry does not lead to an understanding of the social, cultural, economic, psychological, and political factors that have a major impact on human health.

Courses in sociology might help pharmacy students understand our consumer society. In my experience, most pharmacists accept our consumer society as inherently logical, a normal progression in the evolution of *Homo sapiens* (wise man) to *Homo economicus* (business man). Courses in sociology might help pharmacists understand that consumer societies exist primarily for the creation of private wealth. Courses in sociology might help pharmacists understand the intense criticism of consumer societies in many quarters of our society, particularly in academia. In my opinion, pharmacists cannot understand pharmacy unless they understand the critique of consumer societies. A pharmacist who understands pharmacy, but nothing else, doesn't really understand pharmacy. Pharmacists are, in my experience, unaware of the critique that the modern drugstore is an example of out-of-control marketing. The modern drugstore is not a physical manifestation of some quantum leap forward in our understanding of human illness. The thousands of products on drugstore shelves do not represent thousands of significant breakthroughs in understanding the human body. The pharmacy superstars such as antibiotics and insulin are few and far-between. A focus on sociology, political science, psychology, and anthropology would reveal the modern drugstore for what it is: the triumph of marketing in the commodification of health.

Chapter 21

Stories from pharmacy school

When I was in pharmacy school at West Virginia University in the 1970s, the medical, dental, pharmacy, and nursing students had all of our classes on the medical center campus. I found a rigid hierarchy among students, based on the status of each profession and the anticipated income of the practitioners in each field. At the top were medical students, followed by, in this order, dental students, pharmacy students, and nursing students. The medical students often had a superior attitude toward all the other students. It was subtle, yet powerful. The medical students seemed to consciously let their stethoscopes dangle over the tops of their white lab coat pockets, on display as if it were a gold medal won at the Olympics.

The medical, dental, and pharmacy students mostly kept to themselves, not intermingling often with students in other health fields. Walking between classes, pharmacy students saw medical and dental students routinely but spoke rarely. Liaisons between professions seemed to be as uncommon as interracial marriages. The main exception at the medical center was the female nursing students who were in active pursuit of marrying first, a doctor, second, a dentist, or third, a pharmacist. Many of the males in my pharmacy school class spoke often to the female nursing students. Interestingly, one attractive female pharmacy student in my class dated an unattractive med student. I predict she wouldn't have given him the time of day if he had been a pharmacy student.

The dean of my pharmacy school was well liked by most pharmacy students because he had a very down-to-earth, relaxed, easygoing personality. He died while I was still in pharmacy school and the collective grief among many pharmacy students was quite touching. If my memory is correct, he taught one class each semester. One day at the beginning of his class, he made a comment that has remained with me thirty-five years later. He said he'd rather be a proctologist than a dentist. He got a big laugh. I've always wondered what prompted him to make that statement. Here was the Dean of the School of Pharmacy at West Virginia University denigrating one of the four major professions at the medical center. He made this comment sound like a joke but I suspect he was disguising serious resentment. I suspect he had become fed up in his interactions with medical and dental faculty, most of whom seemed to routinely look down on pharmacy faculty as an inferior class of health professionals.

All graduates of pharmacy school must now have a doctorate degree (Pharm.D). It is no longer possible to become a pharmacist with a bachelor's degree in pharmacy (B.S. Pharm). Some pharmacy commentators have stated that pharmacy faculty promoted the requirement for a doctorate because these faculty members wanted to be able to say to medical and dental faculty "All of our graduates must now have doctorates just like your graduates" (i.e., like physicians and dentists).

Pharmacy students shared a class one semester with dental students. In this class, we had a different medical school professor speak on a different topic each class. For example, one day a cardiologist came with an overhead projector that displayed a recording of the markedly different coronary blood flow in an actual patient before and after coronary bypass surgery. On another day we had a physician who began his topic with what I assume was an olive branch. He said something like "Physicians and dentists are colleagues in equally important professions." He was, I assume, trying to smooth over the resentment that many dentists have toward the arrogant attitudes of physicians. But this physician apparently was not adequately informed that he would be speaking in front of both dental students and pharmacy students. Apparently this physician was trying to be collegial toward dental students, not realizing that half the students in the auditorium that day were pharmacy students. I looked around at my classmates but I couldn't really tell whether they realized the implications of his comment. I doubt that this physician would have said "Physicians and pharmacists are colleagues in equally important professions."

I would say that around half of the students in my class were serious students and the other half seemed to be interested in doing only the minimum required to get a pharmacy degree. I once worked with a pharmacist who seemed to have a similar view. He attended the University of North Carolina at Chapel Hill. He told me that the good students in his class were known as the "A-Team" (after the popular TV show in the 1980s) and the slackers were known as "Skid Row."

I don't know how common the use of marijuana is today on college campuses, but I know that it was widespread when I attended college in the early 1970s. Perhaps I should not have been surprised to see that marijuana use was common among many of my pharmacy school classmates. I remember thinking in pharmacy school that the common use of marijuana among many of my classmates was interesting in light of the fact that these students would, as pharmacists, soon have easy access to a wide variety of prescription drugs. I remember thinking that the admissions committee didn't even try to weed out applicants who were regular users of marijuana. Of course, I have no idea how the admissions committee could have gone about trying to weed out these students. I don't know whether pharmacy students who use marijuana are more likely to take advantage of our easy access to drugs like Vicodin and Xanax. From reading pharmacy magazines, however, it is clear that drug abuse is a big problem among pharmacists.

Another incident that occurred in pharmacy school perhaps illustrates my belief that half of my classmates seemed to be interested in doing only the minimum required to get a degree. There were seventy students in my pharmacy school class. I think it was my junior year when all the students in my class took turns—in groups of seven or eight—touring the hospital lab at the West Virginia University hospital. For some reason each group was accompanied by a chaperone from the senior class. I found the tour of the hospital lab fascinating. I was especially interested to see the huge automated equipment that was able to quickly analyze massive numbers of blood samples. In the middle of our lab tour, our senior class chaperone suggested that we simply skip out. He suggested that we could unobtrusively just walk away and no one from the lab and none of the pharmacy faculty would know. It was like we were being naughty in playing hooky from school. He seemed to be saying, "Let's see if we can skip out of here without anyone noticing." None of the other half-dozen or so of my classmates complained (including me), so we just walked away during a lull in the tour. The funny thing is that the lab tour was strictly voluntary. None of our pharmacy faculty was present to see who took the tour and who didn't. I remember thinking how childish it was for our senior chaperone to suggest this. Maybe he wanted the afternoon off to go play golf. Who knows? But I regret that we were not able to continue this fascinating tour of the hospital lab. I have never again had a chance to tour a hospital lab so I regret this lost opportunity. I should have spoken up and said, "No. I'd like to finish the tour." But my classmates seemed contented to go along with the chaperone and skip out of the tour. So off we went. I now wish I had had the fortitude to stand up and point out how ridiculous it was to skip out of a voluntary tour.

One of my classmates was the starting safety on the West Virginia University football team. He was a smart guy and a very good athlete. Another of my classmates told me that this football player possibly could have made it as a professional if he were bigger. One day in physiology lab, I heard one of our professors tell the football player something like "You are to be congratulated for being a good football player and a good pharmacy student. You probably don't have much time to do anything else." When the professor walked away, I heard the football player say, "He's right. I don't have time to wipe my ass."

Another lab incident that stands out in my mind is the day that several dogs were sacrificed to demonstrate the pharmacological effects of various drugs. As best as I can recall, our class of seventy was divided into three groups. Three perfectly healthy and happy dogs were brought into the lab. Our instructor said at the outset that these dogs came from the dog pound and they would have eventually been put to sleep anyway so their fate at the end of the lab exercise (death) was no different from what would have happened to them anyway. The dogs were tied down on their backs and various drugs were injected during our two or three hour lab. I can't remember precisely what was measured but I assume we were shown the effects of various drugs on blood pressure, heart rate, breathing, urinary output, etc. I was sad during the entire lab because I felt this was a cruel way for the dogs to end their lives. I think I could have easily learned as much from a book.

My first year in pharmacy school included human anatomy. One day the professor was discussing the retina, which is part of the eye. The retina contains two types of photoreceptors, known as "rods" and "cones." Rods help us see things at night. I remember the professor said something like, "When you go out at night, you use your rods." That got a big laugh from the class.

When I was in pharmacy school, only medical students and physical therapy students dissected cadavers. One day in anatomy class, the professor said that we would take a tour of the anatomy lab. But before we took the tour, the professor asked all of us to please be careful in our comments (i.e., hold the jokes) after the tour because members of the general public could overhear our conversation and decide against donating their body to the medical school. I found the tour fascinating. There were no students actively dissecting the cadavers during our tour but the cadavers (a couple dozen, I guess) were in plain view, most of which were fully uncovered. The sight of these cadavers up close, in various stages of dissection, was a memorable event, much like viewing someone in a casket at a funeral home, but a more intense experience. I remember that one of my friends had a dreadful expression on his face during the entire tour. My reaction was that this is an interesting part of life and it shows how fragile life is.

Pharmacy school consisted of very little instruction on nutrition, other than the courses we had on the biochemistry of the various vitamins. I recall that we did have only one class on nutrition *per se*.

The instructor was a member of the medical faculty who had been invited to speak to our class. I recall that I rarely approached professors immediately after class to ask questions. But I did feel compelled to stay after class and make a comment to this professor. I told her that I felt that proper nutrition is extremely important and that I don't know why there isn't more focus on nutrition in pharmacy school, and that I felt that people would be much healthier if they ate nutritious foods. The instructor was very pleased that I felt that way about nutrition. She said something like "I hope that someday you have the biggest drugstore in America." I presume she was saying that I would thereby be in a position to promote nutrition. I remember thinking that her comment to me was absurd because modern drugstores are about pills—not prevention, not nutrition.

At my pharmacy school in the early 1970s, pharmacy students were given the opportunity for several weeks to tag along with medical students, interns, residents, and the attending physician as they made their rounds on the hospital floors. We pharmacy students rarely had anything critical to add as the group of six or seven visited several patients. Pharmacists are trained today to be much more competent in this setting, but back then pharmacy students rarely contributed much significant. I recall one exception. A classmate of mine named Bob Yost actually contributed something very important. One of the patients that Bob's group visited had been diagnosed with a very serious blood disorder called aplastic anemia. We had recently learned in class that aplastic anemia is a notable potential adverse reaction to the antibiotic chloramphenicol. As I recall the incident, the medical team had indeed asked the patient whether he had taken chloramphenicol. Supposedly the patient answered no. Apparently Bob was sufficiently curious to visit the patient by himself, i.e., outside the normal group setting. Bob engaged the patient in a relaxed conversation and was able to discover that the patient had indeed taken chloramphenicol. Apparently the patient was so overwhelmed by the medical staff that he wasn't able to recall having taken chloramphenicol. I can't recall whether Bob told a member of the pharmacy faculty or whether Bob told a member of the medical team. But Bob became the hero of our class for a few days. Our instructors praised Bob in class for being an example of how pharmacists can make a valuable addition to the medical team. As I said, pharmacy students today are trained much more intensely for situations like this, but back in the 1970s, this incident stood out as a superior contribution by a pharmacy student. This incident illustrates to me how easy it is to fall through the cracks in our medical system. Here were all these hot shot medical students and doctors who had done a poor job in ascertaining the patient's medical history. The medical staff couldn't figure out why the patient had aplastic anemia. But my classmate solved the puzzle.

I've now forgotten many of the names of my classmates from pharmacy school, but I do remember the name of one physician who was part of the medical staff when my classmates tagged along with the medical staff as they made rounds on the hospital floors. Many of my classmates commented that one doctor, in particular, had the coolest name. His name was Dr. Weiser. Thus it is not surprising that his nickname was "Bud." My classmates loved it every time the hospital operator paged Dr. Weiser. The hospital operator would say, "Paging Doctor Weiser, Doctor Bud Weiser."

At some time during the two years of my college pre-pharmacy curricula, many students on campus developed a bad case of diarrhea. Even though many of my classmates visited the on-campus student health service for whatever ailed them, I went to the student health service only twice during my five years in college. One of these visits was because of this diarrhea. I remember asking the physician who saw me if he knew what was causing the diarrhea. He said something like "It's a bug going around." Only several months later did I read in a newspaper that some organism had been discovered in the municipal water supply. It appears that the more water students drank, the worse was their diarrhea. As I look back on this experience, I am surprised that the water supply was not everyone's focus at that time. Perhaps in a year or two, after learning more about human health, I would have reached that conclusion myself. But I was not yet informed enough to make the connection. This was around 1972 at West Virginia University in Morgantown, West Virginia. Theoretically, Morgantown had the highest concentration of smart people in the state but, even with the faculty at the medical school, I still don't understand why the connection to the water supply was not made sooner. Anyway, the physician at the student health service gave me a prescription for Lomotil, the leading drug at that time for diarrhea. I don't believe I had that prescription filled because I think I was looking for an explanation for the cause of the widespread diarrhea, rather than a pill to stop it. I think that, intuitively, it did not make any sense to try to stop that diarrhea because I felt surely my body was trying to get rid of some noxious substance or organism. I think that the absence of fever caused me to question whether this diarrhea was due to "a bug going around."

When I was at West Virginia University from 1970 to 1975, the pre-pharmacy curriculum consisted of two years (four semesters) and pharmacy school consisted of three years (six semesters). All applicants to pharmacy school were required to sit for an interview. As I recall, the interview usually had one or two members of the pharmacy school faculty and one student who was already in pharmacy school. As best as I can recall, approximately half the students applying to pharmacy school were accepted.

One day while I was in pharmacy school, one of our professors mentioned to the class that he had just come from an interview with an applicant who showed up wearing a T-shirt. It was customary for male applicants to wear a tie for the interview. This professor told the class that the applicant had mentioned that he had already been accepted at another pharmacy school. This professor told us that even though the applicant had a very high grade point average and would have been admitted, the applicant was rejected because wearing a T-shirt to the interview showed disrespect. This professor appeared to have enjoyed voting for rejection of the applicant, in retaliation for the applicant's disrespect.

As I recall, each interview took perhaps a half hour, but it took several weeks to interview all the applicants individually. As it turns out, I was lucky that my interview was not one of the earlier ones. Applicants who were interviewed early in the process were grilled by other applicants regarding the questions that were asked during the interview. I knew many of the applicants to pharmacy school because we shared many classes (mainly chemistry and physics) in the two years of pre-pharmacy curricula.

Here is the reason that I was lucky in having an interview that was not one of the earlier ones. It turns out that one of the primary questions asked by the pharmacy faculty members was whether the applicant hoped to eventually go to medical school. The rumor (apparently true) quickly spread that if pharmacy applicants answered "Yes," those students were rejected. I would have assumed that answering "Yes" implied that the pharmacy student was ambitious and driven, qualities that I assumed would be admired. Applicants to pharmacy school who were interested in eventually going to medical school were rejected apparently because the pharmacy faculty felt it was their duty to train pharmacy students to be pharmacists. It was apparently viewed as wasting a spot on someone who might not end up as a pharmacist. If my interview were one of the first ones, I assume I would have been rejected because I would probably have answered that, yes, I had aspirations of going to medical school. I felt that the interviewers would be impressed by my ambition, even though I wasn't really interested in going to medical school. Having heard from earlier applicants about the "aspirations for medical school" question, I told my interviewers that I had no desire to go to medical school when, sure enough, I was asked.

Perhaps being rejected by the interviewer would have forced me to choose a different major. And perhaps I would have been happier in that other major. I had five official and distinct majors while in college. I started out in Humanities, then switched to General Studies, then switched to General Engineering, then switched to Civil Engineering, then switched to Pharmacy. Perhaps I was one major shy of finding a good fit.

As I write this, I'm fifty-nine years old and I still don't know what major/career/job would have made me happy. Expecting college freshmen to know what career will make them happy for the next 40-plus years is, in my opinion, a tall order. Knowing what I know now, I would certainly not have been happy as a physician. That's because our medical system is about illness and pills, not health. I was very uneasy during my entire time in pharmacy school. I think I intuitively understood that I was learning how disease is treated, not how health is maintained. There was very little in pharmacy school about health and prevention. Pharmacy school was mainly about chemistry and pharmacology.

When I was in pharmacy school, an entire course one semester was devoted to the subject of pharmacy law. There's more to pharmacy law than the public probably realizes. Since pharmacists routinely dispense drugs classified as controlled substances, it is not surprising that there are lots of regulations governing how pharmacists handle these drugs. The category of drugs known as controlled substances consists mainly of drugs with an abuse or addiction potential and a street value. Some well-known controlled substances are the pain killers Percocet, Demerol, Vicodin, and morphine; the anti-anxiety drugs Xanax and Ativan; the sleeping pills Ambien and Sonata, the attention deficit/hyperactivity drugs Ritalin and Adderall, and diet pills such as phentermine.

Government rules require that pharmacists keep strict records for purchases of these drugs. Failure to follow regulations governing these drugs can result in a number of financial penalties and/or suspension of the pharmacist's license to dispense controlled substances. There are also major penalties for unlawfully distributing these substances (for example, selling these drugs to drug dealers).

The professor who taught pharmacy law when I was in pharmacy school is probably deceased now, judging by his age thirty-five years ago. So perhaps I can now safely say that this professor was not one of the better professors at my pharmacy school. The disrespect for this professor among some students in my class was palpable. After 35 years, I still recall certain parts of his exam on controlled substances.

In pharmacy school, one must make judgments about how to allot one's time in studying for the various courses. This sometimes involves the risky business of trying to guess what material is likely to be covered on our exams. For our exam on controlled substances, I predicted that surely this professor would focus on our understanding of the various regulations, rather than on the monetary penalties that accompanied failure to follow these regulations. Surely the professor would realize that students would quickly forget whether violating this or that regulation carried a $500.00 fine, or a $750.00 fine, or a $1,000.00 fine, etc.

I guessed wrong. Out of a total of say, fifty questions, this exam contained perhaps eight or ten multiple choice questions in which memorization of the monetary penalty was required to answer these questions correctly. I remember thinking how useless it was to memorize the monetary penalties rather than understand the stipulations of the various regulations. Thus these eight to ten questions ended with something like: *The monetary fine for violating this regulation is* : a) $200.00 ... b) $250.00 ... c) $500.00 ... d) $750.00 ... e) $1,000.00. I can't recall the precise fines but I know they were significant in the mid 1970s. Worse than the fine was the possibility that the pharmacist would lose his license to dispense controlled substances.

Perhaps this professor simply found it easier to prepare such pointless questions rather than try to determine whether students actually understood the regulations. Would a pharmacist be less likely to violate a regulation if he remembered that the penalty was $750.00 rather than $500.00? I seriously doubt it. But I had made a choice to ignore the monetary penalties while studying for this exam and I got burned as a consequence.

Most of my exams in pharmacy school consisted of multiple choice questions, with five possible answers, i.e., **a, b, c, d, e**. I remember one exam in another class—pharmacology—in which a young instructor put students through hell. As I recall, his exam consisted of approximately ten possible answers for each question. For example:
a…..b…..c…..d…..e…..a,c…..b,d…..b,e…..c,d,e…..a,b,d,e

There was such an uproar as a result of this exam that, as best as I can recall, one of the senior members of the pharmacology faculty told this young instructor to stop playing with students' brains with such an idiotic and mind-bending assortment of answers.

Chapter 22

The effects
of pharmacy school
in the long run

Forgetting most of what we learned in pharmacy school

I recall one of our professors stating that we would forget somewhere north of ninety-five percent of the information we learned in pharmacy school. Here are some examples of information we learned in pharmacy school that is often quickly forgotten:

I remember spending a huge amount of time in pharmacy school memorizing the spectrum of microorganisms killed by the various antibiotics. Retail pharmacists forget this information quickly because we rarely—if ever—use it. That's because doctors specify the precise antibiotic that we should dispense. Doctors do not, for example, write the following on a prescription, "Mary Jones has a Chlymydia infection. Dispense an appropriate antibiotic of your choice." I'm sure I've forgotten almost all the microorganisms killed by the various antibiotics.

Pharmacists forget nearly one hundred percent of what seems like a few hundred drug structural formulas that we learned in pharmacy school. That has had absolutely no effect on my competence as a chain pharmacist. I absolutely do not need to know the structural formula for any drug for any prescription I dispense. A rare exception: It would be nice to be able to recall which drugs contain a sulfur atom in their structural formula, because the sulfur atom can cause serious problems in people who have an allergy to such "sulfa" drugs. But pharmacists don't need to rely on our memory of structural formulas since the pharmacy computer flags drugs that can cause reactions in people with sulfur allergies.

Pharmacists forget many of the drug interactions that we learn in pharmacy school. That would be bad were it not for our pharmacy computer which is programmed for far more interactions than I could ever remember. The pharmacy computer is far more competent than most pharmacists in screening for drug interactions. Pharmacists routinely see our computer flagging an endless number of potential drug interactions among the prescriptions we fill. As a result, most pharmacists probably have retained a higher level of competence in assessing drug interactions than, say, in recalling long lists of potential drug side effects.

Retail pharmacists surely forget the overwhelming majority of the drug side effects that we memorized in pharmacy school. Luckily there are lots of readily available sources for pharmacists to look up potential side effects to answer customers' questions. I usually grab one of the "professional inserts" that are attached to (or folded and stuffed inside) our stock bottles. These professional inserts are reprints of the official prescribing information approved by the Food and Drug Administration.

On the other hand, pharmacists are more likely to remember the most serious drug side effects or sometimes we remember unusual side effects. I recall that "gingival hyperplasia" (overgrowth of the gums in the mouth) is a possible side effect of the anti-seizure drug Dilantin (phenytoin). I remember that "hearing loss" is a possible side effect with the antibiotics such as streptomycin, neomycin, kanamycin, vancomycin, gentamycin, and tobramycin. I remember that a side effect of the antibiotic tetracycline can be a permanent unattractive gray discoloration in the teeth when this drug is prescribed to children. I remember that all the anti-cancer drugs and many of the drugs for rheumatoid arthritis can have devastating side effects.

Because of constant repetition in attaching "May Cause Drowsiness" stickers to anti-anxiety drugs like Valium, Ativan, and Xanax, and to narcotic pain relievers like Vicodin, Tylenol w/Codeine, Percocet, and Demerol, most pharmacists can never forget that drowsiness is a common side effect associated with these drugs.

Pharmacists forget most of the information we learned in pharmacy school on the subject of compounding and I don't know of any easy way to regain that lost knowledge. I haven't found reference books that are particularly helpful in compounding the products that I come across in the real world. Many pharmacists simply don't use our compounding knowledge enough in the real world to maintain it at a high level.

When I was in pharmacy school, most professors posted our exam scores on the wall adjacent to their office door. To protect students from being embarrassed, the scores were posted by social security number rather than by name. As best as I can recall, the class average on a typical exam was usually somewhere around 87 percent. This means that lots of students scored 97 percent but it also means that lots of students scored 77%.

The wide variability in exam scores among pharmacy students has implications in the real world. Take, for example, pharmacy compounding. I am sure that all of my classmates did not receive a score of one hundred percent on all the medications we compounded in pharmacy school. So it is reasonable to assume that medications compounded in the real world will be done so correctly in less than one hundred percent of the time, and I predict that the success rate in the compounding of drugs decreases sharply after pharmacy school. (See chapter on *pharmacy compounding* for details about a study showing rapid decreases in compounding skills after those skills are taught in pharmacy school.)

Consequences of pharmacy schools misrepresenting the real world

"Clinical pharmacy" is an inside-the-profession term that means a pharmacist utilizing his knowledge about drugs to optimize drug ther-

apy just as a physician uses his "clinical medicine" skills to optimize the diagnosis and treatment of disease.

"Alma mater" is Latin for "nourishing mother" or "fostering mother." We were coddled in pharmacy school by professors who were protective of us, as if they were our second mother or substitute parents. Sure, we had to study hard to graduate, but once we were accepted into pharmacy school, our professors seemed to feel it was their duty to help us become pharmacists. The big chains have no similar protective view toward pharmacists.

Teachers and professors in all fields are accused of building the self-esteem of students to sky-high levels, almost to the point where high school and college graduates view themselves as the center of the universe. Pharmacy professors convince students that they will be valued for their drug knowledge when, in fact, the big chains are contemptuous of the product of today's pharmacy schools, the Pharm D. The big chains were happy with BS pharmacists, or even techs or robotics. Pharmacy professors don't level with students and tell them that the model they're pushing in pharmacy school is completely unrealistic in the real world of chain drugstores.

Psychologists say that humans replay in our minds the audio recordings that our brains make of our conversations with our parents. Ideally, our parents are our moral compass. From them we learn compassion and right from wrong. We replay those recordings in our brains for the rest of our lives.

Similarly, pharmacy professors imprint in the minds of young, naïve, impressionable students a model of pharmacy that, in reality, reinforces the occupational and intellectual interests of those professors far more than it does the needs of pharmacists in the trenches. I view the switch to the PharmD degree as a turf grab by pharmacy professors concerned about their academic standing among university faculty who wanted to be able to tell medical and dental professors that the pharmacy curriculum is equal because our entry level degree is now a doctorate just like theirs.

For the rest of their careers, pharmacists ask themselves, "Where is the clinical nirvana that I was promised in pharmacy school?" We graduate from pharmacy school and never recover from the fact that our alma mater wasn't honest with us in describing the real world. It is too painful for us to accept that our pharmacy professors sold us a bill of goods about what pharmacy is really like.

Over the course of my career in chain drugstores, I've heard it said many times (only half-jokingly) that pharmacists need to bring a class action lawsuit against the pharmacy schools in America for misrepresenting the real world. In pharmacy school, our young minds are imprinted with a professional model of the pharmacist that simply does not (and, I predict, never will) exist in the chain drugstore setting.

Pharmacy students graduate with a view of themselves as skilled professionals and experience profound culture shock in the real world in which they don't even have time to eat or go to the bathroom. How could our alma mater have misled us so fundamentally during our college years about the nature of pharmacy in the real world?

Pharmacy students graduate with a belief that they're god's gift to the world of health care, that their drug knowledge will be highly valued in our health care system. That naive view puts them at a severe disadvantage when it comes to dealing with our employer. We see ourselves as professionals while our employers see us as disposable wage laborers. The unspoken corporate attitude toward pharmacists seems to be, "Burn 'em out and hire someone younger." So pharmacists are unprepared to fight the big chains with the only thing they understand: power. We tell ourselves, "True professionals don't need unions."

Acknowledging the real world (i.e., that we need a union) is just too painful for precious young graduates who've been led to believe they will be the savior of our health care system. Pharmacists prefer to carry around in our heads a view of ourselves as highly trained professionals. The big chains are happy that we view ourselves as professionals who are above unions. That's because the biggest thing that scares the chains is powerful unions.

Students' brains are filled with a vision of clinical nirvana, a carrot that has been dangled in front of students at least since I graduated in 1975. From the perspective of a chain pharmacist, I would say that the average chain pharmacist is no closer to the clinical model today than when I graduated 35 years ago. Pharmacy professors are afraid to level with students about real world working conditions out of fear that those students will begin wondering whether pharmacy is the right choice. For their own job security, professors fear declining enrollments in pharmacy schools.

The current pharmacy school model stressing a professional role for the pharmacist does a disservice to new graduates when they enter the real world of retail pharmacy. In the real world, newly minted PharmDs are in for a rude awakening as they quickly discover that they're being paid to use their hands and feet, not their brains. They quickly discover what veteran pharmacists have known for decades: the chains have always been antagonistic to the concept of clinical pharmacy.

I don't like the phrase "pharmacy practice" because I feel that it is pompous and pretentious. A "practice" is something that professionals engage in. If a pharmacist doesn't have time for bathroom breaks or meal breaks, I do not consider him to be a professional. I consider him to be a wage laborer. Who are we kidding in calling ourselves professionals if we don't even have rights that most other employees take for granted? Until we recognize the cold and hard facts about our working conditions, we will be easy prey for the corporate bosses who play hard ball with us, while we consider it beneath us to stand up to these playground bullies.

We need to realize that retail pharmacy is a distributive enterprise, not a cognitive enterprise. Until pharmacists realize that our employers are playing hard ball with us, we will be unable to take the actions required to ameliorate our pathetic working conditions. The big employers treat us arrogantly as wage laborers while we view ourselves as professionals who are above unions.

If our professors had accurately described us as wage laborers, pharmacy students would realize that our best ally is aggressive labor leaders, not ivory tower academicians who fill our heads with subjects like chemistry that we never use in the real world.

PART VII

DRUG SAFETY, EFFECTIVENESS, AND RATIONALITY

Chapter 23

How good are generic drugs?

The issues surrounding generic drugs are endlessly fascinating. Pharmacists like generic drugs because the mark-up is better than on brand name drugs. Insurance companies love generic drugs because generics save the companies a ton of money. As a taxpayer, I'm happy that federal and state governments embrace generic drugs. I'd hate to be taxed to pay for exclusively brand name drugs for Medicare Part D, and for the Veterans Administration, and for Medicaid programs, etc. I like the fact that the government embraces generic drugs because that holds down my taxes. But as a consumer, I prefer brand name drugs when these drugs are used to treat very important medical conditions or when the manufacturing process involves a higher level of expertise (for example, in the case of some long-acting drugs). I take very few drugs myself but when I had an abscessed tooth in 2010, I did opt for a generic amoxicillin, in part because Publix Supermarkets dispense this and a few other antibiotics at no charge. I also opted for the generic form of Vicodin for pain.

One of the fundamental tenets of capitalism is that price determines quality. You get what you pay for. That's why tires for your car with a 75,000-mile tread life warranty cost much more than tires with a 25,000-mile warranty. I equate generic drugs with "no-name" or "store brand" canned vegetables that are available in supermarkets across America. When you go to a supermarket, do you buy the store brand of green beans or canned corn or do you prefer Green

Giant or DelMonte? Are you happy when your automobile mechanic uses a brand of motor oil you've never heard of, or do you prefer that he uses Valvoline or Havoline? Do you prefer Exxon, Mobil, and Shell gasoline, or are you satisfied with discount brands? Do you prefer brand name auto parts like AC-Delco (General Motors) and Motorcraft (Ford), or are you content with names you may not have heard of? If you need a pacemaker for your heart, wouldn't you want the absolute finest on the market? If you need a drug to control a heart arrhythmia, would you be wise to accept a generic? The examples are endless but the point is the same. Can you be assured of quality when the cost of a generic product is some fraction of the brand name? Are generic drugs a rare exception to the fundamental tenet of capitalism that price is the primary arbiter of quality?

Joe and Teresa Graedon, authors of *The People's Pharmacy* books, have been enthusiastic supporters of generic drugs for decades. As a consequence of a growing number of letters they've received from readers of their nationally syndicated newspaper column, they have lately begun to have second thoughts. I haven't seen a clearer critique of the controversy with generic drugs anywhere other than in their book *Best Choices from the People's Pharmacy* (Rodale, 2006, pp. 11-36). The Graedons point out that the FDA is grossly understaffed and that the chances are frighteningly small that the FDA will actually test a sample of a given drug. The Graedons state (p. 24):

Most worrisome of all, the FDA's random testing system is a joke. Although a few bottles are selected for analysis each year, they amount to a relative handful. The FDA says it analyzes about 300 "finished dosage forms" annually, including both branded and generic medicines. That represents approximately 0.00001 percent of the 3 billion-plus prescriptions filled in community pharmacies each year. If you thought your chances of getting a speeding ticket were 1 in 10 million, you probably would not worry very much about obeying the speed limit. Compare that to your lifetime risk of being struck by lightning, which is estimated at just 1 in 3,000. If you were a less than honorable generic drug manufacturer or wholesaler, you would not have to worry much about getting caught by the FDA.

Belief in the quality of generic drugs is, in my opinion, based more on faith than science. Too many powerful groups have a vested interest in the perception that generic drugs are as good as brand name. I'm not making the case that we as a society embrace brand name drugs and discard generics. Quite to the contrary. Americans are grossly overmedicated, in no small part as a consequence of direct-to-consumer drug advertising on TV and in newspapers and magazines. Americans would do well to embrace prevention and let pharmaceuticals return to their proper role in society, important but far more limited.

The FDA implies that consumers are simply imagining differences in effectiveness between brand name drugs and generics. In my 25-year career as a pharmacist, I've noticed that a large number of customers complain because their insurance company or government program pushes them to accept generics. In my experience, customers who feel forced or coerced into accepting generic drugs are more likely to be skeptical of generics. State Medicaid laws often force Medicaid recipients to accept generic drugs. Sometimes I have the impression that some Medicaid customers are against generic drugs because they resent being forced to accept generic drugs, not necessarily because of any bad experience that these customers may have had with generic drugs. Customers with private insurance coverage for drugs often resent the fact that their insurance plan requires a much higher co-pay for brand name drugs than generic drugs. In my experience, some people with private insurance don't think it is fair that their insurance company is coercing them into using generic drugs. They interpret this as their insurance company pressuring them into accepting an "inferior" product.

The Graedons relate stories from readers such as the following: Patients who are well-controlled on the anti-seizure drug Dilantin suddenly begin having seizures when switched to the generic phenytoin. Men taking the brand name Hytrin for enlarged prostate begin having more difficulty urinating when switched to the generic terazosin. Mothers complain that their child's behavior worsens when switched from the brand name Ritalin to the generic methylphenidate. Patients taking the brand name Synthroid complain that they begin experiencing thyroid symptoms when switched to the generic levothyroxine. Patients on the brand name blood thinner Coumadin have more difficulty keeping their clotting in the target range when switched to the generic warfarin. And so on.

The Graedon's cite the following letter from a registered nurse who works with the blood thinner Coumadin, a "narrow therapeutic index" (NTI) drug that needs precise dosing. NTI drugs have a narrow margin between effective dose and toxic dose. (*Best Choices From The People's Pharmacy*, Rodale, 2006, p. 21):

I'm an RN working full-time in a Coumadin clinic. We monitor and adjust the blood thinner Coumadin for over 3,000 patients and I can assure you generics make a difference.

We had patients who had been in target range literally for years as long as they were on Coumadin. When they started taking generic warfarin we found they needed 20 to 30 percent more drug and were much harder to keep in range.

Those who went back to Coumadin went right back on their previous dose and stayed in target.

Generics may be "equivalent" but in a drug with a narrow therapeutic index they sure are not equal.

Another controversial issue with generic drugs regards inactive ingredients. Are they always indeed "inactive"? A good way to test this belief is with drugs used in the eye since the eye is composed of especially sensitive tissues. One eye doctor (ophthalomologist) who is not a big fan of using generic drugs in the eye is Dr. Roger Steinert, Professor and Chair of Ophthalmology at the University of California-Irvine and Director of the Gavin Herbert Eye Institute. He has found that inactive ingredients in generic eye drops can cause irritation to the eye. He prefers brand name eye drops. (Roger F. Steinert, M.D., "Generic vs. Brand-Name Drugs: An Ongoing Debate," *Medscape.com*, April 13, 2012
http://www.medscape.com/viewarticle/761706?src=ptalk)

In ophthalmology we have a very special situation. We are talking largely about eye drops and the effect that they can have on a very sensitive part of the body.

When the US Food and Drug Administration (FDA) allows a generic drug to be marketed, the manufacturer has to use the same concentration of active ingredient and the same route of administration as the branded drug that was previously approved by the FDA. But that is the only requirement. There is no review, no burden of proof, no burden of testing the so-called "inactive ingredients," which include things like the preservatives and other components that can have a significant effect on the eye.

Probably the most famous instance of this issue occurred in 1999 when a number of corneal melts were recognized and ultimately tracked to generic diclofenac, a nonsteroidal agent. This problem was not occurring with the brand-name drugs, and ultimately the problem was attributed to variations in a so-called inactive ingredient (except with respect to the eye, where it apparently was quite active) that was in the generic drops....

From our point of view as practicing ophthalmologists, we have to be sensitive and aware that our patients may not be getting what we think they are getting, and keep an ear tuned to complaints about stinging and burning that we didn't formerly hear with respect to a particular class of medication. If necessary, we can try to force the use of a branded medication, although in many cases the third-party payers simply won't pay for the brand name even if you specify it; it can be quite a battle to justify it and get them to pay for it. We want to avoid sight-threatening complications. It is bad enough to have unnecessary discomfort, but if we get into more situations like corneal melting, we are going to see even more issues related to generics vs brand-name drugs.

Lesley Alderman writes in the *New York Times* that some neurologists are concerned about generic drugs used to prevent seizures (Lesley Alderman, "Not All Drugs Are the Same After All," *The New York Times*, December 18, 2009
http://www.nytimes.com/2009/12/19/health/19patient.html?pagewanted=all)

Some specialists, particularly cardiologists and neurologists, are concerned about generic formulations of drugs in which a slight variation could have a serious effect on a patient's health. The American Academy of Neurology has a position paper that says, in part, "The A.A.N. opposes generic substitution of anticonvulsant drugs for the treatment of epilepsy without the attending physician's approval."...

Two studies published last year in the journal *Neurology* found that patients who switched from a brand-name product to a generic one had more seizures or higher hospitalization rates.

"For many drugs, generics are just fine," said Kimford Meador, a professor of neurology at Emory University.

"But when you're taking a seizure medication, the therapeutic window is narrow," Dr. Meador said. "If the absorption of the drug is slightly different between brand and generic or between generics, then the patient could have a seizure, and that seizure could lead to serious injury or perhaps even death."

Topamax is a drug used for several conditions, including seizures and as a mood stabilizer for people with bipolar disorder. One pharmacist blogs on PharmQD that, at his facility, those patients prescribed this drug for seizures are given the brand name, whereas those patients prescribed the drug for mood stability are given the generic. The implication is that the dose is considered to be more critical for the prevention of seizures than for stabilizing mood. (http://www.pharmqd.com/forum/topic/questions-patients-generic-drugs)

Generics are widely used at our facility but we do have several patients that have to have specifically name brand drug. Topamax patients that have seizures have to have name brand, but Topamax patients that have mood instability get generic.

I once had a customer tell me that he had to get up four times every night to urinate while taking the brand name diuretic Lasix. He told me that he had to get up only twice at night while taking the generic furosemide. Should I conclude that this man is not telling me the truth? Should I conclude that he has been unduly influenced by major brand name companies that generics are inferior? Pharmacists frequently hear complaints from the mothers of children who are on a generic form of Ritalin. Mothers often complain that their child does not do as well on the generic form. As a pharmacist for 25 years, I would like to propose that *Consumer Reports* conducts a major analysis of generic Lasix (furosemide) and generic Ritalin (methylphenidate), for starters.

On October 12, 2007, ConsumerLab.com reported that its tests of a generic version of the popular antidepressant drug Wellbutrin showed differences between the generic and original that might explain recent consumer complaints about the generic product. In February, 2007, readers of *The People's Pharmacy* syndicated newspaper column began reporting problems with a generic version of once-a-day Wellbutrin XL 300. The ConsumerLab.com report shows that the generic product released drug at a very different rate than the original Wellbutrin XL. Tod Cooperman, MD, President of ConsumerLab.com, stated that "This information shatters the myth that generics are always identical to the original and it questions the belief that generics are always equivalent. Even if the active ingredient is the same, releasing it at a different rate may alter a drug's effects." He added, "Generic drugs are essential to keeping medical costs down, but consumers and healthcare providers need to be aware of the potential differences among products otherwise thought to be the same. Generics are not clinically tested for safety and efficacy, so the consumer will be the first to find out if there is a problem." The testing was funded by ConsumerLab.com without drug company involvement.(http://www.peoplespharmacy.com/archives/generic_drug_p roblems/generic_drug_equality_questioned.php *The People's Pharmacy*, "Generic Drug Equality Questioned," October 12, 2007)

It is not rare that pharmacists hear complaints from our custom ers that generics do not perform as well as brand name drugs. Many pharmacists dismiss such complaints outright. Other pharmacists are beginning to wonder if there may be some truth in our customers' complaints. Pharmacists certainly aren't impressed when we receive bottles of a hundred, or five-hundred, or a thousand tablets from a generic manufacturer and we see lots of powder at the bottom of the bottle as a result of too many broken tablets. This tells pharmacists that quality control at the manufacturing plant is not the best. Pharmacists see powder and broken tablets far less often with brand name tablets.

People used to think that generic drugs were made in a bathtub in someone's back yard. That's not the case. Some brand name manufacturers do, in fact, make generic drugs. But I have serious doubts whether, in general, there is as much quality control with generic drugs compared to brand name. For example, when I read advertisements for generic drugs in my pharmacy magazines, I am struck by the fact that the number one theme of these advertisements is QUALITY. Why are all these generic manufacturers trying so hard to convince pharmacists that their generic products are of high quality? If the FDA says that all generic drugs are as good as brand name, why are the generic manufacturers still obsessed with convincing pharmacists about the quality of their generic products? My conclusion is that the makers of generic drugs know that quality is not consistent throughout the industry. For example, here are several excerpts from generic drug advertisements illustrating the common use of the word *quality*. All of these examples are taken from *Generic Drug Review*, a June 2011 supplement to *U.S. Pharmacist*:

AMNEAL PHARMACEUTICALS: **We are passionate and fully-committed to quality. We make each and every product with the care we'd put into making it for our own loved-ones. (p. 7)**

X-Gen PHARMACEUTICALS: **At X-Gen Pharmaceuticals, Inc. we are committed to providing hospitals, surgery centers and other inpatient health-care facilities the indispensable products they rely on for high-quality and low-cost patient treatment. (p. 15)**

PAR PHARMACEUTICAL: **Driven by one principle—Quality. By living this commitment to quality each day, Par Pharmaceutical brings a level of excellence to the pharmaceutical industry that distinguishes it from the competition. Uncompromised quality for patients and our customers. (p. 21)**

GREENSTONE: **Trusted generics from a partner with a solid reputation. Behind every trusted Greenstone product is a commitment to quality and affordability, backed by decades of responsive customer service and supply-management expertise. (p. 27)**

CAMBER PHARMACEUTICALS: Commitment Quality Continuous Supply …That's Camber (p. 30)

ACTAVIS: Quality generics from the ground up. Around the world, there's a growing demand for high-quality, lower-cost alternatives to brand name pharmaceuticals. At Actavis, we're at the forefront of meeting that need. (p. 38)

LUPIN PHARMACEUTICALS: Quality products. Outstanding service. At Lupin Pharmaceuticals, we're committed to being a leader in high-quality generic medications trusted by healthcare professionals and patients across the world. (p. 41)

TEVA PHARMACEUTICALS: Your source for high quality, affordable medicine. …We produce life-saving drugs at tremendous value to consumers—making quality healthcare accessible. (p. 42)

RANBAXY: Ranbaxy is committed to providing high quality, affordable and accessible medicines to patients, doctors and pharmacists alike. (p. 46)

On October 5, 2007 I received an online "Generic Products Survey" from the publisher of *Drug Topics* magazine, sponsored by Mylan Pharmaceuticals, a major manufacturer of generic drugs. (Advanstar Communications Research Services, http://www.snap-surveys.com/advanstar/DT%20Generic%20products%20survey/).
The survey consisted of eighteen questions. The survey began, "Please help us learn more about your perceptions of generic manufacturers and their products." The first four questions were:

Please describe your pharmacy:
• Single outlet store
• 2-3 store units
• Chain store of 4 or more units

How many prescriptions does your pharmacy fill in an average day?
• 1 - 74 per day
• 75 - 149 per day

• 150 - 249 per day
• 250 or more per day

When you think of quality, which generic company comes to mind first?
(Please list your first preference.) [fill in the blank]

How would you rate the following companies with regard to the quality of their generic products, on a scale of 1 to 10? [10 is excellent, 1 is poor]
Actavis... Amide... Andrx... Apotex... Aurobindo... Barr... Caraco... Dava... Dr. Reddy's... Endo... Eon... Ethex... Greenstone... Ivax... Mylan... Par... Pliva... Prasco... Purepac... Qualitest... Ranbaxy... Roxane... Sandoz... Taro... Teva... URL/Mutual... Warrick... Watson... Other

My point is: Why is Mylan Pharmaceuticals, one of the largest generic manufacturers in the world, asking pharmacists about our perceptions of the quality of the products made by twenty-eight generic manufacturers when, according to the FDA, **QUALITY IS NOT AN ISSUE?** My belief is that pharmacists do indeed have differing opinions about the quality of generic drugs made by various generic companies. In my experience, Mylan has a good reputation with pharmacists, so I suspect that Mylan sent this survey to pharmacists with hopes of advertising the results.

My views on generic drugs were first influenced by lab exercises in pharmacy school. In one such lab exercise, students examined pills for variation in "friability" (*friable* means *fragile* or *easily crumbled,* i.e., how easily tablets are broken into pieces). Friability affects how easily tablets dissolve in the stomach and intestines. Tablets that are hard as a rock may end up in your toilet without any of the active ingredient being absorbed into your bloodstream. As part of this lab exercise, students were given different brands of aspirin. I remember we examined Bayer aspirin, Lilly aspirin, and various store brands like those from Rite Aid, Eckerds and K-Mart. Students were each given a small supply of one brand of aspirin and were told to swallow one pill at set intervals at home (i.e., at our dormitory or apartment). We urinated into separate containers every few hours. Each student brought his urine samples to school the next day where we analyzed them for aspirin byproduct. The point of this lab exercise was to demonstrate the wide variation in the speed with which different brand and generic tablets dissolve, as indicated by the length of time it took the aspirin by-product to show up in our urine samples. Tablets must dissolve before they can be absorbed from the intestines into the bloodstream. A tablet that's very hard is much less likely to dissolve as quickly as a soft tablet. But a tablet that's too soft will break up before it arrives at your local drugstore.

Our pharmacy school had a tablet pressing machine, a smaller version of that which the big drug manufacturers use when they press tablets. Students were shown how compression settings have a dramatic effect on the speed with which tablets dissolve. If tablets are pressed with too much pressure (compression), they will take a very long time to dissolve in the gut. If tablets are pressed with too little pressure, they will dissolve more quickly in the gut but they will break up too easily in the bottles in which they are sent to pharmacies. If too much compression is used in pressing tablets, the resultant tablet can be so hard that it never dissolves in the gut (or only partly dissolves) and it ends up in your toilet essentially in the same condition as when you swallowed it.

Pharmacy students learn that there are many factors that can adversely affect the quality of tablets when they're manufactured. That's why we're sometimes wary of generic drugs. Since we sometimes see a much larger quantity of broken tablets and powder in the bottom of our stock bottles of generic tablets than we see with brand name tablets, we may conclude that the manufacturer took very little care in manufacturing the generic tablets. This sometimes causes pharmacists to question other things about generic tablets, like whether the tablets have the stated amount of active ingredient. The FDA routinely assures the public that generics are as good as brand name, but many pharmacists remain skeptical. If we receive bottles in which there are lots of broken tablets and powder, it doesn't do much to inspire the pharmacist's confidence that it's a quality product.

Some tablets are manufactured with a thin shiny film coat. Coated tablets seldom arrive at the pharmacy with a small pile of powder at the bottom of stock bottles. But coated tablets can present their own problems. If the coating is too thick or doesn't dissolve properly, the patient will end up with this tablet in his toilet, with no effect from the drug against the target disease or symptom. The situation with capsules is entirely different. With capsules, the speed with which they dissolve in the stomach and intestines is dependent on the characteristics and quality of the wax gel that makes up the capsule. So pharmacists don't usually find powder in the bottoms of our stock bottles containing capsules. Thus the issue whether generic capsules are equivalent to brand name capsules is not influenced by the pharmacist seeing lots of powder at the bottom of our stock bottles containing capsules.

In my opinion, assessment of the quality of generic drugs is something that should be based on independent lab analysis. But politics has intruded into this issue because state and federal governments and insurance companies have an incentive to say that generic drugs are as good as brand name. The use of generic drugs is the main method that governments utilize to hold down drug budgets. Insurance companies strongly encourage generic drugs to save money for the insurance company and its subscribers. Brand name manufacturers sometimes try to convince Congress that generics lack quality. But many brand name companies also manufacture generics, so, for this reason, and because Big Pharma's criticism of generics looks heartless, the brand name drug companies seem to be criticizing generics less lately.

If I were to need a drug for a condition like heart disease or hypertension, I would probably want a brand name drug. If I were to need a pain medication, I would probably be more likely to accept a generic because people who take pain medication should be able to objectively determine whether the generic pain pills are working adequately, i.e., the pills relieve the pain. Many pharmacy customers adamantly refuse to accept generic pain pills, saying they simply aren't as effective as brand name. In some cases, I suspect the customers actually intend to sell the pills. These people know they can get a higher price on the street for the brand name drug. In this case, the "effectiveness" argument is a ruse. In the case of drugs like antibiotics, when used for important infections like pneumonia, I would want a product made by a manufacturer with a good reputation.

Drug Topics reported the results of a survey on consumer attitudes toward generics: "When it comes to serious medical conditions, some consumers still prefer a brand name medication to a generic. According to the results of a survey conducted on behalf of Medco Health Solutions Inc. by the market research firm ReedHaldyMcIntosh, 79% of patients would take a generic medication to treat a cold or flu, and 76% would turn to a generic to address heartburn. But only 56% would use a generic drug to treat a more serious ailment such as asthma, and only 52% would opt for a generic to treat diabetes. When it comes to heart disease, the percentage of consumers who would accept a generic agent fell even further—to less than 50%." (Anthony Vecchione, "Brand drugs have edge over generics for serious medical conditions," *Drug Topics Generic Supplement,* August 2004, p. 38s)

It is difficult for me to make a blanket condemnation of generic drugs. From years of dealing with these products, pharmacists sometimes get the impression that some generic drugs from some manufacturers seem to be cheaply made. I would have to decide on whether to accept a generic product based on the seriousness of the condition being treated and the (admittedly subjective) impression that I have of the manufacturer of the generic drug. Of course, you can't judge a book by its cover just like you can't judge a generic drug totally by its appearance and the extent that it breaks up in our stock bottles.

If you were to ask your pharmacist what he thinks about the quality of generic drugs, you are likely to get a reassuring answer like: "The government tests generic drugs to assure that they are as good as brand name drugs." The more politically sophisticated pharmacists are, in my opinion, less likely to believe this even though they may indeed say it.

If you are a pharmacist who thinks that government regulators do a satisfactory job in every area (Securities and Exchange Commission, Environmental Protection Agency, Occupational Safety and Health Administration, Consumer Product Safety Commission, etc.), then you are probably more likely to believe that the government has adequate staff and resources to assure the quality of generic drugs. If, however, you think that the government has inadequate budgets for inspections in general, then you are less likely to be swayed by FDA assurances that generic drugs are as good as brand name. My impression is that there are few, if any, government agencies that have adequate resources for thorough inspections, whether it involves examining meat-packing plants, monitoring the exposure of factory workers to toxic chemicals, or testing fruits and vegetables for hazardous pesticide residues, etc. The media routinely exposes government waste and ineptitude (for example, the Pentagon spending a few hundred dollars for a toilet seat or hammer). The fact that such reports of over-spending, lack of accountability, and sheer incompetence never seem to end makes me skeptical about the effectiveness of governmental oversight in any field, not just pharmaceuticals. The FDA agrees that the agency is understaffed. The FDA agrees that they have found many violations in their inspections of both brand name and generic manufacturers. Yet the FDA insists that generic drugs are still as good as brand name.

The pharmacy magazines rarely, if ever, present detailed coverage of the debate over the quality of generic drugs. This is because generic manufacturers have lots of advertising in these pharmacy magazines. So, if pharmacists depend on pharmacy magazines for an unbiased assessment of the quality of generic drugs, I predict these pharmacists will remain uninformed of the nuances in the debate.

I wish *Consumer Reports* would conduct a massive study of the quality of generic drugs. I would trust *Consumer Reports* to be objective far more than I would trust the FDA. No matter how strongly certain people at the FDA may question generic drugs, the FDA Commissioner and the Administration set the general tone that generic drugs are as good as brand name. I suspect that lower level employees at the FDA would be pressured to keep quiet if they had serious questions about the quality of generic drugs.

Most pro-consumer advocacy groups are strong proponents of generic drugs as a way for people to save money. In this environment, it is not politically correct for a pro-consumer person such as myself to question generic drugs. But I am simply skeptical that the pharmaceutical industry can always deliver a quality generic product at a rock-bottom price. I am certain that there are many generic drugs that are equal to brand name. (Brand name drugs themselves vary from batch to batch.) However, I am unconvinced that, in every case, generic drugs are as good as brand name. The problem is that you have no accurate way of knowing if the generic drug you receive at your local pharmacy is as good as the brand name product.

Lots of groups benefit from the widespread use of generic drugs: 1) Insurance companies push generic drugs in a big way to save money. In fact, promoting the use of generic drugs is the primary strategy employed by insurance companies to save money on drugs. Higher customer co-pays for brand name drugs hold down costs for insurance companies. The co-pays for brand name drugs are usually substantially higher than for generic drugs. 2) Pharmacists prefer to dispense generic drugs because the markup is better on generic drugs compared to brand name drugs. With decreasing profits from managed care, pharmacists often feel pushed to buy generics based on price rather than on some subjective assessment of quality or the reputation of the manufacturer. Because of the influence of managed care, which typically puts a cap on third party reimbursements, and declining profitability of their business, pharmacists might choose a generic with the best price even though they may have some qualms about doing so. 3) State Medicaid programs usually mandate generic drugs to save taxpayers money. For state Medicaid programs, the states depend on the FDA's assurances of quality. State Medicaid drug programs depend heavily on generics. 4) The federal government pays for drugs for veterans (in VA hospitals and through the mail) and for hospitalized patients on Medicare, and via Medicare Part D. 5) We as taxpayers save with generic drugs. Our taxes would increase if generic drugs didn't exist.

If the FDA concluded that generic drugs are sometimes inferior, state governments would be placed in the hard-to-justify position of embracing generic drugs while the FDA has questions about those drugs. Abandoning generic drugs would place a huge burden on already-strained state budgets that rely very heavily on generic drugs in state Medicaid programs. If the FDA expressed skepticism about generic drugs, that would open a huge can of worms adversely affecting governmental budgets, insurance company profits, and drugstore profits. The drug companies that market brand name drugs would use this as an opportunity to raise the prices of their already-over-priced drugs. The existence of viable generic alternatives puts pressure on brand name companies to hold down prices. The FDA has a strong incentive to approve generic drugs because the more generic competitors, the greater the pressure on the price of the original brand name drug (*Associated Press* on-line, "FDA: Generic Drugs Can Help Slash Prices," April 4, 2006):

Prescription drug prices soften dramatically even with moderate competition, the Food and Drug Administration said Tuesday in an analysis that shows the arrival in the marketplace of just two generic versions of a brand-name medicine can nearly halve the price consumers pay.

When a brand-name drug faces just one generic competitor, that challenger typically sells for 94 percent of the cost of its branded rival. More competition quickly widens that discount: Once a second generic manufacturer appears, the average price of a generic drug drops to just 52 percent of the brand-name version's cost per dose, according to the analysis posted on the FDA web site.

Prices continue to tumble, albeit more slowly but almost without exception, as more manufacturers join the market, the analysis shows. By the time nine manufacturers are producing generic versions of a drug, their products typically sell for just 20 percent of the price of the brand-name medicine, according to the federal analysis of 1999-2004 retail sales data on single-ingredient drug products collected by IMS Health Inc.

Release of the analysis comes amid ongoing criticism that the FDA is slow to approve generic versions of brand-name pharmaceuticals. The agency has a backlog of roughly 800 generic drug applications.

In May of 2007, *The People's Pharmacy* began inviting visitors to that website (www.peoplespharmacy.com) to share their experiences with generic drugs. As of February 26, 2011, the website contained 1,356 (one thousand three hundred and fifty-six) comments. (http://www.peoplespharmacy.com/2007/05/21/report-generic/) Most people relate their experiences in which a generic drug is less effective or has more adverse effects than the brand name version they were on previously. Conditions that were well-controlled on a brand name medication often become less well-controlled when switched to a generic. The Graedons introduce this massive compilation of patient stories as follows (http://www.peoplespharmacy.com/archives/generic_drug_problems /report_generic_drug_problem.php):

> **In the field of pharmaceuticals, Americans have been told that price doesn't matter. Generic drugs are supposed to be identical to their brand name counterparts. For nearly 30 years, we believed this argument. We encouraged people to save money by insisting that their physicians prescribe generics whenever they were available.**
>
> **All that changed several years ago when some pharmacists started telling us they had doubts about the quality of certain generic products. We also began getting letters from readers who had trouble with their generic prescriptions. Readers have shared their disappointment with generic pain relievers, antidepressants, blood pressure medicines and diabetes drugs. The generic drug manufacturers discount these reports.**

Spend a few hours reading these stories and decide for yourself whether the issue of generic drugs is as simple as the FDA says.

On April 14, 2008, *Drug Topics* revealed the results of their survey of pharmacists on the subject of generics. (Martin Sipkoff, "Exclusive survey of R.Phs. [registered pharmacists] reveals their hopes, fears about generics," *Drug Topics Generic Supplement*, April 14, 2008, pp. 14s-15s). The FDA constantly reassures the public that generic drugs are as good as brand name, yet pharmacists still consider "quality" a very important issue as regards generic drugs. One pharmacist commented, "Generic manufacturers need to be aware that patients do tell us the difference in products and many times refuse to take a particular one. Drug companies need to make sure their products are of the highest quality." The article contains two charts, both of which focus heavily on the issue of the quality of generic drugs. The first chart is titled "The top 15 generic companies by pharmacist votes". The short introduction to this chart states: *Which generic manufacturers provided pharmacists with the highest quality products and best customer service? Here are the top 15, based on responses from pharmacists:*

Company	% of respondents choosing this company
Mylan	65%
Teva	53%
Watson	48%
Sandoz	38%
Greenstone	36%
Barr	29%
Apotex	25%
Ranbaxy	17%
Qualitest	17%
Ethex	16%
Dr. Reddy's	16%
Actavis	14%
Roxane	14%
Endo	13%
Purepac	9%

The second chart is titled "Which factors are important when deciding which company's generic products to stock?" As regards factors that are "extremely important" to pharmacists, notice that "Quality of generic product" is rated the highest.

Factors	Extremely important
Quality of generic product	75%
Product availability	57%
In-stock consistency	51%
Company's reputation	44%
Net price	39%
Customer service	24%

It is important to note that pharmacists' determination of "Quality of generic product" is based mainly on our perception. Our perception is based on factors such as the whether the tablets or capsules look like they're cheaply made, whether we've received feedback from our customers about certain products, whether the manufacturer has few instances in which the product is unavailable due to recalls or manufacturing snafus or a backlog of orders. Many generic tablets and capsules look like they were produced in a haphazard manner, with lots of crumbled tablets and powder in our stock containers.

My purely subjective guess as to why Mylan ranks high among pharmacists is that their products always look like they are well made. And Mylan seems to vary the size, shape, and color among their different products in a very appealing manner, giving each generic product an individual identity, whereas many of the other generic manufacturers seem to produce garden variety white tablets that don't look as distinctive as the products made by Mylan. Mylan seems to take more pride in the appearance of their products. I don't recall seeing lots of broken tablets in the products we received from Mylan. (I don't own any stock in Mylan or in any other drug company.) The fact that readers of *Drug Topics* frequently see advertisements for Mylan products in that magazine may have influenced the results.

It should be noted that Mylan was the target of an unsettling exposé in the *Pittsburgh Post-Gazette* in 2009 in which some employees claimed that the company sometimes sacrificed quality. (Patricia Sabatini and Len Boselovic, "Mylan workers overrode drug quality controls: Internal report detailed 'pervasive' practice of ignoring safety procedures," *Pittsburgh Post-Gazette,* July 26, 2009 http://www.post-gazette.com/pg/09207/986516-455.stm)

When I was in pharmacy school at West Virginia University in Morgantown during the early 1970s, Mylan's plant was in easy walking distance from our classrooms. I always found it strange that our instructors did not arrange a tour of the plant for pharmacy students. One day in pharmacy school I asked one of our instructors why such a tour had not been arranged for students since the plant was so close by. As best as I can recall, the instructor said something like, "You think that would be a good thing to do?" and then he shrugged his shoulders.

Pharmacy students are taught a great deal about the dissolution of tablets and capsules. I still recall the big tablet-pressing machine on the bottom floor of the School of Pharmacy. It was there solely to demonstrate to students how tablets are pressed and why such factors as compression are so important for proper dissolution. So I think it would have been very instructive for students to take advantage of having a large generic manufacturer such as Mylan so close by. I don't recall any other students in my class wondering why such a tour was never arranged.

Perhaps I am being unfair in assuming that the reason the tour was never arranged was because pharmacy instructors prefer to live in the world of theory. Perhaps the theoretical world is far more appealing to instructors than the real world. But I would have loved to tour the Mylan plant.

On December 8, 2011, I received an e-mail from *FDA News—Drug GMP Report*. *FDA News* (fdanews.com) is a provider of regulatory, legislative and business news for executives in industries regulated by the FDA. The e-mail was titled, "FDA Moving to Ensure Uniformity of Generics from Different Makers." The e-mail essentially states that FDA realizes that generics are not uniform from different manufacturers:

> The FDA is eyeing additional steps to ensure uniform quality of the same generic drug produced by different manufacturers, and between different lots of the same product produced by a drugmaker, Keith Webber, acting director of the Office of Generic Drugs (OGD), says.
>
> The agency may examine different ways to ensure product quality, including looking at how well a manufacturer's production process can conform to a drug's design specifications, Webber said last month at the Generic Pharmaceutical Association—FDA Fall Technical Conference in Bethesda, Md. The OGD can also take a closer look at product design, sampling and testing.
>
> Current specifications are not enough to ensure generic drugs are uniform, as the same product could be manufactured to design specifications under separately approved ANDAs but may not prove the same, Webber said.

Of course, you should never judge a book by its cover, just as you should never judge a generic drug solely by its appearance. Obviously pharmacists in the real world don't test the potency or dissolution of the products we dispense, nor do we experiment using ourselves as guinea pigs to see which products are the best at treating the target condition. So we rely on our perceptions, and, admittedly, our perceptions may not necessarily be accurate.

In my experience, most pharmacists are very reassuring when customers ask us "Is the generic as good as the brand name?" Nevertheless, my perception is that many pharmacists privately are not quite as confident that the issue of generic drug effectiveness is as cut and dried as the FDA says. On the other hand, I am sure that there are lots of pharmacists who routinely recommend generic drugs for members of their own family. And I am sure that there are lots of pharmacists who routinely choose to take generic drugs themselves for any and all medical conditions.

Our pharmacy customers prefer simple answers like "Generic drugs are good" or "Generic drugs are bad." In my opinion, the correct answer is much more nuanced. Our customers seem to interpret nuance as indecisiveness.

There are other issues with generic drugs that are completely unrelated to the quality of the product. For example, generic drugs can be a big source of confusion.

Identifying generic drugs used to be much more difficult (for pharmacists and consumers) than identifying brand name drugs. Generic drugs are very often garden variety white tablets, i.e., they have few, if any, unique distinguishing characteristics that make them readily identifiable except for the product number which may be too small to read easily. The manufacturers of brand name products seem to take more pride in the appearance of their tablets and in making sure that the tablets don't crumble too easily. Brand name products are intentionally made with a unique appearance to gain patient loyalty and expectation. Customers ask the pharmacist, "I've been on this light blue blood pressure pill for two years. Why did you refill my prescription with red pills? Did the pharmacy make a mistake?" Sometimes the highly embarrassing answer is *yes.*

If all the tablets in the pharmacy were round and white like many generics, errors would probably be more frequent. The endless variation in shapes, sizes, and colors helps pharmacists and techs cut down on pharmacy errors. Customers often ask the pharmacist to identify a tablet. Tablets that are easy to identify are more likely to have a unique appearance. It is obviously helpful to have the name of the manufacturer on the pill. Most pills are imprinted with a product number. Some pills are imprinted with the brand name of the product, a practice which I wish all companies would adopt. In general—but certainly not always—generic names are longer than brand names. This makes it more difficult to stamp long generic names like hydrochlorothiazide, methocarbamol, amitriptyline, or cyclobenzaprine on small tablets. Thus, it is often easier to identify brand name pills than generics. Generic tablets are much more likely to be unremarkable in appearance. Many generic pills are, however, quite distinct in their appearance.

In the last few years, websites have become available that greatly simplify the process of identifying tablets and capsules, whether they are brand name drugs or generics. Search Google for *pill identifier* and you will find several websites. For example: 1) drugs.com, 2) rxlist.com, 3) webmd.com, 4) healthline.com, 5) healthtools.aarp.org

Usually all that you have to do to identify your tablets and capsules is enter the numbers, letters, or words on those pills. Even though my mother died over ten years ago, I have kept all the pills that she was prescribed during her treatment for colon cancer that spread to her liver. I grabbed ten of those pill bottles containing mostly generic drugs and entered the numbers, letters, and words into the appropriate fields on the drugs.com website. I was quickly given the precisely correct identity of each pill. Below you will see the info I entered and the results:

1. 54 543   Ccorrectly identified as Roxicet
2. Mylan 155   Correctly identified as generic Darvocet
3. SP 4220   Correctly identified as Niferex-150
4. Endo 602   Correctly identified as Endocet
5. INV 276 10   Correctly identified as prochlorperazine 10 mg
6. M 15   Correctly identified as generic Lomotil
7. Watson 349   Correctly identified as generic Vicodin
8. KU 108   Correctly identified as generic Levbid
9. MP 85   Correctly identified as generic Septra DS
10. OC 20   Correctly identified as Oxycontin 20 mg

It is not rare that adults ask pharmacists to identify some tablet or capsule found at home. In my career, sometimes I had the impression that this was a parent who had discovered that pill in his or her child's room or in the child's clothing while emptying pockets before doing laundry. I was somewhat uncomfortable under these circumstances because I suspected that if the pill I identified were a controlled substance, the son or daughter would soon be in for a world of hurt, i.e., confronted by a very angry parent.

Another issue regarding confusion with generic drugs involves what is known as "therapeutic duplication." It is extremely important that consumers learn both the brand and generic names of all their drugs so that they don't end up taking the exact same drug under two different names. For example, if you were taking the generic thyroid hormone levothyroxine and your doctor wrote you a prescription for Levothroid, Levoxyl, Euthyrox, or Synthroid, would you know that all of these are simply brand names for levothyroxine? If you were taking generic theophylline for asthma, and your doctor wrote you a prescription for Slo-Phyllin, Slo-bid, Theo-Dur, Theo-24, or Uniphyl, would you know that these are simply brand names for theophylline? If you were taking generic lithium carbonate for manic depression and your doctor wrote you a prescription for Cibalith, Eskalith, Lithobid, Lithotabs, or Lithonate, would you know that these are simply brand names for lithium carbonate? If you were taking Lanoxin for your heart and your doctor wrote you a prescription for digoxin, would you know that these are the same drug? If you were taking the blood thinner Coumadin and your pharmacy filled a new prescription for warfarin, would you know that these are the same drug?

Reports of concurrent use of digoxin and Lanoxin have been reported in the past, sometimes with unfortunate outcomes. Such situations tend to occur when the same medication is prescribed by brand name by one physician and by generic name by another physician, or when the medications are dispensed from different pharmacies. This problem is becoming more common as healthcare becomes increasingly fragmented. Dupont, manufacturer of the blood thinner Coumadin, says that several cases of therapeutic duplication have been reported to the company. In one case, a 69-year old female inadvertently taking both warfarin and Coumadin was admitted to the hospital with massive rectal and nasal bleeding and an international normalized ratio (INR) of 30.9. During her hospitalization, she suffered a myocardial infarction that was attributed to her blood loss. In another case, a patient received prescriptions for Coumadin from one physician and generic warfarin from another. She ended up hospitalized as a result of "bleeding from her ears and eyes." Fortunately, treatment with vitamin K resolved the patient's symptoms and she was subsequently discharged. (Susan Proulx, "Medication Errors," *U.S. Pharmacist*, June 1998, p. 95)

Whenever you receive a prescription for a drug that you're not familiar with, you should never assume that your doctor has put you on an entirely different medication. It could be the same drug under a different name. Pharmacists see many instances in which customers are not aware that indapamide is the same as Lozol, alprozolam is the same as Xanax, lorazepam is the same as Ativan, atenolol is the same as Tenormin, furosemide is the same as Lasix, gemfibrozil is the same as Lopid, piroxicam is the same as Feldene, methocarbamol is the same as Robaxin, etc.

Trying to decide whether you have a generic drug by comparing it to the brand name is usually a bad idea. Sometimes the generic name does resemble the brand name in some ways. For example, digoxin sounds somewhat like Lanoxin. Naproxen sounds a lot like Naprosyn. Cefaclor sounds like Ceclor. Clonazepam sounds a little like Klonopin. Roxicet and Percocet share "cet" (denoting aCETaminophen). Amoxicillin, Trimox, and Amoxil all share "mox." But in most cases, the generic name does not look anything like the brand name. For example, ranitidine shows absolutely no resemblance to Zantac. Guanfacine shows absolutely no resemblance to Tenex. Glyburide shows no resemblance to Diabeta or Micronase. Ketoprofen shows no resemblance or Orudis. Nortriptyline shows no resemblance to Pamelor.

Here's an actual case illustrating the confusion that can be caused by generic names. Attorney Dan Frith from the Frith Law Firm in Roanoke, Virginia, writes: ["Pharmacy Mistakes Kill," February 13, 2008 (Accessed Feb 28, 2008) http://roanoke.injuryboard.com/medical-malpractice/pharmacy-mis-takes-kill.php?googleid=14934]

My law firm is getting ready to try a case against a local pharmacy which filled and dispensed a doctor's prescription for medication to which our client was allergic. You may ask, "Why did the client take a medication to which she knew she was allergic"? The answer is that she was given the generic form of the drug—the pills did not look the same and the generic name was nowhere close to the name of the medication to which she was allergic. The prescribing doctor has accepted his responsibility and paid money damages to our client but the pharmacy has not.

Here is a comment I posted on *The People's Pharmacy* website as part of a discussion on the quality of generic drugs (April 12, 2011):

For many years, I have wanted to believe that generics are as good as brand name drugs. I have been appalled by the prices of brand name drugs and the profits of Big Pharma. I wanted to be able to tell customers that generics are as good as brand name products because that would have been a good way for me to take a stand against the greedy brand name drug companies.

But, like every pharmacist, I kept hearing a significant number of stories from customers who said that the generic was not as good as the brand name. For years I dismissed these complaints outright. But I began to wonder: "Can all these customers who complain be crazy? Can they all be simply imagining that the generic is not as good?"

No matter what city I worked in, it was not rare that I would encounter customers who would say that a generic was not as good as the brand name version. Of course, customers don't like having a co-pay that is so much higher for brand name drugs compared to generics. They feel their insurance company is coercing them into accepting generics. Can those higher co-pays account for all the complaints about the quality of generic drugs? Are these customers just mad at their insurance company?

Every pharmacist has heard many stories from customers telling us things like how often they would have to urinate while taking the brand name diuretic Lasix in comparison to the generic furosemide.

Every pharmacist has heard lots of stories from mothers who tell us that their child's behavior worsened when switched from the brand name Ritalin to the generic methylphenidate. Some customers tell us that their depression symptoms worsened on a generic antidepressant, or that they experienced more side effects on the generic. Other customers say their doctor has a harder time keeping their clotting in the target range with the generic for Coumadin. And the examples go on and on. What is a pharmacist to make of all of this? Are all of these customers simply imagining these differences between branded drugs and generics?

We hear that the FDA has inadequate resources to inspect the drug companies in this country, much less those in countries like India, China, and Mexico. We go to the FDA website and look under RECALLS and find a very unsettling number of recalls at both brand name companies and generic companies.

In 2009, the *Pittsburgh Post-Gazette* did an expose' on the huge and well-regarded generic manufacturer Mylan, whose plant is in Morgantown, West Virginia, which is not far from Pittsburgh. Mylan is always rated very high among pharmacists in polls in magazines like *Drug Topics* that regularly ask pharmacists to rate generic manufacturers according to our perceptions of the quality of their products. The reporters who did this expose' interviewed many Mylan employees who said that short-cuts were taken too often, that satisfying production goals too often interfered with quality control. (Patricia Sabatini and Len Boselovic, "Mylan workers overrode drug quality controls: Internal report detailed 'pervasive' practice of ignoring safety procedures," July 26, 2009   http://www.post-gazette.com/pg/09207/986516-455.stm)

The cover story for the March 31, 2011 issue of *Bloomberg BusinessWeek* is about the "Quality Catastrophe" at Johnson & Johnson, a company that previously had a stellar reputation.

Yet, somehow, even with all these questions about quality control in plants in this country and around the world, the FDA still tells us that the end product on pharmacy shelves is just fine. Out of a system in chaos, somehow, magically, the end product is just fine. When there are so many questions about quality control in the pharmaceutical industry, how can we as pharmacists act as if there is no controversy here? Are we being honest with our customers? Any pharmacist who takes the time to investigate this issue comes away scratching his head, wondering whether the FDA does indeed have a good handle on the issue.

Many pharmacists seem to have almost a religious belief that all generics are as good as brand name drugs. Attempting to tell these pharmacists otherwise is like criticizing their religion. They get very upset and defensive.

During my career as a pharmacist, I wish I could have had complete faith in all of the generic drugs I dispensed. I wish I hadn't heard customer complaints about the quality of generic products. I wish I hadn't seen so many articles and news releases about major quality control issues in the pharmaceutical industry in this country and around the world. I always hated Big Pharma for their outrageous pricing of drugs, so I would have had a great way to get back at them by strongly recommending generic alternatives. But, intellectually, I was being dishonest with myself and with the customers for whom I filled prescriptions.

As a consequence of news stories in the mass media regarding quality control problems at manufacturing facilities around the world, a pharmacist named Sam blogged on PharmQD that he decided to collect one day's worth of prescription stock bottles to be able to show customers that pills are made at some surprising places. ("Questions from Patients on Generic Drugs," http://www.pharmqd.com/forum/topic/questions-patients generic-drugs)

[On] Friday, I saved every bottle dispensed made in a different country for show and tell. There was Canada, Israel, France, Germany, Sweden, Italy, Slovania, Croatia, India, United Kingdom, England, Switzerland, Puerto Rico, China, Japan, Singapore, I think Brazil was in there too. This is just from a small rural independent pharmacy.—Sam

It is a fact that there is a wide variety of opinions among pharmacists about the quality of generic drugs. Some pharmacists are huge fans of generic drugs as an alternative to the price gouging by Big Pharma. Other pharmacists are not so sure that the race to find the lowest-cost suppliers necessarily delivers a product of top quality. It is a fact that the confidence level among pharmacists about generic drugs covers a wide spectrum.

If Johnson & Johnson, a brand-name company that once had a stellar reputation, has serious problems with quality control, why should we as pharmacists assume that drugs manufactured WHO KNOWS WHERE by other brand-name and generic companies are fine? What do we base that on? Here's one paragraph from the *Bloomberg BusinessWeek* cover story on Johnson & Johnson (David Voreacos, Alex Nussbaum and Greg Farrell, "Johnson & Johnson's Quality Catastrophe," March 31, 2011):

The DuPuy crisis is one of more than 50 voluntary product recalls that J&J has issued just since the start of 2010, covering brand name drugs that read like an inventory of the family medicine cabinet. Tylenol and St. Joseph Aspirin were recalled for foul odors people said made them sick. Benadryl and Zyrtec were recalled for botched amounts of ingredients. Rolaids were recalled for containing bits of wood and metal. Most of these drugstore stalwarts come from J&J's McNeil Consumer Healthcare unit, which has been plagued by dismaying revelations about the conditions and lax controls at its factories in the U.S. It shuttered one factory in Fort Washington, Pa., for a quality overhaul. Under a Mar. 10 consent decree, the plant and two others—in Lancaster, Pa., and Puerto Rico—will remain under Food and Drug Administration (FDA) oversight for five years. J&J McNeil faces fines of $10 million per year if the agency isn't satisfied with its progress.

Timeline for some of Johnson & Johnson's major recalls

Johnson & Johnson said that Chief Executive William Weldon would step down from the post in April, 2012, after 10 years at the helm of the diversified healthcare company.

In the past two years, Weldon faced massive recalls of products, from artificial hips to children's Tylenol, that challenged his leadership and hurt J&J's reputation as a provider of high-quality products. Below is a timeline of some of the major recalls:

Feb 17, 2012: Products: 574,000 bottles of the grape-flavored **Tylenol**. Problem: flaws in a new bottle design.

Jan 27, 2012: Products: 2,000 tubes of **Aveeno Baby Calming Comfort Lotion**. Problem: excessive levels of bacteria in a product sample.

Dec 21, 2011: Products: 12 million bottles of **Motrin** pain relievers. Problem: caplets may dissolve too slowly, delaying pain relief.

Sept 23, 2011: Products: Two batches of **Eprex** anemia drug in 17 countries. Problem: inconsistent potency.

April 14, 2011: Products: 57,000 bottles of epilepsy drug, **Topamax**. Problem: foul odor.

March 29, 2011: Products: 700,000 bottles of **Tylenol** and other consumer medicines. Problem: musty or moldy odor.

March 8, 2011: Products: five lots of **insulin pump cartridges**. Problem: potential leaks.

March 2, 2011: Products: 107 batches of **surgical sutures** (recalled in December). Problem: potential sterility problems.

Feb 11, 2011: Products: 70,000 syringes filled with the antipsychotic drug **Invega**. Problem: cracks in the syringes.

Jan 14, 2011: Products: 50 million bottles and packages of various kinds of **Tylenol, Benadryl, Rolaids** and other consumer products. Problem: lax cleaning procedures at manufacturing plant.

Dec 9, 2010: Products: All lots of **Softchews Rolaids** antacids. Problem: wood and metal bits in the tablets.

Dec 2, 2010: Products: 12 million bottles of **Mylanta** and almost 85,000 bottles of **AlternaGel** liquid antacid. Problem: small amounts of alcohol from flavoring agents was not noted on product packaging.

Dec 1, 2010: Products: 492,000 boxes of **1 Day Acuvue TruEye** contact lenses. Problem: consumer complaints of stinging pain.

Nov 24, 2010: Products: 9 million bottles of **Tylenol**. Problem: inadequate warning of trace amounts of alcohol used in the product flavorings.

Oct 18, 2010: Products: One lot of adult **Tylenol** caplets. Problem: musty or moldy odor.

July 8, 2010: Products: Twenty-one lots of **Tylenol** for children and adults, several forms of **Benadryl** and **Motrin** sold in the United States, Fiji, Guatemala, the Dominican Republic, Puerto Rico, Trinidad and Tobago and Jamaica in expansion of Jan. 15 recall. The company has said this action affected 2.5 million bottles of medicines. Problem: musty or moldy odor detected in earlier recall.

June 15, 2010: Products: Four lots of **Benadryl** and **Extra Strength Tylenol** gels sold in the United States, Trinidad and Tobago, Bermuda and Puerto Rico in expansion of Jan. 15 recall. The company has said 500,000 bottles were affected. Problem: musty or moldy odor detected in earlier recall.

April 30, 2010: Products: Forty products including liquid infant and children's pain relievers, **Tylenol**, and **Motrin** and allergy medications **Zyrtec** and **Benadryl**. About 135 million bottles were affected, according to congressional investigators. Problem: Manufacturing deficiencies that may have affected the quality, purity or potency of the medicines.

Jan 15, 2010: Products: Fifty-three million bottles of over-the-counter products including **Tylenol, Motrin, Rolaids, Benadryl** and **St. Joseph's Aspirin**, involving lots in the Americas, the United Arab Emirates and Fiji. Problem: Unusual moldy, musty or mildew-like odor linked to chemical in wood pallets used to store and ship products.

Dec 2009: Product: Expands November recall of **Tylenol Arthritis Pain Caplets**. Problem: Consumer reports of unusual moldy odor with the 100-count bottles.

Nov 2009: Product: Five lots of **Tylenol Arthritis Pain Caplets**. Problem: Reports of an unusual musty or mildew-like odor that was associated with nausea, stomach pain, vomiting and diarrhea.

Sept 2009: Products: Some lots of infants' and children's **Tylenol**. Problem: Possible bacterial contamination.

July 2009: Product: **Motrin** tablets sold mostly at convenience stores. The recall is the subject of a congressional probe into what some Democratic lawmakers say was a stealthy effort to buy back the drug rather than recall it. J&J has said FDA knew of their actions, while FDA has said as soon as it found out, it sought a recall. Problem: Problems with dissolving. (Anand Basu, Reuters Health Information, "Timeline: Johnson & Johnson Product Recalls," Feb. 22, 2012 http://www.medscape.com/viewarticle/759067?src=mp&spon=18)

Chapter 24

How good are drugs compounded by pharmacists?

What is compounding? The following description of compounding is taken from The International Academy of Compounding Pharmacists' website (http://www.iacprx.org/site/PageServer?pagename=What_is_compounding):

Pharmacy compounding is the long-established tradition in pharmacy practice that enables physicians to prescribe and patients to take medicines that are specially prepared by pharmacists to meet patients' individual needs. A growing number of people have unique health needs that off-the-shelf prescription medicines cannot meet. For them, customized, compounded medications prescribed or ordered by licensed physicians or veterinarians and mixed safely by trained, licensed compounding pharmacists are the only way to better health. Pharmacists are the only health care professionals that have studied chemical compatibilities and can prepare alternate dosage forms. In fact, each state requires that pharmacy schools must as part of their core curriculum instruct students on the compounding of pharmaceutical ingredients. Because every patient is different and has different needs, customized, compounded medications are a vital part of quality medical care. Physicians often prescribe compounded medications for reasons that include (but are not limited to) the following situations:

• When needed medications are discontinued by or generally unavailable from pharmaceutical companies, often because the medications are no longer profitable to manufacture;
• When the patient is allergic to certain preservatives, dyes or binders in available off-the shelf medications;
• When treatment requires tailored dosage strengths for patients with unique needs (for example, an infant);
• When a pharmacist can combine several medications the patient is taking to increase compliance;
• When the patient cannot ingest the medication in its commercially available form and a pharmacist can prepare the medication in cream, liquid or other form that the patient can easily take; and
• When medications require flavor additives to make them more palatable for some patients, most often children.

This description of compounding sounds impressive but, in the real world, most of the products that pharmacists compound are done so for much less important reasons. Even though there are cases in which a custom-made drug is needed, many pharmacists wonder why, with thousands of products on the market, doctors can't simply pick one of those rather than have the pharmacist do some kind of mixing of ingredients, modifying of available dosages, etc. Most of the products I compounded in my 25-year career (in many different cities) seemed to be to satisfy the quirky preferences of some local dermatologist.

Some pharmacists compound products on such a large scale that the FDA feels these pharmacists have crossed the line into manufacturing. The FDA feels these large-scale pharmacist compounders should be held to the same rules as manufacturers.

In my experience, most pharmacists do not enjoy the process of compounding mainly because it is so time consuming compared to filling other prescriptions. Many pharmacists view compounding as burdensome and a throwback to pharmacy a hundred years ago when snake oils, tinctures, salves, potions, purges, leeches, and high-alcohol-content tonics were standard practice. In my opinion many pharmacists view compounding as a bit silly. Pharmacists who are strong believers in science sometimes have a hard time feeling comfortable using the mortar and pestle, that outdated and quaint icon of pharmacy.

I think it is fair to say that many pharmacists are skeptical of the quality of products we compound because we sometimes lack confidence in our knowledge of compounding. Proper compounding sometimes requires a level of expertise that many pharmacists do not feel they possess. I consider my compounding classes in pharmacy school to have been inadequate. These classes did not leave me with a feeling of confidence in my ability to compound products that required more than an average amount of expertise.

The degree of complexity involved with compounding varies tremendously among different products. For example, compounding is simple when two commercially available creams are mixed together, or when two commercially available liquids are combined. Adding a powder to a cream is a little more time consuming. Powders are usually dissolved in an appropriate liquid before being added to a cream. During my 25-year career, I was never absolutely certain regarding the liquid I should utilize to dissolve the powder when preparing some product used for a dermatological condition.

My attitude toward compounding dermatological products was formed when I read a critique of dermatology. I read that dermatology is a good specialty for doctors because there are "no cures, no kills, and no night calls." "No cures" refers to the fact that patients keep coming back to dermatologists since many of the products don't really cure the disease, i.e., they simply relieve symptoms. "No kills" refers to the fact that dermatologists (and the products they prescribe) rarely kill patients, thus making for a less stressful practice. "No night calls" refers to the fact that dermatologists have fewer middle-of-the-night emergencies than most other medical specialists. With that view toward dermatology, I usually had a laid-back attitude toward the skin creams I compounded for conditions like dermatitis. Perhaps I compounded one or two such products per week. I'm not proud of my attitude in this regard and I confess that my attitude was wrong. However, in my experience, a large number of pharmacists seem to have a similar attitude, viewing the compounding of creams for common skin conditions as a lingering remnant of the snake oil era. Of course, there are obviously some skin products, such as antibiotics used topically to treat skin infections, that are very important but most pharmacists do not compound antibiotic creams.

Here is an example of what I mean by not knowing enough to properly compound a product. It was 1975 or 1976 and I was working in a small town in West Virginia for a large national drugstore chain. I had been out of pharmacy school for less than a year. A customer brought in a prescription to be compounded. I was not familiar with how to compound the product so I sought guidance in a reference book that I used in pharmacy school. I can't recall the product I was attempting to compound, but I do remember it was intended to treat a skin condition of some type. The reference book recommended that one substance be dissolved in ether before being incorporated into another substance. I don't think I handled any ether while compounding products in pharmacy school. But I figured: *What the hell. I'll give it a try. I've just graduated from pharmacy school with honors so supposedly my instructors think I'm a competent pharmacist and that I know what I'm doing.* In fact, I didn't know what I was doing and I had no business attempting to compound that product. I ordered a small can of ether to use in compounding the medication. But here's the interesting part. I didn't realize that I needed special equipment or a special room (with controlled air flow) to work with the ether. So here I was working with ether in the pharmacy and I had no idea what I was doing. I remember becoming quite nauseous. Then it dawned on me that I was anesthetizing myself with ether. Soon the entire pharmacy smelled like ether. The two technicians assumed I knew what I was doing but they were wrong. The smell of ether soon became quite powerful.

It so happens that this drugstore was in a two-story building. Above the drugstore were two apartments, one of which I lived in. I told the two technicians that I thought I'd better go upstairs and lie down for a while. I was feeling quite nauseous. It is highly unusual for a chain pharmacist to leave work and go home (in this case upstairs) under circumstances like this. We had customers waiting for prescriptions so my leaving the drugstore was not a good thing to do. But I felt I was going to pass out. So I went upstairs and lay down on my bed. I was quite frightened because I felt like I did when I was undergoing anesthesia for surgery as a child. The ether was putting me to sleep just like I was in surgery. So I lay down not knowing how much sleepier the ether would make me. I did not know whether I would become completely unconscious for a minute or five minutes or twenty minutes or an hour, or…who knows? Luckily I began to feel better after lying down for maybe twenty minutes. I think I returned to the drugstore maybe within a half hour. The two technicians looked at me like "Wow, Dennis. This is strange." Anyway, I recovered fully from the ether maybe within an hour or two. But this was possibly the most bizarre and stupid thing I did in my entire career as a pharmacist. I felt that, since I had just graduated from pharmacy school, surely I was a competent pharmacist. But I had no business working with ether under those circumstances.

I can't remember what excuse I gave the customer, but I think I somehow told him or her that I would not be able to compound that product and that he or she would need to take it elsewhere. Attempting to compound that product with ether was one of the dumbest things I've ever done in my life. I am not claiming that any other pharmacist in America would have been as stupid as I was that day. But I do claim that many pharmacists lack adequate skills to compound every prescription that they attempt to compound. Of course, a pharmacy customer has no way of knowing whether the compounded product his or her doctor prescribes requires more than an average amount of skill on the part of the pharmacist. For some compounded products, clearly it is safer to take those prescriptions to pharmacies that specialize in compounding. In general, chain drugstores do not specialize in compounding.

The filling of most prescriptions is a rather straightforward activity, not complex at all in most cases. The difficult part about pharmacy is not the filling of prescriptions, but the pressure on pharmacy staff to fill prescriptions at lightning speed. The compounding of prescriptions is an exception to this generalization that most prescriptions are easy to fill. Many pharmacists (including myself) hope that all prescriptions that must be compounded are brought in by customers during our partner's shift because compounding can take time that we don't have. *Better that my partner suffers the burden of compounding than me!* Among the pharmacists I've worked with, it has been an unwritten rule that a medication that must be compounded is the responsibility of the pharmacist who is on duty when that prescription is presented. We are not supposed to dump these prescriptions into the lap of the next pharmacist on duty.

Most chain pharmacists don't compound drugs very often so our skills in combining certain drugs may become rusty. Moreover, since we do so few pharmaceutical calculations, our calculating skills in preparing compounded prescriptions can become rusty. Sometimes I ask my partner to look at my calculations when compounding an unusual prescription. I'll ask my partner, "Do you agree with my calculations?"

A study carried out by two pharmacy school professors showed that compounding skills diminish rapidly after those courses are taught to pharmacy students. In a 2006 study by Eley and Birnie [John G. Eley and Christine Birnie, "Retention of Compounding Skills Among Pharmacy Students," *American Journal of Pharmaceutical Education* 2006; 70 (6) Article 132], students were given an identical compounding exercise in two successive years. The results indicated an alarming loss in compounding skills one year after those skills were taught.

It is, therefore, not hard to imagine that compounding skills can be a matter of serious concern after a few decades out of pharmacy school. The study by Ely and Birnie was designed to determine how well pharmacy students retain compounding skills after only twelve months, i.e., from the first year in pharmacy school until the second year. The study had second-year pharmacy students prepare a strength of the beta-blocker metoprolol that is not on the market. The authors tested the performance of second year pharmacy students in remembering the skills they learned as first year pharmacy students in preparing precisely the same strength of metoprolol. Students were told to prepare capsules containing 15 mg of metoprolol. From the article:

Significant differences in scores on a laboratory exercise conduced one year after completing the same exercise as part of a compounding course suggest that pharmacy students do not adequately retain compounding knowledge and skills.

If our hypothesis is extrapolated from compounding capsules to other compounding procedures, a significant number of pharmacy students do not retain the expected and required level of professional competency in pharmaceutical compounding one year after their formal training. …Inevitably a certain amount of knowledge is lost over time, but it was not apparent that such a dramatic decrease in knowledge would occur after only twelve months.

Compounding errors are an emerging and serious problem particularly in the larger chain community pharmacies where the workload is high and mistakes are more likely to occur.

The Food and Drug Administration (FDA) has shown concern that compounded prescriptions are likely to be of lower quality than manufactured medicinal products.

In my opinion, this lab exercise illustrates how out-of-touch many pharmacy professors often are. Metoprolol is readily available on the market in strengths of 25 mg, 50 mg, and 100 mg. How likely is it that a real-world patient would need a 15 mg dose? In the real world, most likely a 25 mg tablet would be split in half if the tablet is grooved for splitting ("scored"), resulting in two half-tablets each containing 12.5 mg. (Please note that not all tablets can or should be split. The manufacturer places a groove in the tablet if splitting is permissible. Some tablets should not be split because splitting will interfere with delayed-release character of those tablets.)

What is the likelihood that there would be a difference of clinical significance between a half-tablet containing 12.5 mg and a capsule compounded by a pharmacist containing 15 mg? Very unlikely. The fact that metoprolol is available in 25 mg, 50 mg and 100 mg tells a lot about the loose dosing of this drug when compared to many other drugs.

Take the blood thinner warfarin (Coumadin) for example. Warfarin is available in 1 mg, 2 mg, 2.5 mg, 3 mg, 4 mg, 5 mg, 6 mg, 7.5 mg and 10 mg. Thus, precise dosing is clearly more critical with warfarin compared to metoprolol. A few milligrams variation with warfarin could be disastrous, resulting in a hemorrhage or blood clot. (Indeed, warfarin is in first place as regards big legal settlements against pharmacists for serious pharmacy mistakes.) The point is that the difference between the 12.5 metoprolol tablet (obtained by splitting a scored 25 mg tablet) and a 15 mg capsule (compounded by a pharmacist) is unlikely to have any clinical significance to the patient.

This example illustrates the marginal benefits that are obtained with many products compounded by pharmacists, i.e., when compared to commercially available products from large pharmaceutical manufacturers.

Consider the case with generic drugs. The FDA specifies that a generic drug must have between 80 percent and 125 percent of the active ingredient compared to the brand name or innovator drug. This means, for example, that, for a 100 mg tablet, the active ingredient in the generic version can be anywhere between 80 mg and 125 mg. Thus, considering the significant leeway that the FDA allows with generic drugs, the difference between splitting a 25 mg metoprolol tablet that is readily available on the market (resulting in 12.5 mg), is highly unlikely to be significantly different from a pharmacist's attempt to compound a 15 mg capsule.

There are, indeed, a few drugs that are very tightly dosed. Most drugs are commercially available in only two or three strengths and that seems to be adequate in most cases. Another prominent example of a drug that is tightly dosed (besides warfarin) is the synthetic thyroid hormone levothyroxine. Levothyroxine is available in a chart-topping twelve strengths: 25 mcg, 50 mcg, 75 mcg, 88 mcg, 100 mcg, 112 mcg, 125 mcg, 137 mcg, 150 mcg, 175 mcg, 200 mcg, and 300 mcg (mcg stands for micrograms, i.e., one-thousandth of a milligram). Suffice it to say that I would be very hesitant to accept a compounded version of warfarin or levothroxine and, as far as I know, none exist.

My point is that dosing is far more critical with some drugs than others. It is unlikely that there is a significant difference between a compounded 15 mg capsule of metoprolol and 25 mg tablet split in half.

I hope this helps to illustrate my point that products compounded by pharmacists very often do not represent significant improvements over products already widely available from large pharmaceutical manufacturers. There are, of course, some exceptions. But when pharmacists compound drugs, there is the very real possibility that something will be done wrong. The greater the complexity in the compounding, the greater chance of error. The study by Eley and Birnie underscores the fact that competence in compounding is not something that the public should take for granted. I would certainly be more likely to trust a moderately-difficult product compounded by a pharmacy that specializes in compounding, as compared to the same product compounded at a large chain drugstore by a pharmacist who, perhaps, does very little compounding in a pharmacy that slings out prescriptions as fast as McDonald's slings out burgers.

From the perspective of a pharmacist worried about liability, one of the few nice things about the compounding of drugs is that it is much more difficult for customers to discover errors in compounded drugs (i.e., in comparison with finding errors in prescriptions consisting of tablets and capsules available from a large pharmaceutical manufacturer). That is because there is no reference book or Internet website that describes what a compounded product should look like. While there are many ways to ascertain the identity of most tablets and capsules on the market, compounded drugs, by their very nature, are much more difficult to verify. For example, there is no easy way for customers to determine that all the proper ingredients are included in products compounded by pharmacists, and there is no easy way to determine that those ingredients were combined in a proper manner. If a pharmacist adds a powder to a cream, there is no way of telling whether the pharmacist first dissolved that powder in an appropriate vehicle before adding it to the cream. If the final compounded product feels quite gritty rather than smooth, it is possible that the powder was added to the cream improperly.

Since pharmacists don't have our pharmacy school instructors looking over our shoulders, we often get a false sense of confidence that we actually know what we're doing when, in fact, sometimes we don't. If I mix two creams together, or I dissolve a powder in a cream, there's no way for the customer to determine whether I've done it correctly—short of taking it to a testing laboratory that is capable of analyzing the amount of each active ingredient in that cream. The customer would likely pay big bucks for such an analysis.

The compounding of drugs is often a hassle since it usually takes more time to prepare these prescriptions than it does for the other products in the pharmacy. This fact often causes pharmacists to wonder why doctors don't simply pick a product that's readily available on the market. Since many pharmacists view compounding as a relic of the past, some pharmacists don't treat compounded drugs with much respect. Some pharmacists view the practice of compounding as a bit silly. Many pharmacists and professors seem to view compounding as an anachronism and therefore worthy of little attention.

There are some instances in which pharmacist compounding is genuinely necessary and important, mainly in the preparation of pediatric dosages, but I can't recall a single instance in twenty-five years in chain drugstores wherein the medication I compounded seemed to be superior to products already in the marketplace, with the possible exception of a product called *Duke's Magic Mouthwash*. With thousands of products in the pharmacy, the pharmaceutical industry would not hesitate to market most products that have the potential to return a profit. The compounding of controversial "natural" female hormones ("bio-identical" hormone replacement therapy) and the compounding of quirky salves for a local dermatologist do not strike me as critical activities, especially in dangerously understaffed pharmacies where each second is precious.

Duke's Magic Mouthwash was commonly compounded in the North Carolina drugstores in which I worked. This liquid product for mouth ulcers is said to have originated at Duke University Medical Center in Durham. Pharmacists prepare this product by mixing a cortisone-type drug with the antifungal drug nystatin and the antihistamine diphenhydramine (Benadryl).

Here's anecdote that may help explain why I feel compounded products represent a unique situation and why, in my opinion, your pharmacist may lack proper compounding skills. When I was in pharmacy school, most professors posted our exam results on the wall adjacent to their office door. To protect students from being embarrassed, the results were posted by social security number rather than by name. As best as I can recall, the class average on a typical exam throughout my entire time in pharmacy school was usually somewhere around 87 percent. This means that lots of students scored 97 percent but it also means that lots of students scored 77%. We never had an exam in which every student scored 100 percent. I recall one of our professors stating that we would forget somewhere north of ninety-five percent of the information we learned in pharmacy school. This estimate undoubtedly includes the compounding of drugs. I am sure that all pharmacy students did not receive a score of one hundred percent on all the medications we compounded in pharmacy school. So it is reasonable to expect that medications compounded in the real world will be done so correctly less than one hundred percent of the time, and I predict that the success rate decreases sharply after pharmacy school. In my opinion, pharmacists simply don't use our compounding knowledge enough maintain it at a high level.

There are lots of differences between pharmacy school and the real world, but here is one that I find especially interesting. Pharmacy students receive regular feedback from our instructors (via exams) about how well we are doing in each of our classes. We receive a numerical grade on each exam. Once we leave pharmacy school, those examinations end. In the real world, when we fill a prescription for the wrong medication, we don't have a professor or his assistant looking over our shoulder. Unless we discover the error ourselves, the only feedback we receive is from customers who return to the pharmacy or call us to inform us that the pills look different from the past. The customers ask "Why do the pills in my bottle look different from the ones I've had in the past? Did I get the wrong medication?"

In twenty-five years as a pharmacist, I can't recall a single instance in which a customer claimed to have received an incorrectly compounded medication. That's simply because such customers usually have nothing to compare it with. For example:

• When pharmacists mix two white creams (most creams are white) together, there is no easy way for the customer to know whether the pharmacist mixed the proper creams.

• When a pharmacist adds two liquids together, there is no easy way for the customer to know whether both liquids were added in proper quantity. (For example, a doctor's prescription may specify that two ounces of Liquid Drug A be added to four ounces of Liquid Drug B.)

• When a pharmacist improperly adds a powder to a cream, there is no easy way for the customer to know unless, perhaps, the cream has a gritty feel when applied to the skin.

So the great difference between pharmacy school and the real world is that pharmacists receive much less feedback regarding errors in the real world. We make errors that our instructors would have caught but our customers usually don't. It is my belief that this leads to a false sense of security among pharmacists. We begin to feel that our accuracy in the real world is much greater than in pharmacy school, because we don't get reports from customers about our accuracy the way we got reports from our instructors in the form of exams. In my opinion, the competence of many pharmacists in compounding in the real world varies as much as it did in compounding exercises in pharmacy school, but pharmacists simply don't get as much feedback about our errors in the real world compared to in pharmacy school.

In my experience the most careless pharmacists make two or three (or more) times as many errors in the filling of all kinds of prescriptions in comparison to the most careful pharmacists. Some pharmacists very rarely make errors. Other pharmacists make more errors than you would believe.

Errors made by pharmacists can be much more difficult to discover than, for example, errors made by a mechanic, a plumber, an electrician, or an accountant. When a mechanic makes an error, our car may not perform as we expect. When a plumber makes an error, we may see a water leak. When an electrician makes an error, a light switch may not work properly or a circuit may trip. When our accountant makes a mistake on our taxes, we may or may not discover that error. When a pharmacist makes an error, it can easily go undiscovered for a long time unless, for example, the tablets or capsules the customer receives look different from what he or she expected. If an infection does not clear up, it may be because the pharmacist mistakenly dispensed a drug totally unrelated to the antibiotic prescribed. If you have a serious respiratory infection and mistakenly receive Prozac instead of an antibiotic, you may begin to ask questions when your lung infection does not seem to be improving.

Even though there was no activity in the drugstore I enjoyed less than compounding, some pharmacists absolutely love to compound drugs and seem to find the process very enjoyable and fulfilling. Some pharmacists have developed a lucrative business in the compounding of drugs, in part because the mark-up on compounded drugs is often better than on products that are ready-made by the big pharmaceutical manufacturers.

Some pharmacists are die-hard believers in compounding "bio-identical" hormones. These products are claimed to be safer than commercially available products like Premarin. That is because the hormones that pharmacists compound supposedly more closely match human female hormones. The hormones in Premarin are isolated from the urine of pregnant horses (mares). Hence the name Premarin comes from PREgnant MARes urINe.

The compounding of drugs by pharmacists has many critics. In my opinion, the FDA rightly observes that the quality of medications compounded by pharmacists is often lower than the quality of medications produced by large pharmaceutical manufacturers who have (hopefully) gained expertise in mass-producing the products they market. Political action by pharmacy associations seems to have been effective, so far, in stalling closer FDA supervision of pharmacist compounding. I predict that the FDA will, at some point, have to assume a greater role in monitoring the quality of products compounded by pharmacists.

Sidney Wolfe, M.D., and his Public Citizen Health Research Group are perhaps the most vocal opponents of pharmacist compounding. They agree with the FDA that there is usually less quality control in the corner drugstore when compared with the big pharmaceutical manufacturers. Wolfe's Health Research Group (HRG) points out that most of the products compounded by your neighborhood pharmacist aren't subjected to FDA standards and FDA inspections. HRG believes, for example, that the so-called bio-identical hormones compounded by pharmacists should be subject to the same FDA approval that Premarin and other "conventional" female hormones must undergo.

In response to many of the controversies surrounding products compounded by pharmacists, *Drug Topics* did a cover story on this issue (Carol Ukens, "Compounding Under Siege," *Drug Topics*, Jan. 6, 2003, pp. 44-49). From the article:

Bad news

In recent years, compounding has been involved in several incidents that captured media attention and triggered calls for more regulation, including the following:
• In North Carolina, one patient died and three became ill from fungal meningitis traced to methylprednisolone compounded by Urgent Care Pharmacy of Spartanburg, S.C. In September 2002, the pharmacy recalled the contaminated product. State and federal inspections found several instances of nonadherence to sterile technique. However, when Urgent Care refused to recall all its compounded products, the Food & Drug Administration issued a national alert advising against use of any products compounded by the pharmacy.
• On Sept. 20, 2002, the FDA put Med-Mart Pulmonary Services of Novato, Calif., on notice that it was operating as a drug manufacturer, not a retail pharmacy. Citing concerns about "large-scale production of massive quantities of inhalation solutions," the FDA threatened actions such as seizure and/or injunction if the firm did not provide a plan to correct numerous operational deficiencies.
• In July 2002, two pharmacists and six healthcare professionals were convicted in Miami of defrauding Medicare of millions of dollars with bogus billing for compounded aerosol medications through South Beach Pharmacy, LaModerna Pharmacy, and/or CDC of South Florida Inc. The compounded drugs contained little or no active ingredients.
• On Sept. 18, 2002, the U.S. Department of Justice sent a letter to Pharmaceutical Compounding Centers of America (PCCA) informing

the Houston firm that the huge volume of chemicals it had supplied to Miami pharmacies should have been a "red flag" that there was Medicare fraud going on. The firm was also informed that its actions "have assisted in the systematic defrauding of the Medicare Trust Fund." PCCA was also the target of an FDA warning letter in July 2001 taking the firm to task for violations of good manufacturing practices, including failure to ensure against cross contamination between cephalosporins and penicillin repackaged on common equipment. The FDA also alleged that PCCA had been repacking and distributing bulk drugs that had been removed from the market, such as phenacetin, dipyrone, and adenosine phosphate.

• On April 10, 2002, the FDA warned three pharmacies that the nicotine lollipops and lip balm they were selling were illegal because they were compounded without an Rx and were made from nicotine salicylate, which is not approved for compounding.

• In June 2002, Portage Pharmacy, Portage, Mich., issued a class I recall of 791 vials of compounded drugs, including methylprednisolone, due to contamination and a class II recall of 175 vials of other compounded medications due to lack of assurance of sterility.

• Two patients in Michigan who had received compounded medication for spinal injection became ill with Chryseomonas meningitis in 2002, according to CDC.

• In March 2001, four Atlanta patients had severe adverse reactions to a compounded thyroid drug prescribed for Wilson's syndrome, a quack diagnosis created by a Florida doctor who lost his license. One R.Ph. was put on probation for five years and the owner-R.Ph. surrendered his license. He had been sanctioned in 1986 for felony convictions for mail fraud and misbranding and adulteration of drugs.

• Thirteen people were hospitalized and three others died from meningitis traced to contaminated betamethasone compounded by Doc's Pharmacy in Walnut Creek, Calif., in May 2001. The pharmacist-owner's license was revoked for one year, but a young pharmacist who co-owned the pharmacy later committed suicide following a 90-day license suspension.

Compounding flunks FDA test

Among 29 samples taken from 12 compounding pharmacies that advertise their wares over the Internet, 10 failed to meet standard quality tests, according to small study by the Food & Drug Administration.

• The 34% failure rate for the compounded samples was "significant," compared with the 2% failure rate among drug manufacturers, according to researchers in the FDA's Center for Drug Evaluation & Research. Nine of the 10 failures were for subpotency; the other was for contamination.

• More than half the samples had less than 70% of the potency stated on the labeling. Three additional samples failed an initial test but there was insufficient product for retesting, so they were not counted among the failures.
(www.fda.gov/cder/pharmcomp/communityPharmacy/default.htm)

EIGHT SERIOUS INCIDENTS INVOLVING PHARMACY COMPOUNDING

1. Compounding pharmacist prepares T3 capsules of varying dosages for Wilson's Syndrome patient, causing thyrotoxicosis—$650,000 settlement in North Carolina

The plaintiff, age forty-five, had a history of cardiac palpitations and shortness of breath. She presented to a physician seeking medical treatment for weight loss. The physician diagnosed her with Wilson's Syndrome, a disorder of peripheral conversion of thyroxin to T3 and ordered thyroid studies.

Though he initially ruled out Wilson's Syndrome, the physician reconsidered based on the plaintiff running an average temperature below 98.6. The physician prescribed T3, to be prepared by the defendant compounding pharmacist. The plaintiff began taking the T3, and four days later began suffering thyrotoxicosis, with symptoms of tachycardia, lightheadedness, insomnia, and itching.

Analysis of the T3 capsules prepared by the defendant pharmacist revealed wildly varying dosages between capsules, with some containing thousands of times the prescribed dosage. The plaintiff continued to experience tachycardia and shortness of breath after being discharged, and was later diagnosed with post traumatic stress disorder.

According to published accounts, the case settled for $650,000. ("Forty-Five Year-Old Female Patient Roe v. Roe Pharmacist, M.D. unknown." Healthcare Providers Service Organization, September 2005 Legal Case Study, Accessed March 9, 2006
http://www.hpso.com/case/cases_prof_index.php3?id=102&prof=Pharmacist)

---

2. Colchicine compounded by Texas pharmacy leads to three deaths

The Oct. 12, 2007 issue of *Morbidity & Mortality Weekly Report* (*MMWR*) describes three deaths attributed to a Texas compounding pharmacy error resulting from an eightfold overdose in patients seeking off-label treatment with IV colchicine for back pain. Toxicology reports showed the colchicine vials contained 4 mg/ml instead of the 0.5 mg/ml indicated on the label; therefore, the intended 2-mg dose was actually 16 mg. Bonnel et. al. (*J Emerg Med*, 2002) showed that deaths have been reported with cumulative doses of colchicine as low as 5.5 mg. According to *MMWR*, the deaths underscore the potentially fatal ramifications of errors by compounding pharmacies, which generally are not subject to the same oversight and manufacturing practices as pharmaceutical manufacturers. In response to the incident, the Texas State Board of Pharmacy, in cooperation with the FDA, issued a recall of all colchicine that had been sold or produced by the compounding pharmacy within the past year.
["*MMWR* reports on colchicine deaths due to compounding error: Three deaths determined to be result of colchicine toxicity," October 15, 2007, *Drug Topics* (Daily News)
www.drugtopics.com/drugtopics/article/articleDetail.jsp?id=465163]

---

3. California pharmacist commits suicide after three deaths and thirteen hospitalizations blamed on compounded betamethasone

A California pharmacist committed suicide in 2002 after a compounding error was blamed for three deaths. The pharmacist was not present when the error occurred in 2001, but he was a co-owner of the pharmacy where the compounding took place. (Carol Ukens, "Compounding case leads to R.Ph. suicide," *Drug Topics*, May 6, 2002, pp. 44, 49)

Jamey Phillip Sheets, 32, apparently could not accept the punishment meted out by the California pharmacy board for a fatal outbreak of meningitis from a drug compounded in the pharmacy he co-owned. A looming license suspension, five years on probation, and a hefty fine were more than the despondent pharmacist could bear. Late last month, he attached 500 mg of fentanyl patches to his neck and chest and lay down to die. ...

The downward spiral that ended in Sheets' suicide began May 2001 when a meningitis outbreak was traced to betamethasone compounded in a pharmacy he co-owned. The contaminated drug mixed in Doc's Pharmacy in Walnut Creek was blamed for three deaths and 13 hospitalizations.

The meningitis outbreak triggered a heavy media barrage and public outrage aimed at the pharmacy and the practice of compounding. And that put the pharmacy board under heavy pressure to discipline those responsible for the contamination. ...

The Sheets suicide is not an isolated incident. For example, about a year ago, an Oregon pharmacist took her life after an error killed a patient. And about five years ago, a Kentucky pharmacist involved in a fatal error was on his way to the pharmacy board to surrender his license. Instead, he stopped his car and stepped in front of a semitrailer barreling down the Interstate. These cases underscore the results of a federal study that found that pharmacists have the second-highest suicide rate in the country (*Drug Topics*, Nov. 6, 1995).

4. Injectable methylprednisolone compounded by pharmacists in southeastern state allegedly results in patients contracting fungal meningitis and some deaths

The injectable dosage form of methylprednisolone was discontinued by a manufacturer, and several medical practices contacted the pharmacy to inquire whether it could compound the product for their use. The pharmacists in a southeastern state responded to this request, preparing more than 1000 vials. Patients who received the injections contracted fungal meningitis, and some died—allegedly as a result of using the medication. The state board of pharmacy conducted an investigation and concluded that a fungus mold linked to spinal meningitis was in the product. (James L. Fink III, B.S.Pharm., J.D., "Pharmacy Law: Liability Coverage for Contaminated Compounds," *Pharmacy Times*, published online Nov. 1, 2008)

5. Five-year-old with attention-deficit hyperactivity disorder given 1000-fold overdose of clonidine as result of compounding error in which *milligrams* substituted for *micrograms*

A 5-year-old child who weighed 17.5 kg received 50 mg of clonidine. The amount ingested was confirmed by analysis of the suspension administered (clonidine HCl 9.78 mg/mL). To our knowledge, this represents the largest ingestion in a child and the largest ingestion on a milligram per kilogram basis in the medical literature. The child's initial presentation included hyperventilation, an unusual feature of clonidine toxicity. The child was discharged without sequela 42 hours after admission. A serum concentration of clonidine 17 hours postingestion was 64 ng/mL, the highest reported to date in a pediatric patient. The intoxication was traced to a pharmacy compounding error in which milligrams were substituted for micrograms. Increased prescribing of clonidine in young children coupled with the requirement to compound clonidine in a suspension and the narrow therapeutic index suggests that the frequency of severe ingestions in children will increase in the future. (M.J. Romano and A. Dinh, "A 1000-fold overdose of clonidine caused by a compounding error in a

5-year-old child with attention-deficit/hyperactivity disorder," *Pediatrics,* 2001 Aug; 108(2): 471-2. PMID: 11483818)

---

6. Florida pharmacy incorrectly compounded supplement given to 21 polo horses that died prior to championship match

---

WEST PALM BEACH, Fla.—An official at a Florida pharmacy said Thursday the business incorrectly prepared a supplement given to 21 polo horses that died over the weekend while preparing to play in a championship match.

Jennifer Beckett of Franck's Pharmacy in Ocala, Fla., told *The Associated Press* in a statement that the business conducted an internal investigation that found "the strength of an ingredient in the medication was incorrect." The statement did not say what the ingredient was.

Beckett, who's the pharmacy's chief operating officer, said the pharmacy is cooperating with an investigation by state authorities and the Food and Drug Administration.

The horses from the Venezuelan-owned Lechuza polo team began crumpling to the ground shortly before Sunday's U.S. Open match was supposed to begin, shocking a crowd of well-heeled spectators at the International Polo Club Palm Beach in Wellington.

"On an order from a veterinarian, Franck's Pharmacy prepared medication that was used to treat the 21 horses on the Lechuza Polo team," Beckett said. "As soon as we learned of the tragic incident, we conducted an internal investigation."

She said the report has been given to state authorities.

Lechuza also issued a statement to AP acknowledging that a Florida veterinarian wrote the prescription for the pharmacy to create a compound similar to Biodyl, a French-made supplement that includes vitamins and minerals and is not approved for use in the United States.

"Only horses treated with the compound became sick and died within 3 hours of treatment," Lechuza said in the statement. "Other horses that were not treated remain healthy and normal."

Lechuza also said it was cooperating with authorities that include the State Department of Agriculture and Consumer Services and the Palm Beach County Sheriff's Office.

Biodyl contains a combination of vitamin B12, a form of selenium called sodium selenite and other minerals. It is made in France by Duluth, Ga.-based animal pharmaceutical firm Merial Ltd. and can be given to horses to help with exhaustion. It is widely used abroad, but not approved in the U.S.

Compound pharmacies can, among other things, add flavor, make substances into a powder or liquid or remove a certain compound that may have an adverse reaction in different animal species. Only in limited circumstances can they legally recreate a drug that is not approved in the U.S., according to the FDA.

Necropsies of the 21 horses found internal bleeding, some in the lungs, but offered no definitive clues to the cause of death.

FDA spokeswoman Siobhan DeLancey said compounding pharmacies cannot legally recreate existing drugs or supplements under patent. In most cases, they are also not allowed to recreate a medication that is not approved for use in the U.S.

On its Web site, the FDA says it generally defers to "state authorities regarding the day-to-day regulation of compounding by veterinarians and pharmacists."

However, the agency says it would "seriously consider enforcement action" if a pharmacy breaks federal law in compounding medications. It isn't yet clear Franck's broke the law. (Brian Skoloff, "Pharmacy Takes Blame in Horses Deaths," *Associated Press*, Apr. 22, 2009 http://news.aol.com/article/horses-die-before-polo-match/435339)

---

7. Tainted ophthalmic solutions from Florida compounding lab left at least 33 people with fungal eye infections

While Franck's Compounding Lab insisted that the source of the tainted ophthalmic solutions that left at least 33 people with fungal eye infections has been fixed, the fallout may be just beginning.

Franck's business manager Stephen Floyd said that the company has "taken appropriate corrective action and now have this issue behind us."

But some say the compounding lab is likely to face serious sanctions from state and federal officials just three years after another mistake by the lab killed 21 prized polo horses.

"You can understand a mistake happening once, but this particular pharmacy has had a series of missteps along the way," said Paul Doering, professor emeritus at the University of Florida School of Pharmacy. "I hate to sound holier than thou, but there is no room for error in the pharmacy business, and this is two huge mistakes for them. I was kind of dumbfounded that this was happening again."

Doering said the state Board of Pharmacy is likely to take "definitive action" against Paul Franck, the owner of the compounding lab, and may even seek to suspend or revoke Franck's pharmacy license.

The tainted products included a dye and a steroid used in eye surgeries. At least 23 of the 33 people who were treated with the products in seven states suffered eye infections that caused vision loss. Twenty four required further surgery.

In the 2009 case, Franck's was cited by the state Department of Health for numerous violations of Florida law covering pharmacies. The state alleged that the lack of experience of Franck's staff contributed to the error in mixing the supplement. A staffer erroneously mixed a high, fatal dosage of selenium into the supplement. [Carlos E. Medina, "Trouble ahead for Franck's?—Second drug controversy in three years could spell problems for Ocala compounding lab," Gainesville.com (The Gainesville Sun), May 4, 2012 http://www.gainesville.com/article/20120504/ARTICLES/120509758?tc=ar]

---

8. Death of 5-year-old Virginia boy after pharmacy technician compounded imipramine solution for bedwetting at five times the dose prescribed by physician

---

A five-year old Virginia boy died as a result of an order entry and medication compounding error that was not caught by the usual verification process. In this case, imipramine was dispensed in a concentration five times greater than prescribed. Imipramine is a tricyclic antidepressant used to treat adults, but it is also used to threat childhood enuresis (bedwetting). An extemporaneous solution was to be prepared at this pharmacy that specialized in compounded prescriptions since a liquid formulation was not commercially available. A pharmacy technician incorrectly entered the concentration of the prescribed solution into the computer as 50 mg/**ml** instead of 50 mg/**5ml**, along with the prescribed directions to give two teaspoonsful at bedtime. He then proceeded to prepare the solution using the incorrect concentration on the label rather than the concentration indicated on the prescription. When the compound was completed, the technician placed it in a holding area to await a pharmacist's verification. At this time, one of the two pharmacists on duty was at lunch and the high workload of the pharmacy made it difficult for the pharmacist to check the prescription right away. When the child's mother returned to pick up the prescription, the cash register clerk retrieved the prescription from the holding area without telling a pharmacist, and gave it to the mother, unaware that it had not yet been checked. At bedtime, the mother administered two teaspoonsful of the drug (500 mg instead of the intended 100 mg) to the child. When she went to wake him the next morning, the child was dead. An autopsy confirmed imipramine poisoning. (Institute for Safe Medication Practices, "Safety Can Not Be Sacrificed For Speed," *North Carolina Board of Pharmacy Newsletter* National Pharmacy Compliance News, April 2006, p. 2.)

On May 31, 2007, the FDA posted the following consumer update, titled "The Special Risks of Pharmacy Compounding" (http://www.fda.gov/ForConsumers/ConsumerUpdates/ucm107836.htm):

Pharmacy compounding is an age-old practice in which pharmacists combine, mix, or alter ingredients to create unique medications that meet specific needs of individual patients.

It's also a practice that is under FDA scrutiny—mainly because of instances where compounded drugs have endangered public health.

"In its traditional form, pharmacy compounding is a vital service that helps many people, including those who are allergic to inactive ingredients in FDA-approved medicines, and others who need medications that are not available commercially," says Kathleen Anderson, Pharm.D, Deputy Director of the Division of New Drugs and Labeling Compliance in FDA's Center for Drug Evaluation and Research (CDER).

Compounded medications are also prescribed for children who may be unable to swallow pills, need diluted dosages of a drug made for adults, or are simply unwilling to take bad-tasting medicine.

"But consumers need to be aware that compounded drugs are not FDA-approved," Anderson says. "This means that FDA has not verified their safety and effectiveness."

Steve Silverman, Assistant Director of CDER's Office of Compliance, says that poor practices on the part of drug compounders can result in contamination or in products that don't possess the strength, quality, and purity required. "And because patients who use these drugs may have serious underlying health conditions," he says, "these flawed methods pose special risks."

Unlike commercial drug manufacturers, pharmacies aren't required to report adverse events associated with compounded drugs. "FDA learns of these through voluntary reporting, the media, and other sources," says Silverman.

The Agency knows of more than 200 adverse events involving 71 compounded products since 1990. Some of these instances had devastating repercussions.

Three patients died of infections stemming from contaminated compounded solutions that are used to paralyze the heart during open-heart surgery. FDA issued a warning letter in March 2006 to the firm that compounded the solutions.

Two patients at a Washington, D.C., Veterans Affairs hospital were blinded, and several others had their eyesight damaged, by a compounded product used in cataract surgery. The product was contaminated with bacteria. In August 2005, FDA announced a nationwide recall of this Trypan Blue Ophthalmic Solution. Contaminated solution had been distributed to hospitals and clinics in eight states.

In March 2005, FDA issued a nationwide alert concerning a contaminated, compounded magnesium sulfate solution that caused five cases of bacterial infections in a New Jersey hospital. A South Dakota patient treated with the product developed sepsis and died.

A Troubling Trend

The emergence over the past decade of firms with pharmacy licenses making and distributing unapproved new drugs in a way that's clearly outside the bounds of traditional pharmacy is of great concern to FDA.

"The methods of these companies seem far more consistent with those of drug manufacturers than with those of retail pharmacies," says Silverman. "Some firms make large amounts of compounded drugs that are copies or near copies of FDA-approved, commercially available drugs. Other firms sell to physicians and patients with whom they have only a remote professional relationship."

FDA highlighted these concerns in August 2006, when it warned three firms to stop manufacturing and distributing thousands of doses of compounded, unapproved inhalation drugs nationwide.

Inhalation drugs are used to treat diseases including asthma, emphysema, bronchitis, and cystic fibrosis. "These are potentially life-threatening conditions for which numerous FDA-approved drugs are available," says Silverman. "Compounded inhalation drugs may be distributed to patients in multiple states, and patients and their doctors may not understand that they are receiving compounded products."

Enforcement

"FDA historically hasn't directed enforcement against pharmacies engaged in traditional compounding," says Anderson. "Rather, we've focused on establishments whose activities raise the kinds of concerns normally associated with a drug manufacturer and whose compounding practices result in significant violations of the new-drug, adulteration, or misbranding provisions of the Federal Food, Drug, and Cosmetic Act."

FDA counts compounded drugs among the new drugs that are covered under the Act. "We consider them new because they're not generally recognized among experts as safe and effective," says Anderson.

She adds that FDA recognizes that states have a central role in regulating pharmacy compounding. "We refer complaints to the states, support them when they request it, and cooperate in investigations and follow-up actions. But there are cases when states are unable to act, and we proceed without them," Anderson says.

Red Flags

In a May 29, 2002, Compliance Policy Guide devoted to human pharmacy compounding, FDA identifies factors that it considers in deciding upon enforcement action. These factors include instances where pharmacists are:
• compounding drug products that have been pulled from the market because they were found to be unsafe or ineffective.
• compounding drugs that are essentially copies of a commercially available drug product.
• compounding drugs in advance of receiving prescriptions, except in very limited quantities relating to the amounts of drugs previously compounded based on valid prescriptions.
• compounding finished drugs from bulk active ingredients that aren't components of FDA-approved drugs, without an FDA-sanctioned, investigational new-drug application.
• receiving, storing, or using drug substances without first obtaining written assurance from the supplier that each lot of the drug substance has been made in an FDA-registered facility.
• failing to conform to applicable state law regulating the practice of pharmacy.

What You Can Do

What can consumers do to protect themselves against inappropriate drug-compounding practices? Ilisa Bernstein, Pharm.D, J.D., Director of Pharmacy Affairs in FDA's Office of the Commissioner, offers these tips:
• Ask your doctor if an FDA-approved drug is available and appropriate for your treatment.
• Check with the pharmacist to see if he or she is familiar with compounding the product in your prescription.
• Get information from your doctor or pharmacist about proper use and storage of the compounded product.

• If you receive a compounded product, ask the pharmacist if the doctor asked for it to be compounded.

• If you experience any problems or adverse events, contact your doctor or pharmacist immediately and stop using the product.

• Report any adverse events experienced while using the product to FDA's MedWatch program.

Chapter 25

Best and worst drugs in the pharmacy

Two rarely-discussed but critical issues are: 1) Not all drugs in the pharmacy are equally safe or effective, and 2) So many drugs in the pharmacy are used to treat conditions that are more logically prevented. Obviously, doctors and Big Pharma would never admit this. Somehow, a large segment of the public seems to think that every drug in the pharmacy is equally safe, effective, and logical. Doctors seldom tell their patients, "Well, the drugs used to treat this condition (Alzheimer's, osteoporosis, psychosis, obesity, many cancers, etc.) aren't really very effective."

This chapter explains my view toward many of the different drugs and classes of drugs in the pharmacy. I've included some of the thoughts that ran through my mind as I dispensed various drugs.

1. Drugs that treat anxiety or depression: I always hated dispensing antidepressants to people who had some obvious physical or mental impairment. Our society is brutally competitive in which winners and losers are inevitable and, in fact, the basis of capitalism. Too often the losers end up taking antidepressants.

I don't want to be involved in any way in dispensing psychoactive drugs (like Ritalin or antidepressants) to children. In my opinion, these children are often the victims of deeply dysfunctional families in a deeply dysfunctional society, or the kids are having trouble in school, or the kids are unattractive, or the kids are doing poorly in athletic competitions, or the kids are not popular. If the number of books on Amazon.com on any given health issue is any indication of the controversy or interest surrounding that issue, then certainly the issue of prescribing drugs like Ritalin to kids is at or near the top. There are perhaps as many as fifty books on Amazon.com in which the authors are strongly opposed to using drugs like Ritalin in kids. (In addition to the subject of treating ADHD without drugs, other controversies that have spawned a huge number of books on Amazon.com are: treating post-menopausal symptoms without drugs, treating depression without drugs, and treating hypertension without drugs.)

For adults, I don't want to dispense pills for anxiety (like Xanax or Ativan), or pills for depression (like Prozac or Paxil), because I feel that people taking these pills need to address the causes of their anxiety or depression rather than seek quick-fix drug solutions. I don't want to be a party to Big Pharma's devious, dubious, and ubiquitous marketing schemes wherein depression is no more than an imbalance of serotonin in the brain.

Whenever I dispense drugs for depression or whenever a customer asks me to recommend something for "nerves," I always think: What's really causing her depression or anxiety? Is she in an abusive relationship? Was she abused or disrespected as a child? Did she have controlling parents? Does her husband beat her? Is she depressed because she's unattractive and consequently she's given a cold reception by our society? Is she depressed because she's married to a jerk? Is she depressed because her job is very unfulfilling? I've never believed Big Pharma's self-serving, mechanistic theory of depression. Big Pharma has a huge financial incentive in promoting depression as a chemical imbalance in the brain. Big Pharma has absolutely no financial incentive to admit that life circumstances are immensely important in causing depression.

Here's an analysis of depression from Andrew Weil, M.D., that absolutely terrifies establishment medicine because it leaves doctors and drugs companies out of the loop. This analysis makes the current focus on brain biochemistry look self-evidently absurd and opportunistic (Andrew Weil, M.D., "Don't Let Chaos Get You Down," *Newsweek*, Nov. 7 & 14, 2011, p. 9):

...there is abundant evidence that depression is a "disease of affluence," a disorder of modern life in the industrialized world. People who live in poorer countries have a lower risk of depression than those in industrialized nations. In general, countries with lifestyles that are furthest removed from modern standards have the lowest rates of depression.

Within the U.S., the rate of depression of members of the Old Order Amish—a religious sect that shuns modernity in favor of lifestyles roughly emulating those of rural Americans a century ago—is as low as one tenth that of other Americans.

Psychologist Martin Seligman, originator of the field of positive psychology and director of the Positive Psychology Center at the University of Pennsylvania, has studied the Old Order Amish, along with other premodern cultures. He concludes: "Putting this together, there seems to be something about modern life that creates fertile soil for depression."

Another prominent researcher whose work I respect, Stephen Ilardi, professor of psychology at the University of Kansas and author of *The Depression Cure*, observes, "The more 'modern' a society's way of life, the higher its rate of depression. It may seem baffling, but the explanation is simple: the human body was never designed for the modern postindustrial environment."

2. Drugs that treat ADHD: One day a man called me to discuss the Ritalin and Dexedrine that his son was taking for hyperactivity. He kept telling me that his son's behavior only became bad when his son started school. It was at school that other kids made fun of his horrendous and heart-breaking birth defect: The child's fingers were attached near his elbow. The man kept telling me that it was the experience of being ridiculed by other kids at school and the bouncing back and forth between divorced parents that surely were the causes of his son's uncontrollable behavior. This man kept repeating this analysis of the situation to me, I assume, in an effort to gain some support from me that his son's behavior might not need a drug solution. But, of course, I can't criticize a treatment that a local doctor has prescribed. This particular doctor truly herds patients through his office. The fact that we get a ton of prescriptions from this doctor guarantees that I'm not going to risk incurring his wrath. As much as I might like, I can't agree with this man that his son may have behavioral problems caused by the birth defect and divorce. I can't question the doctor's diagnosis of a brain malfunction (hyperactivity) and the subsequent prescribing of Ritalin and Dexedrine.

3. Drugs that treat what Pharma calls "disorders": I always hated dispensing drugs for conditions for which Big Pharma appends the term "disorder": seasonal affective disorder (the "winter blues"), obsessive compulsive disorder (e.g., excessive handwashing), attention deficit hyperactivity disorder, premenstrual dysphoric disorder, generalized anxiety disorder, social anxiety disorder (shyness), bipolar disorder, compulsive gambling disorder, compulsive shopping disorder. Here are two disorders you may not have heard of: 1) temper dysregulation disorder, which the American Psychiatric Association is recommending as a new diagnosis, and 2) oppositional defiant disorder (ODD). It's as if Big Pharma is so insecure about the legitimacy of all these diagnoses that they feel compelled to append the term "disorder" to gain public acceptance. Yet we don't hear cancer *disorder*, diabetes *disorder*, pneumonia *disorder*, AIDS *disorder*, etc., because the public is convinced these are legitimate diagnoses.

4. Drugs that treat shyness: I don't feel that shyness should be medicated. I don't want any part of Big Pharma's medicalization of shyness into "social anxiety disorder." There are lots of understandable causes of shyness (excessive criticism from parents, a physical handicap, being involved in an abusive relationship, unattractiveness, etc.) that should not, in my opinion, be medicated with drugs. I don't like dispensing pills to people who are shy as a consequence of their depressing life circumstances. I don't like medicating introverts because they're quiet. I'd like to medicate extroverts who won't shut up!

5. Drugs that treat psychosis: I always hated dispensing anti-psychotic drugs because I am a big fan of Thomas Szasz and others who write about "the manufacture of madness."

6. Drugs that treat obesity: I hated dispensing weight-loss drugs because it is my feeling that at least ninety-five percent of the people taking these drugs simply need to learn to walk away from the kitchen table. To increase the legitimacy of the widespread use and acceptance of these drugs, Big Pharma exaggerates a genetic component in obesity and also exaggerates concepts like a metabolic disorder causing obesity.

According to an article in *Newsweek,* Cleveland Clinic president and CEO Dr. Delos M. Cosgrove, a former cardiac surgeon, "has not backed down from his belief that obesity is a failure of willpower, which can be attacked by the same weapons used to combat smoking: public education, economic incentives, and sheer exhortation." (Jerry Adler and Jeneen Interlandi, "The Hospital That Could Cure Health Care," *Newsweek,* Dec. 7, 2009, p. 53) Nevertheless, Big Pharma wants you to believe that most cases of obesity are due to biochemical and molecular defects or to genetic factors.

One of the most frequently asked recommendations of pharmacists is for products that will help the customer lose weight. These people definitely do not want to engage in a discussion of the necessity of simply eating less food. Over my 25-year career as a pharmacist, I suspect that I've had a thousand overweight females ask me for a product to help them lose weight. Oftentimes, I've thought she's getting criticism at home from her husband for being overweight. So she comes to the drugstore for a quick-fix. Do pharmacists find it fulfilling when we are supportive of medications prescribed for obesity, rather than state the obvious: Obese people need to learn to eat less.

7. Drugs that treat post-menopausal symptoms: I always hated dispensing drugs like Premarin. Even back in the 1970s when I was in pharmacy school, the potential for post-menopausal estrogens to cause uterine cancer was well known. So I have been afraid of this class of drugs for over thirty-five years. Each year seems to bring more bad news about the adverse effects of these drugs, including breast cancer and cardiovascular complications.

8. Drugs that treat cancer: I don't want any part in legitimizing a focus on treating cancer rather than preventing it. Age-adjusted cancer rates vary widely around the world. (*Cancer Rates and Risks,* National Institutes of Health Publication No. 96-691, May 1996) Our focus should be primarily on exploring and publicizing the reasons for this, rather than on seeking new cancer drugs and on improving existing chemotherapy. *The Merck Manual* (17th edition, pp. 2591-2) essentially states that up to 90% of cancer is preventable: "Environmental or nutritional factors probably account for up to 90% of human cancers. These factors include smoking; diet; and exposure to sunlight, chemicals, and drugs. Genetic, viral, and radiation factors may cause the rest."

9. Drugs that treat cough and cold: I don't enjoy recommending products for coughs and colds because I don't feel that these products do much good. In my opinion, the best treatment for coughs and colds is "tincture of time." In other words, get plenty of rest and let the condition run its course—unless the cough and cold are serious and you are in some otherwise weakened state that could lead to complications.

10. Drugs that treat intestinal gas: I don't like recommending products for intestinal gas. Most people seem to view intestinal gas as a medical condition rather than simply a consequence of eating certain foods that produce gas (e.g., bananas).

11. Products that treat constipation: I don't enjoy selling laxatives because I feel that, after millions of years of evolution, the bowel surely knows how to function on its own with adequate fiber in the diet. Eating adequate fiber is a much better approach than the use of laxatives. I am embarrassed to be in a profession that does not roundly criticize the widespread use of laxatives.

12. Products that decrease stomach acid: Modern medicine assumes that the design of *Homo sapiens* is fundamentally flawed, requiring constant shoring up by doctors. Take, for example, the wholesale attack on stomach acid. Big Pharma wants you to believe that stomach acid needs frequent curtailing with antacids, H2 antagonists, and proton-pump inhibitors (PPI's). Like all physiology in the animal kingdom, human digestion has been fine-tuned over millions of years of evolution. Yet leave it to Big Pharma to focus on the molecular and cellular basis of digestion rather than on our modern diet of heavily processed foods, all-you-can-eat buffets, supersized portions, etc. Heartburn is a huge market for drugs, yet this condition is mostly preventable with a change in diet and the will-power to avoid overeating.

Whenever a customer asks me for a recommendation for heartburn (like Maalox, Mylanta, Tagamet HB, Zantac 75, Axid AR, Pepcid AC, Prilosec OTC, etc.), I rarely have the time to discuss possible causes of heartburn, nor do I suspect that most customers care to discuss causes. They simply want a quick fix. Most heartburn is preventable. Heartburn can be caused or exacerbated by coffee, alcohol, fats, chocolate, smoking, and drugs like aspirin, ibuprofen, and iron. It can be caused by lying down too soon after eating or drinking, or simply by eating too much. I occasionally get heartburn after pigging out at all-you-can-eat buffets. I know two obese people who tell me they have great difficulty sleeping unless they take their heartburn medication each night before bedtime. Raising the head of the bed about six inches can help prevent heartburn that occurs while sleeping. Pants that are too tight can also contribute to heartburn. Stress can aggravate heartburn.

In recent years, the Food and Drug Administration has issued numerous warnings about proton pump inhibitors (drugs like Prilosec, Nexium, Prevacid, Aciphex, and Dexilant), saying long-term use and high doses have been associated with an increased risk of bone fractures and infection with a bacterium called *Clostridium difficile*. Studies have shown long-term PPI use may reduce the absorption of important nutrients, vitamins and minerals, including magnesium, calcium and vitamin B12, and might reduce the effectiveness of other medications. Other research has found that people taking PPI's are at increased risk of developing pneumonia. But while using the drugs for short periods may not be problematic, they tend to produce dependency, experts say, leading patients to take them for far longer than the recommended 8 to 12 weeks; some stay on them for life. *The New York Times* quotes several physicians on the potential risks of PPI's (Roni Caryn Rabin, "Combating Acid Reflux May Bring Host of Ills," *The New York Times*, June 25, 2012 http://well.blogs.nytimes.com/2012/06/25/combating-acid-reflux-may-bring-host-of-ills/?partner=rss&emc=rss):

"Studies have shown that once you're on them, it's hard to stop taking them," said Dr. Shoshana J. Herzig of Beth Israel Deaconess Medical Center in Boston. "It's almost like an addiction." ...

"When people take P.P.I.'s, they haven't cured the problem of reflux," said Dr. Joseph Stubbs, an internist in Albany, Ga., and a former president of the American College of Physicians. "They've just controlled the symptoms."

And P.P.I.'s provide a way for people to avoid making difficult lifestyle changes, like losing weight or cutting out the foods that cause heartburn, he said. "People have found, 'I can keep eating what I want to eat, and take this and I'm doing fine,' " he said. "We're starting to see that if you do that, you can run into some risky side effects."

Many patients may be on the drugs for no good medical reason, at huge cost to the health care system, said Dr. Joel J. Heidelbaugh, a family medicine doctor in Ann Arbor, Mich. When he reviewed medical records of almost 1,000 patients on P.P.I.'s at an outpatient Veterans Affairs clinic in Ann Arbor, he found that only one-third had a diagnosis that justified the drugs. The others seemed to have been given the medications "just in case."

"We put people on P.P.I.'s, and we ignore the fact that we were designed to have acid in our stomach," said Dr. Greg Plotnikoff, a physician who specializes in integrative therapy at the Penny George Institute for Health and Healing in Minneapolis.

Stomach acid is needed to break down food and absorb nutrients, he said, as well as for proper functioning of the gallbladder and pancreas. Long-term of use of P.P.I.'s may interfere with these processes, he noted. And suppression of stomach acid, which kills bacteria and other microbes, may make people more susceptible to infections, like *C. difficile.* ...

Most physicians think that GERD is a side effect of the obesity epidemic, and that lifestyle changes could ameliorate heartburn for many.

"If we took 100 people with reflux and got them to rigidly follow the lifestyle recommendations, 90 wouldn't need any medication," Dr. Castell said. "But good luck getting them to do that."

13. Drugs that treat insomnia: Customers frequently ask pharmacists for products to help them sleep. A surprising number of our customers do not know that taking a nap during the day can make sleep at night much more difficult. Many customers do not know that caffeine in soft drinks, coffee, and medications can make sleep difficult. My aunt once told me that she had extreme difficulty falling asleep at night. I asked her whether she consumed any soft drinks or coffee within several hours of her bedtime. She told me that she routinely had a cup of tea before bedtime for years. I suggested that she discontinue the tea at night since it contains caffeine. She told me that eliminating the tea allowed her to fall asleep much more easily. Of course, pharmacists rarely have time to discuss causes of insomnia with our customers.

I have a neighbor who recently had a double bypass. This neighbor asked me to drive him to his doctor for a routine follow up a few days after being released from the hospital. He also asked me to accompany him in the examining room, hoping that I could help him remember the doctor's instructions. My neighbor mentioned to the doctor that he was having trouble sleeping since the surgery. I was absolutely thrilled that this heart surgeon recommended against the use of sleeping pills. The surgeon discouraged my neighbor by saying that sleeping pills induce a sleep that is not natural and, therefore, not as restorative as normal sleep. (Am I being too cynical in suggesting that surgeons are more likely to criticize pills than other doctors—like internists and cardiologists—whose practices consist largely of prescribing pills?)

When doctors phone prescriptions to the pharmacist, most doctors don't comment on why they're prescribing a particular drug. I recall two instances in which a local doctor did make such a comment, and, in both cases, I have a philosophical disagreement with his use of medication. One time this doctor commented to me something like, "Jane Smith's mother just died. She needs something to help her sleep. Give her ten Halcion."

14. Drugs that treat anxiety: On another occasion, this same doctor commented to me something like, "Mary Jones is very anxious while she's studying for her bar exam. Give her fifteen Xanax." I guess I feel that adversity builds character, so I don't really like people depending on drugs to assist them in overcoming the normal hurdles in life. In the 1970s Helen Reddy sang about "wisdom borne of pain."

15. Pain killers: In my opinion, pain (both physical and psychological) can be a great teacher. Pain should force us to try to examine its causes. Instead, we seek to kill pain. Pain teaches us about the fragility of life and our own mortality. From my perspective, nothing sums up the superficial nature of modern medicine more than that class of drugs popularly referred to as "pain killers," not because the pain isn't real but because "killing pain" without examining its causes is as illogical as killing terrorists without examining why they choose to terrorize us. Any new pain should prompt us to explore its causes, rather than reflexively seek to kill it.

In their July 31, 2011 editorial for *The People's Pharmacy*, Joe and Teresa Graedon discuss "Will Your Painkiller Kill You?" (www.peoplespharmacy.com/2011/07/31/will-your-painkiller-kill-you/ Accessed November 11, 2011)

When ibuprofen (Advil, Motrin IB) was initially introduced as an over-the-counter pain reliever in 1984, it was advertised as "advanced medicine for pain." The implication was that this drug, previously available only by prescription, was better than the currently available pain relievers. Aspirin had been around since the turn of the 20th century, and acetaminophen (Tylenol) went over the counter in 1955.

In 1994, when naproxen was switched from prescription (Naprosyn) to nonprescription status (Aleve), it was advertised with the slogan "all day long, all day strong." The pitch was effective; Aleve has become a household name, just like Advil, Motrin IB and Tylenol.

By the way, none of these drugs has been proven more effective than the lowly aspirin when it comes to easing pain.

Americans swallow a lot of pain pills. Over 20 million take an over-the-counter NSAID (nonsteroidal anti-inflammatory drug) every day. Millions more take prescription products like celecoxib (Celebrex), diclofenac (Cataflam, Voltaren) or meloxicam (Mobic). Do people realize the risks they are taking along with their pills?

Too many of us assume that if the FDA has decided a drug should be available over the counter, it is safe enough to take without any concern. Studies have shown that many people taking OTC pain relievers are unaware of any risks and not worried that they will experience side effects (*Journal of Rheumatology*, Nov. 1, 2005; Proceedings of the National Academy of Science of the U.S.A., April 21, 2009).

Even doctors don't always know just how risky such drugs might be. A recent study published in the *BMJ* (online, July 4, 2011) shows that NSAIDs can increase the chance of developing heart rhythm disturbances called atrial fibrillation and atrial flutter.

The extra cases (4 to 7 per 1,000 patients) may not seem like a lot, but the additional risk could add up to as many as 200,000 people each year developing atrial fibrillation. This heart rhythm abnormality can lead to strokes, and heart failure, and significantly increases the risk of dying prematurely (*Journal of the American Medical Association*, May 25, 2011).

The *BMJ* study of NSAIDs is not the only one showing that these drugs may disrupt heart rhythms. A study of British patients last year also showed a 44 percent increase in the risk of atrial fibrillation among people taking NSAIDs (*Archives of Internal Medicine*, Sept. 13, 2010).

Taking an NSAID pain reliever, whether prescription or over the counter, also increases the likelihood that a person with high blood pressure or heart disease will have a heart attack or a stroke (*American Journal of Medicine*, July, 2011).

Unfortunately, older people with arthritis often have heart problems or hypertension. This poses a terrible double bind. Do they put up with pain that seriously impairs their quality of life, or do they take a painkiller that threatens to shorten their lives?

16. Drugs that treat diarrhea: At some time during the two years of my college pre-pharmacy curricula, many students on campus developed a persistent problem with diarrhea. Even though many of my classmates visited the on-campus student health service for whatever ailed them, I went to the student health service only twice during my five years in college. One of these visits was because I, too, had this persistent diarrhea. I remember asking the physician who saw me if he knew what was causing the diarrhea. He said something like "It's a bug going around." Only several months later did I read in a newspaper that some organism had been discovered in the municipal water supply. It appears that the more water students drank, the worse was their diarrhea. As I look back on this experience, I am surprised that the water supply was not everyone's focus at that time. Perhaps in a year or two, after learning more about human health, I would have reached that conclusion myself. But I was not yet informed enough to make the connection. This was around 1972 at West Virginia University in Morgantown, West Virginia.

Theoretically, Morgantown had the highest concentration of smart people in the state but, even with the faculty at the medical school, I still don't understand why the connection to the water supply was not made sooner. Anyway, the physician at the student health service gave me a prescription for Lomotil, the leading drug at that time for diarrhea. I don't believe I had that prescription filled because I think I was looking for an explanation for the cause of the widespread diarrhea, rather than a pill to stop it. I think that, intuitively, it did not make any sense to try to stop that diarrhea because I felt surely my body was trying to get rid of some noxious substance or organism. I think that the absence of fever caused me to question whether this diarrhea was due to "a bug going around."

Even today there is a big debate about when diarrhea should be treated and when it should be allowed to run its course. Diarrhea in children can be very serious due to the possibility of dehydration. That's why many doctors feel that the best way to approach diarrhea is to focus on adding fluids like Pedialyte, rather than on anti-diarrheal products like Donnagel or Imodium. Diarrhea occurs for a reason and that reason is usually because the body is trying to get rid of some nasty substance or organism. So the widespread use of products to halt diarrhea is often irrational, unless there is a chance that the person could become dehydrated, a potentially very serious consequence. Unfortunately most pharmacy customers don't seem to be interested in the nuances of this debate. Most customers just want to stop the diarrhea without understanding its full significance. Let me emphasize that, in serious cases of diarrhea, fluids must be maintained to avoid dehydration.

17. Drugs that treat fever: A debate similar to that of routinely treating diarrhea involves the routine treatment of fever. Should fever always be treated? Some health professionals view fever as a distinct medical condition. Others view fever as a natural defense mechanism used by the body to fight off infection. According to *The Merck Manual of Medical Information—Home Edition* (Whitehouse Station, New Jersey: Merck Research Laboratories, 1997, pp. 843, 845):

Fever, an elevation of body temperature above 100 degrees F. (as measured by an oral thermometer) is actually a protective response to

infection and injury. The elevated body temperature enhances the body's defense mechanisms while causing relatively minor discomfort for the person. ...Because of the potential benefits of fever, there is some debate as to whether it should be treated routinely.

Like the controversy over the routine treatment of diarrhea, many pharmacy customers are not interested in the nuances in the debate regarding the routine treatment of fever. Many customers want to treat all fevers, even mild ones that may assist in fighting off whatever unwelcome organism is present. I hated dispensing fever reducers like Children's Motrin because mild to moderate fever is often a natural defense mechanism to fight off infection. But keep in mind that high fever can be dangerous.

18. Products that treat jock itch: As I look back on my career, I recall very few encounters with customers that I found fulfilling. One example of a fulfilling encounter stands out in my mind. One summer a young man in his twenties approached me and asked me to recommend a non-prescription product for jock itch. I was able to walk with him to the shelf where this product was located. During our brief conversation, he told me that he worked outdoors most of the time in construction. I asked him if he sweated a lot during his work outside. He said that on hot summer days, he sweated tremendously. I asked him if this sweat included the genital area, i.e., the location of the jock itch. He said yes. I told him that trapped moisture is the number one culprit with jock itch. I explained that jock itch is a fungus that loves to grow in a warm and moist environment. I asked him if he wore heavy jeans at work like the ones he was wearing as I spoke with him. He said yes. I explained that he needed to wear clothes at work that allowed greater circulation of air in the genital region. I said that he needed to avoid synthetic and heavy-weight fabric and that he should change into clean dry pants as soon as he arrived at home after work each day. I said that, if possible, he should consider wearing shorts at work on hot summer days. I told him that he would not get rid of the jock itch as long as he continued to sweat in the genital area at work and as long as this moisture was trapped from lack of air circulation in that area. I found it fulfilling to teach him to prevent jock itch. Unfortunately, pharmacists too often are so overwhelmed with prescriptions that conversations like this with customers do not occur.

19. Drugs that treat toenail fungus: My mother developed toenail fungus for the first time in her life upon retiring in Florida. She informed me of this only after she had her toenails drastically trimmed in an effort to get rid of the fungus. In my opinion, she did not know how to prevent the toenail fungus. She used to walk a mile or so every day, outside, in the morning. In south Florida, it is hot even in the morning. I suspect that she did not realize the role that sweat played in her developing toenail fungus. She used to wear heavy white socks and tennis shoes that did not allow adequate ventilation. I feel that her toenail fungus was totally preventable if she had understood the role of moisture and lack of ventilation for that moisture. Many doctors prescribe oral antifungal drugs for patients with toenail fungus. These drugs can cause serious liver damage.

20. Drugs that treat blood pressure and Type II diabetes: I once had an obese customer ask me an endless number of questions about her blood pressure medications. She appeared to be skeptical of the need for those medications. Finally, in total exasperation (I had a pile of prescriptions waiting to be filled), I said to her, "You know, in many people, the single best thing they can do to decrease their need for blood pressure drugs is to lose weight." A previously cordial conversation immediately became uncomfortable. She implied that her weight was none of my business and she walked away. That was the first time I ever mentioned the need to lose weight to a customer who was clearly overweight. And it was also the last time.

The Merck Manual (16th edition, p. 984) says that most cases of hypertension and Type II diabetes are preventable: "Thus weight reduction will lower the BP [blood pressure] of most hypertensives, often to normal levels, and will allow 75% of Type II diabetics to discontinue medication." Ninety percent of diabetics fall under Type II.

21. Sunscreens: A growing body of research seems to suggest that sunscreens are not as effective in preventing skin cancers as is implied by the manufacturers of these products. The advertising seems to lull people into believing that they are fully protected with these products when that may not be the case. My feeling about sunscreens: "Is *Homo sapiens* the only species on the planet that seeks prolonged sun exposure (from sunbathing) during the part of the day that the sun rays are the most damaging?"

According to *Associated Press* writer Linda A. Johnson ("Sunscreens Faulted on Cancer Protection," June 25, 2006):

> Think slathering on the highest-number sunscreen at the beach or pool will spare you skin cancer and premature wrinkles? Probably not, if you're in the sun a lot. That's because you don't need a sunburn to suffer the effects that can cause various types of skin cancer.
>
> Sunscreens generally do a good job filtering out the ultraviolet rays that cause sunburn—UVB rays. But with sunburn protection, many people get a false sense of security that keeps them under the harsh sun much longer. That adds to the risk of eventual skin cancer—both deadly melanoma and the more common and less-threatening basal and squamous cell cancers.
>
> And most sunscreens don't defend nearly as well against the UVA rays that penetrate deep into the skin and are more likely to cause skin cancer and wrinkles. That's ture even for some products labeled "broad-spectrum UVA/UVB protection."

22. Drugs that treat migraine: I don't enjoy dispensing anti-migraine drugs to relieve headaches caused by stress. The focus should be on addressing the causes of the stress, rather than on killing the pain from the migraine.

23. Products that treat acne: Drugstores sell lots of products for acne. But if acne comes with a Western diet, wouldn't it be more logical to focus on the diet rather than focus on products that treat acne? According to *Reuters Health* writer Jacqueline Stenson ("Western Culture May Be Culprit Behind Acne: Theory," Dec. 20, 2002):

> Calling into question the current medical belief that diet does not affect acne, a new report suggests that regularly eating breads, cakes, chips and other staples of Western culture may promote the skin condition.
>
> Dr. Loren Cordain, a professor of health and exercise science at Colorado State University in Fort Collins, and colleagues arrived at their concluson after studying two non-Westernized populations: the Kitavan Islanders of Papua New Guinea and the Ache hunter-gatherers of Paraguay.

In the December [2002] issue of the *Archives of Dermatology*, the study authors report that they found no evidence of acne among 1,200 Kitavan Islanders aged 10 or older, including 300 of them between 15 and 25. They ate primarily fruit, fish, tubers and coconut but almost no cereals or refined sugars.

The researchers also saw no acne among 115 Ache hunter-gatherers, including 15 aged 15 to 25. Their diet consisted mostly of the root vegetable sweet manioc, peanuts, maize and rice, as well as some wild game. About 8% of their diet was made up of Western foods such as pasta, sugar and bread. Previous studies also have found that acne is rare or nonexistent in people living in non-industrialized cultures but tends to appear when they transition to a Western way of life, the report indicates.

In Western cultures, studies have indicated that acne affects 79% to 95% of adolescents and persists into middle age in 12% of women and 3% of men.

24. Drugs that treat asthma: The rapidly increasing incidence of asthma suggests that environmental triggers may play a big role. The pharmacist's job is to dispense drugs that treat and prevent this condition. In my 25-year career as a pharmacist, I don't believe I ever spoke a single word to a customer about the non-pharmacological prevention of asthma.

According to Joe and Teresa Graedon in *The People's Pharmacy*: "A hundred years ago, the pre-eminent physician of that time, Sir William Osler, wrote that asthma was almost never fatal. These days, however, thousands of people die from acute asthma attacks each year. Why has asthma become both more common and more deadly?" (http://www.peoplespharmacy.com/2011/08/27/826-asthma/ Aug. 27, 2011)

The Merck Manual states: The prevalence of asthma has increased continuously since the 1970s, and it now affects an estimated 4 to 7% of people worldwide. About 4000 deaths occur from asthma annually in the US. However, the death rate is 5 times higher for blacks than for whites. Common triggers of an asthma attack include: environmental and occupational allergens, infections, exercise, inhaled irritants, emotion, aspirin, and gastroesophageal reflux. Inhaled irritants, such as air pollution, cigarette smoke, perfumes, and cleaning products, are often involved. Emotions such as anxiety, anger, and excitement sometimes trigger attacks.

(http://www.merckmanuals.com/professional/pulmonary_disorders/
asthma_and_related_disorders/asthma.html?qt=asthma&alt=sh)

See also: Ellen Ruppel Shell, "Does Civilization Cause Asthma?",
The Atlantic, May 2000
(http://www.theatlantic.com/past/docs/issues/2000/05/shell.htm)

25. Vitamins: A rather common scenario is that a customer asks
a pharmacist to recommend a vitamin that would be good for "lack
of energy." I usually want to tell such people that they're asking too
much of vitamins, but I usually just recommend Centrum because
people who ask pharmacists for recommendations for vitamins do
not usually want to receive a lecture from those pharmacists about
the limitiations of vitamin supplements. What I'd prefer to tell these
people is that they should instead focus on a nutritious diet, adequate
sleep at night, perhaps a job that is less exhausting, etc. There is no
quick-fix vitamin solution for "lack of energy."

Some pharmacists are strong advocates of vitamins whereas other
pharmacists do not feel that vitamins do much good in most cases.
There is a wide range in the level of enthusiasm among pharmacists
for vitamins. From my experience, I would say that most pharmacists probably feel that the focus should be on eating a balanced diet
rather than on fine-tuning ones choice of vitamin supplements. Perhaps the skepticism of many pharmacists toward vitamin and mineral
supplements is more a matter of pharmacists being taught in school
that *potent pharmaceuticals* are what pharmacy is all about, whereas
supplements are wimpy substances in comparison to "real" drugs
that directly alter or manipulate some physiological or pathological
process.

Throughout evolution, *Homo sapiens* obtained vitamins and
minerals as natural constituents of whole foods. The ingestion of vitamin and mineral supplements in pills is a phenomenon of the last
hundred years or so. Even though supplement enthusiasts vehe-
mently disagree, in my opinion the human body cannot handle these
vitamin and mineral supplements as safely and effectively when
they're in pills as compared to when they're in whole foods. In my
opinion, taking vitamin and mineral supplements represents reductionism, whereas a focus on eating nutritious foods represents

wholism. Even though many people take supplements as an "insurance policy" because they fear that their diet is not ideal, in my opinion these people should spend their money on nutritious foods rather than on these pills. There is a saying that goes something like this: *A poor diet plus vitamins is still a poor diet.*

Supplement enthusiasts frequently claim that the human body can't tell the difference between vitamins and minerals ingested in foods and those ingested in pills. Yet there is no precedent in the evolution of *Homo sapiens* for obtaining ones vitamins and minerals in the pure, refined form. The human body is an infinitely complex and highly refined product of the natural world. It is not a machine as Big Pharma implies. The human body has evolved to handle whole foods efficiently. It has not evolved to efficiently handle vitamins and minerals from pills or from "fortified" foods and drinks. In my opinion, processed foods fortified with vitamins and minerals are a poor substitute for fresh whole foods eaten in the same form as they exist in nature.

Many supplement enthusiasts correctly state that our health care system focuses too heavily on drugs. These supplement enthusiasts feel they are taking a stand against Big Pharma by choosing to take vitamin and mineral supplements, and they feel they are focusing on health rather than on disease. I'm all in favor of focusing on health rather than disease, but I feel that the ingestion of these supplements is a milder example of the same reductionism that is what the pharmaceutical industry is all about.

The best in-depth examination of the vitamin and supplement industry is, in my opinion, Dan Hurley's *Natural Causes: Death, Lies, and Politics in America's Vitamin and Herbal Supplement Industry* (New York: Broadway Books, 2006). Here is a sample of Hurley's discussion of the issue regarding whether people should take supplements:

...no major medical group or government agency actually recommends the routine use of multivitamins for otherwise healthy children or adults, with only a few particular exceptions. While single, targeted vitamins or minerals are recommended for particular ages or ailments, the idea that everyone needs the "nutritional insurance" of a daily multivitamin has no

basis in science or any official guidelines. Indeed, according to the American Academy of Pediatrics, for children between the ages of five and twelve, "supplements are rarely needed." The American Medical Association's only official policy on vitamins is that women of childbearing age take a folic acid supplement to prevent birth defects, and that newborns receive a onetime dose of vitamin K within one hour of birth to prevent a rare bleeding disorder. The U.S. surgeon general Richard H. Carmona, in designating 2005 as the "Year of the Healthy Child," had only one vitamin recommendation: that every woman of childbearing age take a folic acid supplement. Even the American Dietetic Association states in a position paper, "There is little scientific evidence of benefit to the average person" from a low-dose multivitamin or multivitamin-mineral supplement. Most recently, a panel of thirteen experts convened by NIH on May 17 and 18, 2006, to resolve some of the confusion over multivitamins concluded, "The state of evidence is insufficient to recommend either for or against the use of multivitramin/multimineral [supplements] by the American public."

"Most of the vitamin supplements consumed in the United States are unnecessary," agrees Benjamin Caballero, MD, PhD, director of the Center for Human Nutrition at Johns Hopkins University in Baltimore and a member of the Food and Nutrition Board at the National Academy of Sciences. "But don't rely on my opinion. Look at the 2005 Dietary Guidelines for Americans. They don't recommend any vitamin supplement for the healthy population consuming a variety of foods."

The guidelines, jointly prepared by the Department of Health and Human Services and the Department of Agriculture, represent the federal government's best effort to give science-based advice on nutrition and physical activity. While the guidelines recommend B12 for adults over fifty and folic acid for women of childbearing age who may become pregnant, nowhere do they recommend a multivitamin for anyone. "Nutrient needs should be met primarily through consuming foods," the guidelines state. "Foods provide an array of nutrients (as well as phytochemicals, antioxidants, etc.) and other compounds that may have beneficial effects on health. Supplements may be useful when they fill a specific identified nutrient gap that cannot or is not otherwise being met by the individual's intake of food. Nutrient supplements cannot replace a healthful diet. Individuals who are already consuming the recommended amount of nutrient in food will not achieve any additional health benefit if they also take the nutrient as a supplement. In fact, in some cases, supplements and fortified foods may cause intakes to exceed the safe level of nutrients."

Another nationally prominent nutritionist who advises against the use of multivitamins is Robert M. Russell, MD, director and senior scientist of the Jean Mayer USDA Human Nutrition Research Center on Aging at Tufts University in Boston. "I don't take them myself," he says. Instead of paying attention to their diet and a mixed variety of foods that they should be eating, people think they're getting everything they need from a multivitamin, which is not the case. If you're just depending on a multivitamin, you're missing out on many, many, many benefits that come from eating a variety of foods." (*Natural Causes*, pp. 165-7)

...Thus we must face an increasingly certain conclusion, unpopular though it may be, that vitamin and mineral supplements, with the possible exception of vitamin D, are not only unnecessary for most people, but in many cases harmful. This is far more disturbing news than the revelation that a drug like Vioxx does more harm than good. Drugs, after all, are not marketed and promoted as essential to everybody's health; to the contrary, they are always sold with a lengthy list of possible side effects. Yet so thoroughly do we believe in vitamins and minerals—so carefully have we been manipulated to believe—that many mothers would consider themselves negligent not to give them to their children.... (*Natural Causes*, p. 181)

Some classes of drugs are far more effective than others

I don't think the public realizes that some drugs are far more effective than others and that there is a wide range in effectiveness among the many classes of drugs in the pharmacy. For example, here are some analogies or comparisons:
• Oral contraceptives are far more likely to prevent pregnancy than bisphosphonates are to prevent osteoporosis or bone fracture.

• Insulin is far more effective in treating type 1 diabetes than an antidepressant is in treating your child's depression.

• Levothyroxine is far more effective in treating hypothyroidism than antipsychotics are in treating psychosis.

• Morphine is far more effective in treating severe pain than Aricept is in treating Alzheimer's disease.

• An antibiotic is much more likely to cure your pneumonia than a weight loss drug is to have a lasting effect on your obesity.

• A diuretic is much more likely to relieve your fluid accumulation (edema) than a muscle relaxer is to relieve your backache.

I wish that people understood that antibiotics are usually very effective (against bacteria) whereas drugs like Aricept (for Alzheimer's) have a hard time demonstrating any effectiveness.

I wish that the drug leaflets dispensed with prescriptions included things like whether the drug actually cures a disease or whether it just relieves symptoms. For example, antibiotics can cure pneumonia whereas drugs like ibuprofen or naproxen only relieve the symptoms of arthritis and do nothing toward "curing arthritis."

From my perspective, the most effective drugs in the pharmacy include analgesics, insulin, levothyroxine, birth control pills, and antibiotics. These drugs usually do what they're prescribed for.

Morphine is highly effective against severe pain and I appreciated its availability when both of my parents were dying from cancer. Hydrocodone is usually quite effective in relieving mild to moderate pain. Aspirin, acetaminophen, and ibuprofen are usually quite effective in relieving mild pain. Nevertheless, millions of people find that analgesics do not relieve their pain.

Insulin and antibiotics are highly effective when prescribed properly. Insulin and antibiotics are, in fact, the two drugs (or classes) that, historically, are most responsible for elevating the reputation of modern medicine. These drugs unquestioningly have saved the lives of people who would have died prior to the development of these drugs. Of course, antibiotics are grossly overprescribed, causing serious problems like resistance.

Birth control pills are usually quite effective in preventing pregnancy, although they carry some cardiovascular and cancer risks. As regards the cancer risk, see the National Cancer Institute: "Oral contraceptives have been shown to increase the risk of *cervical cancer.* The risk of *liver cancer* is increased in women who take oral contraceptives and are otherwise considered low risk for the disease. Some studies have shown an increased risk of *breast cancer* in women taking oral contraceptives, while other studies have shown no change in risk." ("Oral Contraceptives and Cancer Risk: Questions and Answers," National Cancer Institute, Accessed January 2, 2012 http://www.cancer.gov/cancertopics/factsheet/Risk/oral-contraceptives)

Levothyroxine, a synthetic thyroid hormone, is usually quite effective in relieving the symptoms of low thyroid (hypothyroidism).

Drugs that lower blood sugar (in type 2 diabetes), blood pressure, and cholesterol often do precisely what they're prescribed for, but I am not a big fan of drugs that are used to treat diseases of modern civilization. In my opinion, the focus of our medical system should be on the prevention of these conditions. Many of these drugs carry significant risks.

In my opinion, the best drugs in the pharmacy meet the following criteria: They have a reasonable benefit to risk ratio and the true incidence of serious adverse effects is well known and not hidden from the public. They are likely to do precisely what they're prescribed for. Any benefit they deliver is not due primarily to the placebo effect. And they are not used to treat diseases of modern civilization.

I wish that the leaflets that are given to pharmacy customers with their prescriptions included a section that compared the safety of that drug with other drugs used for the same condition. And I wish there were some way to indicate whether that drug was in a class of drugs that is generally recognized as safe, or whether it is in a class of drugs that has serious risks.

For example, on a scale of one to ten, anti-neoplastic (anti-cancer) drugs would be given a ten for being the least safe drugs in the pharmacy. Methotrexate for rheumatoid arthritis would be maybe a nine. Coumadin can be life-saving but, used in the wrong dose, it can kill you. Coumadin is the drug most often involved in huge settlements against pharmacists for dispensing errors. One pharmacy legal consultant offered this warning for pharmacists, "You should be careful with every drug you dispense, but the hair on the back of your neck should absolutely stand on end every time you dispense Coumadin."

Some drugs such as fluoroquinolone antibiotics are usually quite effective but carry significant risks. I don't know if anyone knows the true incidence of tendon rupture from fluoroquinolones, but the incidence of rupture should not, in my opinion, be the deciding factor. The severity of this side effect, not necessarily the incidence, is what scares me. My next door neighbor developed severe tendon problems after taking Levaquin. Tendon damage and tendon rupture are well-recognized risks with taking drugs in this class. In the case of my neighbor, the tendon pain went away, then came back, then went away and, so far, has stayed away. I doubt seriously that my neighbor would have agreed to take this drug if he had fully understood the possibility that he would develop the severe tendon problems that he did. Search YouTube for *Levaquin tendon* for some shocking videos of people who have experienced serious tendon problems from drugs in this class.

Most people don't realize that, as a result of pressure from Congress, the FDA approves too many drugs, with the excuse that all the (known) potential hazards are listed in the labeling. Thus the FDA is heavily dependent on doctors carefully weighing all the FDA-approved prescribing info. But that is unrealistic because too many doctors have a simplistic view toward the safety of drugs. Too many doctors feel that if a drug is on the market, it is essentially safe. So neither the FDA nor doctors are doing the job that each expects of the other, and that the public assumes. The result is that many of the drugs on pharmacy shelves are potentially significantly more hazardous than most people realize.

Reading the warnings, precautions, etc. in direct-to-consumer drug advertisements in magazines like *Time* and *Newsweek* should cause people to perhaps increase their general level of skepticism toward pharmaceuticals. But Big Pharma has lulled people into ignoring potential adverse effects in print advertisements and on television. The public assumes that if a drug is on the market, it is essentially safe. On the other hand, I hear lots of people saying that these advertisements scare the hell out of them. They say things like, "Yeah.

When you listen carefully to the side effects, you hear that the drug can nearly kill you." This is often accompanied by a little nervous laughter.

When people purchase electronic devices such as cell phones, iPads, iPhones, computers, etc., the date these products were introduced onto the market is very important to these people because innovation in electronic devices is at a dizzying pace. Understandably, people want to have the latest version. In contrast, the pharmaceutical industry is opposed to listing the introduction date on printed information such as the official prescribing information used by doctors and also on the leaflets given to pharmacy customers with each prescription. The pharmaceutical industry apparently feels that people will be fearful of drugs that have not been on the market for a long time. Apparently having the latest drugs is not as desirable to people as having the latest electronic devices. The drug companies are afraid that the public will fear that newer drugs don't have a track record of safety.

What theory in biology states that it is safe to introduce into the human body synthetic chemicals unique to human evolution for the purpose of disrupting delicate molecular processes and biochemical pathways—and not expect adverse effects, some of which can be serious? Just because we call these synthetic chemicals "pharmaceuticals" and just because they're being employed ostensibly to help people alleviate some disease or symptom, doesn't make Mother Nature less cautious. Mother Nature does not consider the motivation behind the introduction of synthetic chemicals into living organisms. Mother Nature essentially views most pharmaceuticals as foreign to human evolution. As the popular saying goes, "The only difference between a drug and a poison is the dose."

I seriously doubt that other pharmacists carry on a debate inside their own heads about the rationality and safety of the products they dispense. I would like to see pharmacists aggressively critique all the products we dispense the same way that many of my male pharmacy school classmates obsessively and enthusiastically critiqued college football and basketball teams across America. In my ideal world, pharmacists would be like a walking *Consumer Reports* magazine. In the real world, pharmacists are piece-workers and production workers at the pharmacy version of McDonald's. Too often, pharmacists function as cheerleaders for the products of a pharmaceutical industry that has repeatedly shown a willingness to lie about the safety and effectiveness of those products.

In my opinion the pharmaceutical industry is no more honest than Wall Street, the oil companies, the defense contractors, the insurance industry, etc. Before I started pharmacy school, I viewed the pharmaceutical industry as a benevolent enterprise working to improve human health. Now I view it as just like any other industry, i.e., quite willing to push the envelope by marketing drugs that are often of questionable safety and effectiveness. It has been a very long time since I felt the pharmaceutical industry had higher ethical standards than other industries.

"There is no such thing as a 'safe' drug."

That statement comes from George Lundberg, M.D., formerly the editor at *The Journal of the American Medical Association*. Here is more of what Lundberg has to say about the pharmaceutical industry (George Lundberg, M.D., *Severed Trust: Why American Medicine Hasn't Been Fixed,*" New York: Basic Books, 2000, p. 152):

We are in genuine danger of overmedicating ourselves in this country, at great cost and often with questionable benefit. It has been found, for example, that overuse of pain medication can rebound and cause the very pain the mediation was designed to control. When people overuse products like Excedrin, Tylenol, and Advil, for instance, to control headaches— and some people take as many as fifteen tablets per day—the medication itself can cause headaches, yet another paradox in medicine.

People also encounter trouble with prescribed products designed to control conditions that may be better addressed by diet or exercise. Many patients have a strong desire to resolve all their health problems with a drop, a pill, or a plaster. That desire goes back to the days of nostrums

and elixirs, only now the medications come with all kinds of scientific assurances. Think of those splashy magazine ads with great graphics and large type on one page, followed by another page of dense type with warnings, precautions, and listings of adverse reactions. The glamour is on one page, and the science is on the other. What looks easy in one place suddelnly looks terribly complicated and difficult in another. How come? The answer is simple: there is no such thing as a 'safe' drug.

Lundberg further states, "To control runaway medical costs, I would begin by banning all direct-to-consumer medical advertising." (*Severed Trust*, p. 18)

Former FDA Commissioner Jere Goyan described himself as a "therapeutic nihilist"

Philip J. Hilts quotes former FDA Commissioner (1980-81) Jere Goyan describing himself as a "therapeutic nihilist" (Philip J. Hilts, *Protecting America's Health: The FDA, Business, and One Hundred Years of Regulation*, New York: Knopf, 2003, p. 207):

In one of his first press conferences as commissioner, he said frankly "our society has become overmedicated. We have become too casual about the use of drugs, and I'm referring to legitimate prescription and nonprescription drugs, not illicit drugs.... Too many people are taking too many drugs without proper understanding of their potential harmful effects.... I'm a therapeutic nihilist. My philosophy is the fewer drugs people take, the better off they are." He added, "I have a strong belief in the patient's right to know. My philosophy on this makes doctors and some of my colleagues uneasy, but in the best interests of public health, it should be mandated."

He believed drug companies tend to emphasize the selling of drugs, not conveying information about them. He believed as well that doctors are inattentive and often give the wrong drug at the wrong time in the wrong amounts, without regard to cost. At one meeting of doctors he said bluntly, "I staunchly refuse to accept the notion that any physician, merely because he graduated from medical school and is currently a card-carrying member of his or her county medical society, is great, or good, or even tolerably competent. Too much of drug therapy has been atrociously irrational."

Pharma's worst nightmare

Pharma's worst nightmare is that doctors start prescribing rationally (i.e., much more conservatively). As it is now, our medical system seems to be based on the idea that more is better—*more pills means better health*. Gordon D. Schiff, M.D. and colleagues wrote a tremendous article in the Sept. 12, 2011 issue of *Archives of Internal Medicine* titled "Principles of Conservative Prescribing" [*Arch Intern Med* 2011; 171(16): 1433-1440] that should be required reading for every physician, pharmacist and Pharma employee. In my opinion, if the recommendations in this article were fully implemented across this country, the number of prescriptions filled annually would drastically (and I mean *drastically!*) decrease. Laurie Barclay, M.D. wrote a very favorable commentary in *Medscape Medical News* (Sept. 16, 2011 www.medscape.com/viewarticle/749804) describing this article:

Judicious prescribing is required for safe and appropriate use of medications, according to a review article published in the September 12 issue of the *Archives of Internal Medicine*. The review authors present a series of principles to guide more cautious and conservative prescribing, based on recent studies demonstrating problems with widely prescribed drugs.

"In striving to relieve suffering and prolong life, we often turn to medications," write Gordon D. Schiff, MD, from the Center for Patient Safety Research and Practice at Brigham and Women's Hospital, Harvard Medical School in Boston, Massachusetts, and colleagues. "This desire to help patients with the 'latest and greatest' drugs is congruent with the messages and interests of the pharmaceutical industry, but there is an alternate paradigm that represents a radical shift in prescribing attitudes and behaviors.... Although others have used labels such as *healthy skepticism, more judicious, rational, careful,* or *cautious prescribing,* we believe that the term *conservative prescribing* conveys an approach that goes beyond the oft-repeated physician's mantra, 'first, do no harm.'"

The principles underlying conservative prescribing include the following:

• Consider nonpharmaceutical interventions, such as nondrug therapy, treatment or management of the underlying causes, and prevention. Various nonpharmaceutical strategies have been shown to be effective for diabetes, hypertension, insomnia, back pain, arthritis, headache, and other highly prevalent conditions. Greater focus on prevention may ultimately reduce the number of prescription drugs needed.

• Practice more strategic prescribing, including deferring or postponing nonurgent drug treatment; avoiding drug switching unless there are clear indications; being cautious regarding unproven drug uses; and initiating therapy with only one new drug at a time, which facilitates identifying the drug responsible for an adverse event. For self-limiting conditions, such as rhinosinusitis, otitis media, and back pain, watchful waiting may preclude the need for drug therapy if there is spontaneous resolution.

• Remain vigilant for adverse drug effects by having a low threshold to suspect drug reactions; being aware of drug withdrawal syndromes, particularly for drugs such as analgesics and proton pump inhibitors; and educating patients to anticipate possible adverse drug reactions.

• Be cautious and skeptical regarding new drugs by researching unbiased information; waiting to prescribe until drugs have been on the market for a sufficient length of time; avoiding reliance on surrogate markers rather than true clinical outcomes; not stretching drug indications; not being unduly impressed by elegant molecular pharmacology; and being aware of selective drug trial reporting. Clinicians should be highly familiar with a smaller number of commonly used drugs and prescribe these rather than a larger variety of drugs about which they are less knowledgeable.

• Collaborate with patients to implement a shared agenda by not automatically agreeing to prescribe requested drugs; considering nonadherence before prescribing additional drugs; not restarting drug treatment that was previously unsuccessful; discontinuing unnecessary medications; and respecting patients' reservations concerning drugs.

• Consider long-term, broader effects of drugs before prescribing, while recognizing that improved systems may outweigh the marginal benefits of new drugs.

"The recent spate of revelations of undisclosed and unexpected adverse effects of drugs in multiple therapeutic categories should serve as wake-up calls for our profession to take a more sober, balanced, and cautious approach to prescribing," the study authors write. "Lest these experiences be forgotten, with the resulting failure to draw more general lessons, we urge clinicians to take a more cautious approach to prescribing and administering chemicals whose effects are imperfectly understood. While clinicians must always weigh the benefits of conservative prescribing against the risks of withholding potentially needed medications, at the very least we should seek to shift the burden of proof toward demanding a higher standard of evidence of benefit before exposing patients to the risks of drugs."

In an accompanying editor's note, Deborah Grady, MD, MPH, refers to a study suggesting that the US public erroneously believes that drugs approved by the US Food and Drug Administration (FDA) are highly effective and safe. ...

"The recommendations by Schiff et al provide a framework for judicious prescribing that should result in significantly less use of prescription drugs (especially new drugs), fewer drug-related adverse effects, and better health outcomes," Dr. Grady writes.

Chapter 26

Two horror stories about drug reactions in people I know

My brother's drug horror story

One day my brother Jeff called me and told me that he was going to a local walk-in clinic because he was experiencing severe cough and chest congestion. He told me that he thought he might end up being admitted to the local hospital with pneumonia. I was then living in North Carolina and Jeff was living on the west coast of Florida, near Tampa. As usual, he was completely lucid in describing his situation. He called me later and said he was indeed admitted to the hospital. I told him I'd call him later on that day or the next day. The year was 1992 and my brother was 42 years old.

The first time I called him at the hospital, he was again completely lucid as he informed me of his status. But the second time I spoke with him, he was a completely different person, unlike anything I had ever seen before. He was completely unable to finish sentences. All he could say on the phone was, "Dennis, this is the deal." To every question I asked him, he replied, "Dennis, this is the deal." He said this maybe fifteen times over a period of perhaps ten minutes. He was unable to actually describe to me what "the deal" was, i.e., what his status was. He kept answering, "Dennis, this is the deal."

I called my parents who were then living on the opposite coast in Florida, approximately a five hour drive from my brother's hospital. I described to my parents this dramatic change from my previous phone conversation with Jeff. My mother told me that she and my father would drive over to be with my brother when he was released from the hospital. She said he would probably need assistance at his home when he was released from the hospital as he continued his recovery from the pneumonia. I said, "No! You need to go there now! He has become incoherent."

I called back to the hospital and asked for the nurse's station and asked the nurse to have my brother's doctor call me. My brother had never seen this doctor before. In fact, he did not have a primary doctor because he had no health problems. So this doctor knew nothing about my brother's normal behavior. When this doctor called me, she said that my brother's white cell count was very high indicating a serious infection. But this doctor had no idea why my brother was incoherent. She asked me, "Has he ever had psychiatric problems before?" I said, "Absolutely not!" She pursued the issue of his sanity by implying that it was possible that the extreme stress from the pneumonia allowed an underlying psychosis to surface. She seemed to be suggesting to me, "How well do you really know your brother?" I told her repeatedly that his incoherence was absolutely atypical of his personality or behavior.

I called my parents back and repeated to them that they needed to go to my brother's hospital NOW and that I was going to make a reservation to fly to Florida on the next available flight.

What I discovered when I arrived at the hospital became the most horrific day in my life. My brother was lying in a hospital bed and he was incoherent. His doctor had ordered a CAT scan and electroencephalograph (EEG) to check his brain. Both turned up normal. My brother's doctor didn't know what to do. She kept trying to tell me and my parents that my brother must be basically a psychotic person and that it took the stress of his pneumonia to bring out a latent psychosis. I kept telling her that he had never acted anything like this before. And I said, "How could he have managed to cover up a psychosis from us all his life?" The doctor again implied, "How well do you really know him? It's possible." The doctor ordered a psychiatric consult. Afterward, this psychiatrist took me out into the hall and somberly yet confidently told me that my brother was schizoid. The psychiatrist prescribed the anti-psychotic drug Haldol.

In addition to being exhausted from being awake all night, my parents and I were in a state of shock during this entire period. We feared that we had, all of a sudden, a brain-damaged member of our family. For this entire period, my brother had a blank expression on his face. He was unable to laugh or smile. At times, he had the appearance on his face that I would clumsily describe as the look of a "thousand-year-old man, a cosmic grimace, an expression lacking all personality." He looked like someone who had known all the pain in the world since the beginning of time.

One of the strangest things of all was that, intermittently, he would speak with a very distinct and clear British accent, something I had never before heard him do. Months later I happened to come across an article that described a rare condition called "foreign accent syndrome" in which people suddenly begin speaking plainly with a foreign accent, sometimes as a consequence of a stroke or serious migraines. I e-mailed that article to my brother and, even though he indeed distinctly recalls speaking with a British accent, he sent me this explanation: "My situation was different. I was interested in accents, heard a British accent many times on radio and TV, and just tried to emulate it. Thus my mental disorder gave me the desire to try to talk that way."

My brother had been prescribed the following drugs during his hospitalization:

1) nafcillin—antibiotic
2) Azactam—antibiotic
3) Organidin—expectorant and breaks up mucous
4) aminophylline—assists breathing
5) acetaminophen—analgesic and fever reducer

Again, my brother's doctor told me that his white cell count was very high, indicating a serious infection. She told me that if his pneumonia were left untreated, it could kill him. She decided to stop all his medications to see whether he was having a bad drug reaction. She emphasized that treatment needed to resume as soon as it was determined to be a drug reaction. Finally, after a period of about eighteen hours on no drugs, my brother regained his normal mental functioning. At that point, he was put on different drugs and happily made an uneventful recovery. But this day was unquestionably the scariest day in the lives of my parents and me. I had arrived at the hospital around 9 PM. My mother and I stayed with Jeff for the entire night. It was not until around 7 AM the next morning that he could speak coherently.

My brother later told me that he was aware of his incoherence during this period, but was unable to overcome it. He was aware of his inability to finish sentences, yet he was helpless to reverse the situation. He knew he was sane during this horrific period, but he was unable to verbalize it.

I can't say whether the arrival of my parents and me at the hospital definitely altered the course of events during my brother's hospitalization. Even though my brother's doctor (and the psychiatrist who examined him) assumed he was basically a psychotic person, I presume and hope that they would have considered the possibility of a drug reaction even if my parents and I had not rushed to the hospital and vigorously protested that Jeff was NOT a psychotic person. I assume and hope that his doctor would have decided to temporarily stop all medications to see whether he was suffering a drug reaction. I don't know whether my presence and the presence of my parents accelerated the decision to stop all medications to see whether he was having a drug reaction. I don't know how much my parents and my own protesting the diagnosis *that my brother was basically psychotic* had on his doctor's decision to stop all meds. So I cannot say with certainty that the outcome would have been any different had my parents and I not rushed to the hospital. Perhaps we accelerated the decision by Jeff's doctor to stop all medications to see whether he was having a drug reaction. Even so, my brother's hospitalization would seem to make the case for the importance of having family members present at times like this.

What was causing Sam's persistent cough?

I worked for a few years in one drugstore in North Carolina with a clerk named Susan. She later became the merchandise manager at this drugstore. Still later she became a pharmacy technician. I came to know Susan fairly well over the years. In 1987 Susan's husband, Sam, developed a persistent cough. Sam went to his local doctor who ordered several tests, including a chest x-ray. Sam's local doctor couldn't figure out what was causing the cough, so he referred Sam to an ear, nose, and throat (ENT) specialist in a nearby town.

This ENT specialist did more tests. He thought Sam had a lung infection so he put Sam on an antibiotic. When the antibiotic had no effect, the doctor suspected that Sam's cough was due to acid flowing up into his esophagus (heartburn or gastro-esophageal reflux disease), so he prescribed Zantac. When the Zantac had no effect, the ENT specialist suggested that Sam see a pulmonary (lung) specialist at Duke University Medical Center, a thirty-minute drive from Sam's and Susan's home.

The Duke doctor, in turn, ordered additional tests, including skin tests for allergy. Sam once spent an entire day at Duke talking to several doctors. Sam ended up making several trips to Duke, necessitating taking several days off from work. During one of the extensive interviews with Duke doctors, Sam mentioned that he and Susan had recently purchased a bird along with a bird cage. The Duke doctor suggested that Sam could be allergic to the bird so he suggested that Sam get rid of the bird. The doctor also suggested that Sam get a humidifier, which he did.

Susan told me that Sam's cough seemed to be particularly bad when she vacuumed the carpet so she said she intended to shampoo the carpet as soon as she could. Susan also told me that she was concerned that Sam had lung cancer. She said that his coughing was so bad that it was keeping them awake at night and that she had encouraged Sam to sleep on the couch in the living room so that she could get a good night's sleep. Susan told me that, even with their health insurance, she was concerned because the twenty-percent for which they were responsible was "starting to add up."

I had remembered that Sam worked for a company that sold and repaired mobile homes. One day I asked Sam whether he had ever come into contact with asbestos insulation while, for example, removing wall panels to repair leaking pipes. At that time, there were many stories in the media about school districts across the country removing asbestosis insulation at great expense. The concern was that asbestos could cause lung cancer. Sam told me that, yes, he had indeed been in contact with a fair amount of insulation while working on mobile homes. I had read that mobile homes often use lots of formaldehyde in the particle board that is very often used instead of real wood. I suggested to Sam that perhaps he was particularly sensitive to the formaldehyde fumes that can be quite powerful in mobile homes, especially in the summer months.

Sam and Susan happened to live in a mobile home themselves. Sam had remodeled that mobile home himself. Susan told me that the home seemed to be absolutely airtight, so I suggested that she and Sam keep at least one window partially open even in the winter to let in fresh air.

Well, it turns out that all the doctors Sam visited were wrong. And it turns out that I, too, was wrong. The other pharmacist (named Bill) at this drugstore had recently attended a continuing education seminar during which the speaker mentioned that one of the side effects of the anti-hypertensive drug Capoten (captopril) is cough. It so happens that Sam was a little overweight and was taking Capoten to lower his blood pressure. Bill decided to call Sam's local doctor to suggest the possibility that the Capoten was the cause of Sam's persistent cough. The local doctor agreed it was worth a try. So Sam was switched to a different drug for hypertension.

To make a long story short, Sam's cough was caused by the Capoten. After five months of coughing, Sam finally stopped coughing. As I said, this incident occurred in 1987. Today, cough is a fairly well-recognized side effect of Capoten and other drugs in the class called ACE inhibitors.

At that time, Sam and his wife blamed me and Bill for not making the connection sooner. And Susan was amazed that all the doctors Sam visited didn't make the connection either. I had tried to explain to Susan that cough is a fairly uncommon side effect for any drug. But her confidence in me was diminished for a period of time since she had regularly kept me up to date with Sam's cough and his visits with local doctors and those at Duke University Medical Center. Susan told me that, for months, she was worried that Sam had lung cancer.

Susan also told me that she was upset that they had to pay so much money and spend so much time at Duke University Medical Center without the doctors there figuring out the cause of the cough. Sam told me that his medical bills related to the cough totaled about two thousand dollars. Since their insurance covered eighty percent, Sam had to pay nearly four hundred dollars. The failure to recognize Sam's cough as a side effect of Capoten cost the insurance company nearly sixteen hundred dollars. There is no question that Sam's cough was due to the Capoten. The last thing Sam told me regarding the situation was, "The doctors at Duke should have had some way to figure this out."

Shockingly, twenty-five years later, despite countless articles in medical publications, *cough* is still too often overlooked as a side effect of Capoten and other drugs in the class called ACE inhibitors. *The People's Pharmacy* still receives a huge number of letters and e-mails describing cough caused by ACE inhibitors that was unrecognized by the doctors who prescribed one of the drugs in that class. Here is a typical question submitted recently to *The People's Pharmacy* on this issue. (Joe and Teresa Graedon, "Horrible Cough from Blood Pressure Pill," *The People's Pharmacy*, April 16, 2012 http://www.peoplespharmacy.com/2012/04/16/horrible-cough-from-blood-pressure-pill/

Question. I was given a prescription for lisinopril last year to lower my blood pressure. During the winter I developed a constant horrible dry cough that just wouldn't go away. One day at work I started coughing and couldn't stop. It was so bad that the secretary called 911. Various doctors tested me for sleep apnea (negative), throat polyps (negative), allergies (none) and lung function (normal). I couldn't quit coughing. On my own I dropped the lisinopril and within a week my cough vanished. I am upset that I was put through so many expensive tests when the real problem was a common drug side effect.

Answer from *The People's Pharmacy*. Hundreds of readers have reported a similar experience with ACE inhibitor blood pressure drugs like benazepril, captopril, enalapril, lisinopril, quinapril and ramipril. Some have lost bowel and bladder control from coughing so hard.

It is disappointing that you saw so many doctors who failed to correctly identify your cough as a common drug side effect. We consider this a major medical mistake. It is one that happens way to often.

It should be possible to control high blood pressure without intolerable reactions. We are still astonished that so many specialists overlooked your medication as a cause for uncontrollable coughing. Every medical student in the country learns that ACE inhibitors like lisinopril can cause a bad cough. Every physician should know this.

If doctors cannot recognize such a common side effect with such a frequently prescribed medication, we shudder to think what else they are forgetting or ignoring when it comes to adverse drug reactions.

The *Physicians's Desk Reference* is not much help to physicians on the issue of ACE inhibitor-induced cough. The official prescribing information in the *PDR* lists the occurrence of ACE inhibitor-induced cough as much lower than seen in the real world. See *The People's Pharmacy* (Joe and Teresa Graedon, "Can You Trust the Drug Label?" *The People's Pharmacy*, Mar. 13, 2011 http://www.peoplespharmacy.com/2011/03/13/can-you-trust-the-drug-label/):

The bible of drug information is the *Physicians' Desk Reference* (PDR). It contains the prescribing guidelines for medications provided by drug companies and approved by the Food and Drug Administration.

All of the data on drugs found in pharmacy leaflets, online resources and consumer publications comes from this source. Doctors rely on the facts they find in the official label to weigh benefits and risks of medications and inform patients about the likelihood of experiencing certain side effects.

What if this document were flawed? The FDA relies on the manufacturer to supply data about side effect frequency during the approval process. Research suggests that the drug label sometimes underestimates how often bad reactions occur. ...

More than 100 million prescriptions are filled each year for blood pressure medicines called ACE inhibitors. These are drugs like benazepril, enalapril, fosinopril, lisinopril, quinapril and ramipril. These medicines are perceived to be highly effective and extremely safe.

ACE inhibitors have a noteworthy side effect, however. These drugs can cause an unrelenting cough. Doctors who count on the FDA's labeling may downplay this risk.

Research comparing the reported incidence of cough in the PDR/drug label with that in clinical trials found that the actual rate of cough for ACE inhibitors was many times higher than the rate quoted in the *PDR* (*American Journal of Medicine*, Nov. 2010). As the authors note, side effect information in the drug label can be deceptive.

ATTENTION: IMPORTANT NOTE TO READERS

This book should not be used as a substitute for professional medical advice or care. The reader should consult his or her physician in matters relating to his or her health. In particular, the reader should consult his or her physician before acting on any of the information or advice contained in this book.

Stopping a medication can be very dangerous. Every reader must consult with his or her physician before starting, stopping, or changing the dose of any medication.

The possibility of adverse effects from a drug or drugs should not cause the reader to overlook the benefits of medication. A reader concerned about adverse effects of medication should discuss with his or her doctor the benefits as well as the risks of taking the medication.

Nothing in this book should be interpreted as stating or implying that the reader should ever discontinue a drug or take it differently from how it was intended by his or her physician. This could have devastating health consequences. Many drugs are absolutely essential and even life-saving. NO ONE should EVER stop taking any medication without careful consultation with a physician and medical supervision. Even potentially dangerous drugs can be essential for health.

Part of the reason for writing this book is to encourage patients to have discussions with their physicians about the risks and benefits of drugs, and about whether there may be (sometimes major) lifestyle or dietary changes that might lessen the need for some drugs. This book is about prevention. This is not a book that advocates taking drugs differently from how they were prescribed by a physician.

One of the risks in writing a book about drugs is that some readers may misinterpret an author's intentions and then do something contrary to his or her health. Indeed, such fear sometimes keeps pharmacists from frankly discussing the pros and cons of drugs with our customers. We live in very litigious times. If you stop taking a drug or take it differently from how your physician intended it to be taken, that is ABSOLUTELY CONTRARY to the purpose of this book.

Chapter 27

Most drugs are surprisingly crude

Every few years, there's a major plane crash and 100 to 200 people die and we call it a tragedy. Every year, 100,000 people die from adverse reactions to drugs and we call it modern medicine. According to a study in the *Journal of the American Medical Assoc.* in 1998 (Pomeranz, et. al., "Incidence of Adverse Drug Reactions in Hospitalized Patients," April 15, 1998, pp. 1200-1205), "The incidence of serious and fatal ADRs [adverse drug reactions] in US hospitals was found to be extremely high." (p. 1200) Adverse drug reactions may rank from the fourth to sixth leading cause of death in this country. Anyone who has any illusions as to the benign nature of pharmaceuticals needs to read this study.

Perhaps our most surprising result was the large number of fatal ADRs. We estimated that in 1994 in the United States 106,000 (95% CI, 76,000-137,000) hospital patients died from an ADR. Thus, we deduced that ADRs may rank from the fourth to sixth leading cause of death. Even if the lower confidence limit of 76,000 fatalities was used to be conservative, we estimated that ADRs could still constitute the sixth leading cause of death in the United States, after heart disease (743,460), cancer (529,904), stroke (150,108), pulmonary disease (101,077), and accidents (90,523); this would rank ADRs ahead of pneumonia (75,719) and diabetes

(53,894). Moreover, when we used the mean value of 106,000 fatalities, we estimated that ADRs could rank fourth, after heart disease, cancer, and stroke as a leading cause of death. [p. 1204]

Investigative journalist Stephen Fried puts the hazards of prescription drugs into perspective in his remarkable exposé of the pharmaceutical industry, *Bitter Pills* (New York: Bantam, 1998). He quotes a former FDA official (p. 122):

A former high-ranking FDA official had recently looked me straight in the eye and insisted that "the amount of preventable harm done by the misuse of drugs and the lack of properly identifying drug side effects exceeds the sum total of all occupational and environmental hazards in the United States."

If someone asks "Is this drug safe?", we pharmacists have learned to minimize the hazards. If someone asks us "What are the possible side effects with this drug?", we have learned to list just a few, even though there may be fifty listed in the *Physician's Desk Reference*. We pharmacists certainly don't mention the most serious side effects. We may say something like, "You may experience a little nausea, vomiting, diarrhea, or headache." We rarely mention liver damage or kidney damage or GI bleeding or serious blood disorders. We usually mention nuisance side effects rather than truly dangerous side effects.

Of course, this attitude among pharmacists regarding adverse effects does not reflect some stated policy that the chain enforces on us. In the real world, the total focus on sales means that pharmacists must internalize the mercantile goals of our employer. To do otherwise would result in our being labeled as rebellious, not a team player, and as someone who needs to be eased out of his job.

The average consumer of prescription drugs needs to start reading the *PDR* and attempting to understand the arcane language. Consumers need to appreciate all the uncertainties and unknowns that are glossed over by professionals as they justify to you (and themselves) the need for a drug. The average person needs to have a context in which to understand drugs. What do all these strange words mean in the adverse reactions, warnings, precautions, and car-cinogenesis sections of the *PDR*? The drug companies hope that you'll be so overwhelmed by the technicalities and long words that you'll throw up your hands and surrender your body and autonomy to professionals.

Most people are unaware of the actual nature of pharmaceuticals. It is important to contrast pharmaceuticals with foods. Foods pro-vide fuel that allows cells and tissues to do what millions of years of evolution have programmed them to do (e.g., repair cellular and tis-sue damage). In contrast, most pharmaceuticals *force* cells, tissues and organs to do things. Diuretics *force* the kidneys to get rid of fluid. Blood pressure drugs *force* blood vessels to relax. Cardiac drugs *force* the heart to beat more regularly or more forcefully. Drugs for angina *force* the blood vessels on the heart to dilate. Asthma drugs *force* the bronchioles to dilate.

My impression is that most people view drugs as benevolent sub-stances that facilitate or encourage cells, tissues, and organs. Before I entered pharmacy school, I had the incredibly naive view that phar-maceuticals were akin to super-potent vitamins that nurtured dis-eased tissues and organs back to health. In reality, most pharmaceu-ticals are substances foreign to human evolution that overwhelm the delicate processes of nature. Most people are not aware that most drugs are synthesized from petroleum. The OPEC oil embargo dur-ing the Carter Administration was, at that time, said to be a potential threat to availability of pharmaceuticals.

If you read any textbook on pharmacology, you will see that most drugs interfere with the nuts and bolts of cells and force some action on those cells. One of the most striking things for me in pharmacy school was the crudeness of most drugs. I assumed that most drugs were highly refined and as impressive as a fine painting. I was surprised to learn that most drugs in reality show more resem-blance to a hammer or a club. That's why each drug in the *PDR* usually has at least fifty potential side effects.

One of the biggest surprises for me in pharmacy school was the tremendous number of unknowns at the molecular level. I was shocked that so much of a drug's actions is understood only on a theoretical basis. Yet these huge gaps in understanding physiology at the molecular and cellular levels don't seem to dampen the enthusiasm of Big Pharma for marketing drugs on a truly massive scale. Big Pharma doesn't necessarily tread cautiously in the face of the unknown, where molecular and cellular actions are poorly understood. For example, an advertisement for Abilify in *Newsweek* (March 26, 2007, p. 67) states, "Abilify may work by adjusting dopamine activity, instead of completely blocking it and by adjusting serotonin activity. However, the exact way any medicine for bipolar disorder works is unknown."

Effexor XR is a popular drug used to treat depression, generalized anxiety disorder, social anxiety disorder, and panic disorder. The official patient information leaflet for Effexor XR includes the following:

How does Effexor XR work? Effexor XR is thought to work by affecting two naturally occurring brain chemicals, serotonin and norepinephrine.

You can get an idea of the tremendous level of uncertainty about the precise way a remarkably large number of drugs work by reading the "Clinical Pharmacology" section in the *PDR*. Very often, you encounter statements such as "The action of this drug appears to be related to the inhibition of...." or "This drug appears to act by blocking the conversion of...."

For example, the Clinical Pharmacology section for Diabeta (glyburide), a popular drug that is used to lower blood sugar in type 2 diabetes, begins (2001 *PDR*, p. 706):

Diabeta appears to lower the blood glucose acutely by stimulating the release of insulin from the pancreas....The mechanism by which Diabeta lowers glucose during long-term administration has not been clearly established.

In addition to its use as an antidepressant, Prozac (fluoxetine) is used to treat obsessive-compulsive disorder and bulemia. The Clinical Pharmacology section for Prozac begins (2001 *PDR*, p. 1127):

The antidepressant, antiobsessive-compulsive and antibulimic actions of fluoxetine are presumed to be linked to its inhibition of CNS [central nervous system] neuronal uptake of serotonin.

Ambien is a popular sleeping pill. The Clinical Pharmacology section for Ambien begins (2001 *PDR*, p. 2973):

Subunit modulation of the GABA$_A$ receptor chloride channel macromolecular complex is hypothesized to be responsible for sedative, anticonvulsant, anxiolytic, and myorelaxant drug properties.

Xanax is a popular drug used to treat anxiety. The Clincial Pharmacology section begins (2001 *PDR*, p. 2650):

CNS agents of the 1,4 benzodiazepine class presumably exert their effects by binding at stereo specific receptors at several sites within the central nervous system. Their exact mechanism of action is unknown.

The oftentimes surprising level of uncertainty in the Clinical Pharmacology section in the *PDR* stands in stark contrast to the soothing and simple way that drugs are portrayed in advertisements on television and in magazines and newspapers.

Most people are surprised to learn that, when someone swallows a drug, in most cases the drug travels to every part of the body. If you have a headache and take an aspirin, the aspirin doesn't know to go directly and exclusively to the brain. Instead, it goes to almost every part of the body, including the brain. If you take ibuprofen for a sprained ankle, you're getting plenty of ibuprofen in most other parts of the body also. The reason that drugs have so many side effects is that the level of sophistication of most drugs is far less than the average consumer assumes. Most drugs do not make a surgical strike on the intended target. Instead, they strike most cells in the body.

Pills cannot replace a few million years of evolution. The human body makes precise amounts of each substance it needs in response to highly complex and interrelated biochemical pathways and continuous internal feedback. This awesome internal regulatory system has been fine-tuned in the long course of human evolution. Every native substance in the human body has endless versatility and interconnectedness.

Most drugs are only available in two or three strengths. Indeed, drugs that need to be prescribed in precise amounts (for example, warfarin and levothyroxine are available in over a half dozen strengths) are seen as disadvantageous by the drug companies. Drug companies prefer something resembling a "one size fits all" approach because it makes the doctor's job easier. If a doctor is given a choice between prescribing a drug that is available in only one or two strengths, he is more likely to prescribe that drug than one requiring careful dosing among several available strengths.

Human health and energy fluctuate every day, yet, for most medications, the patient takes the same dose every day. Shouldn't the dose of medications fluctuate every day to mirror the constantly changing physiology, especially as regards conditions like hypertension, elevated cholesterol, and type 2 diabetes? The fact that they don't indicates the crudeness of most drug therapies.

The extreme fluidity of human physiology contrasts sharply with the extreme rigidity of most drug therapies. For example, some days I have a voracious appetite; other days I eat very little. Some days I have tremendous energy; other days I don't want to get out of bed. Some days I feel fine with seven hours of sleep; other days I need nine hours. In contrast to ever-changing human physiology, the dosing of drugs is surprisingly rigid. For most drugs, you take the same dose every day regardless of the season, the weather, the time of day, your energy level, etc. Big Pharma implies that taking drugs is the same as putting gasoline in your car's gas tank. But *Homo sapiens* is an extraordinarily complex living organism with constantly changing needs. Taking the same dose of a drug every day is contrary to biology. Do you drink precisely the same amount of fluids each day or eat precisely the same number of calories? The human body is continuously adjusting and fine-tuning itself in response to highly sophisticated feedback. The rigid nature of drug therapies for "chronic" conditions contrasts sharply with the highly refined feedback that our organs send to our brain on a constant basis.

Do you believe that human health results from encouraging and facilitating nature? Or do you believe that human health results from coercion of cells, tissues, and organs with powerful drugs? Is human health something that is nurtured with proper nutrition, or is it something that is imposed with potent drugs?

The pharmaceutical industry routinely utilizes war metaphors which imply the need for a steady supply of pharmaceuticals to ward off disease. (Examples: "war" on cancer, "fight" arthritis, "neutralize" excess acid, "kill" cancerous cells, "battle" high blood pressure, "overcome" depression, "control" cholesterol.) There is no concept that resonates deeper in the human psyche than war. Big Pharma taps into our reptilian brains by describing *Homo sapiens* as being in a constant battle against illness, requiring the weaponry available at the local drugstore. Big Pharma's marketing juggernaut has convinced Americans that health is dependent on *potent drugs* that fight disease, rather than on *education* that might prevent disease. Big Pharma is opposed to prevention the same way that the military-industrial complex prefers weaponry over diplomacy. In this society, the use of potent drugs is seen as masculine, powerful, and decisive, whereas prevention is seen as feminine, wimpy, and touchy-feely. Even though Big Pharma is completely invested in the belief that the attainment of health depends on a war on disease, there is one battlefield metaphor that Big Pharma avoids at all costs: referring to side effects of drugs as "collateral damage."

Big Pharma has absolutely no reverence for the endless complexity of the human body, preferring to promote the idea that human physiology is not very sophisticated, when, in fact, it has been fine-tuned over the millennia. The message of Big Pharma is that modern pharmaceuticals are more advanced than Mother Nature, when, in fact, precisely the opposite is true.

Pharmacy shelves consist in very large part of potent drugs that are classified as "blockers," "antagonists," or "inhibitors." These drugs block, antagonize, or inhibit delicate physiological processes and complex biological pathways, rather than actually heal some defect. Molecular and cellular processes that have been refined over the long course of human evolution are forced into submission with powerful drugs. The drug industry's justification for this mechanistic orientation presumes there are a large number of errors in human evolution that need correcting with potent pharmaceuticals. Some examples:

Antagonists:
1) Angiotensin II antagonists
2) 5-HT3 antagonists
3) Histamine-2 (H2) receptor antagonists

Blockers:
1) Alpha blockers
2) Beta blockers
3) Calcium channel blockers
4) Angiotensin receptor blockers
5) Neuromuscular blockers

Inhibitors:
1) Proton-pump inhibitors
2) COX-2 inhibitors
3) ACE inhibitors
4) Serotonin specific reuptake inhibitors
5) HMG-CoA reductase inhibitors
6) Phosphodiesterase inhibitors
7) Angiogenesis inhibitors
8) Monoamine oxidase inhibitors (MAO inhibitors)
9) Carbonic anhydrase inhibitors
10) Gonadotropin inhibitors
11) Cholinesterase inhibitors
12) Catechol-O-Methyl Transferase Inhibitors (COMT-inhibitors)
13) TNF-alpha inhibitors

If you look in the Product Category section in the *Physicians Desk Reference*, you will see that the overwhelming majority of drugs are *anti* drugs. These are drugs that fight some biological process. The pharmacy consists mainly of drugs that are *anti* disease rather than *pro* health. Some examples of categories of drugs in the *PDR* :

Anti-acne: Accutane, Benzac, Benzamycin, Cleocin T, Retin-A

Anti-anginal: Calan, Cardizem, Corgard, Inderal, Isoptin, Isordil

Anti-arrhythmics: Inderal, Norpace, Betapace, Procan SR, Quinidex

Anti-arthritics: Naprosyn, Orudis, Motrin, Clinoril, Indocin, Voltaren

Anti-asthma: Brethine, Ventolin, Proventil, albuterol, TheoDur, Slo-bid

Anti-coagulant: Coumadin, warfarin

Anti-depressants: Prozac, Zoloft, Wellbutrin, Desyrel, Elavil, amitriptyline

Anti-diabetic: Diabeta, Micronase, Glucotrol, Glipizide, Glyburide

Anti-diarrheals: Lomotil, Imodium, Pepto-Bismol, Donnagel, Kaopectate

Anti-enuresis (bedwetting): Tofranil

Anti-histamines: Claritin, Zyrtec, Benadryl, Tavist, Allegra

Anti-hyperlipidemics (cholesterol): Zocor, Lipitor, Pravachol, Mevacor, Crestor, Lopid, gemfibrozil, Questran

Anti-hypertensives: Calan, Capoten, Lopressor, Procardia, Vasotec, Tenormin

Anti-inflammatory: aspirin, ibuprofen, naproxen, Aristocort, Azmacort, Beconase, Lidex, Vancenase

Anti-migraine: Imitrex, Migranal, Cafergot, Inderal, Midrin, Wigraine

Anti-motion sickness: Dramamine, Bonine, Phenergan, Transderm-Scop

Anti-nauseants: Antivert, Atarax, Compazine, Thorazine, Tigan, Phenergan

Anti-neoplastics (cancer): Nolvadex, tamoxifen, Adriamycin, Cytoxan, fluorouracil

Anti-obesity: Fastin, Tenuate, Ionamin, Dexedrine, Meridia, Xenical

Anti-perspiration: Drysol

Anti-pruritics (itching): Aclovate, Atarax, Diprolene, Lotrisone, Topi-cort, Valisone

Anti-psoriasis: Balnetar, Denorex, Estar, Sebutone, Temovate, Zetar

Anti-psychotics: Haldol, Mellaril, Navane, Prolixin, Stelazine, Thorazine

Anti-pyretics (fever): aspirin, Tylenol, acetaminophen

Anti-seborrhea: Denorex, Ionil, Sebulex, Sebutone, Sulfacet-R, Pentrax

Anti-spasmodics: Bentyl, dicyclomine, Donnatal, Levsin, Librax

Anti-tussives (cough): Tussionex, Phenergan, codeine, dextromethor-phan

Perhaps nothing illustrates the crudeness of drugs more than their potential to cause liver damage and their potential carcinogenicity or mutagenicity.

Liver damage caused by drugs

The human body views most pharmaceuticals quite differently from the way in which it views foods. The human body views most pharmaceuticals as foreign and toxic substances that need to be detoxified by the liver and then eliminated via the kidneys (into the urine) and via the intestines (into the feces). The kidneys and the liver are the organs that suffer the brunt of the damage in the process of eliminating pharmaceuticals from the body. Greg Critser describes the damage that pharmaceuticals cause to the liver (*Generation Rx: How Prescription Drugs Are Altering American Lives, Minds, and Bodies,* Boston and New York: Houghton Mifflin Company, 2005, pp. 173-4):

But one thing is clear. In the new age of pharma, the liver is under attack, perhaps as no time in modern history, and some of the most respected voices in toxicology and hepatology have stepped forward to sound the alarm. While complete liver failure is still somewhat rare in the United States, liver injury is soaring, and drugs comprise an increasing percentage of the assault. As John. R. Senior, a veteran FDA expert on the subject, put it recently, "People are taking more and more drugs, both under prescription and by personal choice of OTC remedies, in addition to dietary or nutritional supplements... Perhaps as a consequence, drug-induced liver injury has become the leading cause for removal of approved drugs from the market, and for acute liver failure in patients evaluated at liver transplant centers in the United States."

Neil Kaplowitz, the co-editor of the most recent, comprehensive medical textbook, *Drug-Induced Liver Disease,* has even more fun news. "In the United States drug-induced liver disease is the most common cause of acute liver failure...a more frequent cause...than viral hepatitis and other causes." He goes on: "The frequency and economic impact...is a major problem for the pharmaceutical industry and the regulatory bodies, especially since the toxic potential of some drugs is not evident in...clinical testing." Kaplowitz, a professor at the University of Southern California, is particularly worried about the need for better testing, to which there are huge barriers. "To identify acute liver failure [in a new drug] with 95 percent confidence," he writes, "would require 30,000 study patients." Today most new drugs get by, thanks to the reforms of the 1980s and 1990s, with about 3,000.

What has been pharma's reaction? The industry is on the record as opposing any major requirement for expansion of trial populations. After all, they like to point out, about half of drug-induced liver injury, DILI for short, is caused by overdose of over-the-counter acetaminophen (like Tylenol), either intentionally (suicidal) or by "therapeutic misadventure" (among people who mindlessly take a handful a day for chronic pain). But that response is at best a dodge of the facts: an increasing percentage of DILI is provoked by prescription drugs, many of them the very prescription drugs for chronic diseases that we increasingly rely upon as lifelong helpmates and that we take properly, according to our doctors' instructions.

Carcinogenicty or mutagenicity of drugs

It should not be surprising that a huge number of drugs in the pharmacy can damage the liver to varying degrees because most of the drugs in the pharmacy are synthetic substances developed in a laboratory and never before seen on this planet. The liver is the primary organ that tries to detoxify these substances. Similarly, it should not be surprising that a huge number of drugs in the pharmacy have shown carcinogenic or mutagenic potential in lab animals. Even worse, some drugs are proven or suspected human carcinogens. See the National Toxicology Program's *Report on Carcinogens* which is updated every few years. (Search Google for *Report on Carcinogens* for the latest edition.)

The carcinogenicity and mutagenicity data in the official prescribing information is something that leaves a lot of health professionals scratching their heads. Why are so many commonly prescribed drugs associated with tumors in lab animals and, in many cases, humans? Thomas J. Moore discusses this issue in some detail in *Prescription for Disaster* (New York: Simon & Schuster, 1998). Moore states:

Despite the complexity of cancer causation, prescription drugs ought to be ranked second only to cigarette smoking as a cancer hazard. While certain industrial chemicals are more potent carcinogens than any drug, there are few chemical agents to which so many people are exposed at relatively high doses for great lengths of time. (p. 96)

...evidence suggests about half of prescription drugs are potentially carcinogenic. (p. 96)

With prescription drugs...animal cancers are often seen near the comparable human dose. This is because animals can rarely tolerate unrealisti-
cally large amounts of potent prescription drugs. With pesticide testing,
animals may not be able to tolerate an enormous dose, but humans
would be exposed to minute trace amounts on fruits, vegetables, or other
produce. However, humans typically ingest a drug continuously for many
years. Thus, when prescription drugs flunk their animal cancer tests, it is
often at exposures in the neighborhood of a typical human dose over
time. For example, salmon calcitonin, now being promoted as a long-
term treatment for osteoporosis in older women, caused cancer in both
rats and mice at lower doses than the manufacturer recommended for
humans. The aggressively marketed new calcium channel blocker Plendil
caused cancers in animals at 2.8 to 28 times the human dose in two years'
time. A typical patient would take Plendil for many years, and thus would
likely exceed the exposure that caused cancer in rats. The epilepsy drug
Depakene produced tumors in rats and mice at less than the human dosage. (pp. 97-98)

Some classes of drugs evidently carry special cancer risks. The survey
[quoted earlier in the chapter] showed that 83 percent of cholesterol-lowering drugs caused cancer in animals; 87 percent of the cancer chemotherapy agents tested were implicated. On the other hand, only half the
antibiotics and about 40 percent of the psychologically active drugs
flunked animal cancer testing. (p. 98)

Sometimes drugs get a clean bill of health on cancer for a dangerous reason: They are too toxic for the animals even at the human dosage. For
example, none of fourteen anti-inflammatory painkillers tested caused
cancer in animals. However, the animal tests had to be conducted at un-
realistically low doses because the drugs were so toxic to the gastrointestinal tract and kidneys—just as they are in humans. For example, Orudis
was so toxic to mice that they could tolerate only half the comparable
human dose. The animal tests for Anaprox, or naproxen, were only at 23

percent of the human dose because of the same toxicity problems. (p. 98)

For millions of people, prescription drugs are their greatest exposure to chemicals with the potential to cause cancer. About half of all approved drugs carry some cancer risk. (pp. 216-7)

Among the top 50 drugs, human evidence of cancer risk is reported for 4 drugs, animal evidence implicates another 12 drugs, and an additional 2 caused cell mutations. Among the best-selling drugs, 19 were apparently not tested for cancer risk. But let's give them the benefit of the doubt, counting only those drugs with scientific evidence of cancer risk. Therefore, 18 of the top 50 drugs have measurable cancer risks. Among the popular drugs with one of the above-noted cancer risks are Premarin, Mevacor, Dilantin, and Prilosec. These drugs provide benefits that may convince consumers to accept these cancer risks (if they even know about he danger). However, we can't call them safe drugs in the sense of being free of the risk of injury. (p. 32)

Chapter 28

When you're confused about medications

Why do my pills look different this time?

In general, when customers question the color or shape of the pills they receive at the pharmacy, the most common answer they're given by pharmacists and techs is that the medication is a generic equivalent or that it is made by a different company. This explanation is usually correct, but there are cases in which pharmacy clerks have given this answer even though they are clearly not qualified to do so.

When your medication looks different from what you were expecting, verify the contents with the pharmacist. Some pharmacy clerks have heard the "generic equivalent" or "different company" explanation so often that the clerks use it themselves reflexively when questioned by a customer. You need to know that newly hired pharmacy clerks may not clearly understand the ramifications of giving this explanation all the time. Many pharmacy clerks clearly do not have the experience or authority to make the determination whether your medication is a generic equivalent, whether it is made by a different company, or whether it is indeed an instance of the pharmacy dispensing the wrong drug. In most cases, the "generic equivalent" or "different company" explanation is correct. However, in some cases the drug the customer has received looks different because it is indeed the wrong medication.

The "generic equivalent" explanation often comes in very handy when there has indeed been a pharmacy error and the pharmacy staff tries to obfuscate this fact. I think it would be fair to say that a large number of pharmacists have used this explanation to cover up what is indeed a mistake. I've used this explanation myself to get out of a fix on more than one occasion. Here's the scenario: A customer brings her container back to me and asks why the pills look different from what she expected. My heart rate immediately goes into the danger zone as I experience another instance that pharmacists have nightmares about: *Another pharmacy error!!*

I have, on occasion, lied to such customers and said that the pills are "a generic." I've seen a few other pharmacists use the same lie. It gets us out of a very touchy situation. Most customers obviously don't know that we're lying to them. They trust us and accept our explanation.

Many pharmacists (myself included) feel that if the corporation provided us with adequate staffing, errors would be a rarity. Therefore, why should we, as pharmacists, offer our head on a platter by admitting an error and thus possibly prompting a lawsuit? It's so much easier to lie to the customer by telling him or her that it's a generic equivalent. Few pharmacists are eager to open a huge can of worms by admitting negligence. Of course, if we perceive that the customer may be at some risk as a result of the wrong medication, we are much less likely to engage in a cover-up. Most pharmacists tell the customer something like "I'll be happy to give you the brand you had before." This is an easy way for us to correct the error without the customer realizing that an error has indeed occurred. Let me emphasize that we do indeed correct the error when it is pointed out to us and, in the most serious instances, we notify the patient's doctor.

Certainly, lying to customers about the occurrence of an error is strictly against corporate policy. Corporate policy states that we should admit our error to the customer, apologize, give the customer a refund for the prescription, and give the customer the proper medication at no charge. Since many pharmacists blame the corporation for the environment in the drugstore that makes errors inevitable, many pharmacists question why should we have to endure the wrath of an angry customer ourselves and why should we make ourselves an easy target for a lawsuit.

I once worked with a pharmacist who was an absolute stickler for rules. He seemed to be one of those people who loved to follow rules to the *nth* degree. But one day I found out that he was actually selective about which rules he enforced. One day I observed him as he spoke with a customer who asked him why her pills looked different this time. He told her that they were a generic equivalent. He said, "They're a generic made by a different company but I'll give you the ones you've had before if you like." She answered "yes". So he gave her the proper pills. After she walked away, this pharmacist passed by me and said something like "Jim [a substitute pharmacist] gave her the wrong pills yesterday but I didn't want to get tangled in a big mess so I just told her that it was a generic." He wasn't necessarily proud of himself for lying but his attitude seemed to reflect the impossible position we pharmacists are placed in.

The point is that it is handy to use the "It's a generic" explanation in instances in which that is indeed the case, and also in instances in which a real error has occurred. William Winsley, executive director of the Ohio State Board of Pharmacy, comments on this tendency to freely use the "It must be a generic" explanation ("Are All Drug Errors System Errors?" *Drug Topics*, April 15, 2002, pp. 18, 20). He says that several cases of severe patient harm have resulted from using this explanation too freely:

When a patient calls the pharmacy and asks if the medication he just received is correct since it has a different color or shape than what he was expecting, the prudent pharmacist reviews the prescription, the patient record, and asks for the color, shape, and identifying marks on the dosage form received by the patient. In several cases this board [the Ohio State Board of Pharmacy] has dealt with, the pharmacist did none of these steps. Instead, he told the patient that the dosage form must have been a generic equivalent and should be safe to take. Several cases of severe patient harm have resulted, followed by board hearings, due primarily to the pharmacist's carelessness.

Here is an actual example of an error that occurred as a result of a pharmacy customer not questioning a change in medication appearance. In this case, methotrexate, an extremely powerful drug used for various conditions (rheumatoid arthritis, some forms of cancer, severe psoriasis), was mistakenly dispensed by a pharmacy instead of the blood pressure drug minoxidil. (Institute for Safe Medication Practices, "Medication Errors," *U.S. Pharmacist*, October 2006, p. 144)

As the number of generic products continues to increase, it seems that both patients and practitioners have become desensitized to changes in medication appearance. Patients may not even question a change, or if they do, practitioners may just reassure them that it was due to a change in manufacturer, without actively investigating the reason. It is not uncommon for ISMP [Institute for Safe Medication Practices] to receive reports from practitioners and consumers that a change in medication appearance was not fully investigated and subsequently contributed to an error.

In one case, a man shared an account of what his 86-year-old father experienced over the course of nine days after his prescription for minoxidil was mistakenly refilled with another medication. He had been taking minoxidil 2.5 mg for years, at a dose of 5 mg (two tablets) twice daily. Due to his failing vision, he did not realize that his minoxidil tablets looked different. His daughter noticed the change but was unconcerned, because the tablets had changed in appearance before. Within a few days, he began to experience a diminished appetite, complained of a sore throat, and felt like he was coming down with a cold. Soon after, he developed a rash on his face, had trouble maintaining his balance, and wished to remain in bed. When a family friend (a nurse) came to see him, she noticed a red, raised rash on his abdomen that looked like a medication rash. She was told that he was not taking any new medications, but that the minoxidil tablets looked different than before. The pharmacy was contacted about the change, and a staff member explained that it was a different generic for minoxidil and that the pills could be exchanged for those that the man usually received. There was no mention of a mistake being made when the medication was exchanged. He was taken to the hospital the next day, when he could barely walk. After the incident was explained to hospital staff, they contacted the pharmacy. It was revealed that the man had been given methotrexate by mistake, because the bottles were stored next to each other. By this time, he had taken

36 methotrexate 2.5 mg tablets, and he was in critical condition. We later learned that he died during the hospital visit.

How could this pharmacy mix-up have occurred? The pharmacy customer was taking minoxidil in the 2.5 mg strength. Sitting on the pharmacy shelf next to the minoxidil 2.5 mg tablets were methotrexate 2.5 mg tablets. Whenever two drug names are somewhat similar, and whenever those two drugs are available in the same strength (in this case 2.5 mg), and whenever those drugs are sitting on the pharmacy shelf next to each other (probably due to these drugs being shelved in alphabetical order), the opportunity for error increases significantly.

Identifying generic drugs is not as difficult as it used to be

Identifying generic drugs used to be much more difficult (for pharmacists and consumers) than identifying brand name drugs. Generic drugs are very often garden variety white tablets, i.e., they have few, if any, unique distinguishing characteristics that make them readily identifiable except for the product number which may be too small to read easily. The manufacturers of brand name products seem to take more pride in the appearance of their tablets and in making sure that the tablets don't crumble too easily. Brand name products are intentionally made with a unique appearance to gain patient loyalty and expectation. Customers ask the pharmacist, "I've been on this light blue blood pressure pill for two years. Why did you refill my prescription with red pills? Did the pharmacy make a mistake?" Sometimes the highly embarrassing answer is *yes.*

If all the tablets in the pharmacy were round and white like many generics, errors would probably be more frequent. The endless variation in shapes, sizes, and colors helps pharmacists and techs cut down on pharmacy errors. Customers often ask the pharmacist to identify a tablet. Tablets that are easy to identify are more likely to have a unique appearance. It is obviously helpful to have the name of the manufacturer on the pill. Most pills are imprinted with a product number. Some pills are imprinted with the brand name of the product, a practice which I wish all companies would adopt. In general—

but certainly not always—generic names are longer than brand names. This makes it more difficult to stamp long generic names like hydrochlorothiazide, methocarbamol, amitriptyline, or cyclobenzaprine on small tablets. Thus, it is often easier to identify brand name pills than generics. Generic tablets are much more likely to be unremarkable in appearance. Many generic pills are, however, quite distinct in their appearance.

In the last few years, websites have become available that greatly simplify the process of identifying tablets and capsules, whether they are brand name drugs or generics. Search Google for *pill identifier* and you will find several websites. For example: 1) drugs.com, 2) webmd.com, 3) healthline.com, and 4) healthtools.aarp.org, and 5) rxlist.com

Usually all that you have to do to identify your tablets and capsules is enter the numbers, letters, or words on those pills. Even though my mother died over ten years ago, I have kept all the pills that she was prescribed during her treatment for colon cancer that spread to her liver. I grabbed ten of those pill bottles containing mostly generic drugs and entered the numbers, letters, and words into the appropriate fields on the drugs.com website. I was quickly given the precisely correct identity of each pill. Below you will see the info I entered and the results:

1. 54 543   Correctly identified as Roxicet
2. Mylan 155   Correctly identified as generic Darvocet
3. SP 4220   Correctly identified as Niferex-150
4. Endo 602   Correctly identified as Endocet
5. INV 276 10   Correctly identified as prochlorperazine 10 mg
6. M 15   Correctly identified as generic Lomotil
7. Watson 349   Correctly identified as generic Vicodin
8. KU 108   Correctly identified as generic Levbid
9. MP 85   Correctly identified as generic Septra DS
10. OC 20   Correctly identified as Oxycontin 20 mg

It is not rare that adults ask pharmacists to identify some tablet or capsule found at home. In my career, sometimes I had the impression that this was a parent who had discovered that pill in his or her child's room or in the child's clothing while emptying pockets before doing laundry. I was somewhat uncomfortable under these circumstances because I suspected that if the pill I identified were a controlled substance, the son or daughter would soon be in for a world of hurt, i.e., confronted by a very angry parent.

Therapy duplication as a result of not knowing brand and generic drug names

Another issue regarding confusion with generic drugs involves what is known as "therapeutic duplication." It is extremely important that consumers learn both the brand and generic names of all their drugs so that they don't end up taking the exact same drug under two different names. For example, if you were taking the generic thyroid hormone levothyroxine and your doctor wrote you a prescription for Levothroid, Levoxyl, Euthyrox, or Synthroid, would you know that all of these are simply brand names for levothyroxine? If you were taking generic theophylline for asthma, and your doctor wrote you a prescription for Slo-Phyllin, Slo-bid, Theo-Dur, Theo-24, or Uniphyl, would you know that these are simply brand names for theophylline? If you were taking generic lithium carbonate for manic depression and your doctor wrote you a prescription for Cibalith, Eskalith, Lithobid, Lithotabs, or Lithonate, would you know that these are simply brand names for lithium carbonate? If you were taking Lanoxin for your heart and your doctor wrote you a prescription for digoxin, would you know that these are the same drug? If you were taking the blood thinner Coumadin and your pharmacy filled a new prescription for warfarin, would you know that these are the same drug?

Reports of concurrent use of digoxin and Lanoxin have been reported in the past, sometimes with unfortunate outcomes. Such situations tend to occur when the same medication is prescribed by brand name by one physician and by generic name by another physician, or when the medications are dispensed from different pharmacies. This problem is becoming more common as healthcare becomes increasingly fragmented. Dupont, manufacturer of the blood thinner Coumadin, says that several cases of therapeutic duplication have been reported to the company. In one case, a 69-year old female inadvertently taking both warfarin and Coumadin was admitted to the hospital with massive rectal and nasal bleeding and an international normalized ratio (INR) of 30.9. During her hospitalization, she suffered a myocardial infarction that was attributed to her blood loss. In another case, a patient received prescriptions for Coumadin from one physician and generic warfarin from another. She ended up hospitalized as a result of "bleeding from her ears and eyes." Fortunately, treatment with vitamin K resolved the patient's symptoms and she was subsequently discharged. (Susan Proulx, "Medication Errors," *U.S. Pharmacist,* June 1998, p. 95)

Whenever you receive a prescription for a drug that you're not familiar with, you should never assume that your doctor has put you on an entirely different medication. It could be the same drug under a different name. Pharmacists see many instances in which customers are not aware that indapamide is the same as Lozol, alprazolam is the same as Xanax, lorazepam is the same as Ativan, atenolol is the same as Tenormin, furosemide is the same as Lasix, gemfibrozil is the same as Lopid, piroxicam is the same as Feldene, methocarbamol is the same as Robaxin, etc.

Trying to decide whether you have a generic drug by comparing it to the brand name is usually a bad idea. Sometimes the generic name does resemble the brand name in some ways. For example, digoxin sounds somewhat like Lanoxin. Naproxen sounds a lot like Naprosyn. Cefaclor sounds like Ceclor. Clonazepam sounds a little like Klonopin. Roxicet and Percocet share "cet" (denoting aCETaminophen). Amoxicillin, Trimox, and Amoxil all share "mox." But in most cases, the generic name does not look anything like the brand name. For example, ranitidine shows absolutely no resemblance to Zantac. Guanfacine shows absolutely no resemblance to Tenex. Glyburide shows no resemblance to Diabeta or Micronase. Ketoprofen shows no resemblance or Orudis. Nortriptyline shows no resemblance to Pamelor.

Here's an actual case illustrating the confusion that can be caused by generic names. Attorney Dan Frith from the Frith Law Firm in Roanoke, Virginia, writes: ("Pharmacy Mistakes Kill," Feb. 13, 2008.

Accessed Feb. 28, 2008. http://roanoke.injuryboard.com/medical-malpractice/pharmacy-mistakes-kill.php?googleid=14934]

My law firm is getting ready to try a case against a local pharmacy which filled and dispensed a doctor's prescription for medication to which our client was allergic. You may ask, "Why did the client take a medication to which she knew she was allergic"? The answer is that she was given the generic form of the drug—the pills did not look the same and the generic name was nowhere close to the name of the medication to which she was allergic. The prescribing doctor has accepted his responsibility and paid money damages to our client but the pharmacy has not.

Falling through the cracks

Both of my parents were simply overwhelmed with the volume of medications their doctors prescribed during the last few months of their lives. When my mother was released from the hospital following colon cancer surgery, she was given a long list of drugs, most of which were simply for relief of symptoms. My mother was one of the most organized people in the world, but the sheer volume of pills she was supposed to take at home was very unsettling to her. She had difficulty understanding what each pill was used for and which ones were strictly for relief of symptoms. At one point as I watched her, she gagged as she was preparing to take more pills. She then told me she was no longer going to take any more of those pills unless they were absolutely critical.

My mother took very few prescription drugs until the few months of her life following her colon cancer diagnosis. Her colon cancer was not diagnosed until it was at an advanced stage and had spread to her liver. Even though many pharmacy customers are very knowledgeable about drug names and drug uses, my mother had little need during most of her life to gain such knowledge. So she was at a disadvantage after her cancer diagnosis when the number of prescribed drugs she was given increased dramatically.

At different points during the last six months of her life, she was prescribed four pain pills—Darvocet, Vicodin, Percocet, and Oxycontin—the first three of which were filled generically, increasing her confusion. The generic Darvocet was labeled PROPO-N/APAP 100-650. The generic Vicodin was labeled HYDROCO/APAP 5-500. The generic Percocet was labeled OXYCODONE/APAP. She did not know that Darvocet was the mildest of the pain pills. She did not know that Vicodin was intermediate. And she did not know that Percocet and Oxycontin were the strongest. She received the generic for Bactrim DS (labeled SMZ/TMP DS 800-160MG) but the label did not tell her that this drug was being used for her urinary tract infection. She received the generic for Levbid (HYOSCYAMINE 0.375 CR) with no indication on the label that these pills were for her stomach spasm and gastrointestinal cramps. She received Actigall with no indication on the label that these pills were being used to decrease her liver enzyme levels. She received the generic for Lomotil (DIPHEN/ATROP 2.5 MG) with no indication on the label that these pills were for diarrhea. She received Cipro with no indication on the label that these pills were for her urinary tract infection. She received Prilosec with no indication on the label that these pills were for stomach acid. She received the generic for Zyloprim with no indication on the label that these pills were being used to counter some of the effects of her chemotherapy.

My mother decided to write the intended use of each medication directly on each bottle. It would, of course, have been so much easier if the pharmacist or tech had typed the intended use on the label. But I do not blame the pharmacists or techs for not indicating on the label the precise use of each medication. If doctors don't specify the precise reason they are prescribing each drug, the pharmacist cannot simply take an educated guess as to why the doctor has prescribed the drug. So the pharmacist cannot add the intended use to the label unless the doctor indicates that on the prescription. For example, Actigall is usually used to dissolve gallstones, rather than to decrease liver enzymes. If the pharmacist had taken an educated guess and labeled the Actigall as being used to help dissolve gallstones, he would have been wrong in my mother's case.

Including the intended use on the label of each medication is not always desired by our pharmacy customers since family members, friends, and neighbors may notice these bottles lying around your house in your kitchen, bathroom, or elsewhere. When the medication is used to treat a sexually transmitted disease, clearly most people would prefer that this detail not appear on the label. I assume that some users of antidepressants don't want the phrase "for depression" on the label. Throughout my entire career, I don't recall ever including any of the following "indications" (intended uses) on customers' labels: "for psychosis," "for shyness," "for attention deficit/hyperactivity," "for excessive handwashing or other obsessive-compulsive behavior," "for AIDS," "for bedwetting," "for lice," "for erectile dysfunction," or "for cancer." Doctors usually specify the more formal "for loose stools" rather than "for diarrhea" and "for nasal congestion" rather than "for runny nose."

Our medical system functions best when patients are highly sophisticated and informed. This system essentially throws potent pills at people and expects everyone to understand their proper use. Yet every pharmacist knows that too many customers take medications incorrectly. For example, pharmacists routinely see customers return for a refill on their medications after, say, fifteen days when these customers were given a thirty day supply with instructions to take one tablet per day.

One Sunday a female customer in perhaps her thirties came to the pharmacy and told me that she was having severe pain in her abdomen. She told me that she had taken a very large number of the non-prescription analgesic Aleve over the previous few days in an attempt to relieve her stomach pain. She told me that she had been released from Duke Hospital in Durham, North Carolina a few days or weeks prior. I think she said she was at Duke for some type of abdominal problem, but I can't recall precisely. It appeared to me that it was possible that her severe abdominal pain could have been caused or exacerbated by her gross overuse of Aleve. Nonsteroidal anti-inflammatory drugs like Aleve and many others are well-known for their potential to cause stomach irritation with ulceration and/or gastrointestinal bleeding in more serious cases. Even though it was a Sunday afternoon, I asked her if it was okay for me to try to reach her doctor at Duke. She said that was okay and luckily her doctor happened to be at Duke when I called. When the switchboard operator connected me with her doctor, I briefly informed her doctor about this young lady's severe abdominal pain, then I handed the phone to this young lady. Her doctor proceeded to tell warn her about the risks of taking too many drugs like Aleve. My feeling was that this young lady needed to head straight for the emergency room. Unfortunately, I don't know how this story turned out but I think it illustrates how poorly so many pharmacy customers understand how easy it is to get into trouble with pharmaceuticals when they're not used properly.

I suspect that many pharmacists have reached the conclusion that it is unrealistic to expect all of our customers to be able to follow the manufacturer's directions on non-prescription labels. Clearly many pharmacy customers have difficulty understanding the directions that pharmacists and techs type on prescription labels. Regardless how much verbal counseling pharmacists provide, and regardless how much written information we provide, some of our customers simply do not seem to be able to manage their medications properly. In the real world, millions of users of prescription drugs have extreme difficulty managing their medications because they have diminished eyesight and mental acuity, because they are marginally literate or illiterate, because English is not their native language, etc.

Pharmaceuticals are potent substances that require competent prescribers and competent patients who are capable of understanding and following directions on labels. We have a sophisticated medical system in this country based on complexity. It appears to me that millions of people in this country fall through the cracks in our complex system every day.

Here's an example from the Institute for Safe Medication Practices of the kind of confusion that pharmacists see all the time, especially among elderly patients. In this example, an elderly patient died after chewing a medication that was not supposed to be chewed. ("To Chew, Or Not To Chew? Patient Dies After Chewing Medication," Institute for Safe Medication Practices, Accessed March 7, 2008 http://www.ismp.org/Newsletters/consumer/alerts/chewable.asp) With the McDonald's model of pharmacy, incidents like this are inevitable.

Some medications should never be chewed, cut, crushed, or diluted. The only way to know is to read label instructions carefully and/or ask your pharmacist or physician how each drug should be taken. Unfortunately, not all patients read the directions or receive and follow this kind of advice from health providers. The following case illustrates the dangers when patients are not given appropriate instructions or do not question how to take medication.

An 83-year-old patient was given Cardizem CD (sustained release diltiazem capsules) for blood pressure control. Because the capsule was too large to swallow, the patient chewed the medication. As a result, her pulse twice slowed to low levels and the family contacted the pharmacist for advice. Upon learning that she was chewing the medication, the pharmacist suggested that the physician substitute immediate release diltiazem tablets, which are easier to swallow. The prescription was changed and the patient did well for several months

Months later the patient returned to her physician for a check up. She was again put on Cardizem CD because the physician apparently did not review the patient's previous medication use and neither the patient nor her caregiver reminded the doctor about the prescription change. Since the patient had either forgotten or never been warned about the danger of chewing Cardizem CD, she again began chewing the larger capsules. She became progressively weaker and died three weeks later. According to her family, the patient had been alert and intelligent but had too much faith in her health providers to question their instructions.

Why does my prescription say simply "Take as directed"?

Have you ever obtained a prescription medication from your pharmacy with the following directions printed on the label that is attached to the vial or bottle: "Take as directed"? These three simple words appear on your prescription label for one of two reasons. The most common reason is because that is precisely what your doctor specified. Supposedly the doctor told you how to use the medication during your office visit, or you've been on the medication for some period and you're familiar with how to take it. But there is also an interesting second reason why the three words "Take as directed" appear on your prescription label. If the pharmacist can't read your doctor's handwriting, and the pharmacist doesn't have the time or desire to contact your doctor's office for clarification, the pharmacist may simply punt and type "Take as directed" on your prescription label.

The nice thing about this, from the pharmacist's perspective, is that it is (or has been—see below) basically legal in addition to being extremely convenient. In other words, "Take as directed" is (or has been) a legally accurate statement in which the pharmacist (if he can't read the doctor's prescription) is telling you *Just take the damn medication like your doctor told you!* I've read a few commentaries written by pharmacists or pharmacy professors stating that use of the "Take as directed" shortcut is not good pharmacy practice and that the pharmacist should make every effort to contact the physician before resorting to the "Take as directed" cop-out.

Of course, when the pharmacist can't read the doctor's directions but goes ahead and types "Take as directed" on your prescription label, the pharmacist is doing you no favor. The pharmacist is attempting to place the ball in your court, hoping that you will call the doctor's office yourself for clarification if you forgot how the doctor told you to take the drug.

When there is grossly inadequate staffing in the pharmacy, the pharmacist's use of "Take as directed" is understandable but, in the eyes of many pharmacists, regrettable. I would predict that nearly every community pharmacist in America has had at least a few instances wherein he or she was so slammed with prescriptions that he or she simply punted and typed "Take as directed" on the prescription label. I've done it myself more times than I am proud to admit—at least once a month, I would guess.

Some pharmacists are uncomfortable punting the ball like this, while other pharmacists seem to be totally fine with it. The latter group rationalizes the situation as follows: *If the doctor doesn't take the time to write clearly and if my employer doesn't provide enough staffing for clearing up problems like this, why should I care?* With adequate staffing in pharmacies, shortcuts like this would be less necessary.

So if you receive a prescription medication from your pharmacy with the directions "Take as directed" on the label and you are confused about this, consider the two major possibilities: 1) Your doctor told you how to take this medication during your office visit and you simply forgot what he said, or 2) Your pharmacy couldn't read your doctor's handwriting and your pharmacist didn't have the time or desire to contact your doctor for clarification.

It appears that the "Take as directed" or "Use as directed" shortcut may indeed get the pharmacist into trouble in the event of a lawsuit stemming from a customer's confusion about how to take or use the prescribed medication. Jesse Vivian, a professor at the Wayne State University Collge of Pharmacy with degrees in pharmacy and law, wrote three full pages on this subject in the February 2012 issue of *U. S. Pharmacist*. Vivian describes a lawsuit against a pharmacist involving the "Use as directed" directions and a customer's confusion and harm after a change in warfarin dosage. Vivian suggests that the courts may be heading toward holding pharmacists partly liable for parroting the doctor's directions and typing on the label, "Take as directed" or "Use as directed." Vivian says the pharmacist should always clarify the directions with the prescriber. He states, "It's time to finally end the confusing practice of putting 'Use as directed' on prescriptions." (page 60). And he concludes by saying "It is way past time for this nonsense to end." (page 67). (See also, David B. Brushwood, "As directed prescription exposes pharmacy to liability," *Pharmacy Today*, 2011; 17(7): 24)

Request a print-out when your doctor transmits your prescription to your pharmacy

Whenever you are at your doctor's office and he tells you that he will transmit your prescription to your pharmacy, you should request a print-out of that prescription so you'll know what to expect when you pick up that medication at the pharmacy. Here is a possible real world scenario from *Pharmacy Times* (Michael J. Gaunt, Pharm.D., "Electronic Prescribing: Potential Areas of Weakness," *Pharmacy*

Times, published online Oct. 15, 2009 http://pharmacytimes.com-
/issue/pharmacy/2009/october2009/MedicationSafety-1009)

A girl was recently taken to a doctor by her parents for evaluation of a skin rash. The doctor prescribed a topical corticosteroid, using a handheld device to place the order electronically. He had asked the couple which pharmacy they'd like to use, which seemed very efficient, except for one issue: the doctor never told the family exactly which drug he was prescribing. He just instructed the parents to pick up the medication at their community pharmacy.

This raises an important question when prescriptions are sent electronically to a pharmacy: How will the patient know what they are supposed to receive, if they are not told the prescribed medication, strength, and directions for use, and given a written copy of the information to compare with the dispensed medication?

In this situation, electronic prescribing (e-prescribing) may lead to an unintended weakness in the system if the patient does not know what to expect when he or she picks up prescriptions at the pharmacy. Ideally, with e-prescribing, patients should receive verbal instructions from the prescriber, be given an opportunity to ask questions, and also be provided with a corresponding voucher listing the prescribed medication, dose, and directions for use. This way, the patient can use the information to check the prescription in the pharmacy by matching the voucher to what he or she actually receives to assure it is correct.

For Spanish-speaking customers, prescriptions translated from English to Spanish can result in dangerous confusion

Here's a common scenario: Say a doctor's prescription for a Hispanic patient has a standard abbreviation that doctors use for all of their patients. Say the doctor indicates on the prescription pad, "1 tab tid." This means "1 tablet three times a day." Most pharmacy computers are programmed to recognize Latin abbreviations like "tid." So, for example, in this case, the pharmacist might enter the following into the computer: "T 1 T TID." The computer will translate this to "Take 1 tablet three times a day" when it prints on the customer's label.

Many pharmacists routinely instruct the computer to translate the directions to Spanish for our Hispanic customers, thinking we're helping those customers. But, according to an article on Health-Day.com, this translation can be unclear, resulting in a hazardous situation. For simple directions like "Take one tablet three times a day," the pharmacy computer probably does a pretty good job in translating this to Spanish. But, in a very large number of cases, the doctor's directions are not so simple and straightforward, resulting in confusing translations.

I was never a big fan of the computer's translation skills when translating from Latin or English to Spanish. I never felt comfortable dispensing a prescription for which I had no idea whether the directions on the label were clear to our customers, or worse, inaccurate. So I think I never translated a doctor's directions from Latin or English to Spanish, even for the simplest directions like "Take one tablet 3 times a day." My hope was that these Hispanic customers would show the label to a bilingual person who could read English directions and translate those directions to Spanish. From the HealthDay News article (D. Thompson, "Prescriptions Translated to Spanish Could Be Hazardous to Health: Computer Translation Programs Give Confusing, Incomplete Instructions, Study Finds," HealthDay.com, April 8, 2010

http://consumer.healthday.com/Article.asp?AID=637694):

Many Spanish-speaking people in the United States receive prescription instructions from the pharmacy so poorly translated that the medications are potentially hazardous to their health, a new study shows.

The errors occur largely because of deficiencies in computer programs that most pharmacies rely on to translate medication information from English to Spanish, said lead researcher Dr. Iman Sharif, chief of the division of general pediatrics at the Nemours/Alfred I. duPont Hospital for Children in Wilmington, Del.

"The technologies that are currently available to produce instructions in the patient's language are inadequate," Sharif said.

Half of the Spanish-language prescription labels reviewed for the study contained errors, and some of those errors could result in life-threatening situations if misinterpreted by the patient, Sharif said.

The study is published in the May [2010] issue of *Pediatrics*.

Of the New York City pharmacies surveyed that provide Spanish-language labels, more than four of every five used a computer program to translate their labels from English to Spanish. Nearly all the pharmacies said they had someone double-check the labels for errors, but researchers found dozens of examples of poorly translated instructions.

A common problem was "Spanglish," Sharif said. The programs produced a mix of English and Spanish on the labels, creating confusing and difficult-to-read instructions.

The use of "Spanglish" also created some potentially dangerous situations. For example, the word "once" means "eleven" in Spanish. "You mean to say 'once,' as in 'take once a day,' and a Spanish-speaking person could interpret that to mean 'eleven,'" Sharif said. Such a mistake could result in an overdose.

Other phrases that weren't accurately translated include "dropperfuls," "apply topically," "for seven days," "for 30 days," "apply to affected areas," "with juice" and "take with food."

Misspellings also created errors. Incorrect use of the word "poca" for the word "boca" meant patients were told "by the little" instead of "by the mouth." One set of instructions included "dos besos," which means "two kisses"; the intended instructions likely were "dos veces," which means "two times."

Poor translations specifically cited in the study included:
• "Take 1.2 aldia give dropperfuls with juice eleven to day."
• "Taking 0.6 mL 2 times to the day by the little with juice."
• "Apply to affected area twice to the indicated day like."

Dr. David Flockhart, director of the division of clinical pharmacology at the Indiana University School of Medicine in Indianapolis, said it's not surprising that these computer-generated errors are occurring.

"Word-for-word, you probably could get it right, but you can't get the entire sense of what's being communicated through a computer program," Flockhart said.

Confusing label directions can be deadly

In my 25-year career as a pharmacist, I saw a huge number of instances in which pharmacists and techs typed unclear or confusing label directions. I blame two factors: 1) Some pharmacists and techs are simply careless and don't really care whether the label directions are easy to follow. These pharmacists and techs see their job as one of quantity rather than quality. 2) The big pharmacy chains and indeed our entire health care system find increased profits in understaffing. This understaffing makes it much more difficult for pharmacists and techs to do our jobs with a degree of professionalism that the public assumes and expects.

Auburn University School of Pharmacy is one of the leading centers in America for the study of pharmacy errors. In 2007 several professors at this pharmacy school cooperated with ABC News' *20/20* in an undercover investigation of pharmacy mistakes. A total of 100 pharmacies in Atlanta, Tampa-St. Petersburg-Clearwater, and New York City-Newark were randomly selected for the study. Trained patient actors presented a new prescription for one of several study drugs to each pharmacy. (E. Flynn, K. Barker, et. al., "Dispensing Errors and Counseling Quality in 100 Pharmacies—Study Summary," Auburn University School of Pharmacy, March 30, 2007 abcnews.go.com/images/WNT/ross_auburn_final_summary.pdf)
With an estimated 3.8 billion prescriptions filled in America each year, the hundred prescriptions filled during this undercover investigation represent an infinitesimally small percentage. Nevertheless, potentially serious errors were discovered in this tiny investigation. For example, out of this sample of a hundred prescriptions, the study found two prescriptions that were filled with directions that were quite unclear and potentially dangerous.

One significant error involved the blood-thinner Coumadin. Coumadin is potentially the most dangerous drug in the drugstore. This drug a) must be dosed precisely by doctors, b) must be filled precisely by pharmacy staff, and c) must be taken by patients precisely according to directions. If the dose of Coumadin is too high, the patient can hemorrhage or bleed to death. If the dose is too low, clotting could occur which could have devastating consequences. The Auburn study noted the following with regard to the unclear directions on the label for Coumadin: "...the instructions on a Coumadin prescription read 'Take 1 tablet by mouth daily as needed' instead of 'Take 1 tablet by mouth every day and as directed.'"

Taking Coumadin "as needed" is absurd and potentially deadly. This is like handing a loaded gun to a patient. Blood thinners like Coumadin are absolutely unlike drugs that can indeed be taken "as needed" such as some pain pills.

Another significant error discovered in this study involved the incomplete or truncated directions that the pharmacy staff typed on the label for the insulin product Novolog:

[Another] significant error was on a label for Novolog Mix 70/30 insulin where the instructions were cut off. The label read "Inject 15 units subcutaneously 15 minutes before breakfast, and 15 units 15 minutes", leaving off "before dinner." The incomplete instructions may result in the patient injecting the second dose at an inappropriate time, leading to high or low blood sugars.

Why were parts of the directions cut off? The most likely explanation is that the directions exceeded the maximum number of characters the computer allows in the "directions" field. Computers are great for many things but they can introduce an entirely new set of potential errors that did not occur twenty or thirty years ago when pharmacists used typewriters to type directions on labels. When pharmacists using typewriters ran out of room on labels, this would be immediately obvious to the pharmacist. However, computers facilitate the filling of prescriptions at lightning speed without notifying pharmacists/techs that the maximum number of characters in the directions has been exceeded. In my experience, the computer merrily proceeds to print the label without informing the pharmacist or tech that part of the directions were cut off. Bells and whistles don't sound when things like this occur.

Here's one example from my career that stands out in my mind. One day a customer returned to the pharmacy for a refill on triamcinolone cream. Triamcinolone is a cortisone-type drug used for a variety of skin conditions. I happened to look at the directions that were typed on the label by another pharmacist who was filling in at our store. It is possible that the directions had been typed by a pharmacy technician and the pharmacist on duty failed to check the directions. (Pharmacists arc responsible for all the work done by technicians.) The pharmacist on duty may have failed to insist that a tech make the directions clearer to the patient. The pharmacy label directions for this triamcinolone cream read *exactly* as follows: "Apply thin film twice daily *times two (2) weeks,* then *as reduce* as tolerated. Avoid mucous *memb* and genitals." I have added bold italic type to indicate the parts that I consider to be unclear or confusing.

Here is how this label should have been typed to be clearer to the customer: "Apply a thin film twice a day for 2 weeks, then reduce as tolerated. Avoid mucous membranes and genitals."

The errors that I find in the original label are as follows: 1) I looked at the doctor's original handwritten prescription. The doctor wrote "X 2 weeks." The pharmacist or tech should have transcribed this as "for two weeks" rather than "times two weeks." It is simply easier to understand "for" rather than "times." 2) The pharmacist or tech has a grammatical error (or typographical error) when he or she typed "then as reduce as tolerated." The first "as" should not have been there. 3) The pharmacist or tech should have typed out the word "membrane" rather than use the shorthand "memb." Not everyone knows what a "mucous membrane" is but even fewer people know what a "mucous memb" is.

What reaction does the customer have when reading this label? Does she know what "times two weeks" means? Does she see the poor grammar? Does she know what "mucous memb" means?

Here are two examples from the *North Carolina Board of Pharmacy Newsletter* in which a pharmacist or tech typed unclear directions. The consequences in these two examples are far more serious than one would expect from confusion in the above example involving triamcinolone cream. A patient died, at least in part as a result of not understanding the directions. The drug involved in this patient's death was methotrexate, a potentially risky drug even when taken properly. (*North Carolina Board of Pharmacy Newsletter,* Item 846–Critical Doses, October 1995, p.4)

A patient received a prescription to treat psoriasis, which was written for methotrexate 2.5 mg with the directions stating, "Two tablets every 12 hours for three doses each week." The patient who was marginally literate had her husband pick up the prescription. He customarily asked store clerks to make out his checks for him, which is one of the cardinal signs of a marginally literate or illiterate patient. …The patient consumed two tablets every 12 hours for six consecutive days until she was hospitalized. She eventually expired.

The patient obviously understood the directions as two tablets every 12 hours each day in contrast to what the physician had intended. The prescriber meant for her to take two tablets one day in the morning, two tablets 12 hours later in the evening, and two tablets the next morning. The directions were obviously unclear and subject to several different interpretations. The patient's death was due, at least in part, to methotrexate toxicity.

The same issue of the *North Carolina Board of Pharmacy Newsletter* describes another incident in which the label directions were incorrectly understood and resulted in another patient's death. This incident involved another powerful drug, melphalan. Melphalan is used to treat multiple myeloma and ovarian cancer. (*North Carolina Board of Pharmacy Newsletter*, Item 846—Critical Doses, October 1995, p. 4)

…a prescription for melphalan whose directions were for the patient to consume six tablets for four days each month was incorrectly understood by the patient. The decedent took two consecutive courses for a total of 48 doses, and expired due to the melphalan overdose.

When you pick up your prescription medications from the drugstore and you look at the directions typed on your label(s) by pharmacists/techs, don't assume that you must be dumb for not clearly understanding how your doctor intends for you to take those medications. Due to the assembly-line nature of pharmacy today, pharmacists and techs too often don't have the time to make sure that the directions are easily understandable. Call the pharmacist and ask him or her to clarify the directions. You're not stupid. Unclear or confusing label directions are much more common than you know. The chains' focus on quantity rather than quality means that too many drugstores in America are an accident waiting to happen.

PART VIII

COMMUNICATION OF DRUG INFORMATION

Chapter 29

Counseling: How much verbal information do you need from your pharmacist?

Try explaining the pharmacy counseling law to a non-pharmacist. Good luck.

A federal law passed in 1990 called the Omnibus Budget Reconciliation Act (OBRA '90) contains a provision stating that pharmacists must offer to counsel our customers on new prescriptions. Here are some questions I commonly get when I try to explain this counseling regulation to family members and non-pharmacist friends.

What does it mean that pharmacists must offer to counsel customers?
We must offer to discuss their medications.

That seems awfully vague. What specifically do you have to discuss?
Here's what a pharmacist-lawyer at the University of Florida College of Pharmacy says (David B. Brushwood, R.Ph., J.D, "The pharmacist's legal duty to counsel patients," *Drug Topics*, April 17, 2006, p. 56):

According to the OBRA '90 standard, pharmacists must offer to discuss prescribed medications with patients or family caregivers. The subject of the discussion is up to the individual pharmacist. The flexible requirement

is that the discussion between the pharmacist and the patient must pertain to matters deemed significant by the pharmacist. These matters may include common side effects, techniques for self-monitoring, and action to be taken in the event of a missed dose, if the pharmacist deems them significant. Patients or their family caregivers may refuse consultation if they wish.

If customers accept the offer to be counseled, we can tell them such things as the purpose of the drug, the most common side effects, how to take the drug (like the number of times per day), whether or not to take it with food, what foods to avoid while on the medication, how to store the medication, what to do if they miss a dose, and things like the necessity to refrigerate, shake well, avoid sunlight, etc.

Sometimes I've concluded that no verbal communication is best. I've always felt that written information is better because most people don't remember what we tell them or they are confused by what we tell them or they mistakenly do precisely opposite what we tell them. For example, some antibiotics are not supposed to be taken with milk. I have felt that some of our customers are so easily confused that, once at home, they'll remember only that I mentioned milk so they'll take it *with* milk. So I've felt sometimes that the best verbal instructions I can give are no verbal instructions. If pharmacists have the right to decide what we deem relevant, it seems to me that we ought to be able to decide when it is best to leave well enough alone. For example, in this case, we usually put a "Do not take with milk" sticker on the prescription vial. The right to tell customers what we feel is best for them should also include the right to *not* counsel customers whom we feel will be confused.

In my opinion, written information in the quiet of the customer's home is the simplest and clearest communication. I've always found written information to be much more helpful than trusting my recollection of what someone tells me. After I speak with a dentist or mechanic, I always write down their recommendations for what work needs to be done. Whenever I call my car insurance agent or bank, I always take notes. I don't recall a customer ever taking notes when I counsel them.

You've told me that you don't have time to eat lunch or go to the bathroom. Do you have time for a discussion with each of your customers?

Absolutely not. And many customers aren't interested anyway. Many customers just want to get their drugs and go home or go to the supermarket or go to work. Most pharmacists just have time to say something like "Be careful. This medication may make you drowsy."

How could the federal government pass a law that's so vague?

Most pharmacists don't realize that the idea for the OBRA counseling regulation originated in the pharmacy community with the National Community Pharmacists Association (NCPA), the trade group that represents independent pharmacists. (The National Association of Chain Drugstores represents the chains.) Contrary to the belief of many pharmacists, the impetus for this regulation did not originate with the federal government. Certain leaders at NCPA approached members of Congress and requested that the offer to counsel become law. Prior to that, the federal government showed no interest in whether pharmacists counseled. NCPA felt that the counseling requirement would give the profession more respect and would help to convince certain payers that pharmacists do much more than transfer pills from big bottles to little bottles. Pharmacists are trying to convince insurance companies and the general public that we should be paid for our counseling, just like you pay a doctor or lawyer for a consultation.

What reaction do customers have when they're asked if they want to be counseled by the pharmacist?

Most customers don't really understand what they're being asked. Often a technician or clerk will simply ask the customer, "Do you have any questions for the pharmacist?" And customers don't understand why we're requiring them to sign a counseling log. They think they need to sign the log to indicate that they've received their prescriptions. Most customers don't know the log has anything to do with accepting or declining the offer to be counseled by the pharmacist.

What if the prescriptions are picked up at the drive thru window?

We have to fight the noise from the car engine, from the car radio, and from the children screaming or crying. Unless we have a secure drive thru with pneumatic tubes like at a bank drive-thru, we end up inhaling a good dose of fumes from the auto exhaust.

What if a 16-year-old son or daughter picks up the prescriptions? How do you counsel them?

We don't. Some pharmacists throw a few words at them like "Tell your mother to take this antibiotic until it's all gone." I don't know whether there are any statistics on this but I bet that around half the time the person picking up the prescription is not the actual person for whom the prescription was filled. It is often the spouse or teen-age son or daughter. Counseling a family member is usually very problematic because that person may have less interest in what I have to say.

Some state boards of pharmacy enforce the counseling law more aggressively than other state boards. Some state boards send under-cover inspectors around to pharmacies to see whether we offer to counsel customers. Pharmacists who don't offer to counsel can be cited by the state board and fined. A pharmacist in Wisconsin sent me an e-mail saying he had just received a citation for failure to counsel. He told me that he was hit with a fine of $250.00 and $400.00 in court costs. He wrote:

When the inspector introduced herself after this so-called violation, I felt like I was caught in an ambush. I was FURIOUS. And like a cornered cat, the hair on my back stood up. I had to calm myself down before calling the prosecuting attorney, so that I would be polite when I informed her that the terms of the citation were not acceptable and I would be seeking legal counsel to fight these charges.

Later this pharmacist e-mailed me:

I did seek the advice of legal counsel. I faxed the info to him and he looked it over. He agreed that it was nitpicking, but he looked up the stat-

ute and stated that "They got you, and while it is a picky little matter, it is their way of showing you that they are in charge." The lawyer also stated that the $400.00 court fee is "made up" and that, if I have a hearing, the court fee will be $1200.00 whether I win or lose!!!

With the slight possibility that an undercover board of pharmacy inspector is watching me, I usually throw a few words at whatever family member happens to pick up the prescription. That is, unless I'm really stressed out, or really exhausted, or mad at the world, or the person picking up the prescription appears highly unlikely to remember a single word I say. I don't really know what the OBRA counseling regulation has to say with regard to what is required of pharmacists when a family member or friend or neighbor picks up the prescription. That is a vague part of a very vague law.

I wonder whether there are lots of other laws that Congress passes that are as vague as the law that requires pharmacists to offer to counsel customers on new prescriptions. Laws like this breed cynicism among pharmacists because we don't have enough staffing to allow us to tell our customers nearly as much as we would like. This is the first law I've ever heard of that requires someone to do what he feels is right, i.e., to tell customers whatever the pharmacist thinks is important. This is like a law for highway safety that states "You are not allowed to exceed the speed limit but you are allowed to determine what the speed limit should be."

Lawyers are having a field day with this law, increasingly accusing pharmacists of negligence for anything negative that occurs as a result of drug therapy. Once we initiate the act of counseling a customer, lawyers say we have a duty to be complete in our answer. For example, if we tell a customer that the medication can cause drowsiness, lawyers will accuse us of negligence for not telling that customer every other possible adverse effect.

Mail order pharmacists are exempt from the requirement to verbally offer to counsel customers—as long as these mail order pharmacists provide their customers with a toll-free number. Many pharmacists wonder why the exemption allowing mail order pharmacists to have a toll-free number doesn't apply to all pharmacists. The law seems to be picking on community pharmacists and giving special leniency to mail order pharmacists. Whatever happened to the "equal protection" clause in the U.S. Constitution which states that all citizens shall be treated equally? Many community pharmacists are angry that mail order pharmacists have this exemption from the counseling regulation. Mail order pharmacists are given this exemption because they obviously can't provide face-to-face communication with someone who lives hundreds or thousands of miles away. I suspect that many pharmacists working for the big chain drugstores feel we deserve an exemption because we're not given enough staffing to allow us time for counseling.

The fact that the trade group representing independent pharmacists pushed for a counseling regulation is a sign of the weakness and vulnerability of community pharmacists. Pharmacists see that mail order pharmacy is growing rapidly. We see that the big pharmaceutical companies and the big drugstore chains would like to decrease the role of pharmacists. We see that the market views pharmaceuticals like widgets. Bruce Roberts, executive VP-CEO of the National Community Pharmacists Association, describes the threat to the future of retail pharmacists (Carol Ukens, "R.Ph.s must act to protect profession," *Drug Topics*, March 20, 2006):

> **Outside forces, including politicians, the government, and pharmacy benefit managers are trying to turn medications into just another commodity and to disenfranchise retail pharmacy, said Roberts. "It's painfully obvious what's up with regard to pharmacy. I don't think we'll be able to continue down this path and have a sustainable model for the long term. Mail order is growing like crazy. People believe that all we're selling is widgets, nothing that inherently needs the guidance of a pharmacist. If we're just a business model competing head-to-head with mail order, it doesn't bode well for the future."**

When an industry or profession finds itself at risk, it often seeks government protection, as NCPA did with OBRA. The community drugstore model is endangered by mail order pharmacies, so NCPA sought to shore up the status of the independent pharmacy by requiring that pharmacists voluntarily offer to counsel our customers. However, many of the state boards of pharmacy were not happy with such an amorphous regulation. Some state boards wanted a regulation with more teeth. Even though NCPA wanted a voluntary regulation requiring the offer to counsel customers, many state boards have aggressively gone after pharmacists who do not offer to counsel customers. Many pharmacists view this as a power play by the state boards to increase their visibility and influence. (Similarly, many pharmacists view the requirement that all graduating pharmacists now have a doctorate as a power grab by the schools of pharmacy.)

The big pharmaceutical manufacturers ("Big Pharma") feel that pharmacists are unnecessary middlemen between the doctor and the patient. Big Pharma prefers the model of mail order pharmacy where prescription drug orders are filled the same way that Amazon.com fills orders for books. To Big Pharma, a pharmacist's advice or guidance are unnecessary. Big Pharma promotes the idea that pharmaceuticals are no different from any other consumer product: no more complicated, no less safe. Big Pharma does not believe that consumers of pharmaceuticals need pharmacists' counseling or drug information leaflets explaining proper use, side effects, etc. Big Pharma thinks that all the customer needs to know is, for example, "Take one tablet three times a day." Possible side effects? Drugs don't cause side effects!!

Many pharmacists feel that the writing is on the wall, that the future of the community pharmacist is in jeopardy, that market forces will continue to minimize the role of the pharmacist, and that we'll end up working as a drone at some huge mail order facility. Even though the big chains are opening up shiny new drugstores on every corner, corporate management at those chains would like to staff the stores with the smallest possible number of pharmacists, preferring less expensive techs and robotics instead. The big chains certainly don't want their pharmacists spending time advising customers. The big chains feel that counseling is a major drag on productivity. The big chain drugstores never embraced the OBRA counseling regulation. The big chains have never felt that they have a duty to educate our customers. When the Wisconsin pharmacist who was cited for failure to counsel wrote to me, he said that when he informed his supervisor of the citation, the supervisor said, "Bullshit."

Counseling in the real world

Let me make it perfectly clear that, if I had adequate staffing, I would be 100% in favor of counseling. All the arguments in favor of counseling are absolutely correct. Counseling saves lives. Lots of errors are caught during counseling. I agree that many customers are in a complete fog about their medications and counseling can clear this up. Pharmacists: How many times have you had a customer ask you, "What's this drug used for?" How many times have you wondered how someone could leave his doctor's office without really understanding the purpose of the medication his doctor has prescribed?

My techs tell me that I spend too much time talking to customers. To be honest, I'd much rather counsel customers than fill prescriptions. Running the computer and counting pills can be boring while counseling can be fulfilling. I'd much rather interact with customers all day than stare at a computer. Unless a pharmacist suffers from what Big Pharma terms "social anxiety disorder" (a.k.a., shyness), counseling is the easiest job in the pharmacy. With each of our customers' patient leaflets in front of us, counseling should be a breeze. I am totally exhausted at the end of most days when I fill two hundred prescriptions, but I bet if I did nothing but counsel all day, I'd feel like I had the day off.

Most pharmacists would desperately love to thoroughly counsel every customer. The boards of pharmacy seem incapable of understanding that basic reality. They seem to be incapable of understanding that the reason we don't counsel is not because we don't want to counsel. It is because, too often, there is simply inadequate time and staffing for counseling. Since counseling is the easiest and most fulfilling job in the pharmacy, it should tell the boards of pharmacy something when they discover instances of "failure to counsel."

Do the boards of pharmacy think we are simply being recalcitrant? Do the boards of pharmacy think we're willfully and wantonly trying to flaunt their counseling regulations? Do the boards of pharmacy think we're akin to misbehaving kids who need to be spanked? Most pharmacists I know would love to do nothing but counsel all day long. When are the boards of pharmacy going to see the real world for what it is? The boards of pharmacy have the luxury of passing regulations while sitting in comfy chairs. At the same time, pharmacists are filling prescriptions as fast as they are physically capable.

The boards of pharmacy are good at passing regulations that don't take into consideration real world working conditions. Boards of pharmacy have shown themselves to be too timid to pass regulations that require safe levels of staffing in pharmacies. I wish the boards of pharmacy would pass a regulation that mandates that pharmacists have enough staffing so that counseling is possible.

We fear the pharmacy boards because of their power to discipline us for failing to counsel. Yet, at the same time, the boards are doing nothing substantial to address our dangerous working conditions. Pharmacy boards say that they can only pass regulations that protect the public safety. But surely unsafe working conditions endanger the public safety.

Many pharmacists are contemptuous of the pharmacy boards for threatening disciplinary action for failure to counsel. The boards readily tell us that our job entails counseling. Yet, when we say the boards should perform their job (protect the public safety by addressing pharmacists' working conditions), we're met with arrogant indifference.

The counseling regulation is unquestionably well intended. In my opinion, pharmacists should counsel because it is the right thing to do, not because it is a regulation passed by the board of pharmacy. In the end, regulations that don't acknowledge the real world breed cynicism.

Our professors in pharmacy school do a brilliant job of preparing us to counsel our customers—in a sterile environment. Don't these professors realize what the real world is like? Professors and boards of pharmacy need to instruct us how to counsel customers in a hyper-stressful environment in which we're running an or hour or two behind, customers are yelling at us, people at the drive-thru window are honking their horns, all four phone lines are for the sole pharmacist on duty, and we haven't had a meal or bathroom break all day. On top of that, customers are telling the clerk at the register, *I've waited long enough! Tell the pharmacist I want my prescriptions back so I can go somewhere else to get them filled!*

Proper counseling technique involves such things as asking open-ended questions. Don't tell the customer what the drug is used for. Instead, ask him if he knows what it's used for. Open the pill container and show the customer the pills. That way we can catch errors. Indeed, most pharmacists would love to practice this type of pharmacy. When we protest that there's simply no time, the boards and professors and legal experts tell us "Well you'd better find the time! It only takes a few seconds." The legal experts tell us "You'd better find the time to counsel because a jury won't believe you when you say you didn't have enough time to tell Mr. Jones that his anxiety medication could make him too drowsy to drive."

It is a sad commentary on the current state of affairs that pharmacists feel we need to minimize customer contact because it slows down production. When we start talking to customers, some of them do indeed have lots of questions. Some of them want to tell us their complete medical history. Some of them want to tell us about their grandchildren. Customers look at the pills we're showing them and say "They're so big they must be horse pills." Or they see us take the lid off the vial and say "I don't want those safety caps! I have to get the kids to take them off for me!" All the questions, comments, and jokes from customers put us even further behind. Unfortunately, we can't catch up by counseling customers. The boards need to acknowledge that there is simply an incredibly powerful conflict between the need to counsel and the need to produce.

In the real world, almost any words spoken to customers seem to pass for counseling. "Call me if you have any questions" probably passes for counseling in some states. "This may cause drowsiness" probably passes and, indeed, this is a very important warning. "Take this until it's all gone" probably passes for antibiotic counseling.

What legally constitutes adequate counseling? If we need to tell the customer the most common uses of the drug, the most common side effects, warnings, and contraindications, the best time to take the drug, and what to do if you forget to take a dose, then the vast majority of pharmacists in America are breaking the law. How many possible side effects do we need to mention? The top two, top five, top ten?

The big chains and managed care are pushing pharmacists in one direction (speedily herding customers) while lawyers are pushing us in the opposite direction (giving more warnings to our customers).

Some chains advertise that their pharmacists are eager to counsel customers about medications. The truth is that the chains don't value pharmacists who spend too much time counseling customers. The chains can tolerate counseling only as long as it doesn't slow our processing of customers. Chains give lip service to counseling, but most pharmacists learn quickly that our No. 1 job (by far) is filling prescriptions as fast as we can (i.e., faster than we should).

When I shop at Home Depot or Office Depot, I am amazed that, most of the time, the salespeople have plenty of time to answer my questions. Pharmacists would love to have as much time to discuss medications with our customers. The difference is that the big pharmacy chains have adopted the fast food model.

Our pharmacy leaders say that pharmacists need to assume more liability through counseling if we want to be recognized by payers (insurance companies, state Medicaid programs, Medicare Part D, etc.) as independent professionals who should be compensated for our cognitive services rather than just for the products we dispense. This means acceptance of a duty to warn customers about potential dangers associated with drug therapy. With an increased counseling role and a duty to warn come increased liability and lawsuits. Even though I am absolutely 100% in favor of counseling, somehow I bet that the people advocating all this increased liability for pharmacists aren't themselves actually filling prescriptions all day long. Educators and boards of pharmacy are good at promoting regulations that affect others, not themselves.

Did our pharmacy leaders understand the extent to which the OBRA counseling provision would increase pharmacists' legal liability? Thanks to aggressive lawyers, in the not-too-distant future, pharmacists may have recurrent nightmares as a result of these three words: "failure to warn."

It used to be that, if the pharmacist dispensed the right drug, the right dose, the right directions, and gave it to the right customer, we were free of liability. Things have become a lot more complicated lately. Our profession has succeeded in tremendously increasing the liability on front line pharmacists. I propose that our educators and associations institute a moratorium on finding new ways to increase pharmacists' liability, unless these advocates of expanded pharmacist liability first figure out some way to fix the horrendous problem of understaffing that endangers the safety of our customers. I think the boards of pharmacy need to acknowledge the real world when they find instances of "failure to counsel." I think that the enormous problem of understaffing needs to be fixed before pharmacists are disciplined.

Some pharmacy leaders believe there's no future in "dispensing" alone, because of mail order mills, robotics, and the tremendous power of insurance companies (also known as pharmacy benefit managers or PBMs). Therefore pharmacists must embrace cognitive roles, i.e., advising customers about the proper use of their medications. Pharmacy associations, pharmacy school faculty, and boards of pharmacy have embraced the expanded cognitive role for pharmacists, but have they fully recognized the legal jeopardy to pharmacists who actually do the dispensing? These groups seem to be completely oblivious to the harsh reality of filling prescriptions at incredible speeds with woefully inadequate staffing.

Most pharmacists have time for, at best, a very few sentences such as "Be careful. This may make you drowsy." Or "Be sure to take this antibiotic till it's all gone." A few words of advice to the customer are usually better than nothing, but I think it needs to be pointed out that this level of communication is nowhere near being adequate in the eyes of aggressive lawyers. Lawyers see pharmacists as tasty targets because our employer has deep pockets. Lawyers often sue everyone they can, including the doctor, the pharmacist, the drugstore, and the drug manufacturer. Lawyers hope something sticks. Pharmacists have made lawyers' jobs easier since we have proclaimed that we want more responsibility in drug therapy management. Lawyers are happy to oblige pharmacists' desire for expanded responsibility. Lawyers will increasingly sue pharmacists when anything goes wrong as a consequence of a patient's drug therapy.

Lawyers envision pharmacists' responsibilities as going far beyond our simple warning to a customer that a medication may cause drowsiness or an antibiotic needs to be taken till it's all gone. Many pharmacists feel if we say something to customers—*anything*—then we've satisfied the OBRA counseling requirement. Lawyers don't look at the situation in such simplistic terms. Even though understaffing forces pharmacists to adopt a minimalist approach to counseling, lawyers will, in court cases, contend that we must have a maximalist approach. Lawyers will claim that our customers deserve no less, i.e., our customers deserve to know every possible adverse consequence of every drug that is being prescribed.

Pharmacists have effectively placed a bullseye on our forehead and it seems clear that lawyers will increasingly take aim at us. Lawyers are ecstatic to see pharmacists embracing a greater role in drug therapy. Doctors, on the other hand, are often leery of pharmacists' expanded roles in drug therapy because doctors often view pharmacists as encroaching on the doctors' turf.

Even though I am one hundred percent in favor of counseling customers about medications, I am also one hundred percent in favor of having adequate staffing so that counseling is possible. I sometimes read "letters to the editor" from pharmacists proudly stating that they counsel every customer. I assume these pharmacists are working in slow stores.

I wonder whether there are other professionals in our society who have so willingly and eagerly exposed themselves to increased liability. It is as if we're saying to lawyers, "Come and get us!" Did the people in pharmacy who eagerly advocated OBRA '90 fully appreciate the extent to which pharmacists would be vulnerable to aggressive lawyers? The desire to move ourselves away from the product has opened a Pandora's box of expanded liability. Did our brilliant leaders fully appreciate the incredible liability this places on the shoulders of pharmacists on the front lines?

While pharmacists on the front lines suffer under the burden of expanded liability, certain groups in pharmacy seem to be quite contented: pharmacy professors, boards of pharmacy, and that small subset of pharmacists who have both R.Ph. and J.D. after their names (i.e., registered pharmacist and attorney). All these groups seem to view the expanded liability very differently from those pharmacists who actually dispense drugs. The professors, the boards, and the pharmacist-lawyers seem to view pharmacists' expanded liability as, perhaps, "deliciously terrible." The expanded liability is terrible for those pharmacists on the front lines but it increases the relevance, visibility, and importance of professors, board members, and R.Ph.-J.D.'s.

Whenever legal experts comment on pharmacy errors, I often wonder what planet they're living on. When, for example, a legal expert asks how it is possible that we placed Coumadin in a bottle labeled Cardura, I often wonder how long it has been since they dispensed drugs themselves, assuming these legal experts were actually pharmacists at some point. Errors often occur while we're running one or two hours behind, while people at the drive-thru window are honking their horns, and while the non-pharmacist store manager is on the store intercom rudely telling us (sometimes almost yelling) that all four phone lines are for the pharmacist. This environment is worlds apart from examining an error in hindsight, after the fact, like during a court case. Of course, in hindsight, we know it's an error. We didn't make the error because we didn't know the difference between Coumadin and Cardura. We made the error because the pharmacy was in chaos from being dangerously understaffed, forcing us to fill prescriptions at lightning speed.

Here are some scenarios that aren't too difficult to imagine in which we will be sued at some point in the not-too-distant future. Pharmacists would love to be able to spend the time with each customer that would allow us to prevent every possible adverse consequence. Unfortunately, the chains don't see things the same way that we do.

The following questions are directed at pharmacists:

1. Can you see yourself being sued for failure to warn a customer and call his or her doctor and emphasize that using albuterol asthma inhaler too often means asthma is out of control? If such a customer were to end up in emergency room, can you see yourself being sued for not notifying the doctor and/or not adequately stressing to the customer the significance of overuse of this inhaler.

2. Can you see yourself being sued for failure to notify all the doctors who prescribe pain medications that their patient is becoming addicted? Every pharmacist has many customers who appear to be addicted to pain pills. Will some lawyer say that you have a duty to

discuss each of these customers in detail with all the doctors who prescribe these pain pills, even when the patient utilizes many doctors to get access to these drugs?

3. Can you see yourself being sued for filling prescriptions with potentially interacting drugs even though you call the prescribing doctor and he says to go ahead and fill them? Here's an instance a neighbor told me about. A doctor prescribed Zocor 80 mg daily, gemfibrozil 600 mg daily, niacin 1000 mg daily, and Zetia 10 mg daily. The *Physicians' Desk Reference* says to use no more than 10 mg of Zocor daily in patients receiving gemfibrozil. It also says that niacin doses of 1000 mg or more increase the risk of muscle damage and that Zetia is not recommended with gemfibrozil. When I showed my neighbor these warnings in the *PDR*, he asked his doctor if there's anything to be concerned about. I was told that the doctor replied, "You've had two heart attacks. We're treating you aggressively." If this patient were your customer and he developed rhabdomyolysis (a serious muscle disorder), would he sue you for continuing to fill these prescriptions?

4. Can you see yourself being sued for filling prednisone prescriptions in the following scenario: A customer with rheumatoid arthritis develops osteoporosis and needs a hip replacement as a result of long term use of prednisone. Will some aggressive lawyer say you should have refused to fill these prescriptions and/or called the doctor to express your concern?

5. Can you see yourself being sued for failure to ask every customer every time for an update on all the over-the-counter medications they're taking so that you can enter that information into your computer in order to screen for possible interactions (like serotonin syndrome from the combination of Robitussin DM and Paxil)?

6. Can you see yourself being sued by a customer with rheumatoid arthritis who develops lymphoma from long-term use of methotrexate? Will some lawyer say you were negligent for continuing to fill methotrexate prescriptions long term, in view of the fact that the link to lymphoma is part of the black box warnings in the labeling?

When we call a doctor about a drug interaction and he tells us to go ahead and fill the prescription, do we need to second-guess the doctor and refuse to fill the prescription? If the customer suffers adverse consequences from the drug interaction, lawyers will say that we as pharmacists should indeed have second guessed the doctor and refused to fill the prescription. In any large statistical sample, some people will experience adverse consequences from a drug interaction, others will not. In my opinion, it should be the doctor's responsibility to make the final decision regarding potential drug interactions, not the pharmacist's.

Legal experts tell us that we need to give our customers what seems like an ever-increasing volume of information. We are told that our medication leaflets need to be the most detailed ones available anywhere. With an oversupply of lawyers in America, pharmacists can count on being sued more often for failure to list less common or rare side effects in our leaflets or for failure to verbally warn customers about these side effects. When customers experience uncommon adverse consequences, pharmacists are being sued for providing lists containing only the most common side effects.

Two separate lawsuits against pharmacists are based on the failure to warn about the risk of priapism (an abnormally persistent erection) from two different drugs: Desyrel and Caverject. In the first case, the patient (who had an erection lasting over four hours after taking the anti-depressant Desyrel), sued the pharmacy, claiming that the pharmacist should have told him about this risk. He literally claimed that the pharmacist had a legal duty to tell patients of risks foreseeable to health care practitioners when ordinary people would not know enough about a drug to know which questions to ask. In this case, the Court of Appeals held that the pharmacist could not be held liable under the circumstances.

In the case involving the erectile dysfunction drug Caverject, the patient injected the medication into his penis as directed, and suffered a severely painful erection that lasted almost 72 hours. On June 3, 2002, the patient underwent surgery to reduce the erection. As a result of the incident, the patient was diagnosed with priapism, resulting in permanent and non-reversible impotence. The patient argued that the law should impose a duty on pharmacists to warn of foreseeable risks known to be associated with the use of particular drugs, and that the failure to do so renders the prescription as not properly dispensed. The court decided that, if the legislature wanted to require pharmacists to warn customers of the side effects associated with prescription drugs, it would have done so by statute.

In commenting on these two cases, pharmacist-lawyer Jesse Vivian, B.S. Pharm., J.D., a professor in the Dept. of Pharmacy Practice at Wayne State University, says that we should "not take this as a free and clear message that pharmacists are legally immune from civil liability for failing to warn about known adverse effects associated with the use of a particular drug. ...there are, in fact, several courts that have come to the opposite conclusion of the judges involved in this case. ...While both of these cases were correctly decided under prevailing laws—especially considering the lack of any discernible legislative intent to the contrary—it is not hard to imagine that sometime in the near future, the courts are going to take judicial notice that the practice of pharmacy is moving away from a strict dispensing of a product model and into an information management model. In this context, courts may well impose new and greater expectations in the context of liability when things happen that could have been easily avoided with just a bit of counseling." (Jesse Vivian, "Legislative Intent, *U.S. Pharmacist,* Nov. 2005, pp. 92-97)

A Texas lawsuit involved a pharmacist's failure to warn about a very uncommon adverse reaction in the death of a 14-year old Austin boy. The lawsuit charged that the pharmacist failed to warn about potential adverse reactions from desipramine. After taking the antidepressant for two years, he developed a chronic allergic reaction to the medication. The suit contended that the pharmacist failed to warn the boy's mother. An expert witness for the dead child's family testified that the pharmacist had a duty to tell the mother more than just that the drug could cause dry mouth or constipation. On appeal, the court ruled for the pharmacist after finding that the adverse reaction was a rare side effect of the medication. (*Drug Topics,* April 19, 1999, p. 43 and *Drug Topics,* Sept. 18, 2000, p. 38)

Nothing makes me angrier than pharmacy "experts" (often a hired-gun pharmacy professor) who testify in lawsuits that pharmacists have a duty to warn the customer about an ever-increasing list of possible adverse consequences. These "experts" are not living in the real world. They are being paid 200 or 300 dollars per hour to testify that pharmacists have a duty to warn. I doubt seriously that these professors would provide more counseling than average when faced with the overwhelming workload that is typical of many drug-stores across this country. I'd like to put my pharmacy professors and heads of boards of pharmacy in a high volume store and see how well they counsel customers. I'd like to see them thoroughly counsel every customer without having a dozen misfills and lines all the way to the parking lot. I'd like to see how well these "experts" tell every customer about every conceivable consequence of every medication. I'd like to see how long chain management tolerates that.

I bet that most pharmacists are more exhausted after a day's work than heads of boards of pharmacy or pharmacy professors. One pharmacist told me that she goes home each day after her shift and sits in a dark room just to decompress. I wonder how many board members and professors do likewise. I wonder how many heads of boards and professors don't have time to eat or go to the bathroom.

If we are forced to defend ourselves in a court case in which a customer is harmed as a result of some drug therapy, we would, of course, like to make the critical point that we'd absolutely love to have the time to tell customers everything they could possibly need to know about the drugs their doctor has prescribed. But lawyers will ask us, "Why have you agreed to work for an employer that does not allow you time to counsel customers? Are you being forced to work for that employer? If you feel that conditions with that em-ployer are dangerous, you have a duty to quit and to report your employer to the board of pharmacy." We reply "But working condi-tions with all the big chains are becoming absurd everywhere. If we report our chain to the board of pharmacy, we fear that our bosses will make life so miserable for us that we will end up quitting. The board of pharmacy will send an inspector to investigate our store only."

Pharmacy school professors seem to think the environment in the drugstore is as relaxed as that at pharmacy school, and that pharma-cists have the time to sit down with each customer for a leisurely conversation, sharing several cups of coffee, maybe a Danish. The professors seem to think we've got an hour to discuss with each cus-tomer their entire medical history and every possible adverse drug effect. The reality is that pharmacists too often have time for only one or two short sentences with customers.

Pharmacy school professors don't seem to realize that most customers simply want to get their prescriptions filled as quickly as possible so they can get out of the drugstore and go home or go to work or to the supermarket. Pharmacy school professors don't seem to realize that many customers don't want a lot of information about their drugs. We know that many customers throw away the drug leaflets we give them without reading a single word. Some customers tell us that they don't want to learn about the drug their doctor has prescribed because they wouldn't want to take the medication after reading all the possible side effects. I have found that nearly 100% of people who look up their drug in the *Physicians' Desk Reference* (at a library or bookstore) become less enthusiastic about taking that drug after they see the list of potential side effects. The list in the *PDR* is usually far more comprehensive than the list we provide our customers in our leaflets.

Our pharmacy professors say they are not expecting us to practice medicine, but that is exactly what they are expecting us to do. When we are responsible for second-guessing every prescription the doctor writes, we are indeed practicing medicine. The individual pharmacist is being forced to play a role that should be played by state medical licensing boards and physician continuing education. Pharmacists don't have the time to second-guess every prescription decision made by every doctor. It seems that, because of OBRA, lawyers are, in fact, expecting us to practice medicine.

I am continually amazed by the huge disconnect between pharmacy school professors and the real world. It is as if the pharmacy school professors have no clue what it's like in the real world, or else they have a tremendous disincentive to acknowledge the real world. Many pharmacists say that pharmacy school professors embraced the counseling requirement to increase the visibility and importance of professors and to justify the requirement that all graduating pharmacists now have a doctorate, known as a Pharm.D. degree. Many pharmacists feel the requirement for a doctorate as the entry level degree was a power grab by the schools of pharmacy.

Do professors realize the absurdity of pharmacy schools producing drug experts in an environment in which the big chains don't want drug experts? The big chains want pharmacists who can dispense at lightning speed. The big chains are dripping with disdain for pharmacists who spend too much time counseling customers. The pharmacy professors are loath to acknowledge the fact that the real world is the opposite of pharmacy school.

The state boards of pharmacy are the governmental regulatory entities that have the responsibility to protect the public safety. So why don't the boards step in and require working conditions that are conducive to the safe filling of prescriptions? In my opinion, the boards of pharmacy have as much backbone as a banana. The state boards of pharmacy appear to be strongly intimidated by the legal and political clout of the big chains. Consequently, the state boards take the wimpish approach of targeting individual stores and individual pharmacists as a result of complaints from the public, rather than targeting the chain drugstore industry as a whole for operating stores in a manner that makes errors inevitable.

I once spoke with the head of one state board of pharmacy. I asked him why the board of pharmacy doesn't do something about pharmacists' working conditions. He told me that if I knew a specific store that had dangerous working conditions, the board would investigate that store. I told him that this misses the point. It is not fair to investigate individual stores because pharmacists' employers (i.e., chain management) would be extremely unhappy if they found out we had reported them to the board of pharmacy. I told him that the board of pharmacy needs to investigate the big chains as a whole. This head of the state board of pharmacy told me that his worst days are when he has to fight the corporate lawyers from the big chains.

Here are two e-mails I received from pharmacists as a result of my editorial in *Drug Topics* titled "Counseling in the real world." (December 8, 2003, pp. 24, 26)

Subj: Counseling in the real world
Date: 1/31/04
From: [Pharmacist M. K.]
To: dmiller1952@aol.com

I just finished reading your "Counseling in the real world" article and I'm really glad someone is finally speaking out. I'm a third year pharmacy student at USC and I'm already feeling very frustrated. This is definitely a catch 22 situation and pharmacists really need to get some support from our employers and the pharmacy boards. I work at Kaiser Permanente and it is an extremely busy place w/the long lines, phones ringing off the hook, etc. Already as an intern I feel I'm being pulled 10 different ways. So I am dreading getting my license and having to worry about the liability.

In school they teach us counseling and, as you said, the professors preach on about the amount of stuff that we must convey to the patient, not realizing that there is just no time. The pharmacy resident who facilitates my discussion group told us that when we counsel patients on their hypertension meds, we must discuss lifestyle changes as well. That discussion should include a detailed exercise regimen like how often they should get on a treadmill, for how long, and at what speed. Isn't that insane? Not only is there not time for that in the outpatient, retail setting, but we do not get trained here at USC on things like physical fitness. I don't even know how long I should be on the treadmill. We also don't get the opportunity to review the patient's chart in an outpatient setting so there's no way we could even comment on that aspect of things (at a hypertension clinic, yes; at the 24 hour outpatient pharmacy, no).

It's so funny that you are comparing pharmacy to fast food. Maybe I'm a little out of the loop here, and maybe this comparison has been made by others but I haven't heard it yet. I thought I was the only one who saw such a similarity between the two. Last week, I went inside the local In & Out (do you have that in Florida?). It was the first time I had been in a fast food joint in a long time. While I was waiting for my order, I watched the workers do their thing and I started to get a bit of anxiety, as it seemed all too familiar, despite the fact that I had never ever worked fast-food before. And then of course it hit me. It reminds me of work at the pharmacy. The fast pace, the long lines, the hierarchy, the audience watching and waiting for their order, the drive through!!! I went home and told my mom that I'm nothing but a glorified fast food clerk. Sometimes I'm even the cook. We do compounding at our pharmacy and the standards we use really suck, just like at a fast food place.

You are so right about the fast food model and I'm so glad someone with your experience and background sees it that way too. I thought I was going nuts. I feel better now. Thank you so much for sharing your insight with the rest of us.

My point is that I completely agree w/everything you said. Professors preach and employers are all about the bottom line. We are getting the short end of the stick here and something has to be done about it. Once again, thank you for speaking up. You said it perfectly. I'm going to send a couple of my profs the link in case they haven't already seen it yet.

Sincerely,
[Pharmacist M. K.]

Subj: Re: Counseling in the real world
Date: 12/31/03
From: [Pharmacist S. T.]
To: Dmiller1952

Thank you for your editorial in *Drug Topics*. You are so right about everything! I just don't understand why pharmacists don't come together and do something about it. In my state, pharmacists are not required to counsel every single patient. However, I still try to counsel patients because it's my duty to counsel as a pharmacist. Unfortunately, after we moved to a new pharmacy, with a drive through, and after the budget cut, I hardly have any time to counsel anymore. Instead, I write down all the important information on the labels and have my tech inform the patients. That's wrong and I know it! But, that's the only way for me to convey my messages to the patients because I am the only pharmacist on duty with only 2 hours of overlap every day. Sometimes things get so hectic that I just want to walk out and quit. I didn't go to school to learn how to fill and verify as fast as I can. Anyway, I do make sure I counsel patients, personally, if they just get out of surgery, or ER, or if they have more than 4-5 prescriptions. I do take the time to make sure they know what they are taking. But you are right, some of the patients don't even want to listen to us. All they want is to get their medications and get out of the pharmacy as quickly as possible! They think we are McDonald's or Burger Kings. Patients need to be educated!

It's very frustrating to be a pharmacist anymore. No lunch, no breaks, and not enough tech help. All we ever hear from our supervisors is the KPI's (don't even know what it stands for anymore). We get graded for things we do such as how fast the scripts go from one station to another station. If we get a D or and F, we get lectured. We always get yelled at about the phone hold time. Don't they see that there is a problem with the pharmacy if we consistently get D's and F's? KPI's should be used as a tool to tell them whether we need more help or not. Well, first of all, there are only 2 people in the pharmacy and there is only so much we can do. We have to fill scripts, ring customers up in the out-window and the drive through. We have to answer questions from customers, we have to get doctor's calls, and we have to check voice mails, etc.! I think it's absurd to grade us on how fast we can fill a script because that's not the only thing I do. I am probably telling you things that you already know. I guess I am just venting. I cried twice last week because of the workload and not enough tech help. Every day I come home, I am so exhausted that I don't even want to do anything else. Most of the time, I just doze off on the couch after work.

I'm sorry for bothering you, but thanks for letting me vent my frustration. My job is eating me alive!

Thank you.
[Pharmacist S. T.]
P.S. I hope I didn't get myself into trouble by whining too much. :)
Thanks for reading.

Chapter 30

When health professionals
are less than candid

When pharmacists are less than candid

At times, I feel that pharmacists have completely bought into the Big Pharma line that pharmaceuticals are great. At other times, I'm not so sure. In general, I would say that a very large number of pharmacists feel that our customers take too many drugs. I would say that many pharmacists wonder why customers take drugs so enthusiastically in light of the huge number of adverse reactions, precautions, and warnings listed in the *Physicians' Desk Reference*.

If you want to put your pharmacist on the defensive, tell him that you read the drug information leaflet provided by the drugstore that accompanied your prescription and the potential side effects scared you. Or better yet, tell him that you went to the library and looked up your drug in the *PDR* and that information really scared you. Pharmacists, including myself, usually begin what I call the "minimization routine" in which we say the drug wouldn't be on the market if the government (Food and Drug Administration) didn't feel it was safe. Many pharmacists, including myself, say this even though we don't necessarily believe it. Many customers naively believe that most of the adverse effects listed in the *PDR* are rare when, in fact, studies have shown that they occur more frequently than implied or stated. Take, for example, the incidence of cough caused by the class of anti-hypertensive drugs called ACE inhibitors. (Joe and Teresa Graedon, "Can You Trust the Drug Label?" *The People's Pharmacy*, Mar. 13, 2011 http://www.peoplespharmacy.com/2011/03/13/can-you-trust-the-drug-label/)

The bible of drug information is the *Physicians' Desk Reference (PDR)*. It contains the prescribing guidelines for medications provided by drug companies and approved by the Food and Drug Administration.

All of the data on drugs found in pharmacy leaflets, online resources and consumer publications comes from this source. Doctors rely on the facts they find in the official label to weigh benefits and risks of medications and inform patients about the likelihood of experiencing certain side effects.

What if this document were flawed? The FDA relies on the manufacturer to supply data about side effect frequency during the approval process. Research suggests that the drug label sometimes underestimates how often bad reactions occur. ...

More than 100 million prescriptions are filled each year for blood pressure medicines called ACE inhibitors. These are drugs like benazepril, enalapril, fosinopril, lisinopril, quinapril and ramipril. These medicines are perceived to be highly effective and extremely safe.

ACE inhibitors have a noteworthy side effect, however. These drugs can cause an unrelenting cough. Doctors who count on the FDA's labeling may downplay this risk.

Research comparing the reported incidence of cough in the PDR/drug label with that in clinical trials found that the actual rate of cough for ACE inhibitors was many times higher than the rate quoted in the *PDR* (*American Journal of Medicine*, Nov. 2010). As the authors note, side effect information in the drug label can be deceptive.

The labeling information for other drugs also may be inaccurate. Antidepressants, for example, often cause sexual side effects. These are far more common in real life than in the prescribing information. The same may be true for muscle pain caused by statin-type cholesterol-lowering drugs.

Incomplete data may give both patients and physicians a false sense of security. This can result in needless doctor visits and unnecessary medications.

For some strange reason, many of our customers seem to think some celestial power has magically set the incidence of side effects at one in a million users. Pharmacists frequently hear comments from our customers such as, "Yeah, one person in a million experienced that side effect so it was included in the list." In fact, the incidence of adverse effects varies tremendously between drugs and between users.

In our hyper-litigious society, pharmacists understandably fear being sued if someone decides to discontinue a drug (or take it at a different frequency from what the doctor prescribed) and, as a result, that person suffers some adverse consequence. So pharmacists largely keep their personal opinions about drug safety to themselves. Many pharmacists are thus, unfortunately, little more than cheerleaders for whatever drugs your doctor has prescribed.

I'm afraid that characterization very often included me. I rarely criticized a drug that a doctor prescribed when a customer asked me some variation of, "Is this drug safe?" Customers expected an honest answer from me, but often did not get it. Even though I may have read articles about growing reports of potential problems with those drugs, I did not tell our customers that I had read such articles. Even though I may have read articles that certain consumer advocates like Sidney Wolfe's Public Citizen Health Research Group had petitioned the FDA to remove a drug from the market because of some health risk associated with that drug, I did not tell our customers about those petitions.

For all the drugs that have been withdrawn from the market over the last several decades, pharmacists often know months or years in advance that that drug is associated with some potentially serious side effects. We've been reading about that drug in our pharmacy magazines for months or years in advance of the addition of a "black boxed" warning or the removal of the drug from the market. As long as a drug was still on the market, I downplayed concerns about the drug out of fear that the customer would stop taking the drug, or would go back to his doctor and say, "My pharmacist says this drug may be withdrawn from the market." I didn't want an angry doctor calling me and yelling at me. Further, with the understaffing that is too common in chain drugstores, I simply did not have time for thoughtful conversations with customers. As much as I regret it, most customers who asked me questions got reassuring answers, even when those drugs had "black boxed" warnings (the most serious category of warnings) in the official prescribing information.

The decision to take a drug should ideally involve the patient having a good understanding of the risks versus benefits of that drug or whether another drug might work as well with fewer potentially serious side effects. But the one- or two-sentence "counseling" that pharmacists undertake often is just a sound bite rather than a real discussion. Most pharmacists simply don't have time for real discussions about drugs. Some pharmacists don't like to speak with customers because those pharmacists are introverted or because speaking with customers slows down our high octane production line that turns prescriptions into a blur as they pass by pharmacists and techs. Finding mistakes in this environment is often like playing a fast-paced video game in which anything less than total concentration can result in a disaster.

Pharmacists vary tremendously in their concern about adverse effects. For example, I would say that around half of the students in my pharmacy school class were serious students and the other half were intent on doing the minimum required to graduate. Of that latter half, I don't think they particularly care whether our customers understand the drugs they're prescribed. I don't think those pharmacists care enough to have frank conversations with customers, or indeed whether those pharmacists know the pertinent information that would be most beneficial to those customers.

There is absolutely no question that some pharmacists stay abreast of the latest drug information far better than others. There are, for example, pharmacists who subscribe to Dr. Sidney Wolfe's *Worst Pills/Best Pills* newsletter. On the other hand, there are pharmacists who have tremendous disdain for Dr. Wolfe, considering him "anti-drug." Moreover, there are a huge number of pharmacists who have no idea who Dr. Wolfe is. As a result of his petitions to—

and lawsuits against—the FDA, Dr. Wolfe may be the single most in-fluential person in this country when it comes to causing the FDA to add warnings to the official prescribing information or indeed in having drugs removed from the market. From my perspective, the FDA would be much more lenient with the drug companies if not for Dr. Wolfe. He is the Ralph Nader for drugs.

Pharmacists working for the big chains too often provide sooth-ing and reassuring answers to our customers who are, in fact, ex-pecting us to be straight shooters. I have tremendous fear of being sued by someone who decides—based on my opinion—to discontinue a drug or to take it at a frequency different from what their doctor has prescribed. Let me emphasize, however, that there is no doubt that there are many drugs that are absolutely essential, absolutely life saving, and that I would take myself if the situation arose when I felt I truly needed it.

Engaging health professionals in a frank discussion of the poten-tial adverse effects of drugs is often not an easy thing to do. After all, filling prescriptions is what pays our salary. It's how we make our living and how we support our families. It's like expecting a car dealer to tell you about weaknesses in the cars he's selling. That's why I feel our health care system should be taken out of the private sector. Health professionals have a tremendous conflict of interest in recommending a pharmacological solution rather than, say, a major lifestyle change. It's not particularly good for business for pharma-cists to focus too heavily on potential adverse effects associated with the drugs we dispense.

How well are pharmacists suited for the task of explaining to our customers the risks and benefits of drugs? Let me explain it in terms of what subjects are likely to engage pharmacists in conversation. What subjects do pharmacists actually like to talk about among themselves? In personal conversations it is usually very easy to en-gage other pharmacists in discussions about our customers and our working conditions. From my experience, pharmacists love to talk about customers who ask (what we view as) dumb questions, cus-tomers who are very impatient and rude, customers who invent all kinds of excuses to explain why we should refill their controlled sub-stances early, customers who can't understand why prescriptions aren't filled as quickly as McDonald's fills burger orders, customers who phone in refill requests and then arrive in the store five minutes later and can't understand why it's not ready, etc.

However, in my experience, engaging a pharmacist in a conversation about the criticism of the drugs we dispense is an entirely different matter. Even though there are perhaps two dozen booklength exposés available about Big Pharma, I just haven't met pharmacists who are interested in discussing what these books have to say.

Top 7 Pharma Exposés

1. ***Overdosed America***: *The Broken Promise of American Medicine* by John Abramson, M.D.

2. ***Prescription for Disaster***: *The Hidden Dangers in Your Medicine Cabinet* by Thomas J. Moore

3. ***Bitter Pills***: *Inside the Hazardous World of Legal Drugs* by Stephen Fried

4. ***The Truth About the Drug Companies***: *How They Deceive Us and What to Do About It* by Marcia Angell, M.D.

5. ***Powerful Medicines***: *The Benefits, Risks, and Costs of Prescription Drugs* by Jerry Avorn, M.D.

6. ***Generation Rx***: *How Prescription Drugs Are Altering American Lives, Minds, and Bodies* by Greg Critser

7. ***Our Daily Meds:*** *How the Pharmaceutical Companies Transformed Themselves into Slick Marketing Machines and Hooked the Nation on Prescription Drugs* by Melody Petersen

---

In addition, bookstores and libraries have lots of books that are critical of psychiatry and its mechanistic view of the brain. There are lots of books available that are critical of pushing hormones on postmenopausal women and pushing drugs like Ritalin on kids. There are lots of books available that offer common sense ways to decrease elevated blood pressure, elevated cholesterol, and elevated blood sugar—all without drugs. But pharmacists just don't seem to be interested. Search books on Amazon.com with the term *without drugs* and you will discover a surprisingly large number of books in a wide array of medical conditions.

Pharma's worst nightmare—a sample of books on Amazon.com having "Without Drugs" in their titles or subtitles

Treat type 2 diabetes without drugs

- ***Diabetes Without Drugs:*** *The 5-Step Program to Control Blood Sugar Naturally and Prevent Diabetes Complications* by Suzy Cohen R.Ph. (Nov 9, 2010)
- ***Dr. Neal Barnard's Program for Reversing Diabetes:*** *The Scientifically Proven System for Reversing Diabetes Without Drugs* by Neal D. Barnard MD (Apr 1, 2008)

Treat depression without drugs

- ***The Depression Cure:*** *The 6-Step Program to Beat Depression Without Drugs* by Stephen S. Ilardi (Jun 1, 2010)
- ***Beyond Prozac:*** *Healing Mental Suffering Without Drugs* by Dr. Terry Lynch (Apr 2005)

Treat elevated cholesterol without drugs

- ***Cholesterol Down:*** *Ten Simple Steps to Lower Your Cholesterol in Four Weeks—Without Prescription Drugs* by Janet Bond Brill (Dec 26, 2006)

Reverse osteoporosis without drugs

- ***7 Secrets to Prevent or REVERSE Osteoporosis and Osteopenia:*** *How I Reversed Osteoporosis Naturally Without Drugs And How You Can Too!* by Muryal A. Braun (Mar 28, 2012)

Treat insomnia without drugs

- ***Get a Good Night's Sleep:*** *How to Conquer Your Insomnia Without Drugs or Medication* by Katherine A. Albert (Dec 15, 1997)

Treat elevated blood pressure without drugs

- *In 12 weeks You Can Control Your High Blood Pressure Without Drugs* by Cleaves M. Bennett (Nov 15, 2010)
- *The Blood Pressure Cure:* 8 Weeks to Lower Blood Pressure Without Prescription Drugs by Robert Kowalski (Apr 7, 2008)
- *Control High Blood Pressure Without Drugs:* A Complete Hypertension Handbook by Robert Rowan and Constance Schrader (May 15, 2001)
- *The Dash Diet for Hypertension:* Lower Your Blood Pressure in 14 Days— Without Drugs by Thomas Moore, M.D. (July 19, 2011)

Treat panic attacks and anxiety without drugs

- *A Life Less Anxious*: Freedom From Panic Attacks and Social Anxiety Without Drugs or Therapy by Steve Pavilanis and Patricia Alma Lee (Nov 11, 2009)

Treat ADHD without drugs

- *ADHD Without Drugs*—A Guide to the Natural Care of Children with ADHD – By One of America's Leading Integrative Pediatricians by Sanford Newmark MD (Apr 30, 2010)
- *Should I Medicate My Child?* Sane Solutions for Troubled Kids With—and Without—Psychiatric Drugs by Lawrence Diller (Apr 15, 2003)

Reverse heart disease without drugs

- *Stress Diet and Your Heart:* A Lifetime Program for Healing Your Heart Without Drugs or Surgery by Dean Ornish MD (Feb 7, 1984)
- *Conquering Heart Disease:* New Ways to Live Well Without Drugs or Surgery by Harvey B. Simon MD (Oct 1, 1995)
- *Healing Your Heart:* Proven Program for Reducing Heart Disease Without Drugs or Surgery by Herman Hellerstein (Feb 1, 2007)

Treat pain without drugs

- *Foods That Fight Pain:* Proven Dietary Solutions for Maximum Pain Relief Without Drugs by Neal D. Barnard MD (2008)

I always felt like a fish out of water in the drugstore because I knew that the subjects that interested me were of very little interest to most pharmacists. In my experience, most pharmacists are very interested in their paycheck (as I was), but little interested in a critique of the products that we dispense.

So if you expect your pharmacist to be the ideal person to give you his or her opinion about the safety and effectiveness of drugs, I think you are in for a disappointment. In my experience, most pharmacists have largely bought the narrative promoted by Big Pharma, i.e., pharmaceuticals are the primary determinant of human health. Many pharmacists are indeed interested in proper nutrition, but somehow they do not see any inconsistency in the view that nutrition is important to prevent diseases, and in the view that human health is proportional to the per capita consumption of pharmaceuticals.

As I've stated many times in this book, pharmacists too often don't have time for significant discussions with customers about possible risks associated with the drugs those customers are taking. In my opinion, the decision to take a drug should involve that patient/customer having a good understanding of the possible risks and benefits associated with taking that drug.

Most pharmacists could write an interesting article on the reactions we receive from our customers regarding the drug information leaflets we include with each prescription we dispense (or after these customers have gone to a library or bookstore and looked up their drug in the *PDR*). Nearly one hundred percent of our customers are less enthusiastic about taking that drug after reading about it. Some customers are mildly concerned about what they read. Other customers call the pharmacist after reading that information and say, "I just read the leaflet you gave me with my prescription and I'm not sure I want to take this drug." A few go even further and ask us if they can return the medication and get a refund.

On many occasions as I've handed the prescriptions to customers, I say, "Hold on just a second. I need to get the drug leaflet from our printer." (Filling a prescription for Drug X automatically prints a leaflet for that drug.) Oftentimes, customers (more likely male) tell me, "Oh. I never look at those leaflets anyway." Or they say, "I just throw those leaflets away without looking at them." Sometimes these customers seem to be implying that they don't want to read the leaflets because they'll be scared. Sometimes the macho male customers seem to be telling us, "I'm not interested in reading your damn leaflets." As you might guess, I view these customers as very naïve about the drugs they're taking, in fact bordering on dangerously ignorant. Some of these customers call the pharmacist a few days after they begin taking the drug and describe some side effect they're experiencing like loss of appetite, nausea, vomiting, diarrhea, abdominal pain, insomnia, constipation, etc. I then print out the leaflet for that drug so I can see for myself what side effects are listed and, sure enough, that side effect is listed. I tell the customer, "Yeah. That side effect is listed in the leaflet we gave you with your prescription." Then the customer very often says, "I threw it away without reading it when I got home."

When drug companies are less than candid

Pharmacists sometimes get a big helping of our own medicine as regards evasiveness about the risks and benefits of drugs. One of the most exasperating experiences in my career was when I called one of the big drug companies and asked a question about one of their drugs. Several years ago a customer brought in two prescriptions for drugs that had a "very significant" interaction potential. I can't recall the two specific drugs involved. I remember one was a brand name drug and the other was a generic, so I called the manufacturer of the brand name drug. The manufacturer of a brand name drug is supposed to be the top expert on that drug since they're the ones who conducted the trials on that drug prior to approval by the FDA. The doctor prescribed "drug B" to be taken immediately after finishing "drug A." Prior to that incident, I had read that a "washout period" of two weeks was recommended between administration of the second drug. In other words, it is recommended that these two drugs not be given within two weeks of each other. The first drug needs to be entirely cleared from the body (via the urine or feces) before the second drug is administered in order to avoid a potentially serious interaction between the two drugs.

So I called the manufacturer of the branded drug and spoke with someone in the "drug information" or "professional information" department. I asked her if she agreed that drug A should be completely washed out of the system (by waiting two weeks) before beginning drug B. She told me that, yes, there is a significant potential interaction between drug A and drug B, but she refused to tell me a specific amount of time that was recommended between finishing drug A and beginning drug B. She handled the entire conversation as if it were a potential lawsuit, giving me legalistic answers to all my questions, rather than just frank and straight-forward answers.

Finally, in exasperation, I told her. "Look, this is not a lawsuit or a potential lawsuit. I'm just wondering what I should do in this situation with the two prescriptions I'm holding. Should I call the doctor and tell him that the patient should wait some period of time before beginning drug B?" This drug information specialist refused to budge or to give me any helpful information about resolving the situation. So I began to return her unhelpful answers with equally unhelpful questions.

Initially I had asked her, "Is it true that two weeks should elapse between finishing drug A and beginning drug B?" She answered, "We can't advise you specifically on that." Then I asked her, "Would it be safe to wait a month?" She answered, legalistically, again, "We can't advise you specifically on that." So I decided to respond to this increasingly absurd conversation by asking increasingly absurd questions. I asked, "Would it be safe to wait two months?" She answered again, "We can't advise you specifically on that." Finally, in complete exasperation, I asked her, "How about waiting a year or twenty years or fifty years? Would that be safe?" She answered again, legalistically, "We can't advise you specifically about that." So I said, "Thank you. Goodbye."

Why did this drug information specialist (probably a pharmacist) not answer my question in a helpful manner? After thinking about it for awhile, I've concluded that her primary objective was to avoid a lawsuit. Therefore she limited her answers strictly to what's included in the "labeling," i.e., the official prescribing information that's approved by the FDA. The labeling is what you see when you open a *Physicians' Desk Reference.* Reading the *PDR* is more like reading a legal document than reading, say, some book hypothetically titled, "Helpful drug information for doctors and pharmacists."

Since the official prescribing information can't realistically answer every possible question (including every possible drug interaction), this drug information specialist was wearing her "legal" hat when I spoke with her, rather than wearing her "helpful" hat. It appears to me that this drug information specialist views all incoming calls as, first and foremost, potential lawsuits, so she responds legalistically rather than helpfully. I strongly suspect she knew the answer to my question, but was afraid to tell me, for legal reasons—not for medical reasons. She could have said, "Yes, waiting two weeks before giving the second drug is advisable." But since details about the specific drug interaction weren't included in the official labeling, she would not answer my question directly.

Today, there's lots of pharmacy software that's very helpful with drug interactions questions. This incident occurred nearly twenty years, i.e., long before drugstores had access to the Internet. Even a Google search today for this interaction would give me far more information about this interaction than I received (i.e., none) in calling the drug company that owns that drug.

Even though I deplore the way that drug information specialist handled that conversation, I am not surprised. Lawsuits against drug companies are common and sometimes very lucrative and warranted. My beef is that our litigious society often makes frank and open discussions about the risks and benefits of drugs impossible because all the parties are afraid of being sued.

When doctors are less than candid

How many potential side effects should your physician tell you when he writes a prescription? From my perspective, doctors downplay the possibility of side effects, fearing the power of suggestion. I also suspect that doctors want to believe the drugs they're prescribing are free from side effects. The doctor's ego may suffer if he acknowledges to his patients (and to himself) that many drugs are double edged swords with significant benefits and risks. Should a doctor mention the most common adverse effects, and/or the potentially most serious adverse effects?

Go to YouTube and/or Google and search for *Levaquin tendon.* The antibiotic Levaquin has the potential to cause serious tendon damage and even rupture which can cause extreme disability. My next door neighbor developed serious Achilles' tendon pain after taking Levaquin for bronchitis. He tells me that his doctor never mentioned "tendon damage" when prescribing that drug. I am certain that my neighbor would not have agreed to take Levaquin if he knew then (when his doctor prescribed that drug) that he could develop such serious tendon problems. Levaquin now carries a black-boxed warning about the possibility of serious tendon problems, including tendonitis and rupture of the Achilles tendon.

Jay S. Cohen, M.D., author of *Overdose: The Case Against the Drug Companies* (NY: Tarcher, 2001), writes on his website (MedicationSense.com, April 26, 2011) about the wall that is erected by doctors when patients ask questions about drug side effects. In this case, an ex-runner asks about the antibiotic Levaquin. Levaquin now carries a black-boxed warning about the possibility of serious tendon problems, including tendonitis and rupture of the Achilles tendon.

Recently, I met with Chris, a 37 year-old man who had developed signs of a peripheral neuropathy including burning and shooting pains in his hands and feet after receiving Levaquin. A runner for many years, he can no longer run because of pain and is in constant discomfort.

Seeking answers, Chris had questions for his doctors. Their reactions surprised him. "I merely asked if my symptoms might be related to the antibiotic. I wasn't seeking to blame anyone. They immediately threw up a wall. I could see their demeanors change. Each doctor rejected outright the possibility that Levaquin could have caused the problem. It was clear they didn't want to talk about it or look at any evidence, even the package insert."

I didn't sense any anger or blame in Chris. He never came across to me as someone full of rage, seeking to pin a lawsuit on a doctor. He was only seeking input and guidance. He didn't get either.

Why is this happening? Perhaps because doctors, like all people, have problems accepting blame. Many doctors over-identify with their medications. After all, the most common action that doctors take is to write a prescription. Doctors write more than 3 billion prescriptions annually, more than 8 million prescriptions every day of the year. However, the personal attachment of some doctors to their medications goes beyond reasonable and becomes pernicious when they become defensive and dismissive about obvious, common side effects.

It is well known that doctors are inadequately trained about medication side effects and how to handle them. Doctors are not adequately taught how to deal with their own emotions when a patient is disabled, hospitalized or dies because of a drug a doctor has prescribed. And of course, there is the constant fear of a lawsuit. Yet, when doctors refuse to look at information brought by patients from package inserts, which are written by the drug manufacturers and approved by the FDA, or articles from respected medical journals, something is very wrong. In this era of "evidence-based medicine," it is absurd when doctors bury their heads in the sand, refusing to even glance at evidence from the drug manufacturers and the FDA, the best source of evidence on medication reactions.

In my opinion, doctors have a tremendous conflict of interest in recommending pills rather than things like lifestyle changes, eating whole foods (not processed foods), maintaining proper weight, etc. The public is in awe of science and doctors are seen as scientists when they prescribe drugs. Few people are willing to pay doctors handsomely for advice about lifestyle changes—advice that they can get from their grandmothers for free. So doctors have a tremendous incentive to exaggerate the benefits of drugs, or, at the very least, be very defensive about drugs. Excepting some specialties, the most common action doctors take is to write a prescription. So it's not surprising they're so defensive about the drugs they prescribe.

Even though most elevated blood pressure and elevated cholesterol and elevated blood sugar (in type 2 diabetes) can be prevented with a major focus on nutrition and weight loss, doctors have a tremendous incentive to prescribe drugs for these conditions since that is what American patients expect. Americans have been so completely sold on pharmaceuticals that they feel short-changed when all they get from their doctor is advice. Therefore, doctors have an incentive to downplay the extent to which most of their patients simply have diseases of modern civilization. If doctors were to acknowledge that fact, patients would realize that the use of potent pharmaceuticals for preventable conditions is profoundly illogical.

PART IX

THE BIG PICTURE

Chapter 31

A brief history of
my disillusionment

In my opinion, when you enter a drugstore you should have the same questioning attitude as when you enter a church. Whenever I'm in a church, I'm overwhelmed with one question: But what if there's no god? In my opinion, when people enter a drugstore, they should have one primary question: Is this the most rational approach to health? Does health have more to do with one's use of medications, or does health have more to do with one's lifestyle and nutrition choices?

Pharmacy has an inglorious history associated with snake oils but, even though a veneer of science covers the products in a modern drugstore, I still wonder whether the modern drugstore is as guilty of exploiting human gullibility today as it was a hundred years ago. The products have changed (becoming more closely associated with the field of chemistry) but human gullibility has remained pretty much constant.

Perhaps my biggest surprise in pharmacy school and in my 25-year career as a pharmacist was that our medical system had so very little to do with health. I was surprised to discover that it is all about using potent pharmaceuticals to overwhelm the delicate processes of nature. Our medical system is primarily about profits, not health.

After graduation from pharmacy school in 1975, I worked for three years for Rite Aid in Summersville, Huntington, and Charleston, West Virginia, and managed to save twenty thousand dollars during that period. My disillusionment was so great that I quit pharmacy after those three years. I really had no choice but to quit. The contradictions were just too great. So I took my twenty thousand dollars and moved to North Carolina in 1978. I wanted to be in a warmer climate where the winters were not quite as cold as in West Virginia. And I wanted to live near some big universities so that I could read about our medical system and try to discover why it had so little to do with health.

This time frame was soon after Ivan Illich's *Medical Nemesis: The Expropriation of Health* was published (Pantheon Books, 1976). I bought a copy of this book soon after reading a review in my hometown newspaper. Illich certainly seemed to be saying what I was thinking, but I couldn't understand everything he was saying. I had graduated from pharmacy school in 1975 with a grounding in drugs, but I had read very little in the field of sociology, or more specifically, medical sociology. I re-read *Medical Nemesis* several times over a period of about two years. Each time I re read the book, I understood a little more of what Illich was saying. I began to understand how an institution like modern medicine could become so huge and powerful and respected despite the fact that much of what passed for scientific medicine was not scientific at all. *Medical Nemesis* was a very important book in academic circles in the mid-to-late 70s, but I don't recall a single mention of it in pharmacy magazines. This was before the Internet so I used the *Readers Guide to Periodical Literature* to find every article I could about Illich and *Medical Nemesis.*

It was also during this time frame that Rick Carlson's *The End of Medicine* was published (John Wiley & Sons, 1975) and Robert Mendelsohn's *Confessions of a Medical Heretic* was published (Contemporary Books, 1979). During this period I spent a huge amount of time in the medical libraries at the University of North Carolina at Chapel Hill and Duke University in Durham. It was in reading periodicals like *International Journal of Health Services* at these libraries that I discovered that the issues that were so important to me were primarily discussed on the political Left. It was only after graduation that I really began to understand politics and political ideology. I had graduated college with very little understanding of political ideology. I knew very little about politics beyond my perception that Republicans are for the rich and Democrats are for working people.

At graduation from pharmacy school, our dean stated what I suspect deans in all disciplines tell students at graduation: "Your education is just beginning." In my case, no truer words were ever spoken. My real education about medicine and health didn't begin until I graduated from pharmacy school. With the Internet today, it is much easier to examine the critique of modern medicine, but back in the seventies and eighties, it took some work at medical libraries. There were tremendous contradictions between what I was taught in pharmacy school, what I experienced working three years as a pharmacist for Rite Aid, and what—after graduation—I discovered in my quest to understand the critique of modern medicine.

I had been doing so much reading about criticism of modern medicine that I finally decided I needed to actually meet in person one of the people who were at the forefront of this critique. I had wanted to meet Ivan Illich but I read somewhere that he was living in Cuernavaca, Mexico. I didn't want to travel to Mexico so, on a lark, I decided to write a brief note to Illich, asking him if he had any plans to be in the eastern United States. I had never mailed a letter to anyone outside the USA, so I doubted seriously that he would receive it or that I would get a reply. I sent him a short note on a 3 X 5 index card. A month or two later, I received a small envelope in the mail. At the bottom of my 3 X 5 index card, he wrote a very brief message. As best as I can recall, he wrote something like, "Have no plans to be in the eastern US in the next six months." I think he signed it "I. Illich."

I was willing to travel anywhere in the eastern US to see Illich but I never considered going to Mexico. So I looked in the acknowledgements section in *Medical Nemesis* and I saw that the two people Illich thanked most prominently were John McKnight at Northwestern University in Evanston, Illinois (near Chicago) and Roslyn Lindheim at the University of California, Berkeley. California was too far away, but I was determined to meet someone who knew Illich well, so I drove all the way to Evanston to meet John McKnight. It was very helpful actually meeting a highly educated person who was not in awe of the institution of modern medicine.

As I said, after graduating from pharmacy school in 1975 and working three years as a pharmacist for Rite Aid in West Virginia, I saved twenty thousand dollars and decided to quit pharmacy. I moved to rural North Carolina to a small town called Apex which is less than a half-hour's drive from the universities in Durham and Chapel Hill. This was my "back to nature" period in my life so I lived on two farms over the next five years. I did my best to stretch my savings as long as I could because I dreaded going back to work as a pharmacist. Even though I was a pharmacist, I took odd jobs during this period so that I could avoid employment in drugstores. I had a part-time job setting up Armstrong ceiling tile displays in hardware stores (mainly Lowe's) in eastern North Carolina. I had a part-time job that consisted of lightly sanding used computer keyboards (with the keys removed) before they were repainted and re-sold. I had a part-time job in which I drove an IBM van to cities like Philadelphia, Baltimore, and Mobile, Alabama. The van contained an experimental computer of some kind. I had a part-time job at a plastics stamping plant. I helped one of my neighbors when he harvested his tobacco crop, and often accompanied him to the tobacco markets in Durham. I managed a small cattle ranch (averaging around seventy Limousin cows at any given time) in Morrisville, North Carolina. These cattle were raised for beef, not milk, so I never milked a cow. The owner lived in Connecticut and had the ranch as an investment. I frequently accompanied a neighbor who was a handyman on various plumbing and electric jobs at farms nearby. Thus I had a variety of jobs that paid roughly minimum wage even though I was a pharmacist. I was so disillusioned that my profession had so little to do with health that I was determined to avoid being a pharmacist for as long as I could. Finally, after five years, all my savings had run out and I was killing myself making a living with these part time jobs, so I very reluctantly returned to pharmacy in 1983, working for Revco (later acquired by CVS) for the rest of my career in the Raleigh-Durham-Chapel Hill area of North Carolina.

During the first half of my pharmacy career in North Carolina, most of the drugstores I worked in were located in strip shopping centers. Most of these strip shopping centers consist of two main anchor stores: a supermarket like Food Lion and a drugstore next door. (Stand-alone drugstores like those owned by CVS and Walgreens are much more common nowadays.) During the many years that I parked my car and walked toward the drugstore to begin my shift, I thought to myself: Here are two opposite models of human health. In one model (the supermarket), there is the fresh produce section (which, unfortunately, contains lots of pesticide residues on the fruits and vegetables). Next door in the drugstore is the opposite model: "better living through chemistry." I now live in a small condo in Florida which is about a mile from a large farmers market. As I walk up and down the aisles of this farmers market, I think to myself: *This is what health looks like.* I've never had that feeling in a drugstore. When I enter a drugstore, I don't think *health.* I think: shelves full of products with catchy packaging containing synthetic chemicals that cover up symptoms, marketing gone mad, a pill for every ill, the commodification of health, P.T. Barnum. And I also ask myself, "Am I the only pharmacist who thinks this way?" Contrary to what the public thinks, the modern drugstore is based far more on marketing than science. Health has been commercialized and commodified in this country much like Christmas. In my opinion, both drugstores and Christmas would be a lot better off with less focus on products.

How can pharmacists find their jobs fulfilling when it consists of pushing the corporate view that claims health is dependent on the consumption of pharmaceuticals? That is an extremely limited and constraining view of health. How can pharmacists go to work every day and immerse themselves in a view of health that completely downplays any relationship between *Homo sapiens* and the planet Earth, and that ignores an endless number of social, cultural, economic, psychological, and nutritional factors? Since most of the prescriptions that pharmacists fill are for diseases of modern civilization, shouldn't the focus of our health care system be on preventing these diseases rather than on attacking them with potent pharmaceuticals? During the years that I lived on the cattle ranch in rural North Carolina, I learned that cattle ranchers take it as a fact that cattle grazing on sub par pastures would not thrive as well as cattle grazing on lush pastures. Not surprisingly the corporate view of health downplays any similar link between the health of *Homo sapiens* and the planet Earth from which we gain our sustenance.

Health care in the USA is based on an outdated Western-style capitalist consumption model which has been superimposed on our society over a more rational model based on the intimate connection between *Homo sapiens* and the natural world. Our medical system is all about using pills to control biological processes that nature had well in hand for millions of years. In my opinion, our medical system is fundamentally dishonest and corrupt because it is based on pills rather than prevention.

Working forty-plus hours a week in a drugstore is, to me, as disorienting as working in a shopping mall. A couple of people have told me that, after a few hours spent shopping in an indoor mall, they are overcome with an urgent need to get away, to get outside to reality. That's how I feel in a drugstore. The modern drugstore is aisle upon aisle of products that, too often, have more to do with profits than health. The modern drugstore is, in my opinion, an artificial reality completely divorced from the natural world. It seems to me that the employees in the farmers market are, somehow, more genuine, earthy, and real in comparison to the employees in drugstores. Is that because the farmers market sells a product that is more genuine, earthy, and real in comparison to what's sold in drugstores? The placebo effect plays an important role in the value (perceived and real) of too many—but certainly not all—products in the drugstore. There are no placebos at the farmers market. Every product in the farmers market is precisely what it is. Too many of the products in drugstores are far less effective (and less safe) than advertised.

The process of filling prescriptions is not an inherently fulfilling activity. It is, from my perspective, as boring as filling burger orders at McDonald's and it is, in fact, quite similar to filling burger orders. The main difference is that the orders we fill at the drugstore are potentially a lot more dangerous than a burger order (unless, for example, the meat is tainted with a pathogenic bacteria and is cooked inadequately). This is not to say that some people don't enjoy filling prescriptions and burger orders. If you're the type person who re-flects a lot about the work you're doing, I suspect that you would be less happy filling prescriptions or burger orders. If, however, you're the type person who works on automatic pilot from the time your shift begins until the time it ends, it is quite conceivable that you could enjoy filling prescriptions and burger orders, even though both jobs appear to be repetitive and mind-numbingly boring.

If you've ever watched greyhounds race around a dirt tract, you see that they chase a fake mechanical rabbit that travels around the railing on the inner perimeter of the track. Occasionally there is a malfunction with the device that propels the mechanical rabbit around the track and the greyhounds catch the fake rabbit. Accord-ing to some web discussions, the greyhounds are useless from that point forward, because once they've discovered that the rabbit is not real, they lose their desire to chase it around the tract.

Some people say this is a myth and that the greyhounds are still good at racing. But let's assume it is true for a moment. I reacted like the greyhound when I realized that most of the diseases in mod-ern societies are Western diseases. I lost any remaining enthusiasm I had for filling prescriptions. If a pharmacist learns that most of the prescriptions he fills are for preventable conditions, how can that pharmacist maintain his enthusiasm for filling prescriptions?

In my opinion, the most devastating critique of modern medicine is not the greed of doctors and drug companies and it is not the mechanistic and reductionistic orientation of modern medicine—even though these are indeed devastating critiques. The most devastating critique of our medical system is that it does not have prevention as its primary focus. Many doctors will admit that, yes, the prevention of diseases is important. Many doctors will admit that, for example, obesity can contribute to a large cascade of health problems. But these doctors often say, "Diets just don't work. People don't stick with diets." That is, in my opinion, a bogus answer. What this soci-ety needs is a fundamental change in the way we look at health and disease, rather than having people "go on a diet." Proper nutrition and disease prevention should be at the center of our health care sys-tem, not at its periphery. When "going on a diet" is seen as just an-other approach to health, the results are too often disappointing.

Proper diet and good nutrition should not be add ons like adding another drug to a patient's regimen. Proper nutrition and disease prevention should replace pills as the primary focus of our our health care system.

The modern drugstore is a model of health based on the complete removal of *Homo sapiens* from the natural world. Most of the products in the modern drugstore are unique to human evolution, never before seen on the face of the earth, synthesized from the same petroleum that fuels your automobile. Most of the products in the drugstore overwhelm the delicate processes of nature as they target symptoms rather than the fundamental causes of the diseases of modern civilization.

Drugstores sell lots of vitamins, dietary supplements, and herbal remedies. I do not consider vitamin supplements to be natural. Prior to the last hundred years or so, *Homo sapiens* was never exposed to individual isolated vitamins. Vitamin supplements represent reductionism, a concept that is foreign to millions of years of evolution.

During the first half of my career, I found most pharmacists to be unenthusiastic or antagonistic toward dietary supplements and herbal remedies. Later on, when management saw the huge profit potential in products like saw palmetto, echinacea, black cohosh and St. John's Wort, these and other herbals began filling our shelves.

A large percentage of the critics of modern medicine (including some pharmacists) are fans of alternative medicine. These critics want a more "natural" approach to health and consider vitamins, herbs, and dietary supplements as filling that bill. I'm as skeptical of the reductionism that characterizes much of alternative medicine as I am of that same reductionism in mainstream medicine. Moreover, there seems to be almost as much hype surrounding vitamins, herbs, and dietary supplements as there is surrounding pharmaceuticals. In my view, the basic determinants of health are quite boring, easily understandable by laymen, and largely independent of drugstores and "alternative" stores specializing in dietary supplements, vitamins, and herbs. There's simply too much hype surrounding everything in drugstores and in stores specializing in alternative remedies.

I want to emphasize that I feel there are many prescription drugs that are absolutely essential and lifesaving, such as insulin, antibiotics, and thyroid hormone. I was very grateful for the availability of morphine for the severe pain in the final days of both of my parents' lives when they were dying from cancer (my mother from colon cancer and my father from non-Hodgkin's lymphoma). I'd be the first in line for an antibiotic if I had pneumonia. If I'm in a serious automobile accident, I want the absolute finest that modern medicine has to offer. Modern medicine is great at handling medical emergencies but, in my opinion, very poor in promoting a healthy lifestyle and in preventing the diseases of modern civilization.

The discoveries of insulin and penicillin were indeed awesome accomplishments which created a wave of optimism among the public that Big Pharma rides to this day. Big Pharma would like you to believe that every product on pharmacy shelves is as effective and important as insulin and antibiotics. Big Pharma continues to get mileage out of the insulin story whenever it can. Many drug companies routinely try to compare their products to insulin, trying to bask in the glory of that pharmacy superstar, even though most of these other products come nowhere near matching insulin's significance.

For example, the manufacturers of antidepressants sometimes try to convince you that taking drugs like Prozac, Paxil, or Wellbutrin for depression is somehow analogous to taking insulin for type 1 diabetes. Big Pharma would like you to believe that all the diseases of modern civilization have solutions as simple and as rational as the use of insulin in type 1 diabetes. Big Pharma would like you to view all the diseases of modern civilization as deficiency diseases that can be reversed with drugs just as scurvy is reversed with Vitamin C. Big Pharma dreams of the day that consumers will actually believe that, for example, depression is due to a deficiency of Prozac, elevated blood pressure is due to a deficiency of Lopressor, and elevated cholesterol is due to a deficiency of Lipitor. This perverse and dishonest conception of human health implies that the well-being of a population is directly proportional to the consumption of pharmaceuticals.

Pharma uses a gargantuan marketing budget to distort public perception of the causes of human illness so that pharmaceuticals seem more rational than they are. In describing *Homo sapiens* in purely mechanistic and reductionistic terms, pharmaceuticals seem to be completely rational. But if the drug industry were to describe *Homo sapiens* as a part of the natural world, the mass prescribing of pharmaceuticals would be seen as enriching doctors and Pharma rather than as addressing human maladaptation in modern societies.

It is immensely important for Pharma to promote a narrative that *Homo sapiens* is a machine apart from the natural world because most pharmaceuticals are synthetic substances, never before seen on the face of the earth, that overwhelm the delicate processes of nature. Therefore Pharma cannot risk leveling with the public about the true nature of most pharmaceuticals. This distortion of the causes of human illness is purposeful and highly sophisticated. Pharma has succeeded beyond even its wildest dreams in promoting a mechanistic view of disease, rather than a natural view of disease. If human health were widely viewed as dependent on the natural world, public enthusiasm for pharmaceuticals would drastically decrease.

Pharma's number one goal is to move *Homo sapiens* from the natural world to a world of molecules, cells, genes and pharmaceuticals. There is no word that scares Pharma more than the word "natural." Pharma does not want you to view health as being a consequence of good nutrition, proper body weight, clean air and water, fulfilling jobs, etc. Pharma has taken a very narrow view of health (based on molecules and cells) and made it look like the only possible model of health. Pharma has produced elaborate and seductive molecular explanations for nearly every medical condition (see the pharmacology section in each drug's official labeling) to legitimize pharmacological management of those conditions, while completely ignoring what is known about the non-drug prevention of those conditions.

Some examples: Pharma has succeeded in defining depression as a consequence of chemical "imbalances" in the brain, rather than as a consequence of one's life circumstances. Pharma has succeeded in defining cancer as a molecular and cellular malfunction based primarily on genes, rather than as a consequence of living in a world of synthetic chemicals. (If the planet Earth could speak, it might say that *Homo sapiens* is the <u>disease</u> and cancer is the <u>cure</u>!) Pharma has succeeded in defining obesity as a molecular and physiological malfunction, rather than as an inability to walk away from the kitchen table. Pharma has succeeded in defining shyness or introversion as a medical condition rather than as one location on the broad continuum of human personality.

My completely unnecessary ear surgery at age nine

Here is a story that doesn't have anything to do with pharmacy or drugs. But it does, in my opinion, illustrate how a certain narrative can become a juggernaut in our medical system.

When I was in the third grade, my teacher informed my mother that I was not pronouncing my "r's" correctly. I was slurring the "r" rather than pronouncing it clearly. For example, when I pronounced the word "roar," it came out sounding something like "war." But if you think about it, it takes a little more effort to crisply enunciate the word "roar" than it does the average word.

My third grade teacher suggested to my mother that I needed to see a speech pathologist. The speech pathologist decided that the reason I was not properly pronouncing words with the letter "r" was because I was not hearing words accurately. So the speech pathologist recommended that I see an audiologist.

I vividly remember the appointment with the audiologist. He placed earphones in my ears and intermittently generated electronic beeps at low intensities. I was told to signal each time I heard a beep. I remember hearing very few beeps during the audiologist's test. But I was so nervous during the test that I don't think I could have heard a jet engine if one were in the same room. So I flunked the audiologist's test, or so he claimed. The audiologist recommended that I see an ear, nose, and throat specialist. The theory was that my ears were full of fluid from having had what I consider to have been a normal number of colds.

But here's the interesting part. I could always hear conversations between people perfectly. I could hear radios and televisions perfectly. I could hear my teachers perfectly. I vividly remember riding in the family car with my parents one day. My mother and father were in the front seat and I was alone in the back seat. I remember my mother talking about my "hearing problem" that had been diagnosed by the speech pathologist and audiologist. I vividly remember my mother telling my father that I couldn't hear their conversation so it was okay to discuss the subject in my presence. But I heard her words perfectly just like I heard all conversations perfectly.

I did indeed end up having ear surgery. I never heard whether the surgeon claimed to have found any fluid accumulated in my ears. I remember screaming as loud as I could as I was admitted to the hospital. I was absolutely horrified because the entire situation made no sense to me.

So why didn't I speak up and tell my parents and my teacher and the speech pathologist and the audiologist that I could hear everything fine? I was too intimidated to speak up. Here were these two professionals saying that I had a hearing problem. So I felt that surely they knew what they were talking about. But I absolutely didn't need ear surgery because I could hear everything normally.

I suspect (but I have no proof) that the audiologist was playing along with the narrative. I don't care what criteria the audiologist used in the hearing test to determine I had a hearing problem. No one had ever mentioned that I had any hearing problem before my third grade teacher told my mother that I didn't correctly pronounce words containing the letter "r." That, in turn, led the speech pathologist to conjecture that the reason I didn't speak those words correctly was because I couldn't hear them accurately.

Unfortunately, my parents were not sophisticated enough in medical matters to tell all these so-called professionals, "This is bullshit. We've never noticed before that Dennis had any hearing problems." My parents were apparently intimidated by the white coats.

So this is what happened in a nutshell. My third grade teacher told my mother that I didn't pronounce words containing the letter "r" properly. I ended up having completely unnecessary ear surgery as a result. My hearing was perfect before the ear surgery and, luckily, it has remained perfect to this day.

The only reason I didn't enunciate words containing the letter "r" properly is because I was pathologically shy as a child. I was so shy as a child that it is surprising I pronounced any words crisply or clearly.

This incident was possibly my first introduction into the view I developed much later that health professionals often go along with certain narratives created by professionals who refer patients. Sometimes they do this for financial reasons. I suspect that sometimes they do it to make themselves and their patients feel they (the professionals) have effective treatments. I can only guess that perhaps the audiologist did not want to essentially declare that the speech pathologist's theory was bogus.

Over the next few years, I gradually began pronouncing my "r's" more crisply because I was older and less shy, not because I was hearing words more clearly.

Chapter 32

Pharma's distorted view of human health

For financial and ideological reasons, Pharma locates human pathology at the molecular and cellular levels. In contrast, evolutionary biology seeks explanations for disease based on the discordance between the genetic make-up of *Homo sapiens* and life in modern societies. Our genes have not evolved to handle the conditions and diet typical of modern societies. Jeffrey Kluger and Elizabeth Dias write in *Time* that "even in desperately poor places [around the world], cheap, processed Western-style fare has wrecked havoc on health." ("Does God Want You To Be Thin?" *Time*, June 11, 2012, p. 53) This statement is extremely embarrassing to doctors and drug companies for pushing pills rather than nutritious foods and the prevention of disease.

Modern medicine is profoundly ideological and reactionary because it explains human disease as a mechanical breakdown in individuals that is devoid of any connection to the environment, the workplace, or the society. Blaming all human disease on defective molecules and cells diverts attention from social pathology. Surely it is intensely ideological to focus on the treatment of cancer, while ignoring the ubiquity of synthetic chemicals and carcinogens in our environment. Surely it is intensely ideological to blame all psychological problems on brain chemistry and leave unexamined our society, our culture, our dysfunctional families, and the abusive relationships in our lives.

As pathology increases in the wider society, the medical profession buries its head deep in the cell in an effort to avoid threatening the status quo and the economic interests of the big corporations. As society becomes more dysfunctional and dystopian, Pharma focuses on molecules and cells rather than on social and economic pathology. The medical profession is richly rewarded for locating pathology in cells rather than in societies.

Pharma is strongly opposed to viewing human disease as a consequence of Westernization, urbanization, and the industrial mode of production. Pharma is strongly opposed to the public understanding that the term "diseases of modern civilization" means most diseases in modern societies are preventable. Pharma is strongly opposed to the public understanding the huge difference between its mechanistic/reductionistic view of human health based on synthetic chemicals (i.e., "drugs"), and a natural view of human health based on the intimate connection of *Homo sapiens* to the natural world.

Pro-business interests want explanations of disease causation that do not blame the workplace. For example, big business does not want doctors to blame cancer on the chemical industry or on worker exposures to hazardous and toxic substances. Big business would rather focus on the treatment of cancer than on the identification and removal of carcinogens. Big business does not want doctors to blame behavioral problems on things like highly stressful workplaces that adversely affect the psychological well-being of workers. When workers bring workplace-related problems home, the psychological well-being of workers' spouses and children can be adversely affected as well. So big business is antagonistic to that medical specialty known as "occupational diseases."

Working for big corporations very often means performing some repetitive task (sometimes deadeningly monotonous, sometimes extremely stressful) in which, for example, the number of units of production per hour is closely monitored (number of prescriptions filled by pharmacists per hour, number of patients seen by doctors per hour, number of airline reservations made per hour, number of tech support phone calls handled per hour, number of smart phones assembled per hour, etc.).

For those people who say that some circumstance in their lives is causing them to be chronically depressed, Pharma wants them to believe: *It's not your life circumstances. It's your brain chemistry.* For those people who say that, for example, the environment may be the cause of their cancer, Pharma wants them to believe: *Cancer is not due to things like chemicals. Cancer is due to genetic flaws or malfunctions in your cells unrelated to the environment.*

Doctors should be at the forefront in fighting for the removal of carcinogens from the environment. But they certainly are not. The American Medical Association is primarily concerned with maintaining and increasing the incomes of physicians, not with addressing the social, cultural, or economic origins of human disease. It is contrary to the economic interests of physicians to acknowledge the fact that the great majority of their patients have diseases of modern civilization for which the focus should be prevention rather than pills. Equally regrettable, the AMA, largely as a consequence of receiving huge advertising revenues from Pharma, fails to take a leadership role in discussions about the safety and effectiveness of pharmaceuticals.

Pharma prefers reductionism

Modern medicine seeks to inhibit enzymes in cells or to block the transmission of nerve impulses, rather than examine disease from a social or cultural context. The modern pharmacy consists in very large part of synthetic chemicals that block or inhibit complex biochemical processes and pathways in an effort to cover up symptoms, rather than address the underlying cause of human disease.

Calcium channel blockers, ACE inhibitors, beta blockers, alpha blockers, angiotensin receptor blockers, etc., are Pharma's solution for diseases of modern civilization such as hypertension and heart disease. HMGCo-A reductase inhibitors are Pharma's solution for elevated cholesterol, a condition of modern societies. Serotonic specific reuptake inhibitors (SSRI's) and monoamine oxidase inhibitors (MAOI's) are Pharma's solution for depression. Angiogenesis inhibitors are one of Pharma's solutions for cancer. Proton pump inhibitors and histamine-2 antagonists are two of Pharma's solutions for heartburn (renamed "gastroesophageal reflux disease" to make it sound more like a medical condition than a result of simple things like overeating or obesity).

Most drugs in the pharmacy exist as a certain number of milligrams of one specific molecule (along with added ingredients like binding agents and fillers). The molecular structure of this molecule can be drawn on a sheet of paper. In contrast to pharmaceuticals, whole foods contain perhaps hundreds of substances, the health benefits of which are continually being proposed.

Whereas nature favors diversity and variety, Pharma prefers uniformity, standardization, and homogeny. Think of the variety of insects, birds, apples, trees, dogs, and even bananas on the planet Earth. According to *Bloomberg Businessweek*, India has 670 varieties of bananas. (June 11, 2012, p. 91) In contrast, most of the drugs in the pharmacy consist of a certain number of milligrams of one specific molecule (plus binders, fillers, etc). Most products in the pharmacy are available as a one (or two or three) size fits all pill. Prozac is available as 10 mg, 20 mg, or 40 mg of fluoxetine, the generic name for this drug. Drugs are also designated by their empirical formula:

This is Prozac: $C_{17}H_{18}F_3NO \cdot HCl$
This is Lipitor: $(C_{33}H_{34}FN_2O_5)_2Ca \cdot 3H_2O$
This is Celebrex: $C_{17}H_{14}F_3N_3O_2S$

The majority (but certainly not all) of the drugs in the pharmacy are synthesized in a laboratory originally from petroleum.[1] Among important exceptions are the pharmacy superstars insulin and antibiotics. Another exception is probiotic supplements. These supplements consist of microorganisms used for the purpose of restoring

---

[1] Many of the small molecues needed to assemble pharmaceuticals come from petroleum.
(http://boards.straightdope.com/sdmb/showthread.php?t=429880)

the normal bacterial population inhabiting the GI tract. The normal GI tract "flora" can become significantly unbalanced as a result of things like antibiotics and/or diarrhea.

Pharma's research interests are limited to the examination of molecules and cells. Excluded are studies comparing disease incidences between industrialized and non-industrialized societies, or between populations that eat whole foods and populations that eat processed foods. Pharma likes to compare its products with placebos rather than with existing drugs that are similar. Pharma doesn't want to conduct clinical trials in which their drug for elevated blood pressure or type-2 diabetes or elevated cholesterol is compared to significant weight loss or a major change in diet. Pharma doesn't want to compare the incidences of disease in *Homo sapiens* with the incidence of disease in wild animals. For example, obesity, hypertension, heart disease, type 2 diabetes, elevated cholesterol, osteoporosis, dental caries, gout, etc., are uncommon in animals living in the wild—as opposed to domesticated animals or those living in zoos. According to Thomas McKeown, "…although non-communicable diseases do occur in animals affected by the manmade environment, in the wild they are very uncommon, particularly in primates." (Thomas McKeown, *The Origins of Human Disease*, New York: Basil Blackwell, 1998, p. 30)

Pharma benefits from describing more diseases as "chronic"

Pharma wants you to believe that an ever-expanding number of illnesses are "chronic" rather than "acute." That gives Pharma long-term patients/customers. Pharma is much more interested in selling depression as a chronic condition rather than as something that can resolve itself if there is a major change in one's life circumstances (for example, finding a fulfilling job, getting out of an abusive relationship in which the other person is dominant and you are subordinate, etc.). I once read that someone who won millions of dollars in a state lottery suddenly lost his shyness. How could that be possible since Pharma defines shyness as a chronic personality disorder?

Indeed, the division of conditions into "acute" versus "chronic" seems to benefit primarily the marketing agenda of Pharma. "Acute" conditions would probably include, for example, infection, the common cold, pneumonia, a sprained ankle, a broken bone or other trauma, etc. But the category consisting of "chronic" conditions is much more subjective and elastic. Certainly conditions like type 1 diabetes, hemophilia, hypothyroidism, multiple sclerosis, Parkinson's disease, and epilepsy would logically fit in the "chronic" category pending the discovery of some previously unrecognized and preventable trigger. If all the following conditions are diseases of modern civilization, is it logical to place them into the "chronic" category: elevated blood pressure, elevated cholesterol, type 2 diabetes, asthma, obesity, depression, osteoporosis, heart disease, etc.? The medical-industrial complex gains a long-term customer by placing all these conditions in the "chronic" category, implying that, once diagnosed, these conditions will be with us for the rest of our lives. We are told that we must consume products of the pharmaceutical industry for the remainder of our lives. We are not told that these are diseases of modern civilization and they are potentially preventable and/or reversible with major dietary and lifestyle changes. One famous example, among many, is *Dr. Dean Ornish's Program for Reversing Heart Disease: The Only System Scientifically Proven to Reverse Heart Disease Without Drugs or Surgery* by Dean Ornish, M.D. (1995).

Thinking back on the days when I watched TV regularly, I don't recall any Pharma advertisements for antibiotics. Why? Because antibiotics are typically used for "acute" conditions. Pharma prefers to market drugs that will be used for years if not decades. There's much more money to be made by labeling conditions "chronic" than there is, for example, with antibiotics used for acute bacterial infections.

Modern medicine is profoundly ideological

People on the political Left might say that the focus on chemistry in pharmacy school and modern medicine reflects a very sophisticated and clever political bias in a capitalist society intended to divert attention from the pathological aspects of capitalism. For example, many people view cancer as largely a consequence of the ubiquity of synthetic chemicals in our air, water, food, and workplaces. *The Merck Manual* (17th edition, pp. 2591-2) essentially states that up to 90% of cancer is preventable: "Environmental or nutritional factors probably account for up to 90% of human cancers. These factors include smoking; diet; and exposure to sunlight, chemicals, and drugs. Genetic, viral, and radiation factors may cause the rest."

If you agree that the environment plays a large role in the causation of cancer, you might agree that corporate America has a powerful incentive to focus on the pharmacological management of this disease rather than on prevention. Corporate America feels threatened by a focus on environmental causes of cancer. Thus corporate America prefers a mechanistic and reductionistic focus on molecules and cells, rather than a focus on cancer epidemiology. This inward focus on research and treatment is financially rewarding to the pharmaceutical industry, and it diverts attention from the corporations that produce and expose us to a wide range of synthetic chemicals that may be responsible for many human cancers. Corporations downplay the role of chemicals in cancer causation and exaggerate the roles played by politically less sensitive factors such as genes, viruses, and aging. Corporations want a focus on cells and molecules, not on the environment or the society.

Some critics on the Left charge that modern medicine is profoundly ideological and that its mechanistic/reductionistic focus based on pharmacology rather than prevention reflects a grand political strategy aimed at obscuring any interpretation of disease origins that threatens the status quo. Accordingly, as the pathology increases in the wider society, modern medicine buries its head deeper and deeper in the cell to avoid threatening the big corporations. Thus the microscope is the most appropriate metaphor for reactionary capitalist medicine because a microscope is incapable of examining the patho logical aspects of capitalism. The microscope provides an infinitesimally narrow view of human illness. In contrast, the field of epidemiology is very threatening to capitalism because this discipline often focuses on things like cancer clusters in communities situated near polluting factories. The field of epidemiology looks at disease from a population perspective rather than from a molecular or cellular perspective. Pharma's success in locating the consequences of social pathology at the molecular and cellular levels in *Homo sapiens* rather than at the societal level is quite remarkable, stunning, and, in my opinion, devious.

The general public is probably shocked when I state that pharmacists in the trenches have very close to zero need for chemistry. As a result of the e-mail feedback I received from pharmacists in response to my editorial in *Drug Topics* on that issue, most pharmacists seem to agree. I would like to propose that a focus on social, cultural, political, and economic factors in the causation of human illness replaces the current focus on chemistry in pharmacy school. Of course, such a focus is likely to be of little direct use to pharmacists in the trenches, but it might help them understand that the pill-for-every-ill orientation of our medical system is absurd.

Pharma is opposed to focusing on social, cultural, political, and economic factors in the causation of human illness even though these factors can be profound. For example, obesity often leads to a cascade of serious health problems, yet obesity may be caused in large part by America's ubiquitous fast food outlets and the by the typical modern American supermarket. Both sell primarily processed foods that are heavily advertised in the mass media. Americans are doing precisely what they're told to do in those advertisements: consume, consume, consume. Thus, in my opinion, obesity has a very prominent social, cultural, and economic cause, i.e., the aggressive marketing of unhealthy foods by huge corporations.

An article in *Bloomberg Businessweek* states that "Kuwait is the second-most obese nation in the world, behind the U.S." The article says that this epidemic of obesity is largely caused by the influx of American fast food outlets that accompanied the buildup to the 1991 Gulf War. (Peter Savodnik, "The Other Gulf War Syndrome," *Bloomberg Businessweek*, June 25, 2012, pp. 83-85)

Kuwait's obesity epidemic—a result of the influx of U.S. fast food— has made the country a global capital of stomach stapling. ...

At least 88 percent of Kuwaitis ... are considered overweight. According to a study published in June [2012] by the London School of Hygiene and Tropical Medicine, using data from the World Health Organization, Kuwait is the second-most obese nation in the world, behind the U.S.

As waistlines in Kuwait and across the Persian Gulf have expanded over the last three or four years, so too has the business of bariatric surgery [stomach stapling as a treatment for obesity]. ...

According to surgeons like Al Senea, the bariatric boom can be traced to the buildup to the 1991 Gulf War. That was when hundreds of thousands of U.S. troops desceneded on the Gulf nation, bringing with them Taco Bell, Hardee's, Baskin-Robbins, and Nathan's Famous hot dogs, among others. ...Andrew Smith, the author of the *Encyclopedia of Junk Food and Fast Food*, says, "The American military went in, and obviouisly they wanted fast food. Therefore, the number of fast-food establishments expanded exponentially." ...

If war introduced fast-food joints to Kuwait City, peace made them a permanent fixture.

In addition to obesity, another example of a medical condition which often has prominent social and economic causes is depression and the resultant suicide. Suicide often results from depression and feelings of hopelessness. According to an article in *Newsweek* (Barbie Latza Nadeau, "Europe's 'White Widows,'" June 25, 2012, p. 36), suicide has greatly increased in Europe as a result of the recent financial crisis. The article discusses the suicide rate in Italy and then states:

Many more have killed themselves in Greece, which once boasted the lowest suicide rate in Europe. There, 1,727 people have killed themselves (or attempted to do so) following the financial strains of the austerity measures since 2009. The ghastly trend is on the rise in Spain, too, where the unemployment rate for people under 25 years old is now more than 50 percent, which helps explain why that age group has the fastest-growing suicide rate in that country. In Ireland, which has been in recession since 2009, deliberate self-harm rates have doubled since the crisis began. In the countries most affected by the euro-zone crisis, depression is on the rise and suicides are spreading.

In my opinion, modern society should not be taken at face value. What attitude should a well-adjusted person maintain toward a society in which living is equated with consuming? Should a well-adjusted person maintain an attitude of hedonism, bemusement or skepticism toward a consumer society? Is it reasonable to feel cynical as a consequence of constant and clever manipulation by people whose financial interests very often conflict with our own best interests? What attitude should people maintain toward a society that is infinitely different from what our genes are prepared for? Pharma clearly has a powerful interest in ignoring the pathology that is evident upon examing the social psychology of modernization.

—Tony Dokoupil writes in *Newsweek* ("Zombie Apocalypse," June 18, 2012, p. 7) "…it is well established that city living—with its constant noise and lack of solitude—is linked to higher levels of insanity…".

—No less an authority than the Unabomber says "[I] attribute the social and psychological problems of modern society to the fact that society requires people to live under conditions radically different from those under which the human race evolved...". ("Ted" Kaczynski, "Unabomber's Manifesto," cyber.eserver.org/unabom.txt)

Obviously, Pharma is not interested in acknowledging that social, cultural, economic and political factors can have a profound effect on obesity, depression, psychosis, and many other health problems. Pharma prefers to focus on molecules and cells, not societies. Over a hundred years ago, Rudolph Virchow discussed the importance of social, cultural, economic, and political factors in the causation of human illness. Virchow (1821–1902) was a prolific and influential 19th–century German physician, pathologist, and anthropologist, and one of the founders of "social medicine." In my opinion his critique is still critically important even though it is conveniently ignored by Pharma.
(http://ocp.hul.harvard.edu/contagion/virchow.html)

Social medicine unites medical and political thought, and, as Virchow stated, "Medicine is a social science, and politics is nothing more than medicine on a grand scale." In his view, medicine and public health practices, applied politically, could transform society; politics and social sys-

tems could have profoundly positive or negative effects on public health; and both the politician and the physician had a moral obligation to heal society.

Virchow believed that all epidemics were social in origin. In his famous report on the 1847–48 typhus epidemic in Upper Silesia—a Prussian province, now within the borders of Poland—Virchow stated that the proper response to the epidemic was political, not medical. The improvement of social conditions, he wrote, would achieve the desired result "far more rapidly and more successfully."

Virchow, like Florence Nightingale, was skeptical of the germ theory because of its potential to deemphasize the social factors that caused disease and to encourage a superficial approach to prevention and cure. He believed that any simple or mechanical explanation of disease was wrong, disagreeing with both Pettenkofer's "three factors" approach and Koch's reductionism. Poverty caused disease as much as germs.

Thus Virchow might agree with Samuel Epstein, M.D., author of *The Politics of Cancer* (San Francisco: Sierra Club Books, 1978), that the proper response to the current cancer epidemic is political, not medical. Virchow might also agree that Pharma's focus on molecules, cells, chemistry, and pharmacology distracts from environmental factors that cause disease. Another excellent source on social, cultural, economic, and political factors in the causation of human illness is a book by David Stuckler titled *Sick Societies: Responding to the Global Challenge of Chronic Disease* (Oxford University Press, 2011).

In my opinion, the best example of how financial interests and ideology influence explanations of disease causation is the field of cancer.

Devra Davis, Ph.D., MPH, is the Director of the Center for Environmental Oncology at the University of Pittsburgh Cancer Institute. The field "environmental oncology" sends shivers down the spine of corporate America. Davis explains how vested interests have opposed a shift toward prevention. (Devra Davis, *The Secret History of the War on Cancer,* NY: Basic Books, 2007, inside front dust jacket):

For much of its history, the cancer war has been fighting the wrong battles, with the wrong weapons, against the wrong enemies. The campaign has targeted the disease and left off the table the things that cause it–tobacco, alcohol, the workplace, and other environmental hazards. Conceived in explicitly military terms, the effort has focused on defeating an enemy by detecting, treating, and curing disease. Overlooked and suppressed was any consideration of how the world in which we live and work affects whether we get cancer. The result is appalling: over 10 million *preventable* cancer deaths over the past thirty years. This has been no accident.

The official cancer effort was directed by leaders of industries that generated a host of cancer-causing materials and products. Their economic interest lay in making the disease less deadly but never in preventing it altogether. *The Secret History of the War on Cancer* shows, decade by decade, how this leadership acted to downplay research on prevention, and kept research on environmental causes from gaining widespread circulation or benefiting the general public—and how this suppression of knowledge continues today.

...this is the story of a major public health effort diverted and distorted for private gain, at a cost of millions of lives.

Pharma wants you to undergo chemotherapy without asking tough questions about cancer causation. Pharma doesn't want you to focus on political activism aimed at eliminating carcinogens from our air and water, decreasing pesticide residues in our foods, lessening exposure to ionizing radiation, etc. Pharma's advertising encourages people to focus on bravery, tenacity and stoicism in fighting cancer (e. g., "Stand Up To Cancer"), rather than on political activism aimed at preventing cancer. Americans are encouraged to donate money for research into the development of new drugs to treat cancer. In my opinion, Americans should be encouraged to donate money to environmental groups that focus on the prevention of cancer, rather than donate money to private corporations that find the treatment of cancer very lucrative financially. Pharma has a huge financial incentive to move the focus away from the prevention of cancer. You'll never hear Pharma admit that most cancers are preventable. See, for example, Samuel Epstein's *The Politics of Cancer Revisited* and four accompanying editorial reviews on Amazon.com.

> *The Politics of Cancer Revisited*
> Samuel S. Epstein, M.D., John Conyers, Jr. (Introduction), David R. Obey (Foreword), East Ridge Press, 1998.

Editorial reviews on Amazon.com:

A unique and superbly documented indictment of the National Cancer Institute and the American Cancer Society for their reckless indifference to cancer prevention, for their incestuous relationship with the cancer drug industry, and for their false claims for miracle cancer drugs and for winning the war against cancer. This is essential reading for every concerned woman and man on how to reverse the cancer epidemic by personal and political initiatives. – *Barbara Seaman, Co-founder, National Women's Health Network and author, "The Doctors' Case Against the Pill"*

Cancer continues to be the scourge of many workplaces; this book is an extraordinary weapon to mount an attack on this deadly disease. It minces no words in indicting the cancer establishment whose misdirected efforts have contributed to the ongoing cancer epidemic. Dr. Epstein's work is a strong rebuttal to the self-interested Pollyannas in the cancer establishment and provides worker advocates with essential knowledge that will serve to protect the lives of those we represent. – *Robert Wages, President, Oil, Chemical, and Atomic Workers Union International Union, AFL-CIO*

Samuel Epstein's book *The Politics of Cancer* blew the lid off the "cancer establishment" when it was published in 1978. Twenty years later, the new "POLITICS OF CANCER Revisited" is a blockbuster. It exposes the rampant industrial pollution that causes many preventable cases of cancer. It also shows the frightening power of industry in keeping us from winning the war against cancer. We all owe Professor Epstein a debt of gratitude for almost single-handedly keeping this issue alive and before the public for all these years. – *Ralph W. Moss, Ph.D., Director, The Moss Reports*

Some twenty years later, we have a most worthy sequel to the ground-breaking "The Politics of Cancer." This work is muscular, relentless, and compelling. Its thesis: billions of public dollars are being misspent in an ill-conceived "war on cancer" – a war we are losing because we are not addressing the increasingly carcinogenic environment that man has created. We have introduced these creations into our water and air, our food chain, our habitation, our workplace, and into the products produced there. In failing to allocate these resources for prevention, we are fighting the wrong war. The author documents that opposition from powerful corporate interests, and their allies in government and the academy, has sustained this strategy. We have here a must-read for the scientist and the citizen concerned with the public's health. – *Quentin D. Young, M.D., President, American Public Health Association*

Chapter 33

The continually-expanding anti-Pharma library

Books critical of Pharma's approach to anxiety, depression and psychosis

1. ***The Emperor's New Drugs***: *Exploding the Antidepressant Myth* by Irving Kirsch (Mar 8, 2011)

2. ***The Myth of the Chemical Cure***: *A Critique of Psychiatric Drug Treatment* by Joanna Moncrieff (Oct 13, 2009)

3. ***Unhinged: The Trouble with Psychiatry***—*A Doctor's Revelations About a Profession in Crisis* by Daniel Carlat (May 18, 2010)

4. ***Manufacturing Depression***: *The Secret History of a Modern Disease* by Gary Greenberg (Feb 8, 2011)

5. ***Crazy Like Us***: *The Globalization of the American Psyche* by Ethan Watters (Mar 22, 2011)

6. ***Blaming the Brain***: *The Truth About Drugs and Mental Health* by Elliott Valenstein (Feb 1, 2002)

7. ***The Medicalization of Society***: *On the Transformation of Human Conditions Into Treatable Disorders* by Peter Conrad (Apr 20, 2007)

8. ***They Say You're Crazy***: *How the World's Most Powerful Psychiatrists Decide Who's Normal* by Paula Caplan
(Mar 4, 1996)

9. Shyness: *How Normal Behavior Became a Sickness* by Christopher Lane (Dec 2, 2008)

10. America Fooled: *The Truth About Antidepressants, Antipsychotics and How We've Been Deceived* by Timothy Scott (Apr 26, 2006)

11. Doctoring the Mind: *Is Our Current Treatment of Mental Illness Really Any Good?* by Richard Bentall (Sep 30, 2009)

12. Mike's Story: *How I Overcame Depression, Bipolar, OCD, Anxiety and Other Issues Without Drugs* by Dr. Roland S Trujillo and Mr. Michael Carlos Simon (Jan 2, 2012)

13. The Depression Cure: *The 6-Step Program to Beat Depression Without Drugs* by Stephen Ilardi (Jun 1, 2010)

14. Beyond Prozac: *Healing Mental Suffering Without Drugs* by Dr. Terry Lynch (Apr 2005)

ALLAN HORWITZ

13. The Loss of Sadness: *How Psychiatry Transformed Normal Sorrow into Depressive Disorder* by Allan Horwitz, Jerome Wakefield and Robert Spitzer (Jun 18, 2007)

14. All We Have to Fear: *Psychiatry's Transformation of Natural Anxieties Into Mental Disorders* by Allan Horwitz and Jerome Wakefield (Jun 1, 2012)

15. Creating Mental Illness by Allan Horwitz (Sep 1, 2003)

JOSEPH GLENMULLEN

16. Prozac Backlash: *Overcoming the Dangers of Prozac, Paxil, and Other Antidepressants With Safe, Effective Alternatives* by Joseph Glenmullen (Apr 17, 2001)

17. The Antidepressant Solution: *A Step-By-Step Guide to Safely Overcoming Antidepressant Withdrawal, Dependence, and "Addiciton"* by Joseph Glenmullen (Jan 9, 2006)

18. Coming Off Antidepressants by Joseph Glenmullen (Jan 26, 2006)

ROBERT WHITAKER

19. Anatomy of an Epidemic: *Magic Bullets, Psychiatric Drugs, and the Astonishing Rise of Mental Illness in America* by Robert Whitaker (Aug 2, 2011)

20. Mad in America: *Bad Science, Bad Medicine and the Enduring Mistreatment of the Mentally Ill* by Robert Whitaker (May 25, 2010)

DAVID HEALY

21. The Creation of Psychopharmacology by David Healy (Sep 15, 2004)

22. Pharmageddon by David Healy (Mar 12, 2012)

23. Let Them Eat Prozac: *The Unhealthy Relationship Between the Pharmaceutical Industry and Depression* by David Healy (Oct 1, 2006)

PETER BREGGIN

24. Medication Madness: *A Psychiatrist Exposes the Dangers of Mood-Altering Medications* by Peter Breggin (Jul 8, 2008)

25. Toxic Psychiatry: *Why Therapy, Empathy, and Love Must Replace Drugs, Electroshock, and Biochemical Theories in the "New Psychiatry"* by Peter Breggin (Aug 15, 1994)

26. Your Drug May Be Your Problem: *How and Why To Stop Taking Psychiatric Medications* by Peter Breggin and David Cohen (Jul 10, 2007)

27. Brain Disabling Treatments in Psychiatry: *Drugs, Electroshock, and the Psychopharmaceutical Complex* by Peter Breggin (Dec 17, 2007)

28. The Antidepressant Fact Book: *What Your Doctor Won't Tell You About Prozac, Zoloft, Paxil, Celexa, and Luvox* by Peter Breggin (Jul 3, 2001)

29. Talking Back to Prozac by Peter Breggin and Ginger Ross Breggin (Jan 19, 2010)

30. Prozac: Panacea or Pandora? *The Rest of the Story on the new Class of SSRI Antidepressants Prozac, Zoloft, Paxil, Lovan, Luvox, and More* by Chase Shephard and Peter Breggin (Jun 1994)

THOMAS SZASZ

32. The Myth of Mental Illness: *Foundations of a Theory of Personal Conduct* by Thomas Szasz (Feb 23, 2010)

33. The Medicalization of Everyday Life: *Selected Essays* by Thomas Szasz (Oct 1, 2007)

34. The Myth of Psychotherapy by Thomas Szasz (Dec 12, 1998)

35. The Manufacture of Madness: *A Comparative Study of the Inquisition and the Mental Health Movement* by Thomas Szasz (Mar 1, 1997)

36. Coercion As Cure: *A Critical History of Psychiatry* by Thomas Szasz (Dec 31, 2009)

37. Psychiatry: *The Science of Lies* by Thomas Szasz (Sep 1, 2008)

Books critical of Pharma's approach to ADHD

1. *ADHD Without Drugs:* *A Guide to the Natural Care of Children with ADHD—By One of America's Leading Integrative Pediatricians* by Sanford Newmark MD (Apr 30, 2010)

2. *Overcoming ADHD Without Medication**: A Parent and Educator's Guide-book by Association for Natural Psychology* (Nov 15, 2009)

3. *The Myth of the A.D.D Child**: 50 Ways to Improve Your Child's Behavior and Attention Span Without Drugs, Labels, or Coercion* by Thomas Armstrong (Sep 1, 1997)

4. *The A.D.D. Nutrition Solution**: A Drug-Free 30 Day Plan* by Marcia Zimmerman (Jun 7, 1999)

5. *ADD/ADHD Drug Free**: Natural Alternatives and Practical Exercises to Help Your Child Focus* by Frank Jacobelli and Lynn A. Watson (Aug 6, 2008)

6. *Overcoming ADHD**: Helping Your Child Become Calm, Engaged, and Focused—Without a Pill* (Merloyd Lawrence Books) by Stanley I. Greenspan and Jacob Greenspan (Aug 11, 2009)

7. *No More Ritalin**: Treating ADHD Without Drugs* by Mary Ann Block (Jun 1, 1996)

8. *Who's Crazy Here?:* *Steps to Recovery Without Drugs for ADD/ADHD, Addiction & Eating disorders, Anxiety & PTSD, Depression, Bipolar Disorder, Schizophrenia, Autism* by Gracelyn Guyol (Aug 24, 2010)

9. *Train Your Brain, Transform Your Life**: Conquer Attention Deficit Hyperactivity Disorder In 60 Days, Without Ritalin* by Nicky Vanvalkenburgh and Dave Siever (Apr 11, 2011)

10. *ADHD Alternatives**: A Natural Approach to Treating Attention Deficit Hyperactivity Disorder* by Aviva J. Romm C.P.M. and Tracy Romm Ed.D. (Jul 1, 2000)

11. *Getting Rid of Ritalin**: How Neurofeedback Can Successfully Treat Attention Deficit Disorder Without Drugs* by Robert W. Hill and Eduardo Castro (Jan 2002)

12. *ADHD**: How to Improve your Child Life Without Drugs* by Haphiza Baboolal (Feb 26, 2012)

13. *Twelve Effective Ways to Help Your ADD/ADHD Child**: Drug-Free Alternatives for Attention-Deficit Disorders* by Laura J. Stevens (Sep 4, 2000)

14. *The ADD and ADHD Cure**: The Natural Way to Treat Hyperactivity and Refocus Your Child* by Jay Gordon and Jennifer Chang (Jul 28, 2008)

15. *Ritalin Is Not The Answer*: *A Drug-Free, Practical Program for Children Diagnosed with ADD or ADHD* by David B. Stein (Jan 29, 1999)

16. *Unraveling the ADD/ADHD Fiasco*: *Successful Parenting Without Drugs* by David B. Stein (2001)

17. *The Ritalin-Free Child*: *Managing Hyperactivity & Attention Deficits Without Drugs* by Diana Hunter (Dec 1995)

18. *Without Ritalin*: *A Natural Approach to ADD* by Samuel A. Berne (May 15, 2006)

19. *Calming the Chaos*: *A Drug-free Program to Eliminate the Symptoms of ADHD* by Sandra Starr Ed.D. (Dec 9, 2009)

20. *Answers To Adult ADD & ADHD*: *Sure Fire Ways To Help Heal The Negative Symptoms of ADD & ADHD And Accomplish Your Goals Without Drugs or Medication* by BuildABetterLife (Jul 25, 2010)

21. *The Ritalin Fact Book:* *What Your Doctor Won't Tell You* by Peter Breggin (Aug 2002)

22. *Should I Medicate My Child?* *Sane Solutions for Troubled Kids with—and Without—Psychiatric Drugs* by Lawrence Diller and (Apr 15, 2003)

Books critical of Pharma's approach to cholesterol

---

1. *The Truth About Statins*: *Risks and Alternatives to Cholesterol-Lowering Drugs* by Barbara H Roberts (Apr 24, 2012)

2. *How Statin Drugs Really Lower Cholesterol*: *And Kill You One Cell at a Time* by James B. and Hannah Yoseph (Mar 12, 2012)

3. *The Great Cholesterol Myth*: *Why Lowering Your Cholesterol Won't Prevent Heart Disease—and the Statin-Free Plan That Will* by Jonny Bowden and Stephen Sinatra (Nov 1, 2012)

4. *Ignore the Awkward:* *How the Cholesterol Myths Are Kept Alive* by Uffe Ravnskov (Jan 10, 2010)

5. *Fat and Cholesterol Are Good for You* by Uffe Ravnskov (Jan 26, 2009)

6. *The Cholesterol Myths:* *Exposing the Fallacy That Saturated Fat and Cholesterol Cause Heart Disease* by Uffe Ravnskov (Apr 2002)

7. *The Great Cholesterol Con:* *The Truth About What Really Causes Heart Disease and How to Avoid It* by Malcolm Kendrick (Oct 1, 2008)

8. *Statin Drugs Side Effects and the Misguided War on Cholesterol* by Duane Graveline (May 21, 2008)

9. *The Statin Damage Crisis* by Dr. Duane Graveline M.D. and Malcolm Kendrick M.D. (Aug 28, 2010)

10. *Lipitor: Thief of Memory* by Duane Graveline, Kilmer S. McCully and Jay S. Cohen (Nov 1, 2006)

11. *The Dark Side of Statins* by Duane Graveline MD MPH and Glyn Wainwright MSc (Oct 15, 2010)

12. *What You Must Know about Statin Drugs & Their Natural Alternatives: A Consumer's Guide to Safely Using Lipitor, Zocor, Pravachol, Crestor, Mevacor, or Natural Alternatives* by Jay S. Cohen (Jan 1, 2005)

13. *Cholesterol Down: Ten Simple Steps to Lower Your Cholesterol in Four Weeks—Without Prescription Drugs* by Janet Bond Brill (Dec 26, 2006)

14. *Hidden Truth about Cholesterol-Lowering Drugs* by Shane Ellison (Nov 1, 2005)

15. *The Great Cholesterol Con* by Anthony Colpo (Feb 25, 2012)

Books critical of Pharma's approach to heart disease

---

1. *Dr. Dean Ornish's Program for Reversing Heart Disease: The Only System Scientifically Proven to Reverse Heart Disease Without Drugs or Surgery* by Dean Ornish MD (Dec 30, 1995)

2. *Healing Your Heart: Proven Program for Reducing Heart Disease Without Drugs or Surgery* by Herman Hellerstein (Feb 1, 2007)

3. *Conquering Heart Disease: New Ways to Live Well Without Drugs or Surgery* by Harvey B. Simon (Oct 1, 1995)

4. *How to Prevent or Even Reverse Heart Disease—Without Drugs or Surgery!* by Robert D. Willix Jr. (Apr 15, 2005)

5. *Stress Diet and Your Heart: A Lifetime Program for Healing Your Heart Without Drugs or Surgery* by Dean Ornish, M.D. (Feb. 7, 1984)

Books critical of Pharma's approach to elevated blood pressure

---

1. *The Blood Pressure Cure: 8 Weeks to Lower Blood Pressure Without Prescription Drugs* by Robert Kowalski (Apr 7, 2008)

2. *The K Factor: Reversing and Preventing High Blood Pressure Without Drugs* by Richard Moore and George Webb (May 1986)

3. **Control High Blood Pressure Without Drugs:** *A Complete Hypertension Handbook* by Robert Rowan and Constance Schrader (May 15, 2001)

4. **In 12 weeks You Can Control Your High Blood Pressure Without Drugs** by Cleaves M. Bennett (Nov 15, 2010)

5. **How to Control High Blood Pressure Without Drugs** by Robert L. Rowan (Sep 13, 1987)

6. **The Dash Diet for Hypertension: Lower Your Blood Pressure in 14 Days—Without Drugs** by Thomas J. Moore M.D., Njeri Karanja and Laura P. Svetkey (Oct 9, 2001)

7. **Lower Blood Pressure Without Drugs:** *Hypertension. the Most Epidemic Medical Condition Known to Man* by Roger Mason (Apr 1, 2009)

8. **Eight Weeks to Lower Blood Pressure:** *Take the Pressure Off Your Heart Without the Use of Prescription Drugs* by Robert E. Kowalski (Sep 2007)

Books critical of Pharma's approach to cancer

1. **National Cancer Institute and American Cancer Society:** *Criminal Indifference to Cancer Prevention and Conflicts of Interest* by Samuel S Epstein (May 17, 2011)

2. **The Politics of Cancer Revisited** by Samuel S. Epstein, John Conyers Jr. and David R. Obey (Oct 1998)

3. **Cancer-Gate:** *How to Win the Losing Cancer War* (Policy, Politics, Health and Medicine) (Policy, Politics, Health and Medicine Series, Vicente Navarro, Series) by Samuel S. Epstein (Feb 28, 2005)

4. **The Secret History of the War on Cancer** by Devra Lee Davis (Feb 24, 2009)

5. **When Smoke Ran Like Water:** *Tales Of Environmental Deception And The Battle Against Pollution* by Devra Lee Davis (Dec 25, 2003)

6. **Living Downstream:** *An Ecologist's Personal Investigation of Cancer and the Environment* by Sandra Steingraber (Mar 23, 2010)

7. **Raising Elijah:** *Protecting Our Children in an Age of Environmental Crisis* (A Merloyd Lawrence Book) by Sandra Steingraber (Mar 29, 2011)

8. **Questioning Chemotherapy:** *A Critique of the Use of Toxic Drugs in the Treatment of Cancer* by Ralph W. Moss (Jul 1995)

9. **The Cancer Industry** by Ralph W. Moss (Oct 1996)

10. *Cancer Wars*: *How Politics Shapes What We Know And Don't Know About Cancer* by Robert N. Proctor (Apr 14, 1996)

Books critical of Pharma's approach to menopause

1. *Menopause Without Medicine* by Linda Ojeda, Ph.D. and Jeffrey S. Bland, Ph.D. (Jun 27, 2000)

2. *AARP Menopause Drug Alternatives*: *All-Natural Options for Better Health Without the Side Effects* by Mark Stengler, Robin Young-Balch and James F. Balch (Nov 11, 2011)

3. *A Seven-Step Program for Getting Through Menopause and Enjoying a Longer, Healthier Life Without Drugs* by Catherine D. Lowes (Sep 1998)

4. *All about Menopause*: *And Its Treatment Without Drugs* by David Potterton (Jan 1996)

5. *What Doctors Don't Tell You:* *Guide to the Menopause*: *Natural Ways to Manage Menopause Without Drugs* by Lynne McTaggart (1997)

6. *Managing the Menopause Without Oestrogen* by Margaret Rees and Tony Mander (Jun 15, 2004)

Books critical of Pharma's approach to osteoporosis

1. *Seven Secrets to Prevent or REVERSE Osteoporosis and Osteopenia*: *How I Reversed Osteoporosis Naturally Without Drugs And How You Can Too!* by Muryal A. Braun (Mar 28, 2012)

2. *Building Bone Vitality*: *A Revolutionary Diet Plan to Prevent Bone Loss and Reverse Osteoporosis—Without Dairy Foods, Calcium, Estrogen, or Drugs* by Amy Lanou and Michael Castleman (May 1, 2009)

Books critical of Pharma's approach to asthma

1. *Instant Asthma Relief*: *Get Relief From Asthma Symptoms Without Drugs or Side Effects* by Jim Patterson and Robin Leigh Cahill (Feb 1, 2012)

2. *How To Cure Asthma Without Drugs* by Rhonda Gessner (Jan 15, 2012)

3. *All About Asthma*: *And Its Treatment Without Drugs* by David Potterton (Jan 1996)

4. *Attack Asthma*: *How to Conquer Environmental Illnesses and Allergies Without Drugs* by William Vayda (Apr 1995)

Books critical of Pharma's approach to type-2 diabetes

1. *Diabetes Without Drugs*: *The 5-Step Program to Control Blood Sugar Naturally and Prevent Diabetes Complications* by Suzy Cohen R.Ph (Nov 9, 2010)

2. *Dr. Neal Barnard's Program for Reversing Diabetes*: *The Scientifically Proven System for Reversing Diabetes Without Drugs* by Neal D. Barnard (Apr 1, 2008)

3. *Reversing Diabetes*: *Reduce or Even Eliminate Your Dependence on Insulin or Oral Drugs* by Julian M. Whitaker (Jun 1, 2001)

4. *AARP Diabetes Drug Alternatives*: *All-Natural Options for Better Health Without the Side Effects* by Mark Stengler, Robin Young-Balch and James F. Balch (Nov 11, 2011)

5. *Natural Diabetes Cure*: *Curing Blood Sugar Disorders Without Drugs* by Roger Mason (Mar 2012)

Books critical of Pharma (not disease specific)

1. *Overdosed America*: *The Broken Promise of American Medicine* by John Abramson, M.D.

2. *Prescription for Disaster*: *The Hidden Dangers in Your Medicine Cabinet* by Thomas J. Moore

3. *Bitter Pills*: *Inside the Hazardous World of Legal Drugs* by Stephen Fried

4. *The Truth About the Drug Companies*: *How They Deceive Us and What to Do About It* by Marcia Angell, M.D.

5. *Powerful Medicines*: *The Benefits, Risks, and Costs of Prescription Drugs* by Jerry Avorn, M.D.

6. *Natural Causes*: *Death, Lies, and Politics in America's Vitamin and Herbal Supplement Industry* by Dan Hurley

7. *Best Choices From The People's Pharmacy* by Joe and Teresa Graedon

8. *Generation Rx*: *How Prescription Drugs Are Altering American Lives, Minds, and Bodies* by Greg Critser

9. *Selling Sickness*: *How the World's Biggest Pharmaceutical Companies Are Turning Us All into Patients* by Ray Moynihan and Alan Cassels

10. *The $800 Million Pill*: *The Truth behind the Cost of New Drugs* by Merrill Goozner

11. *The Big Fix*: *How the Pharmaceutical Industry Rips Off American Consumers* by Katharine Greider

12. *Protecting America's Health*: *The FDA, Business, and One Hundred Years of Regulation* by Philip J. Hilts

13. *The Merck Druggernaut*: *The Inside Story of a Pharmaceutical Giant* by Fran Hawthorne

14. *Inside the FDA*: *The Business and Politics Behind the Drugs We Take and the Food We Eat* by Fran Hawthorne

15. *The Whistleblower*: *Confessions of a Healthcare Hitman* by Peter Rost, M.D.

16. *Big Pharma*: *Exposing the Global Healthcare Agenda* by Jacky Law

17. *On The Take*: *How Medicine's Complicity with Big Business Can Endanger Your Health* by Jerome Kassirer, M.D.

18. *Critical Condition*: *How Health Care in America Became Big Business—and Bad Medicine* by Donald L. Barlett and James B. Steele

19. *Poison Pills:* *The Untold Story of the Vioxx Drug Scandal* by Tom Nesi (Sep 16, 2008)

20. *Hard Sell*: *The Evolution of a Viagra Salesman* by Jamie Reidy

21. *Hope or Hype*: *The Obsession with Medical Advances and the High Cost of False Promises* by Richard A. Deyo, M.D., and Donald L. Patrick, Ph.D.

22. *Last Well Person*: *How to Stay Well Despite the Health-care System* by Nortin M. Hadler, M.D.

23. *Severed Trust*: *Why American Medicine Hasn't Been Fixed* by George Lundberg, M.D.

24. *Worst Pills, Best Pills:* *A Consumer's Guide to Avoiding Drug-Induced Death or Illness* by Sidney Wolfe, M.D., and the Public Citizen Health Research Group

25. *Disease Mongers:* *How Doctors, Drug Companies, and Insurers Are Making You Feel Sick* by Lynn Payer

26. *Our Daily Meds:* How the Pharmaceutical Companies Transformed Themselves into Slick Marketing Machines and Hooked the Nation on Prescription Drugs by Melody Petersen

27. *What Doctors Don't Tell You*: The Truth About the Dangers of Modern Medicine by Lynne McTaggart

28. *Top Screwups Doctors Make and How To Avoid Them* by Joe and Teresa Graedon

29. *Overtreated:* Why Too Much Medicine Is Making Us Sicker and Poorer by Shannon Brownlee

30. *Worried Sick:* A Prescription for Health in an Overtreated America by Nortin M. Hadler, M.D.

31. *Overdiagnosed:* Making People Sick in the Pursuit of Health by H. Gilbert Welch, M.D.

32. *How We Do Harm:* A Doctor Breaks Ranks About Being Sick in America by Otis Webb Brawley, M.D.

33. *The Healing of America:* A Global Quest for Better, Cheaper, and Fairer Health Care by T. R. Reid

34. *Confessions of an Rx Drug Pusher* by Gwen Olsen

35. *Death by Prescription:* The Shocking Truth Behind an Overmedicated Nation by Ray. D. Strand, M.D.

36. *White Coat, Black Hat:* Adventures on the Dark Side of Medicine by Carl Elliott

37. *Pharmageddon* by David Healy

38. *The Risks of Prescription Drugs* by Don Light

39. *Blood Feud:* The Man Who Blew the Whistle on One of the Deadliest Prescription Drugs Ever by Kathleen Sharp

40. *Cured to Death:* The Effects of Prescription Drugs by Arabella Melville and Colin Johnson

41. *Modern Medicine Is Killing You* by Niraj Nijhawan (Nov 1, 2010)

42. *Dispensing With the Truth:* The Victims, the Drug Companies, and the Dramatic Story Behind the Battle Over Fen-Phen by Alicia Mundy (Aug 20, 2002)

43. *Heart Failure:* A Critical Inquiry into American Medicine and the Revolution in Heart Care by Thomas J. Moore (Sep 1990)

44. *Deadly Medicine:* Why Tens of Thousands of Heart Patients Died in America's Worst Drug Disaster by Thomas J. Moore (Mar 1, 1995)

45. *Are Your Meds Making You Sick*? *A Pharmacist's Guide to Avoiding Dangerous Drug Interactions, Reactions, and Side Effects* by Robert S. Gold (Dec 13, 2011)

Chapter 34

We need more prevention—
not more pills

—*You are what you eat.*

—*An ounce of prevention is worth a pound of cure.*

—*An apple a day keeps the doctor away.*

—*Early to bed, early to rise makes a man healthy, wealthy, and wise.*
(Ben Franklin)

—*Walking is a man's best medicine.* (Hippocrates)

—*All health begins with a good night's sleep.* (Irish proverb)

—*Every human being is the author of his own health or disease.*
(Buddha)

—*The art of medicine consists in amusing the patient while nature cures
the disease.* (Voltaire)

—*Insanity: a perfectly rational adjustment to the insane world.*

—*If all of medicine were sunk to the bottom of the ocean, it would be
all the better for humanity and all the worse for the fishes.* (Virchow)

One of the original ideas behind managed care was that, by stressing prevention, people would be healthier and medical bills would be lower. The reality with managed care is that doctors don't have enough time to teach their patients about preventing diseases. In the real world, doctors and pharmacists are forced to herd patients. So if doctors, pharmacists, insurance companies, and drug companies don't teach people about prevention, who will?

Pharmacists: Do you believe that Americans abuse their bodies for 30 to 40 years and then expect a pill to reverse all the damage? Do you ever wonder whether most of your customers could prevent their conditions with the proper knowledge? Does the subject of prevention interest you or would you prefer to stick with drug therapy issues? What role should pharmacists play in encouraging and educating our customers about ways to remain healthy and to prevent disease? Has American medicine become such an assembly line that the notion of prevention today is simply too idealistic and "pie-in-the-sky"? Is the ideal of prevention a quaint throwback to simpler times? Indeed, are pharmaceuticals so effective that there's no need for our medical system to stress prevention?

Maintaining ideal body weight throughout life is an example of the primary prevention of heart disease. Early treatment of hypertension is an example of the secondary prevention of heart disease. There are many things pharmacists can do to promote the primary prevention of disease—by encouraging our customers to lose weight, avoid tobacco and alcohol, etc. Clearly primary prevention is superior to secondary prevention. Surely it's better to totally prevent a condition than rely on pharmaceuticals to moderate the worsening of that condition.

I once had an obese customer ask me an endless number of questions about her blood pressure medications. She appeared to be skeptical of the need for those medications. Finally, in total exasperation (I had a pile of prescriptions waiting to be filled), I said to her, "You know, in many people, the single best thing they can do to decrease their need for blood pressure drugs is to lose weight." A previously cordial conversation immediately became uncomfortable. She implied that her weight was none of my business and she walked away. That was the first time I ever mentioned the need to lose weight to a customer who was clearly overweight. And it was also the last time.

Pharmacists occasionally ring up customers at the register when we don't have a cashier or tech available. Over the years, I have seen a small number of pharmacists mention to customers the hazards of smoking (by utilizing a bit of sarcasm) as they ring up a pack or carton of cigarettes. This conversation with the customer always gets my attention because I'm always curious to see how the customer will react. It's always an awkward situation. I haven't yet seen a customer tell the pharmacist that it's none of his business, but that seems to be what's on the customer's mind. I've always viewed those pharmacists as having more guts than me, and possibly stepping over the line, but maybe they're the ones with the right idea.

Do pharmacists have a role in helping our customers prevent disease by lifestyle changes? Or is our only role in giving advice about pharmaceutical approaches?

Should pharmacists remind obese customers that losing weight is often the best way to get their blood pressure under control? This is clearly a valuable piece of advice, but it has a tendency to upset these people. Should we leave that task to their doctor?

Do we, as pharmacists, have a duty to encourage our customers to quit smoking or is that something that only their doctor should do?

Granted, these types of conversations with customers can be very uncomfortable. And, of course, how would pharmacists find the time (and privacy) for these conversations?

Drugstores have a bit of an image problem with regard to the subject of prevention of diseases, i.e., we sell tobacco, alcohol, and candy.

Do hospitals sell cigarettes or alcoholic beverages in their gift shop or cafeteria? Then why should pharmacies? Is there any hypocrisy in selling cigarettes and also selling nicotine patches and gum to aid in smoking cessation, or, worse, filling prescriptions for medications to treat lung cancer caused by smoking? Is there anything hypocritical about pharmacies selling alcoholic beverages? Alcohol is associated with countless deaths each year from auto accidents, liver cirrhosis, etc.

Americans associate holidays with candy. The drugstore aisles overflow with candy each Halloween, Easter, Mother's Day, Valentine's Day, and Christmas. As everyone knows, candy causes dental caries and contributes to obesity, which, in turn, contributes to Type II diabetes and hypertension. Is it hypocritical for us to sell candy in the front of the store and fill prescriptions (Xenical and Meridia) for obesity in the pharmacy?

We also fill countless prescriptions for acetaminophen w/codeine and penicillin VK as a result of the dental caries caused by candy. Is it strange that many public schools are prohibiting soft drink and candy vending machines while pharmacies sell lots of soft drinks and candy?

Pharmacists should realize that the potential for prevention is profound. *The Merck Manual* (16th edition, p. 984) says that most cases of hypertension and Type II diabetes are preventable: "Thus weight reduction will lower the BP [blood pressure] of most hypertensives, often to normal levels, and will allow 75% of Type II diabetics to discontinue medication." Ninety percent of diabetics fall under Type II. *The Merck Manual* (17th edition, pp. 2591-2) essentially states that up to 90% of cancer is preventable: "Environmental or nutritional factors probably account for up to 90% of human cancers. These factors include smoking; diet; and exposure to sunlight, chemicals, and drugs. Genetic, viral, and radiation factors may cause the rest."

According to Bradley Willcox, M.D., D. Craig Willcox, Ph.D., and Makoto Suzuki, M.D. (*The Okinawa Program*, NY: Clarkson Potter, 2001),

In Okinawa [Japan], the occurrence of heart disease is only one fifth that of American levels. The rate of breast, ovarian, and prostate cancers is less than a quarter of American levels. And the number of centenarians per hundred thousand is six times that of the United States. Most important, Okinawans have the world's longest disability-free life expectancy.... Heart disease is minimal, breast cancer so rare that screening mammography is not needed, and most aging men have never heard of prostate cancer. In fact, as a group, the three leading killers in the West—coronary heart disease (CHD), stroke, and cancer—occur in Okinawa with the lowest frequency in the world ... To understand the magnitude of this health phenomenon, imagine a typical town of 100,000 inhabitants. If the town were located in Okinawa, only 18 people would die from coronary heart disease in a typical year. If the town were in the United Sates, 100 people would die.

Since pharmaceuticals are readily available in the USA, consumers here probably think we're inevitably the healthiest country in the world. Not so. In 2000, the World Health Organization issued life expectancy rankings for countries based on the expected number of years to be lived in what might be termed the equivalent of "full health." Using this new system, the USA ranked 24th in the world, behind such countries as Spain, Italy, Greece, Monaco, and Andorra. This means that the availability of the most innovative pharmaceuticals is not the primary determinant of life expectancy.

Prevention can be easily understood by most people, but doctors embrace pharmaceutical solutions because the public has been conditioned to value high-tech approaches more than common sense prevention. Nevertheless, the potential for prevention is profound. For example, John Abramson, M.D., currently on the clinical faculty at Harvard Medical School, writes in *Overdosed America* (New York: HarperCollins, 2004):

...the evidence from study after study, including gold-standard randomized clinical trials, shows that we can usually do a great deal more to maintain our own health than the medical industry, particularly the drug industry, promises it can do for us. (p. 210)

...physical fitness, smoking cessation, and a healthy diet trump nearly every medical intervention as the best way to keep coronary heart disease at bay. (p. 222)

...why does the decision to start a cholesterol-lowering statin drug [e.g., Lipitor, Zocor, Mevacor, Pravachol, Crestor] dominate our preventive medicine strategy when healthy lifestyle changes have been shown to be so much more effective? (p. 202)

The only reasonable conclusion from the best scientific evidence available is that taking a statin while ignoring routine exercise, a healthy diet, and the dangers of smoking may be good for drug company profits but is not good for your health. It's not uncommon to hear doctors say that we should "just put statins in the water." Wherever that phrase came from, it is certainly not from unbiased research. The narrow focus on cholesterol levels, statins, and cardiac tests and procedures has succeeded in drawing attention away from far more effective lifestyle changes that cost little more than a shift toward vegetables, whole grains, and unprocessed foods at the supermarket; and a pair of sneakers for a walk or jog around the park or a workout at the gym. (p. 225)

According to Temple and Burkitt, many, if not most, of the diseases filling hospital beds and doctors' offices in North America are potentially preventable (Norman J. Temple, Ph.D., and Denis P. Burkitt, M.D., *Western Diseases*, Totowa, New Jersey: Humana Press, 1994, p. viii). That's why I find my job to be so unfulfilling.

Doctors are not trained to confront disease with the outlook of Louis Pasteur, who remarked, "Whenever I meditate on a disease, I never think of finding a remedy for it, but rather a means of preventing it." It will require a whole change of outlook for the question: "How can this be prevented?" to acquire anything like equal prominence with: "How can it be cured?"

This book is an attempt to draw attention not only to the fact that a huge proportion of diseases responsible for death and suffering in the Western world are potentially preventable, but also, in several instances, are actually reversible without recourse to drugs or surgery.

Cancer is an immensely lucrative disease but it, too, is largely preventable. From the liberal/left perspective, the best way to address the cancer epidemic is to fight corporate polluters, fight for clean air and water, fight for tougher environmental laws, and fight for funding for research into the prevention of cancer. The political Left wants the National Cancer Institute to focus on the prevention of cancer. The NCI appears to have largely adopted the view of the drug industry by focusing on finding new drugs to treat cancer instead of focusing on non-drug measures to prevent cancer. The Left says that the medical-industrial complex has a huge vested interest in exaggerating the roles of genes, viruses, and aging as factors in cancer causation. Focusing on genes, viruses, and aging takes the heat off the corporations responsible for our exposure to carcinogens and other toxic chemicals. From the right-wing perspective, the best way to address the cancer epidemic is to look for newer and better drugs. The political Right expects Big Pharma to cure cancer.

Big Pharma does not like a focus on the ubiquity of synthetic chemicals in our surroundings because such a focus implies that most cancers are preventable. Big Pharma doesn't want people to realize that most cancers are preventable because people would begin asking why the focus in America is on treating cancer rather than preventing it. Consequently, the public would be much less willing to undergo treatments with toxic chemotherapy for a condition that is largely preventable. The National Cancer Institute has been politicized into accepting the focus of Big Pharma on chemotherapy the same way that the FDA focuses on drug treatments rather than prevention. It is pure politics to treat cancer with drugs rather than seek to prevent it. A health care system that focuses on drug treatments rather than prevention is concerned about private financial gain rather than public health.

The pill focus defines modern medicine: *Why prevent cancer when there's much more money in treating it?* Chemotherapy for advanced cancers is much more financially lucrative than advice from doctors to avoid prolonged exposure to the sun, to quit smoking, to limit air and water pollution, to wash pesticide residues from fruits and vegetables, to limit exposure to ionizing radiation and suspected carcinogens, etc. Cancer provides lots of jobs for oncologists treating cancer, for radiologists diagnosing cancer, for pharmacists dispensing cancer drugs, for nurses caring for patients with cancer, for lab technicians testing blood so that doctors can monitor the results of chemotherapy. Cancer provides lots of jobs for people at drug companies who look for new cancer drugs. Lots of hospitals are needed to care for people with cancer. Cancer is an immensely profitable disease for our health care system.

In my opinion, prevention should occupy the dominant position in our approach to cancer that chemotherapy now enjoys. Of course, some cancers are more difficult to prevent than others. Viruses, for example, do cause some cancers. Human papilloma virus can cause cervical cancer. But viruses (plus molecular dysfunctions, aging, and genetics) provide a convenient scapegoat for a drug industry that does not want to admit that most cancers are potentially preventable and that the ubiquity of synthetic chemicals in our surroundings may be responsible for a huge number of human cancers.

Devra Davis, Ph.D., MPH, is the Director of the Center for Environmental Oncology at the University of Pittsburgh Cancer Institute. The field "environmental oncology" sends shivers down the spine of corporate America. Davis explains how vested interests have opposed a shift toward prevention. (Devra Davis, *The Secret History of the War on Cancer*, NY: Basic Books, 2007, inside front dust jacket):

For much of its history, the cancer war has been fighting the wrong battles, with the wrong weapons, against the wrong enemies. The campaign has targeted the disease and left off the table the things that cause it–tobacco, alcohol, the workplace, and other environmental hazards. Conceived in explicitly military terms, the effort has focused on defeating an enemy by detecting, treating, and curing disease. Overlooked and suppressed was any consideration of how the world in which we live and work affects whether we get cancer. The result is appalling: over 10 million *preventable* cancer deaths over the past thirty years. This has been no accident.

The official cancer effort was directed by leaders of industries that generated a host of cancer-causing materials and products. Their economic interest lay in making the disease less deadly but never in preventing it altogether. *The Secret History of the War on Cancer* shows, decade by decade, how this leadership acted to downplay research on prevention, and kept research on environmental causes from gaining widespread circulation or benefiting the general public—and how this suppression of knowledge continues today.

...this is the story of a major public health effort diverted and distorted for private gain, at a cost of millions of lives.

Big Pharma does not want you to know that (as previously noted) the conservative *Merck Manual* (17th edition, pp. 2591-2) states that up to 90 percent of human cancers can be prevented: "Environmental or nutritional factors probably account for up to 90% of human cancers. These factors include smoking; diet; and exposure to sunlight, chemicals, and drugs. Genetic, viral, and radiation factors may cause the rest." Big Pharma wants you to undergo chemotherapy without asking tough questions about cancer causation. Big Pharma doesn't want you to focus on political activism aimed at eliminating carcinogens from our air and water, pesticides from our foods, etc. Big Pharma's advertising encourages you to focus on bravery, tenacity and stoicism in fighting cancer, rather than on activism in preventing cancer. Big Pharma has a tremendous financial incentive to move the focus away from the prevention of cancer. You'll never hear Big Pharma admit that most cancers are preventable.

The urgent need for a paradigm shift to prevention has been advocated by some people for many years. Back in 1997 John Bailar, M.D., Ph.D. and Heather Gornik, M.H.S. gave a bleak assessment in *The New England Journal of Medicine* of the progress in the war on cancer. ("Cancer Undefeated," *The New England Journal of Medicine*, May 29, 1997, pp. 1569-74):

The war against cancer is far from over. ...The effect of new treatments for cancer on mortality has been largely disappointing. The most promising approach to the control of cancer is a national commitment to prevention.... [p. 1569]

Will we at some future time do better in the war against cancer? The present optimism about new therapeutic approaches rooted in molecular medicine may turn out to be justified, but the arguments are similar in tone and rhetoric to those of decades past about chemotherapy, tumor virology, immunology, and other approaches. In our view, prudence requires a skeptical view of the tacit assumption that marvelous new treatments for cancer are just waiting to be discovered. ...it is now evident that the worldwide cancer research effort should undergo a substantial shift toward efforts to improve prevention. [p. 1573]

A national commitment to the prevention of cancer, largely replacing hopes for universal cures, is now the way to go. [p. 1574]

Pharmacy students are likely to be disappointed and disillusioned in pharmacy school—and indeed in their entire careers—if any of the following apply: (1) they are very interested in prevention, (2) they reject the view that *Homo sapiens* is apart from nature, (3) they are inclined to believe that most of the diseases in modern civilization are, in fact, lifestyle diseases that can be prevented, and (4) they reject the notion that the human body is poorly designed and constantly prone to breakdown. Such pharmacy students are likely to be disappointed with the completely mechanistic focus of pharmacy school on molecules and cells rather than on the discordance between our genes and life in modern societies. As pharmacists, they will find their careers unfulfilling because the focus is on addressing symptoms of disease rather than on the ultimate causes of those diseases. Medicine and pharmacy today are obsessed with interrupting biochemical pathways and covering up symptoms. Our health care system should instead be focused on the causes and prevention of disease.

Chapter 35

Diseases of modern civilization

Even though my skepticism toward many pharmaceuticals began in pharmacy school, it was not until after graduation that I discovered the significant body of literature in what is known as "Western diseases" or "diseases of modern civilization." The fact that so many drugs in the pharmacy are less safe and less effective than advertised is enough reason to be concerned. But the additional fact that most of the drugs (but certainly not all) are used to treat diseases of modern civilization certainly made me even less enthusiastic about the drugs I was dispensing.

"Diseases of modern civilization" means that these are preventable diseases. So this begs the question: Why is our medical system spending tens of billions of dollars treating diseases instead of preventing them? The short answer is that there's very little money in prevention. Our medical system is primarily about profits, not health. Thus my disillusionment toward pharmacy stems in large part from the fact that so many of the drugs pharmacists dispense are less safe and less effective than advertised, and from the fact that most of these drugs are used for preventable conditions.

There is some disagreement regarding what is the best term for these diseases: *Western diseases, diseases of civilization, diseases of urbanization and industrialization, diseases of advanced societies, diseases of modernity, diseases of modern civilization, etc.* Here are three (partial) lists of such diseases which I've compiled from the three books I've found most informative on this subject:

---

1. Norman J. Temple, Ph.D., Denis P. Burkitt, M.D., *Western Diseases*, Totowa, New Jersey: Humana Press, 1994, pp. 24-25.

The diseases listed below are those for which Temple and Burkitt feel there is strong evidence that they should be considered as Western diseases.

A. Diseases for which specific causes, mainly dietary, have been postulated, and in many cases demonstrated.
Coronary heart disease
Cerebrovascular disease (one consequence of which is stroke)
Essential hypertension
Deep vein thrombosis
Pulmonary embolism
Varicose veins
Obesity
Type II (noninsulin dependent) diabetes
Cholesterol gallstones
Kidney stones
Osteoporosis
Gout
Constipation
Hiatus hernia
Appendicitis
Diverticular disease
Hemorrhoids
Colorectal polyps
Colorectal cancer
Breast cancer
Prostate cancer
Lung cancer
Uterine cancer
Ovarian cancer
Dental caries

B. *Diseases of obscure etiology*
Type I (insulin dependent) diabetes
Crohn's disease
Celiac disease
Pernicious anemia
Ulcerative colitis
Multiple sclerosis
Rheumatoid arthritis

**2. Noel T. Boaz, Ph.D., M.D., *Evolving Health:*
The Origins of Illness and How the Modern World Is Making Us Sick,
New York: John Wiley & Sons, 2002**

Allergies p. 58
Cancer p. 75
Breast cancer pp. 89-90
Prostate cancer p. 93
Cancer of the gastrointestinal tract pp. 175 6
Heart disease pp. 97, 103
Hypertension and heart disease p. 113
Gout p. 146
Back pain pp. 149-153
Hip, knee, and foot bony ailments pp. 153-155
Varicose veins and hemorrhoids pp. 155-156
Carpal tunnel syndrome p. 158
Fibromyalgia pp. 159-60
Diverticulitis p. 171
Appendicitis p. 171
Tooth decay p. 171
Irritable bowel syndrome pp. 171-2
Peptic ulcer p. 172
Inflammatory bowel disease p. 173
Depression and suicide pp. 181-5
Eating disorders p. 188
Anorexia and bulimia pp. 188-9
Attention deficit hyperactivity disorder pp. 189-191
Obesity chapter 9

3. S. Boyd Eaton, M.D., Marjorie Shostak, and Melvin Konner, M.D., Ph.D., *The Paleolithic Prescription*, New York: Harper & Row, 1988

Atherosclerosis p. 47
Hypertension p. 49
Type II diabetes p. 50
Chronic obstructive lung disease p. 51
Cancer p. 53—colorectal cancer, breast cancer, lung cancer
Osteoporosis p. 56
Hearing loss p. 57
Dental caries p. 58
Alcohol-related diseases p. 59
Diverticular disease p. 61
Obesity p. 63

Other books that discuss diseases of modern civilization include:
• Staffan Lindeberg, *Food and Western Disease*, Chichester, West Sussex (United Kingdom): Wiley Blackwell, 2010.
• Teresa Pollard, *Western Diseases: An Evolutionary Perspective*, New York: Cambridge University Press, 2008.
• Jennie R. Joe and Robert S. Young (eds), *Diabetes As a Disease of Civilization: The Impact of Culture Change on Indigenous Peoples*, Mouton de Gruyter, 1993.
• Brian Inglis, *Diseases of Civilization: Why We Need a New Approach to Medical Treatment*, Academy Chicago Publishers, Ltd., 1999.
• Mark Nathan Cohen, *Health & the Rise of Civilization*, New Haven: Yale University Press, 1989.
• Thomas McKeown, *The Origins of Human Disease*, New York: Basil Blackwell, 1988.
• Michael Pollan, *In Defense of Food*, New York: The Penguin Press, 2008.

Most prescriptions pharmacists fill are to treat "diseases of modern civilization." These are diseases that are new from an evolutionary perspective. Pharmacists fill what seems like an ever-increasing, never-ending, overwhelming onslaught of prescriptions. Some pharmacists may be tempted to step back and scratch their heads and wonder: Why do such massive numbers of people in our society have angina, hypertension, heart disease, type 2 diabetes, asthma, obesity, osteoporosis, depression, breast cancer, prostate cancer, colon cancer, etc.?

Are these conditions simply a symptom of increases in average life span in the last hundred years? Are these conditions for which a genetic predisposition simply manifests itself as we grow older? Has diagnosis of disease improved dramatically allowing doctors to diagnose these conditions more readily? Has direct-to-consumer advertising brought more people into doctors' offices, allowing doctors to find disease that might not have been found otherwise?

Are pharmacists filling more prescriptions for these conditions as a result of the growth in prescription drug coverage? As people get drug coverage from their jobs or from some governmental entity, do these people naturally increase their use of prescribed drugs? There is a joke about prescription drug insurance: "The card made me sick." In other words, people seem to use more prescription drugs when they get drug coverage. They seem to be telling themselves, "I've got the card so I may as well use it."

Allow me to make the case that the most common diseases for which pharmacists fill prescriptions are primarily a consequence of such things as our modern diet of highly processed foods; obesity; sedentary lifestyles; environmental and workplace contaminants; alcohol and tobacco use; stresses and pathology that accompany urbanization, industrialization, wage labor and a hyper-consumption society; etc. Let's examine the evidence that the most common diseases in modern societies are indeed preventable and that the widespread occurrence of these diseases is new from an evolutionary standpoint, i.e., these diseases are not due to the fact that people are living longer.

Unquestionably, there are genetic diseases which may be largely unavoidable. But I submit to you that, for the most common diseases in America, for which pharmacists fill the great majority of prescriptions, the basic etiology is not genetic and is not a consequence of aging. The incidences of these diseases have skyrocketed in the last hundred years or so. Clearly our gene pool cannot have changed this rapidly in such a short time span. It is commonly accepted that it takes thousands of years for the genetic makeup of a population to evolve. The dramatic increase in these diseases in the last hundred years means that these diseases cannot be genetic. Our gene pool cannot possibly have changed so dramatically in the course of one century.

As a pharmacist for twenty-five years, I often sought an explanation for why people in modern societies have so many medical conditions. In searching for an answer to this question, the first book I found that seemed to address this question head-on was *Western Diseases* (edited by Norman J. Temple, Ph.D., and Denis P. Burkitt, M.D., Totowa, New Jersey: Humana Press, 1994). The numerous contributors to *Western Diseases* are strong advocates of the view that the most common diseases in advanced societies are indeed preventable and are not inevitable manifestations of increasing lifespans in the last hundred years. The editors have named these diseases of modern civilization "Western diseases," even though they admit that this term results in much confusion:

The term "Western" encompasses that large group of disorders that currently have their highest incidence rates in more affluent Western countries yet are still rare, or even unknown, in rural communities throughout the Third World. ...The designation of "Western" is not entirely satisfactory, since these disorders are becoming more common in more affluent societies in the East and Middle East. ..."Related to Western lifestyle" might be the most appropriate term, but it is too cumbersome, and so "Western" is the term now generally used. (Denis P. Burkitt, M.D., p. 15)

To make the case that the vast majority of prescriptions that pharmacists fill are for "Western" diseases or "diseases of modern civilization" (and are therefore largely preventable), here are the major points for you to consider:

A. There is a profound mismatch between our genes and our lifestyles.

B. Western diseases are essentially new diseases.

C. The best way to examine the preventability of diseases is to examine their wide variation in incidence throughout the world. Another good method is to ask if wild animals develop these diseases since wild animals are not exposed to the lifestyle and dietary changes that have been so remarkable in modern societies. As it turns out, animals living in the wild rarely get cardiovascular disease and cancer.

D. Contrary to popular opinion, these diseases are not occurring simply because people are living longer.

E. No alternative hypothesis consistent with the epidemiological evidence has been put forward.

F. The striking variations in the incidences of these diseases around the world are not due to underreporting from undeveloped societies.

G. The incidence of hypertension, breast cancer, colon cancer, prostate cancer, depression, type 2 diabetes, asthma, osteoporosis, and dental caries varies widely around the world.

The sources noted in sections A thru G below are the four books I have found most insightful on the subject of diseases of modern civilization:
- Norman J. Temple, Ph.D., Denis P. Burkitt, M.D., *Western Diseases* (Totowa, New Jersey: Humana Press, 1994)
- S. Boyd Eaton, M.D., Marjorie Shostak, and Melvin Konner, M.D., Ph.D., *The Paleolithic Prescription* (New York: Harper & Row, 1988)
- Noel T. Boaz, Ph.D., M.D., *Evolving Health: The Origins of Illness and How the Modern World Is Making Us Sick* (New York: John Wiley & Sons, 2002)
- Thomas McKeown, *The Origins of Human Disease* (New York: Basil Blackwell, 1988)

A. The most common diseases in industrialized societies reflect a profound mismatch between our genes and our lifestyles

Drs. Boyd Eaton, Marjorie Shostak, and Melvin Konner believe that the major chronic illnesses which afflict humans living in affluent industrialized Western nations are largely the result of a mismatch between our genetic constitution and a variety of lifestyle factors.

...with genetic makeups essentially out of synch with our lifestyles, an inevitable discordance exists between the world we live in today and the world our genes "think" we live in still. This mismatch...can account for many of our ills, especially the chronic 'diseases of civilization' that cause 75 percent of the deaths in industrial societies. (Eaton, Shostak and Konner, p. 43)

B. Western diseases are essentially new diseases

In *The Origins of Human Disease* (New York: Basil Blackwell, 1988), Thomas McKeown says that Western diseases are essentially new diseases:

Perhaps the most persuasive evidence that the non-communicable diseases are essentially new diseases is the observation that they are rare in populations which have retained their traditional way of life, but begin to appear when they change to the Western lifestyle. ...While there may be differences of opinion about the acceptability of some of the conditions as Western diseases, the general conclusion that they are appearing in developing countries where formerly they were rare is not in doubt. (McKeown, pp. 152-3)

See also *Western Diseases*:

The common factor in all these situations is that populations living in an environment little removed from that in which they have evolved have low prevalences of Western diseases, whereas those who alter their culture and diet become prone to all the diseases of Western culture. (Burkitt, p. 23)

C. Animals living in the wild rarely get cardiovascular disease or cancer

In addition to citing epidemiological data on the wide variation in international incidence of disease, McKeown buttresses his argument for Western diseases by making the important observation that animals living in the wild rarely get cardiovascular disease or cancer:

...although non-communicable diseases do occur in animals affected by the manmade environment, in the wild they are very uncommon, particularly in primates. Because of its bearing on the problems of human health, [this conclusion] is of great interest, particularly in relation to the most common causes of death in developed countries, cardiovascular disease and cancer. ...the evidence suggests that spontaneous tumors of free-living wild animals are also rare. (McKeown, pp. 30-31)

Homo sapiens may be fundamentally maladapted to life in industrialized and urbanized societies. Burkitt agrees with the evidence in wild animals: "An argument in favor of this maladaptation hypothesis is the rarity of all these diseases in wild animals." (Burkitt, p. 17)

D. These diseases are not occurring simply because people are living longer

---

Eaton, Shostak and Konner refute the widely cited belief that these diseases are occurring simply because we are living longer:

One common suggestion is that traditional people do not contract these diseases simply because they do not live long enough to get them. Reasonable though this argument may seem, recent studies have refuted it. Young men in industrialized societies show early signs of many of these illnesses—atherosclerosis, hypertension, and obesity, for example—while young men from technologically simple societies do not. In addition, even people aged sixty and above in traditional groups continue to avoid these diseases. This is not true for their Western counterparts who—even if they have no symptoms—still show silent but ominous evidence of the key disease processes. (Eaton, Shostak, and Konner, p. 45)

E. No alternative hypothesis consistent with the epidemiological evidence has been put forward

Modern humans are believed to be adapted to the hunter-gatherer environment in which our ancestors lived for tens of thousands of years in the distant past. Western humans have made more changes to our life-style, particularly our diet, in the last 200 years or eight generations since the Industrial Revolution than our ancestors made in the previous 20,000 years. ...

Although some may reject the argument that these diseases must have a basic shared cause in Western lifestyle, no alternative hypothesis consistent with the epidemiological evidence has been put forward during the two decades or more that this hypothesis has been discussed. (Burkitt, p. 17)

F. The striking variations in the incidences of these diseases around the world are not due to underreporting from undeveloped societies.

These striking contrasts have been observed throughout the world and can no longer be a matter of dispute. The argument that they might be common but remain undetected in less developed populations is no longer tenable. Despite the profuse literature on the subject that has appeared over the last two decades, these diseases have rarely been reported as having a high prevalence in any community that has not radically changed its lifestyle during the past few generations. (Burkitt, p. 18)

G. The incidences of hypertension, breast cancer, colon cancer, prostate cancer, depression, type 2 diabetes, asthma, osteoporosis, obesity, and dental caries vary widely around the world.

The following three sentences from Noel Boaz, M.D., Ph.D., are enough to put most drugstores out of business (*Evolving Health: The Origins of Illness and How The Modern World Is Making Us Sick*, New York: John Wiley & Sons, Inc., 2002):

In hunter-gatherer societies around the world, old people do not gain weight as they age. Starting out as fit, physically strong adults, they maintain good muscle mass, strength, and low fat-to-muscle ratios into advanced age. They do not suffer from diabetes, high blood pressure, heart attack, stroke, osteoporosis, inflammatory bowel disease, cancers, or the myriad of other standard ailments that affect aged Westerners. (Boaz, p. 221)

Let's examine each disease individually.

1. Hypertension does not exist in all societies

New York Times medical writer Jane Brody puts hypertension in perspective: ("Personal Health," *The New York Times*, May 18, 1994, p. B7):

That hypertension is preventable In the vast majority of people is obvious from one universal fact: only in industrialized countries does blood pressure rise with age. In less developed countries where few people are overweight, where the diet does not promote clogged arteries, where daily physical activity is routine, where heavily salted processed foods do not overload the body with sodium and where heavy drinking of alcoholic beverages is uncommon, blood pressure does not creep up and up as people get older, and hypertension is not a national epidemic.

Also, see the Special Report "Nonpharmacological Approaches to the Control of High Blood Pressure" in the journal *Hypertension* (*Hypertension* 8: 444-467, 1986). The incidence of hypertension is not a result of increased life spans in advanced societies:

Evidence from studies worldwide strongly supports the conclusion that arterial pressure does not increase with age in populations in which body weight does not increase with age. (p. 445)

See *The Paleolithic Prescription* (page 49):

What is clear is that hypertension is widespread in industrial societies such as ours, and rare in technologically simple ones. Furthermore, blood pressure commonly increases with age in our society.... Among people such as the San (Bushmen), the Eskimo, the Australian Aborigines, the Zairian Pygmies, the Tanzanian Hadza, and many other preindustrial groups, blood pressure remains low throughout life.

2. Eighty percent (or more) of heart disease is preventable. Heart disease increases with a Westernized diet.

A healthy lifestyle—including a low-fat, high-fiber diet, exercise, and moderate alcohol intake—can dramatically reduce the risk of heart disease, according to findings from the Nurses' Health Study. The study suggests that a healthy lifestyle can cut heart risk by as much as 80%. Dr. Frank B. Hu of Harvard University describes the impact of lifestyle on heart disease as "profound," and speculates that the effects of diet and exercise on heart disease could be even greater. He says that the nurses in the lowest risk category followed guidelines for moderate risk reduction. With stricter guidelines, including an even lower fat intake and eating more fruits and vegetables, risk could drop even lower, Hu predicts. ("Healthy lifestyles could prevent 80% of heart disease," *Reuters*, November 8, 1999)

Atherosclerosis is not the inevitable result of the aging process: (See Hans Diehl, *Western Diseases*, 1994)

In the United States, as in many industrialized Western countries, almost every second man and woman dies from degenerative vascular disease related to atherosclerosis, a process that expresses itself most frequently as coronary artery disease, with angina and myocardial infarction as its classical manifestations. The disease is so prevalent that it has often been assumed to be a natural concomitant of the aging process. (p. 237) ...and yet atherosclerosis is not natural, nor is it the inevitable result of the aging process. Large populations in the world are clinically unaffected by it. (p. 239)

3. Cancer incidence varies widely around the world with highest incidence in industrialized countries. This suggests that cancer is largely a preventable disease.

The sixteenth edition of *The Merck Manual* (Rahway, New Jersey: Merck Research Laboratories, Sixteenth Edition, p. 2644) strongly suggests that cancer is a preventable disease:

It is generally accepted that environmental or nutritional factors account for as much as 90% of human cancers. The factors include smoking, dietary habits, and exposure to sunlight, chemicals, and drugs. Genetic, viral, and radiation factors are estimated to cause the remaining 10%.

The tremendous variation in the incidence of cancer around the world implies that most cancers are preventable and that it is not a result of the fact that lifespan is greater in westernized nations or that cancer is inevitable as we grow older. The World Health Organization says that cancer is increasing around the world as industrialization increases (*World Health Report 1998 Executive Summary*, http://www.who.org/whr/1998/exsum98e.htm):

In many parts of the world, dramatic shifts in cancer occurrence are being observed. In several newly industrialized regions, cancer has become, unexpectedly quickly, one of the leading causes of death. Cancer of the breast, colon and prostate have emerged in several countries in which they were hardly known 20-30 years ago.

...In developing countries, as their economies grow, noncommunicable diseases will become more prevalent, largely because of the adoption of "western" lifestyles and their accompanying risk factors—smoking, high-fat diet, lack of exercise.

Sandra Steingraber, Ph.D., a biologist, summarizes the wide variation in cancer incidence around the world as a consequence of industrialization (*Living Downstream: An Ecologist Looks at Cancer and the Environment*, Reading, Mass: Addison-Wesley, 1997, p. 59):

Industrialized countries have disproportionately more cancers than countries with little or no industry (after adjusting for age and population

size). One-half of all the world's cancers occur among people living in industrialized countries, even though we are only one-fifth of the world's population. Closely tracking industrialization are breast cancer rates, which are highest in North America and northern Europe, intermediate in southern Europe and Latin America, and lowest in Asia and Africa. Breast cancer rates are thirty times higher in the United States than in parts of Africa, for example. Breast cancer incidence in the United States is five times higher than it is in Japan, but this gap is rapidly narrowing. Of all the world's nations, Japan has the most rapidly rising rate of breast cancer.

Among the nations of the developed world, similar time trends are in motion for a number of major cancers. Mortality rates of breast cancer and prostate cancer are rising in almost all industrialized countries. The accelerating U.S. rates of brain cancer, kidney cancer, multiple myeloma, non-Hodgkin's lymphoma, and melanoma are replicated in France, West Germany, England, Japan, and Italy. Increased access to health care, improved diagnostic techniques, and a greater cultural willingness to write the word "cancer" on a death certificate account for some, but not all, of these increases.

4. Breast cancer incidence varies widely around the world

White women in the San Francisco Bay Area of the United States have an age-adjusted breast cancer incidence of 104.2 per 100,000. In contrast, the age-adjusted breast cancer rate among women in The Gambia (a country in western Africa) is only 3.4 per 100,000. This means that there over 30 times as much breast cancer among white women in the San Francisco Bay Area compared to women in The Gambia. (National Cancer Institute, *Cancer Rates and Risks*, NIH Publication 96-691, 1996, p. 27)

According to the National Cancer Institute, breast cancer rates in the United States are among the highest in the world. From 1973 to 1991, invasive breast cancer incidence in the United States increased 25.8 percent in whites and 30.3 percent in blacks, or roughly 2 percent per year. The NCI further states that the increased rates cannot be completely explained by increased use of mammography, suggesting that changes in other breast cancer risk factors may be occurring. Studies of migrants who emigrate from low-incidence areas to high-incidence areas have found that the rates of breast cancer increase to that of the new country, reflecting changes in lifestyle and environmental factors, showing that international differences in rates are not due to genetic factors. (National Cancer Institute, *Cancer Rates and Risks*, NIH Publication 96-691, 1996, pp. 120-1)

One of the biggest misconceptions about the alarming incidence of breast cancer is that it is largely due to genetic factors. In fact, "only between 5 and 10 percent of all breast cancers seem to be due to an inherited mutation." (*Cancer Rates and Risks*, p. 120)

5. Prostate cancer rates vary widely around the world

Age-adjusted prostate cancer rates for black men in Atlanta, Georgia are estimated at 102.0 per 100,000. For men in Qidong, China, the age-adjusted rate is only 0.8 per 100,000. This means that there is 127 times as much prostate cancer among black men in Atlanta compared to men in Qidong, China. (National Cancer Institute, *Cancer Rates and Risks*, NIH Publication 96-691, 1996, p. 25)

6. Colorectal cancer

Colorectal cancer incidence and mortality vary at least ten-fold between countries with the highest and those with the lowest rates. The highest incidence and mortality rates are seen in the more industrialized countries of North America, Northern and Western Europe, and New Zealand; the lowest rates are in Asia and Africa. A rapid rise in colorectal cancer rates in a particular area signals the action of environmental factors. Such a rapid increase has been observed in Japan, where from 1969 to 1981 colorectal cancer mortality increased 44 percent in men and 40 percent in women. (Arthur G. Schatzkin, "Colon and Rectum," *Cancer Rates and Risks*, National Cancer Institute Publication 96-691, p. 130)

7. Dental caries or "cavities"

Caries is rare among nonindustrial peoples unaffected by modernizing influences. ...The absence of tooth decay in these populations is well documented, as is its dramatic rise following the introduction of widespread sugar consumption. Unlike most of the diseases of civilization, the absence of caries has been documented directly in populations of our ancestors. The best preserved of human remains, teeth have been shown over and over again to be relatively little affected by decay in a variety of archaeological and paleontological populations. (S. Boyd Eaton, M.D., Marjorie Shostak, and Melvin Konner, M.D., Ph.D., *The Paleolithic Prescription* (New York: Harper & Row, 1988, , pp. 58-59)

8. Osteoporosis

[Osteoporosis] was rare among our remote ancestors, but is common in modern populations. (Eaton, Shostak, and Konner, p. 57)

9. The incidence of depression varies around the world

Is it our society that is dysfunctional rather than the individual? Is depression the result of a biochemical imbalance in the brain, or is the result of one's life circumstances? Writing in *Time*, Robert Wright summarizes the issue: ("The Evolution of Despair," Aug. 28, 1995, pp. 52, 53):

Rates of depression have been doubling in some industrial countries roughly every 10 years. ...What isn't natural is going crazy—for sadness to linger on into debilitating depression, for anxiety to grow chronic and paralyzing. These are largely diseases of modernity. When researchers examined rural villagers in Samoa, they discovered what were by Western standards extraordinarily low levels of cortisol, a biochemical by-product of anxiety. And when a Western anthropologist tried to study depression among the Kaluli of New Guinea, he couldn't find any.

10. Type 2 diabetes increases with industrialization

• The incidence of type 2 diabetes has risen sharply in recent decades. It now afflicts more than 3 percent of Americans, up from less than 1 percent in 1958. By 2025, the number of adults with diabetes is expected to reach 300 million worldwide—more than twice the number estimated to have the disease in 1995.

• Americans who are overweight are nearly three times as likely as people of normal weight to develop diabetes.. The recent rise in diabetes can be traced to a rise in obesity, a result of increasing inactivity without a compensating decrease in caloric intake.

• According to Dr. Michael P. Stern of the Univ. of Texas Health Science Center in San Antonio, a 9% increase in type 2 diabetes has been noted every year in the 10 years before 1996. ("Diabetes increasing in US adults," *Reuters*, June 16, 1998)

• Dr. James R. Gavin III, senior scientific officer at the Howard Hughes Medical Institute in Chevy Chase, Md., notes that type 2 diabetes "virtually disappeared during World War II" because "there was no food and no gasoline." Studies have shown that regular physical exercise helps to normalize blood sugar levels. (Jane Brody, "Type 2 diabetes increasingly common killer, crippler," *The Herald-Sun*, Durham, North Carolina, Nov. 19, 1995, p. G2)

• In major urban areas such as New York City, diabetes has undergone a dramatic upsurge, increasing in prevalence tenfold from 1866 through 1923 and continuing that trend to the present. This pattern reflects the fact that diabetes is expressed primarily in persons who have adopted a Western, industrialized society diet. Only a small proportion of indigenous peoples who generally have maintained a high fiber, low fat diet have this disorder. (Marc Lappe, *Evolutionary Medicine: Rethinking the Origins of Disease*, San Francisco: Sierra Club Books, 1994, p. 165)

• According to Dr. Aila Rissanen of the obesity research unit at Helsinki University Central Hospital, "If we were able to prevent obesity from occurring, we could prevent up to 80 percent of cases of diabetes." (Denise Mann, "Few Know of Obesity-Diabetes Link, Survey Shows," *Medical Tribune* online, July 21, 1997)

• A World Health Organization report predicts that diabetes will reach epidemic proportions in the world during the first quarter of the 21 st century. Developing countries will see the greatest increase in the number of adult diabetes patients. In emerging nations, the number of adults with the disorder will rise 170%, from 84 million in 1995 to 228 million in 2025. By comparison, the number of adults with diabetes will increase 42% in industrialized nations, rising from 51 million in 1995 to 70 million in 2025. ["Worldwide diabetes 'epidemic' predicted," *Reuters* online, Sept. 8, 1998]

• There has been a sharp increase in type 2 diabetes among China's under-40 population. "We have a huge emerging problem not just in Hong Kong but in the whole of Asia," said Dr. Clive Cockram of the Chinese University of Hong Kong and Prince of Wales Hospital. According to Cockram, "In Hong Kong, our children are rapidly becoming obese, they have one of the highest cholesterol levels in the world...they engage in sedentary pursuits...computer games, TV, and study...and very little personal play." ("Diabetes increasing in young Chinese," *Reuters*, Feb. 5, 1999)

To underscore the fact that diabetes is a disease of Western industrialized societies, see the following chart "Prevalence of Diabetes in Different Societies." (Marc Lappe, *Evolutionary Medicine: Rethinking the Origins of Disease,* San Francisco, Sierra Club Books, 1994, p. 166). Compare the incidence in traditional societies versus a sample of westernized societies (Canada, Australia, USA, and Japan).

Prevalence of Diabetes in Different Societies

Major nutrient source	Population Group	Prevalence
Gatherers	African nomadic Bryoas	0.0%

Hunters and gatherers	Alaskan Athabaskans	1.3%
	Greenland Eskimos	1.2%
	Alaskan Eskimos	1.9%
Vegetarians and fish eaters	New Guinea Melanesians	0.9%
	Loyalty Island Melanese	2.0%
	Malaysia, rural villagers	1.8%
Grain, fish, and meat eaters	India, rural villagers	1.2%
	Israel, Yemenites	0.1%
	New Caledonians	1.5%
	Polynesia, Pukapuka	1.0%
	Fiji Islanders	0.6%
Industrialized westerners	Australians, Canadians, Americans, and Japanese	3.0% to 10.0%

11. Asthma incidence varies widely around the world and increases with industrialization.

• The highest prevalence of asthma is in the United Kingdom, Australia, New Zealand and Ireland. In the United States, which is in the top 10 of countries surveyed in a major study of asthma prevalence, self-reported cases of asthma rose 75% between 1980 and 1994. The countries with the lowest asthma prevalences include several Eastern European countries, Indonesia, Greece, China, Taiwan, Uzbekistan, India and Ethiopia, according to the first results from the

International Study of Asthma and Allergies in Childhood (ISAAC), published in the April 25, 1998 issue of *The Lancet*. Overall, the prevalence of asthma was 20 to 60 times higher in some countries compared with others. Dr. Richard Beasley of Wellington Asthma Research Group in Wellington, New Zealand, who led the study, noted that the variation in symptom prevalences among various centers throughout the world is "striking."

• In the United States, asthma rates have risen dramatically since 1980, according to a report issued April 24, 1998 by the Centers for Disease Control and Prevention (CDC). ("Asthma Varies Widely Around the World," *Reuters* online, April 24, 1998) The death rate for children aged 19 years and younger due to asthma rose by 78 percent between 1980 and 1993. ("US Says Asthma Cases Up 75 Percent Since 1980," *Reuters* online, April 23, 1998)

• International studies in adults and in children in which meticulous attention has been given to methodological detail support the clinical impression that differences in asthma occurrence between countries are real. In addition there is evidence of an increase in prevalence of asthma, particularly in children, in industrialized and in industrializing countries. For instance, in Great Britain, one in seven children is now thought to have asthma, whereas in sub-Saharan African countries, where the disease was non-existent in the 1960s, asthma rates are similar to those in many industrialized countries. [Margaret R. Becklake and Pierre Ernst, "Environmental Factors," *Lancet* 1997; 350 (suppl II): 10-13]

• Asthma is on the rise among people of all ages. The recent dramatic increase in the incidence of asthma cannot be blamed on genetics. "The genetic makeup of the population couldn't have changed enough to see the increases in asthma that are being seen in many developed countries. So there's got to be some kind of environmental exposure, but exactly what that is really isn't known," says Dr. Stephen Redd of the U. S. Centers for Disease Control and Prevention (CDC). ("U.S. Doctors Mystified By Increase in Asthma," *Reuters* online, May 7, 1998)

• Dr. Irwin Redlener, president of the Children's Health Fund, New York, says that factors in the increase in cases may include everything from outdoor air pollutants to cockroaches, dust mites and tobacco smoke. Redlener says that asthma shows a predilection for affecting people in large cities across the country. ("U.S. Doctors Mystified by Increase in Asthma," *Reuters* online, May 7, 1998)

Asthma isn't usually a problem in preindustrial societies, regardless of their natural surroundings. But when development sets in, asthma quickly follows. Dr. Hal Nelson of Denver's National Jewish Medical center cites a 1991 study of children in Zimbabwe. Only one in 1,000 of those living in rural villages suffered from obstructed airways. Yet asthma plagued one in 17 (5.8 percent) of those in a prosperous section of the capital, Harare. Researchers have documented the same pattern among Aboriginal people in Kenya, South Africa, Papua New Guinea, New Zealand and Australia. Even within Western societies, increasing urbanization seems to make people more and more vulnerable. The United States has an overall asthma rate of about 5 percent, says Dr. Irwin Redlener of New York's Montefiore Medical Center. But the rate is 8.4 percent in New York City, and it can reach 25 percent among kids in the poorest urban neighborhoods. [Geoffrey Cowley, Anne Underwood, et. al., "Why Ebonie Can't Breathe," *Newsweek*, May 26, 1997, p. 61]

I quit pharmacy after twenty-five years because I felt my job as a pharmacist was often unfulfilling because I spent all day filling prescriptions for diseases that are largely preventable. If the diseases that make up the largest numbers of visits to doctors in the USA are related to our diet and lifestyle, it would seem logical that the greatest improvements in health would result from basic preventative efforts rather than from a focus on drug development and genetic research. Surely it is better to prevent disease than to treat it.

Doctors are fond of saying that patients have a very hard time making major changes in their diets and lifestyles. Implied in this observation is the assumption that since these major changes are very difficult to realize in the real world, a reliance on pills is unavoidable. I agree that getting Americans to make major changes in their diets and lifestyles is very difficult. It is in no small part made more difficult by the saturation of our society with advertisements for the products of the pharmaceutical industry. Pharma has done a masterful job in convincing Americans to accept the quick-fix pill-for-every-ill outlook. But here is my point: If messages about the critical importance of prevention saturated our society as effectively as advertisements for pharmaceuticals (or, better yet, if direct-to-consumer drug advertisements were banned as they are everywhere except in the USA and New Zealand), then Americans would be far healthier than any level of pill consumption could ever accomplish. Let's ban those direct-to-consumer drug advertisements and replace them with messages stressing the critical importance of major changes in diet and lifestyles. Messages about the critical importance of diet and lifestyles should saturate our society instead of messages to take pills. But I can't see this happening in my lifetime because there's no money in prevention.

The concept of "diseases of modern civilization" is not immediately obvious to everyone. Understanding this concept takes a little understanding of human health combined with a little understanding of society. For most people, modern societies and modern diets are taken at face value because that's all we've known for our entire lives. To understand diseases of modern civilization, one must be willing to look at society critically and to compare modern societies with those that are less modern. We must also be willing to compare human health with the health of animals living in the wild. Domesticated animals and animals living in zoos do indeed develop many of the same health problems as *Homo sapiens*.

For a population that has grown up eating the highly-processed foods commonly found in the modern supermarket, it is a somewhat radical concept to say that the typical American diet is killing us. It is almost un-American. But I wonder: Shouldn't Americans be uneasy that it nearly requires a degree in chemistry to understand all the synthetic substances listed on typical food labels?

Obesity and dental caries are the two most obvious examples of diseases of modern civilization. It should not be too difficult for most people to connect obesity and dental caries to the standard American diet. From my perspective, modern lifestyles, modern diets, and modern societies cause as much havoc to the human body as the modern diet causes to our teeth.

Dentists make a very nice living treating the adverse consequences of the modern American diet. Fillings, crowns, dentures, and implants make dentistry a very lucrative enterprise. Yet our ancestors from a few centuries ago had very little need for dentists. Animals living in the wild do not need dentists.

PART X

ISSUES

Chapter 36

Decoding pharmacy jargon

In my criticism of jargon, I want to emphasize that I recognize the importance of precise language in medicine and pharmacy. I am not opposed to precise words. I *am* opposed to the use of overly technical and pompous words in instances in which more widely understood words would do just as well. If pharmacists have as their goal an increase in our customers' understanding of drugs and medical conditions, is it not possible for us to sacrifice a slight bit of precision for the sake of comprehension? Perhaps pharmacists need to examine our motivations when we use fancy words. Language should be used to communicate. It should not be used to intimidate or to minimize the potential risks of drugs and medical treatments. Let me make the case that many words commonly used in medicine and pharmacy are unnecessarily technical and in some cases even pretentious.

The drug information that we give customers with the prescriptions we dispense usually includes only a small fraction of the long list of side effects in the official prescribing information approved by the FDA (the "professional labeling"). Therefore, if one of our customers wants a complete list of side effects, he either has to ask us for a copy of the professional labeling (also known as the "professional insert") or he needs to consult a copy of the *Physicians' Desk Reference (PDR)* at his local library or bookstore. Consequently, shouldn't the FDA require that the language in the professional labeling be more understandable to laymen? More specifically, shouldn't the FDA make an attempt to do away with unnecessarily technical terms in the "adverse effects" section of the professional labeling? There are dozens of examples in the professional labeling in which a term familiar to laymen could be substituted for a technical term. In my opinion, there is no justification for using a technical term for a side effect when a commonly understood term would do just as well. Examples of medical and pharmacy jargon:

adipose tissue—fat tissue

alopecia—hair loss

amenorrhea—failure of menstruation

anorexia—loss of appetite

anorgasmy—failure to have an orgasm

antiemetic—drug that treats nausea and vomiting

antineoplastic—drug that treats cancer

antipyretic—drug that treats fever

antitussive—drug that treats cough

anxiolytic—drug that treats anxiety

arthralgia—painful joint

asthenia—weakness

ataxia—lack of muscle coordination

axilla—armpit

bradycardia—slow heart rate

caries—dental cavities

cerebrovascular accident—stroke

cerumen—ear wax

climacteric—menopause

cognitive impairment—impaired thinking

dependence—addiction

dermatologist—skin specialist

dysmenorrhea—painful or difficult menstruation

dyspepsia—indigestion

dysphagia—impaired swallowing

dysphonia—impaired voice

dyspnea—shortness of breath
edema—fluid accumulation
enuresis—bedwetting
epistaxis—nosebleed
etiology—cause
flatulence—gas
gingival hyperplasia—overgrowth of gums
gynecomastia—enlargement of breasts in males
hematuria—blood in the urine
hepatic—liver
hepatologist—liver specialist
hirsutism—excessive hair growth
hypercholesterolemia—elevated cholesterol
hyperkalemia—elevated potassium
hypernatremia—elevated sodium
hypertension—high blood pressure
hypotension—low blood pressure
indications—approved uses
insomnia—sleeplessness
mastication—chewing
mastitis—inflammation of the breast
menarche—onset of first period
myalgia—muscle pain
myocardial infarction—heart attack
nocturia—getting up at night to urinate
oncologist—cancer specialist
ophthalmic—eye
ophthalmologist—eye specialist
otic—ear
otorhinolaryngologist—ear-nose-throat specialist
parasthesia—burning or tingling sensation
polydipsia—excessive thirst
polyphagia—excessive eating
polyuria—passage of large quantities of urine
pruritus—itching
pulmonary—relating to lung

pulmonologist—lung specialist
renal—kidney
somnolence—sleepiness
stomatitis—mouth inflammation
syncope—fainting
tachycardia—rapid heart rate
tinnitus—ringing in the ears
umbilicus—belly button or navel
urticaria—hives
vertigo—dizziness

Do these technical terms illustrate the need for precision in medical communication? Or are these examples of words that are used to make the public feel inferior? When I was in pharmacy school, I remember discussing the following scenario with a classmate: *What would we do if a customer asked us a question that we could not answer?* My classmate told me, "Just throw a few long words at them and they'll shut up!" We both laughed.

Many times a customer shows me a skin rash and asks me to recommend a non-prescription cream. Since I don't know much about skin conditions, I often suggest that the customer see a dermatologist. Believe it or not, I often wonder whether many customers know what a "dermatologist" is. So I recommend "a dermatologist—a skin doctor." My brother read this and told me that I shouldn't underestimate the intelligence of pharmacy customers. That's when I told him that one day a customer asked me how to pronounce "CVS" (as in the pharmacy chain known as "CVS"). The intelligence of pharmacy customers spans a very wide spectrum.

If you look in the Yellow Pages in the phone book under "Physicians," you see the following categories: **Pulmonologist, Oncologist, Nephrologist, Hepatologist, Ophthalmologist, Otorhinolaryngologist**, etc. Why not simply identify each specialty as lung, cancer, kidney, liver, eye, ENT (ear, nose, and throat), etc.?

The use of Latin abbreviations is another example of communication that is meant to impress or intimidate or increase awe. Customers who see strange abbreviations like **PO** (by mouth), or **QD** (daily), or **BID** (twice a day), or **TID** (three times a day), or **PC** (after meals), or **AC** (before meals), or **HS** (at bedtime), often feel ignorant. Sometimes it looks like modern medicine does its best to make the public feel stupid.

Customers frequently call the pharmacist and describe a symptom and then ask if the symptom can be a side effect of a drug. The pharmacist grabs a copy of the official labeling that is attached to the product. We quickly scan the long list of side effects. I can never remember the definition of words like **epistaxis** (nosebleed), **urticaria** (hives), **stomatitis** (mouth inflammation), **ataxia** (lack of muscle coordination), **syncope** (fainting), **asthenia** (weakness), **dysphagia** (impaired swallowing), etc. I have twenty prescriptions waiting to be filled and I have to hunt for my medical dictionary so that I can answer the customer's question correctly. Many times I've been tempted to say (and I've observed other pharmacists saying) "No, that side effect is not listed." In fact, it may very well be listed but we've forgotten the definition of some of these unnecessarily technical terms. With dangerous understaffing in many pharmacies, pharmacists often don't have adequate time to answer customers' questions about side effects. Technical language makes a bad situation worse.

Here are some more of my favorite examples:
• "Hypertension of unknown cause" is referred to as **idiopathic hypertension.**
• "Hospital acquired infection" is referred to as **nosocomial infection.**
• Symptoms associated with the menopause are referred to as **vasomotor symptoms.**
• **Dysfunction** is a more impressive word than "malfunction."
• In the professional labeling, "approved uses" would be more widely understood than **indications.**
• If a layman picks up a copy of the *PDR*, does he know what the word **contraindication** means? Why not use "strongly advised against" instead?

Professionals have a tendency to use long and complex words to impress laymen. Appending the term "disorder" or "syndrome" makes a condition sound more serious and legitimate. Some critics say medical professionals are medicalizing or pathologizing normal human experience with the following diagnoses:
• **attention deficit disorder**—poor grades in school

- **hyperactivity disorder**—unruly behavior in children
- **obsessive-compulsive disorder**—excessive handwashing, etc.
- **social anxiety disorder**—shyness
- **generalized anxiety disorder**—a broader form of shyness
- **premenstrual dysphoric disorder**—a more severe form of premenstrual syndrome
- **seasonal affective disorder**—the winter blues
- **body dysmorphic disorder**—a negative image of one's body
- **panic disorder**—panic attack
- **road rage syndrome or intermittent explosive disorder**
- **restless leg syndrome**
- **shift work sleep disorder**—Nuvigil is a drug promoted for use by people who work the overnight shift and have trouble staying awake. A less expensive approach and one with fewer potential side effects is coffee.

Other disorders on the horizon:
- **temper dysregulation disorder**
- **oppositional defiant disorder (ODD)**
- **compulsive shopping disorder**
- **compulsive gambling disorder**
- **binge-eating disorder**—eating until feeling uncomfortably full
- **hypersexual disorder**—sex addiction

Is Pharma so insecure about the legitimacy of all these diagnoses that their marketing people feel the necessity to append the term "disorder" to gain public acceptance? Yet we don't hear cancer *disorder*, diabetes *disorder*, pneumonia *disorder*, AIDS *disorder*, etc., because the public is convinced these are legitimate diagnoses.

Here are some terms that I wish psychologists and psychiatrists would use to examine their own motivations for constantly expanding the universe of billable diagnoses:
- **diagnostic inflation**
- **medical imperialism**
- **disease mongering**
- **overdiagnosis**
- **medicalization**
- **pathologization**—e.g., the pathologization of ordinary behavior such as sadness over a spouse's death

More examples of my least favorite terms in medicine and pharmacy:

Pruritis: I once received a prescription in which the doctor's directions stated, "Take one tablet daily for pruritus." I didn't know if I should replace "pruritus" with "itching." Did the customer know the definition of "pruritus"? Why in the world would the doctor want the word "pruritus" on the patient's label rather than itching? Pharmacists are not normally supposed to change key words in the doctor's directions unless there is a compelling reason to do so. Maybe this doctor was trying to impress the patient with the word "pruritus." Maybe the doctor felt that the patient would view the office visit more favorably if it resulted in a fancy diagnosis of "pruritus" rather than merely "itching."

Edema: Doctors like to use the word "edema" when it would be more meaningful to use "fluid accumulation." Many times I've typed "Take one tablet daily for edema" when I possibly should have substituted "fluid accumulation." Should health professionals have a duty to communicate using language understandable to the layman?

Anxiolytic: One of my favorite examples of an unnecessarily technical word is "anxiolytic." This word comes from "anxiety" and "lysis" (decline of a disease process). This is a ten dollar word for the class of drugs used to treat anxiety (Valium, Ativan, Tranxene, Xanax, etc.). Other drug class names that strike me as unnecessarily technical are "antipyretic" (treats fever), "antineoplastic" (treats cancer), "antitussive" (treats cough), and "antiemetic" (treats nausea and vomiting)

Adjunct: One of my least favorite words is *adjunct*. I graduated from pharmacy school without a clear understanding of what an *adjunct* professor is—possibly because there were none (as far as I know) at the pharmacy school I attended. I knew there are assistant professors, associate professors, and full professors, but I did not know what an *adjunct* professor is. Several years later I happened to read that an *adjunct* professor is a part-time professor who is hired on a contractual basis, rather than being given tenure and a permanent position. Pharmacy professors and pharmacy magazine editors frequently write things like "Drug X is used as an *adjunct* to diet and exercise in the management of type 2 diabetes." Here *adjunct* means "something that is joined or added to another thing." *Adjunct* is one of the most pompous words that I know. I don't know anyone who uses this word in everyday conversation. I would be embarrassed to use this word in public.

Suicidal ideation: A side effect of some antidepressants is "suicidal ideation." This is a sanitized version of "thoughts of suicide." Another fancy word for this is "suicidality."

Polypharmacy: Commonly used in pharmacy magazines and journals, "polypharmacy" is a sanitized version of "overmedication." Since many pharmacy magazines and journals receive most of their revenue from pharmaceutical industry advertising, it is not surprising that these publications seem to have a very hard time admitting that Americans may be overmedicated. Thus, use of the term "polypharmacy" is less likely to anger advertisers. I am exaggerating only slightly in stating it is the dream of Big Pharma that every human being on this planet is drugged to the gills. Substituting the sanitized word "polypharmacy" for "overmedication" is almost as Orwellian as adopting the moniker "Clear Skies Initiative" for George W. Bush legislation that eased up on air quality standards.

Misfill: When I first heard the word "misfill," I thought this was a peculiar word. I remember the occasion vividly. The year was 1983 and my district supervisor was standing near me. As he prepared to leave, he mentioned that he was headed to another store in his district where he had to deal with a pharmacist's "misfill." "Misfill" is a sanitized version of "mistake."

Habituation: The word "habituation" (e.g., "This drug may cause—or result in—habituation.") is used instead of "habit-forming" in an attempt to obfuscate the risk. Similarly, "dependence" and "drug-seeking behavior" are somewhat less scary than "addiction." Addiction implies moral weakness or lack of will power.

Medical misadventures, untoward effects, adverse events: People in the military frequently speak of "taking out" enemy "combatants" rather use the more precise term: "killing" them. Similarly, in an effort to sanitize the loss of life, pilots say they "took out several enemy positions." We say that a friend or relative "passed away" or "passed on" rather than say he or she "died." In the world of pharmaceuticals, there is a similar effort to soften or obfuscate the potential adverse consequences of prescription drugs. I am struck by how routinely drug advertisements on television are successful in making potentially frightening side effects sound almost desirable or appealing. Doctors, drug companies, and pharmacists refer to side effects and adverse effects as "adverse events," "untoward effects," and "medical misadventures." Melody Peterson writes in *Our Daily Meds* (New York: Farrar, Straus, and Giroux, 2008, p. 298):

> **In the medical literature, these maladies are broadly called "drug-induced disorders" or "adverse drug reactions." Industry scientists writing in medical journals often refer to them simply as "events." Many physicians and pharmacists prefer to call them "medical misadventures," as if someone has suffered an unlucky mishap like wandering off a path in the woods. The euphemism has helped create a false perception that these are unfortunate occurrences in the practice of medicine that no one can do anything about. Stripped of all such embellishments, these "events" are the serious injuries and deaths caused by prescription drugs.**

"May": In my opinion, *may* is the most loaded and most misleading word used by Big Pharma. Based on very preliminary research, often in mice or rats, drug companies frequently say that Investigational Drug X *may* be effective against, for example, various types of cancer. The implication here is that the claim is *probably* true but the drug company is simply being cautious or conservative. Often the opposite is true. The drug company is often hyping very preliminary results and the investigational drug is never approved. Whenever you hear a drug company say that Investigational Drug X *may* be effective in Treatment Y, you should be highly skeptical and view this as highly preliminary. The word *may* is also used often to explain how a drug works when no one really knows for sure how it works. For example, drug advertisements on television say that depression *may* be caused by a chemical imbalance in the brain. The ads then proceed to state that their antidepressant helps correct that imbalance. The viewer is left with the impression that depression is *probably* due to a chemical imbalance in the brain even though this is a highly controversial point. It is pure speculation according to many critics of psychiatry. For example, the patient leaflet for Abilify, a drug that treats bipolar disorder, states, "Abilify *may* [my emphasis] work by adjusting dopamine activity, instead of completely blocking it and by adjusting serotonin activity. However, the exact way any medicine for bipolar disorder works is unknown." (*Newsweek*, March 26, 2007, p. 67)

Medicines: Pharmaceutical marketers are highly proficient in the use of language to manipulate consumers. Perhaps it's just quirkiness on my part, but I especially dislike the way the pharmaceutical industry refers to drugs as "medicines." Medical writers and laymen are often unknowingly guilty of the same practice. Use of the term "medicines" irritates me the same way as the sound of chalk screeching across a blackboard. That is because when Big Pharma uses this term, I view it as heavy-duty manipulation. Whereas the term *drugs* often conjures up an image of "street drugs" like crack cocaine and heroin, the term *medicines* conjures up heroic images from the past such as penicillin curing life-threatening infections or insulin saving the lives of diabetics. Even though the drug companies routinely refer to drugs as *medicines* in direct-to-consumer advertisements, pharmacists rarely use that word. For example, pharmacists might say to a technician, "Mrs. Smith wants to get her blood pressure *pills*." In my experience, it is extremely rare that a pharmacist would tell the tech, "Mrs. Smith wants to get her blood pressure *medicine*." The clever use of language is just one more example of the endless tactics that the pharmaceutical industry employs to distort the nature of pharmaceuticals and to gloss over the many potential risks associated with these substances. Read almost any direct-to-consumer drug advertisement in magazines like *Time* or *Newsweek* and you will see these products referred to with the soothing word "medicines." From my experience, pharmacists would almost always use the words "pills" or "drugs" instead. As I write this in 2007, here are several examples from my current issue of *Newsweek* (March 26, 2007) of what I consider to be cleverly manipulative wording: (I have italicized the word "medicine" or "medicines" in each example below.)

• Lunesta belongs to a group of *medicines* known as "hynotics" or, simply, sleep *medicines*.

• Avandia works differently than other diabetes *medicines* by helping your body use its own natural insulin better.

• Zetia is different than the most common cholesterol-lowering *medicines*, called statins.

• Boniva is a prescription *medicine* used to treat or prevent osteoporosis in women after menopause.

• Vytorin is a *medicine* used to lower levels of total cholesterol, LDL (bad) cholesterol, and fatty substances called triglycerides in the blood.

• Abilify is a prescription *medicine* used to treat patients with an acute manic or mixed episode associated with Bipolar 1 Disorder.

Meds: I don't like referring to medications as "meds". Pharmacists often say something like this to techs: "Mrs. Smith wants us to refill all her meds." Or "Mrs. Smith wants us to refill all her pills." I prefer "Mrs. Smith wants us to fill all her prescriptions." Nor do I like the word "scripts," as in "How many scripts did you fill today?" I prefer "How many prescriptions did you fill today." I'm not trying to be pretentious. I just feel the terms "meds" and "scripts" imply a very casual attitude toward medications and prescriptions, trivializing the many serious issues (adverse effects, overmedication, medicalization, dependency, etc.) surrounding the products pharmacists dispense. It is as if the products on our shelves are as non-controversial and straight-forward as the health benefits of fresh fruits and vegetables. It reminds me of my college years in which students referred to sociology as *sosh*, psychology as *psych*, and political science as *poli-sci*. I respect the fields of sociology, psychology, and political science because these disciplines have the potential to explain the deep pathology in modern societies. Referring to these college courses as *sosh, psych,* and *poli-sci* trivializes the examination of our lives and society. I agree with the axiom that "the unexamined life is not worth living." From my perspective, a majority of college students prefer to live in a world of hedonistic consumption and materialism. In the world of pharmacy, I don't feel that prescription drugs are trivial substances. I feel that people should view prescription drugs with a sober, dispassionate evaluation of risks versus benefits. Big Pharma is spending massive sums of money to convince the public that prescription drugs are safe as candy. Therefore, in my opinion, consumers need to maintain a healthy level of skepticism. Using the affectionate terms *meds* and *scripts* implies that medications and prescriptions are akin to an adorable little puppy or kitten. These terms ignore the serious critique of pharmaceuticals that is readily available, for example, by reading any of a couple dozen books critical of the drug industry, or by reading customer reviews of these books on Amazon.com or BarnesandNoble.com. A great many of these customer reviews show a higher level of sophistication in understanding the critique of Big Pharma than I've seen among the many pharmacists I know. Pharmacists' routine use of words like *meds* and *scripts* and *nerve pills* and *druggies* implies to me a superficial, anti-intellectual, unquestioning, naïve, facile attitude toward pharmaceuticals. In my opinion, comedian/social critic Bill Maher, the Mark Twain of today, has a much more sophisticated understanding of the critique of Pharma than the vast majority of pharmacists I know.

Nerve pills: An extremely common occurrence in the pharmacy is when customers tell us they want their *nerve pills* refilled. Or a tech tells us, "Mrs. Smith says she wants her *nerve pills.*" Perhaps I'm over-reacting again but I feel that the serious cultural implications of the widespread use of anti-anxiety drugs in our society are trivialized by referring to this class of drugs as *nerve pills*. Nerve pills like Xanax and Ativan and antidepressants like Prozac and Paxil are viewed in America as reasonable ways to address the deep pathology in modern society.

"Druggies": Many pharmacists refer to drug abusers as "druggies." In my opinion, this term trivializes the serious problem of drug abuse in our society just as the word "nukes" trivializes the problem of nuclear proliferation. The words "druggies" and "nukes" almost imply some level of affection. Perhaps pharmacists find some level of enjoyment or entertainment in the endless number of stories and creative excuses drug abusers invent in an effort to get early refills on controlled substances such as Vicodin, Lortab, Xanax, and Ativan.

"Genetic" drugs: A large number of pharmacy customers are illiterate or poorly literate. Many pharmacy customers routinely refer to "generic" drugs as "genetic" drugs. This may seem like a minor slip of the tongue but, to me, it indicates a fundamental misunderstanding of two totally different words. "Generic drugs" have nothing to do with genes. Pharmacists often wonder how our customers can fully understand their medications when many customers clearly don't know that generic drugs have nothing to do with genetics.

Pharmacy "patients": I understand the desire of pharmacy magazine editors to elevate the professional status of pharmacists by referring to our clientele as "patients." However, I feel that "customers" is a more honest term. From my experience in the real world, chain drugstore pharmacists almost never refer to our clientele as "patients." Such a pharmacist would, in my opinion, be viewed by his colleagues as quite naïve and as someone who too unquestioningly accepted the model of pharmacy sold to us in pharmacy school. Among pharmacists who actually work in chain drugstores, the term "patient" is used only when referring to a doctor's patient (e.g., "Dr. Smith's patient"). It is unimaginable that our district supervisors or bosses further up the corporate ladder would refer to our clientele as "patients." Perhaps most chain pharmacists adequately understand that using the term "patients" is too pretentious for a workplace in which we feel utterly powerless against the rigid chain hierarchy, where taking a bathroom break seems to be viewed by the corporation as something that only a slacker would do. The attitude of upper management seems to be: *Real pharmacists don't need bathroom or meal breaks!*

Pharmacy "practice": If pharmacists have a drive-thru window where they work, and they don't have time to rest or eat or go to the bathroom, I consider it pompous for those pharmacists to say that they "practice" pharmacy. In reality, they "practice" fast food. Only once can I recall hearing a pharmacist asking another pharmacist, "Where do you practice?" I remember it sounded extremely hokey. Pharmacists living in the real world ask simply "Where do you work?" For the many pharmacists who feel they work at the pharmacy equivalent of McDonald's, the term "pharmacy practice" is laughable.

The Pill: Birth control pills have a special status in the pharmacy lexicon. Whenever someone says "The Pill," we all know that means birth control pills. Whenever a tech tells the pharmacist that a young female "wants a refill on her pills," we know that means birth control pills. I used to work with one tech who always referred to birth control pills as "party pills." This tech would say something like "Mary Jones wants to get her party pills." Perhaps I'm being too much of a curmudgeon, but I feel that the term "The Pill" doesn't convey that oral contraceptives are a serious class of drugs with some potentially risky cardiovascular side effects clearly listed in the *Physicians' Desk Reference*.

Chapter 37

How accurate are expiration dates?

When I graduated from pharmacy school, the pharmacist was not required to type the expiration date of the medication on the label. Adding the expiration date to the label is a good thing but it is not always accurate, for many reasons. In a pharmacy that's woefully understaffed, checking the expiration date on products takes only a few seconds, but when we're absolutely overwhelmed with prescriptions and running an hour or two behind, the accuracy of the expiration date is sometimes a casualty.

In general, I would say that the stock bottles (each containing, say, 30 or 100 or 500 or 1000 pills) that we receive from our warehouse have an expiration date of two to three years. State law in some states requires that pharmacists print on the prescription label a maximum expiration date of one year from the date the prescription was filled. In other words, say a pharmacist fills a prescription for some medication that has an expiration date of two or three years down the road. Since most of the products sitting on pharmacy shelves at any given time do indeed have a manufacturer's expiration date that is more than a year down the road, the pharmacy computer has been programmed to print, by default, an expiration date on the label that is one year after the date the prescription is filled. This is done primarily in recognition of the fact that once a stock bottle has been opened by the pharmacist, or once a medication has been dispensed to a customer, the rate of deterioration of that product is subject to many factors.

Eyeballing every single product on our pharmacy shelves every few months (two or three thousand containers I guess) is an extremely time-consuming and boring process. Consequently, I have seen many instances in which expired drugs are sitting on pharmacy shelves. Some of these drugs end up being dispensed to customers. Of course, if we had adequate staffing, there would be more time to regularly check our shelves for expired products. Thus, if your pharmacist or technician is overwhelmed with prescriptions, he or she may just allow the pharmacy computer to print the default expiration date (one year down the road) without actually looking to see what expiration date is actually stamped by the manufacturer on the stock bottle.

Having expired products sitting on pharmacy shelves is not an unusual thing at all. In my experience, it is rare to walk into a pharmacy and find no expired drugs on the shelves. The same thing holds true for all the non-prescription drugs on the sales floor. That's why you should always check the expiration date every time you purchase a product for cold or cough or pain or whatever.

Upon retirement in Florida, I fractured a tooth and developed significant pain in that tooth. It was a weekend so I went to a local drugstore, a major national chain, to buy a bottle of Advil. I briefly considered the store brand ibuprofen which was directly adjacent to the Advil. I picked up the ibuprofen while trying to decide whether to buy the Advil or the store brand. I happened to notice that the brand name Advil had a good expiration date (like two years down the road), but the store brand ibuprofen was four or five months out of date. I wasn't really surprised. That's because, from my experience, the non-pharmacist store manager (who is responsible for checking store shelves for expired non-prescription drugs) is usually in the same boat as the pharmacy manager. Like the pharmacist, the non-pharmacist store manager's staffing is tightly controlled by corporate so pulling expired products from the sales floor is very often not a high priority. The big chains simply don't provide adequate staffing to run drugstores like the public assumes. Newspapers occasionally run articles about an undercover reporter or state inspector finding large numbers of expired products on drugstore shelves. The bad publicity for the drugstore and hefty fine imposed by state inspectors don't, in my experience, usually result a long-term change in behavior. In my experience, expiration dates simply aren't usually seen as a high priority in understaffed drugstores.

The entire issue of expiration dates is very interesting. There is tremendous disagreement about how realistic expiration dates are, given the wide variety of ways in which medications are handled. For example, most drugs are shipped to chain drugstores from the chain warehouse which may be a few hundred miles away. And, in my experience, most of the time, the drugs are shipped in eighteen-wheel trucks that are not climate controlled. When I worked in Summersville, West Virginia, I recall receiving a pint bottle of Dimetapp, completely frozen. (Dimetapp, a drug used to treat symptoms of the common cold, required a prescription at that time. It is now available without a prescription.) The glass container was broken but the liquid contents hadn't made a big mess because it was still frozen when I unpacked the entire warehouse order, probably within an hour of receiving it.

In my mind I can still see that glass bottle with several large cracks in it. What happened to this pint bottle of Dimetapp was exactly what would happen if someone placed, for example, a bottle of Coca Cola in his or her freezer. Since liquids expand when they freeze, they crack glass bottles. So the Dimetapp was unusable. I guess I could have theoretically separated the frozen contents from the broken glass and allowed it to thaw in a bowl and then poured the melted contents into an empty pint bottle. But that wasn't really an option because I had to assume there could be glass particles mixed in with the frozen Dimetapp. So the easiest and safest thing to do was to throw the broken bottle and its frozen contents into the trash. That's exactly what I did and what I hope most pharmacists would do.

In general, the two most common storage recommendations with drugs are 1) keep in a cool dry location away from direct sunlight and 2) do not freeze. Drugs are clearly subject to freezing while being shipped to drugstores in the winter. And they can be exposed to extremely high temperatures in the summer while being shipped in these eighteen-wheelers that are typically not climate controlled.

There have been a number of articles written about the subject of expiration dates of medications. Search Google for *drug expiration dates.* In addition to the issue of these drugs being sent to drugstores in the cold of winter or the heat of summer via eighteen-wheelers, there is the issue of medications received in the mail from distant mail order operations. Say you have a 9 to 5 job and your mail is delivered at 10 AM each day. This means that your medication will be sitting outside in your mail box during the hottest part of the day. There have been a few studies that have examined the stability of drugs under such temperature extremes and the results haven't been too bad, but I don't really have a lot of confidence that these studies have given a definitive answer to the issue of drug stability under temperature extremes. The private companies involved certainly don't have a financial incentive to find something wrong.

Another important factor regarding expiration dates is how the medication is stored once inside your home. The medication should be kept in a cool place, out of the sunlight, and away from moisture. The medicine cabinet in the bathroom is actually one of the worst possible places to keep medications. That's because the exposure of medications to the warm moist air from the bathtub or shower accelerates the deterioration of those medications.

So the expiration date on your prescription vial or bottle may or may not be an accurate reflection of the real world. Indeed, one of the most common questions pharmacists get from customers involves expiration dates. Here's a very common scenario. We receive a phone call from a customer who says, "I have a bottle of [Drug X] and it says the expiration was a couple of months ago. Is it still good?" You're likely to get slightly different answers to this question from different pharmacists. Some pharmacists say, "Yeah, it's probably still good." Other pharmacists say, "No. I'd throw it away." Since we live in such a litigious society, I usually answer this question by telling the customer that it would probably be a good idea to throw away the medication. But I usually add, just as an aside, that the expiration of medications is something that usually occurs gradually. Some people seem to think that if a medication has an expiration date of, say, May 3, 2012, then it is perfectly fine on the day before and useless or harmful on the day after. That's not the case. The way you store the medication and the way that it was shipped (exposed to extreme temperatures or not) are important things to be factored in when looking at expiration dates.

Do pharmacists ever knowingly dispense drugs that have expired and place a false expiration date on your prescription label? Here's a scenario. A customer comes to the drugstore and presents you with a prescription. You go to the pharmacy shelves and think to yourself, "Hmm. I haven't dispensed this drug in a long time. I wonder if it's still in date." So you look at the expiration date and notice that it's a few months out of date. Rather than tell that customer that the drug we have sitting on our shelves is out of date, most pharmacists would probably tell the customer that we are out of stock of the drug and that we can have it from a local supplier the next day (unless it's a weekend).

Sure enough, the customer arrives the next day to pick up his medication. But guess what? I forgot to order that drug from our local supplier so I can't fill the prescription. I have a few alternatives. I can lie and tell the customer that our supplier was out of the drug and I had no way of knowing that when I told him the day before that we would have it the next day. I can then tell the customer that even though our local supplier is out of stock, I can call around to a few drugstores in the area to see if they have the drug on hand. The vast majority of customers will be satisfied that the pharmacist is doing all he can. But there are a few customers who are your worst nightmare: loud, rude, arrogant, aggressive, and even threatening. Say this customer happens to be of the "worst nightmare" variety. There are some pharmacists who—in order to avoid what they know will be a terrible confrontation with the customer—will act like the drug did indeed arrive from our supplier. These pharmacists will go ahead and fill the prescription with the expired drug that has been sitting on our shelves for a long time. The pharmacist will not inform the customer that the drug has expired. The pharmacist will put a safe expiration date on the label.

The pharmacist has several ways to rationalize this unethical behavior. The pharmacist says to himself, "If I hadn't bothered to even look at the expiration date yesterday, I wouldn't actively be doing anything wrong." Or the pharmacist can rationalize dispensing an expired drug by saying to himself, "If this customer weren't such a complete asshole, I would tell him the truth that I forgot to order the drug. He's only getting what he deserves. I'm not going to give this customer a chance to tear me apart for not having the drug as I told him I would." Knowingly dispensing an expired drug to a customer is a serious breach of pharmacy practice. However, in the real world of dealing with oftentimes impossible customers in a dangerously understaffed pharmacy in which we're running an hour or two behind, rules are broken to avoid being verbally abused by such customers.

Upon retirement, I moved to Florida. One day I did a neighbor a favor by picking up her prescription at a local chain drugstore. The medication was Aggrenox, a drug that is used to reduce the risk of stroke in people who have had blood clots. I noticed that the pharmacist's prescription label indicated, "Exp. Date: See Product Pkg." I don't think this would have been legal in North Carolina, the state in which I worked for most of my career. In North Carolina, the pharmacist was required to place a specific date on the prescription label. In this case, the pharmacy label was attached directly to the manufacturer's box containing 60 capsules. Upon looking closely at the expiration date stamped on manufacturer's box, I see simply "Nov 12." I can see that this could be very confusing to the average pharmacy customer. I predict that the average pharmacy customer would interpret this as indicating that the Aggrenox expires on the twelfth day of November, whereas it is, in fact, saying that this drug expires in November of 2012.

Chapter 38

The case against anti-depressants

When I became a pharmacist, one of the things that surprised me most was the huge number of people in our society who are taking antidepressant drugs, even many of my neighbors. At what point does one begin to examine this from a sociological perspective? Does this say something about us as a nation? Or is the brain chemistry of millions of Americans simply defective?

Whenever I fill a prescription for an antidepressant, I often wonder what it is in the customer's life that makes her so depressed and I wonder whether she has made the effort to examine her life circumstances or whether she is looking for a quick fix in a pill. I wonder: Is it her job? Is it her spouse? Problems with the kids? Financial problems? When I fill an antidepressant prescription for a child, I wonder what his/her home life is like. Are parents placing too much pressure on kids to excel at school and in sports? Are kids depressed when they're not socially popular?

Have we as a nation gone overboard in blaming all depression on brain neurochemistry rather than on the everyday reality of people's lives that is, well, depressing? I once read that someone lost his severe shyness when he won a state lottery. If shyness were due to a chemical imbalance in the brain (as Pharma claims when it recommends drugs like Paxil as a solution), then shyness would be unaffected by winning a state lottery. I once heard, jokingly, that most of the people for whom we fill antidepressant prescriptions don't have any problem that a hefty pay raise wouldn't solve. I have imagined what would happen if the people who are depressed because of financial circumstances were to win a multi-million dollar state lottery. Would their depression disappear? If so, doesn't that prove that their depression was caused by their life circumstances, not a brain chemical imbalance?

I've filled antidepressant prescriptions for people who are physically very unattractive. I know that beauty is only skin deep, but our society seems to accept that dictum in theory but not in practice. Our society too often gives a cold shoulder to people who are not attractive. Is an antidepressant appropriate when someone's depression and social isolation are caused by a physical appearance that no cosmetic or wardrobe makeover can overcome?

Are pharmacists prime candidates for depression because of our working conditions? Almost any article on job satisfaction says that employees need a feeling of control over their work. Most chain pharmacists are utterly powerless to increase the level of staffing set by corporate. Pharmacists have incredibly high workloads, with disastrous consequences if we make a mistake, yet we have no power to correct the dangerously low staffing that jeopardizes the safety of our customers. Pharmacists see this as a prescription for burnout, disillusionment, and depression.

Even though many people claim that antidepressants make them feel better, that doesn't prove that depression is caused by a chemical imbalance in the brain. Many studies show that antidepressants are no more effective than a placebo in treating mild to moderate depression. Joe and Teresa Graedon write (*Top Screwups Doctors Make and How To Avoid Them*, New York: Crown Archetype, 2011, p. 87):

> **Over 100 million prescriptions are written each year for drugs like citalopram (Celexa), escitalopram (Lexapro), fluoxetine (Prozac), paroxetine (Paxil), and sertraline (Zoloft). A 2010 review of multiple studies concluded that such drugs were helpful for severe depression, but when it comes to mild to moderate depression, the benefit of antidepressant medications "may be minimal to nonexistent." In fact, they were no bet-**

ter than sugar pills for relieving the symptoms of the mild to moderate depression for which they are frequently prescribed.

Even though I try to limit my consumption of caffeine, this drug almost always improves my mood, energy level, stamina, and felling of well-being. Whenever I'm totally exhausted in the pharmacy, caffeinated soft drinks almost always make me feel better. Does the fact that caffeine improves my mood prove that my mood was caused by a chemical imbalance? In my career of 25 years as a pharmacist, caffeinated soft drinks have been nearly as common in the pharmacy as pill bottles. Caffeine seems to be pharmacists' drug of choice to get us through a grueling day. Do pharmacists have a chemical imbalance that we treat with caffeine?

In a *Time* essay ("The Art of Unhappiness," Jan. 17, 2005, p. 74), James Poniewozik ponders the relentless pursuit of happiness in our society: "What is the one modern form of expression almost completely dedicated to depicting happiness? Advertising. ...Today the messages we're bombarded with are...relentlessly happy. 'Celebrate!' commanded the ads for the arthritis drug Celebrex, before we found out it could increase the risk of heart attacks. It gets exhausting, this constant goad to joy. If you're not smiling—after we made all those wonderful pills and cell-phone plans!—what's wrong with you? Not to smile is un-American. You can pick out the Americans in a crowd of tourists by their reflexive grins."

Did you ever notice that there are a lot of conditions around lately that are somewhat suspiciously labeled "disorders" to make the use of antidepressants seem reasonable? Capitalization of the name of the disorder often lends legitimacy to the diagnosis. The "winter blues" is now called "Seasonal Affective Disorder." Shyness is now called "Social Anxiety Disorder." A broader form of anxiety is now called "Generalized Anxiety Disorder." People who are unhappy with the appearance of their body are said to suffer from "Body Dysmorphic Disorder." People who wash their hands excessively are said to suffer from "Obsessive Compulsive Disorder." People who get very angry on the highway are said to suffer from "Road Rage Syndrome" or "Intermittent Explosive Disorder." A severe form of premenstrual syndrome (PMS) is now "Premenstrual Dysphoric

Disorder" (PMDD). "Compulsive Gambling Disorder" and "Compulsive Shopping Disorder" are now promoted as legitimate reasons for taking a SSRI-type antidepressant.

Under what circumstances is taking an antidepressant logical? Psychiatrists prefer a mechanical view of depression (an imbalance in serotonin). Psychologists prefer to examine one's life circumstances (family dynamics, childhood, parents, spouse, job, etc.). Sociologists would probably say that our society is the source of the pathology, not the brain.

The act of taking an antidepressant medication tells the user that something is wrong with himself, that his body is somehow defective or inferior, or, more specifically, that his brain chemistry is out of whack. This locates the pathology within the individual which is less threatening than blaming our spouse, our family, our job, our boss, our culture, etc.

Some psychiatrists admit that depression can be divided into two categories: 1) that which is caused by life circumstances (e.g., abusive parents, abusive husband, abusive supervisor, a deadeningly repetitive production job, an unhappy marriage, problems with the kids, being fired from ones job, etc.) and 2) that which is caused by a biochemical imbalance in the brain. I have a big problem with the second category. I do not believe that depression is a condition that lends itself to a mechanistic explanation. According to Big Pharma, the relationship between serotonin and depression is as clear as the relationship between insulin and diabetes. Big Pharma would prefer to ignore the fact that depression can be caused by one's relationships or by social pathology. Our society force feeds us war, religion, and relentless consumption. A society that values people for their wealth rather than for their character will inevitably cause depression in a significant portion of the population. Big Pharma would never entertain the possibility that consumer societies are inherently superficial and unfulfilling. Big Pharma prefers to stick its head in the sand by examining molecules and cells rather than by examining the pathology in our culture and society.

The use of antidepressants is, in my opinion, indicative of the quick-fix approach with much of modern medicine in which root causes of conditions are avoided for the simple reason that certain people have a vested interest in avoiding the discussion of root causes. Corporate polluters don't want to discuss air and water pollution as an important cause of cancer. The big food processors don't want to admit that their products and advertising encourage obesity. Abusive parents or spouses don't want to discuss abuse as a cause of depression. Modern medicine is an exercise in avoiding discussions of root causes of illnesses. It is quite remarkable that the drug industry has succeeded so completely in convincing people that their depression is caused by a chemical imbalance in the brain rather than by the depressing circumstances in their lives.

Modern medicine and psychiatry have long been accused of reinforcing the status quo, of providing diagnoses that don't make waves and don't offend the people who are the ultimate cause of the problem. If parents were to send a child to a psychiatrist and that psychiatrist were to conclude that the parents are the problem, do you think that the psychiatrist is going to embark on the dangerous task of criticizing or blaming the parents? It is much easier for psychiatrists to simply prescribe an antidepressant for the child. Of course, managed care finds that antidepressant drugs are a cheaper quick-fix than years of psychotherapy.

Millions of people say they feel better on antidepressant drugs. But my question is: What does this tell us about a society that prefers quick-fixes over substantial examination of root causes? At what point does one begin to focus on society itself rather than on the brain chemistry of individuals? Explaining depression as a defect in brain biochemistry lessens *Homo sapiens* to the level of a simple machine. Can we ever hope to become a more civilized species if we believe that we are nothing more than machines? How can we dream of taming our basest instincts if we view ourselves as programmed for wars, aggression, and apathy toward suffering?

Whatever became of the notion that learning to overcome ones problems on ones own builds character? Is it possible that depression is a teacher just like pain is a teacher? Pain somewhere in our body tells us that we are doing something wrong or that something *is* wrong. Depression is a teacher that tells us something is wrong in our relationships with people, or that we need to examine why our lives are so unfulfilling, or that we need to examine whether our society is pathological.

If someone finds a lifetime of pursuing material goods (a bigger house, a more expensive car, etc.) unfulfilling and becomes depressed in a trivial materialistic world, should this person take an antidepressant? Antidepressants have the effect of homogenizing us into a nation of hedonistic affable air-head consumer automatons who do not reflect on our existence.

There is a saying that it is necessary for one to experience the "lows" in life in order to be able to appreciate the "highs." You cannot fully appreciate the joy in life without knowing the pain. Modern medicine seeks to eliminate physical pain as well as psychic pain and the pain of living ones life.

There is also a popular saying about "wisdom born of pain." President Johnson was said to have suffered extreme anguish over the Viet Nam War. From that anguish, he possibly realized that Viet Nam was a mistake. In contrast, President George W. Bush never seemed to have any self-doubt about the wisdom of the War in Iraq. Do you prefer presidents who anguish over decisions, or do you prefer presidents who don't seem to lose any sleep over decisions? If antidepressants erase the anguish from life, will we as a species be less wise?

There are those who say that the unexamined life is not worth living. Modern psychiatry does not promote the examination of our lives. There is another saying that the world is a nice place until one reads a newspaper. Modern medicine seeks to remove us from any examination of our existence, our relationship with our society, and, in general, anything other than molecules, cells, genes, viruses and pharmaceuticals. The cell is the focus of modern medicine rather than the society.

The drug companies often begin their TV commercials for antidepressants by saying that depression "may be caused by a chemical imbalance in the brain. Zoloft [or Prozac, Paxil, etc.] helps treat this imbalance." But what if depression is caused by one's life circumstances? Big Pharma certainly prefers a cellular focus toward depression rather than the big picture outlook expressed in this *Time* article

(Gregg Easterbrook, "The Real Truth About Money," Jan. 17, 2005, pp. A32-A34):

...if you charted the incidence of depression since 1950, the lines suggest a growing epidemic. Depending on what assumptions are used, clinical depression is 3 to 10 times as common today than two generations ago. ...In nations with high levels of income equality like the Scandinavian countries, well-being tends to be higher than in nations with unequal wealth distribution such as the U.S. ...Psychology and sociology aside, there is a final reason money can't buy happiness: the things that really matter in life are not sold in stores. Love, friendship, family, respect, a place in the community, the belief that your life has purpose—those are the essentials of human fulfillment, and they cannot be purchased with cash. Everyone needs a certain amount of money, but chasing money rather than meaning is a formula for discontent. Too many Americans have made materialism and the cycle of work and spend their principal goals. Then they wonder why they don't feel happy.

Here are two brief anecdotes involving two of my neighbors. I feel that these two ancedoctes illustrate how our medical system pushes antidepressants too easily.

I have a neighbor in her early eighties who I have gotten to know fairly well. Her husband died recently. She told me that when she visited her internist for a routine check-up, she mentioned to him that she was having difficulty coping with the loss of her husband. The internist prescribed the antidepressant Zoloft. My neighbor told me that she dreads her next appointment with her internist because, she says, he will be angry with her for deciding against taking the Zoloft. I told her that he should be proud of her for having the will-power and determination to work through her grief without an antidepressant. She told me, "I need to cry my way through this" in learning to cope with the loss of her husband. I repeated to her that the doctor should be proud of her determination to work through the grieving process unmedicated. She said somewhat sarcastically, "Well, we'll see whether he's proud of me or not."

I have another neighbor in his early eighties who just had coronary bypass surgery on two blocked arteries. A few days after he was discharged from the hospital, I happened to be at his apartment when a home-care registered nurse arrived to check on him. My neighbor commented that he was depressed after the surgery. I was struck by how quickly the home-care nurse determined that surely my neighbor needed an increase in the dose of his antidepressant Celexa. The nurse said something like, "Well your doctor may need to increase the dose of your antidepressant." In my opinion, the nurse should have encouraged my neighbor by stressing that recovery would be a slow process and that it was just two weeks post surgery. The nurse's knee-jerk conclusion that my neighbor needed a higher dose of antidepressant struck me as very facile.

Before: Blame your cold mother
Now: Blame your brain chemistry

For an excellent description of how American psychiatry changed from blaming one's cold mother to blaming one's brain chemistry, see Elliot S. Valenstein, Ph.D., a Professor Emeritus of Psychology and Neuroscience at the University of Michigan (*Blaming the Brain: The Truth About Drugs and Mental Health*, New York: The Free Press, 1998, pp. 1-2.):

American psychiatry is said to have changed from blaming the mother to blaming the brain. It was not so very long ago that the cause of mental disorders was thought to be rooted in early experiences within the family, but now it is widely believed by most authorities and the public alike that the cause is a chemical imbalance in the brain. Today, schizophrenia is commonly claimed to be caused by an excess of the neurotransmitter dopamine and depression by a deficiency of serotonin, while anxiety and other mental disorders are attributed to other neurotransmitter abnormalities. Brain chemistry is believed to be not only the cause of mental disorders, but also the explanation of the normal variations in personality and behavior. How did these radical changes occur within the span of a few decades and does the evidence really support these new theories? Whose interests are served by promoting drug treatment and biochemical explanations and how are these interests advanced? What are the long-range implications of the biochemical theory of mental disorders and the growing reliance on drugs to treat all psychological and behavioral problems? This book attempts to answer these questions and to provide a long-overdue examination of the assumptions fundamental to current biochemical theories.

From about 1945 through 1960, most people had very different ideas about the cause of mental disorders. Although orthodox psychoanalytic therapy was practiced by only a small percentage of mental health professionals, psychoanalytic explanations of the causes of different mental disorders and the best way to treat them dominated the field. In 1950, it was rare that someone not committed to psychoanalytic theory would head a major psychiatry department. Psychotherapists in private practice often spent years trying to discover the repressed causes of their patients' mental disorders. The value of this approach and the theory underlying it is now widely questioned, if not totally rejected, by most mental health professionals. Today, the disturbed thoughts and behavior of mental patients are believed to be caused by a biochemically defective brain, and symptoms are not "analyzed," but used mainly as a means of arriving at the diagnosis that will determine the appropriate medication to prescribe. Almost all current chairmen and the majority of the staffs of psychiatry departments are committed to a biochemical approach to mental illness.

How radically our ideas have changed is indicated by the fact that most psychiatric residents no longer receive any instruction in intensive psychotherapy, and many complete their training without meeting regularly with a single patient in psychotherapy sessions. During the 1950s, any research on schizophrenia was considered unethical if it included a control group given drugs without complementary psychotherapy. By 1970, however, the situation had reversed, and it was considered unethical to have a group that received only psychotherapy and no drugs.

Certain jobs are more likely to cause depression

If depression is caused by a chemical imbalance in the brain, why is it that certain jobs are more likely to cause depression? According to a report from the Substance Abuse and Mental Health Services

Administration (Kevin Freking, "Report ranks jobs by rates of depression," *The Associated Press*, October 13, 2007
http://news.yahoo.com/s/ap/20071013/ap_on_go_ot/depressing_jobs;_ylt=AhaaQr_722NJnSC8U9MxhSh34T0D):

> People who tend to the elderly, change diapers and serve up food and drinks have the highest rates of depression among U.S. workers. Overall, 7 percent of full-time workers battled depression in the past year, according to a government report available [October 13, 2007]. Women were more likely than men to have had a major bout of depression, and younger workers had higher rates of depression than their older colleagues. Almost 11 percent of personal care workers—which includes child care and helping the elderly and severely disabled with their daily needs—reported depression lasting two weeks or longer. ...Workers who prepare and serve food—cooks, bartenders, waiters and waitresses—had the second highest rate of depression among full-time employees at 10.3 percent. In a tie for third were health care workers and social workers at 9.6 percent. The lowest rate of depression, 4.3 percent, occurred in the job category that covers engineers, architects and surveyors. Government officials tracked depression within 21 major occupational categories. They combined data from 2004 through 2006 to estimate episodes of depression within the past year. That information came from the National Survey on Drug Use and Health, which registers lifetime and past-year depression bouts. ...Depression leads to $30 billion to $44 billion in lost productivity annually, said the report from the Substance Abuse and Mental Health Services Administration. The report was available [October 13, 2007] on the agency's Web site at http://oas.samhsa.gov. Just working full-time would appear to be beneficial in preventing depression. The overall rate of depression for full-time workers, 7 percent, compares with the 12.7 percent rate registered by those who are unemployed.

**The incidence of depression varies
considerably around the world**

If depression is caused by a chemical imbalance in the brain, why is it that the incidence of depression in certain countries is much higher than in other countries? A study by Weissman, et. al., in the *Journal of the American Medical Association* ("Cross-national epidemiology of major depression and bipolar disorder," *JAMA*, July 24, 1996, http://jama.ama-assn.org/cgi/content/abstract/276/4/293) found high variability in rates around the world in the incidence of major depression. Population-based epidemiological studies using similar methods from ten countries (United States, Canada, Puerto Rico, France, West Germany, Italy, Lebanon, Taiwan, Korea, and New Zealand) found:

...The lifetime rates for major depression vary widely across countries, ranging from 1.5 cases per 100 adults in the sample in Taiwan to 19.0 cases per 100 adults in Beirut. ...In every country, the rates of major depression were higher for women than men. ...The differences in rates for major depression across countries suggest that cultural differences or different risk factors affect the expression of the disorder.

Having a subordinate position in a social hierarchy can lead to depression

Here is an explanation of depression based on evolutionary psychology that I find very reasonable and logical. Explanations of depression based on factors such as social hierarchy make the drug industry's explanation of depression based on a "chemical imbalance" look extremely suspect.

There is often a strong correlation between depression and low social status. According to Wolpert and Evans, the manifestations of melancholic depression and, conversely, euphoric mania are typical of people occupying omega and alpha status roles. Evolutionary psychology suggests that depression is part of an adaptive coping process. It involves passive submission to a prolonged or uncontrollable stress. The persistence into the post-hunter-gatherer era of depressive states continues to foster (relatively) stable hierarchies of social dominance. Dominance and submission relationships have been characteristic of humanity, whereas compassion develops later than the will to dominate. Pecking orders may be an immutable law of nature. See Lewis Wolpert and Dylan Evans (Chapter 4: Self-Infliction, Social Adaptation or Biological Destiny? Models of Psychopathology and Their Relationship to Stigmatization. (c) 2001 Lewis Wolpert and Dylan Evans. In: A H Crisp (ed) *Every Family in the Land: Understanding prejudice and discrimination against people with mental illness,* Sir Robert Mond Memorial Trust, September 24, 2001, http://www.stigma.org/everyfamily/lwolpert.html):

The best known evolutionary hypothesis about depression is the social competition hypothesis. This hypothesis sees depression as an adaptive response to finding oneself in a subordinate position in the social hierarchy. The idea was first stated explicitly by the British psychiatrist John Price and has since been developed by others. The hypothesis states that depression is an adaptation whose function is to inhibit aggressive behavior to rivals and superiors when one's status is low. Depression is considered to preserve the stability of the group by preventing constant struggles for status in the social hierarchy. Many animals display submission cues to [an] ... aggressor who appears bigger and stronger. These submission cues usually prompt the aggressor to terminate the attack. The social competition hypothesis views depression in humans as homologous with these "involuntary yielding strategies."

Yielding prevents the aggressor from being more aggressive and promotes behavior which encourages acceptance of a subordinate position and also enables the individual to conserve resources. According to the social competition hypothesis depression will, in general, occur when the individual's perception of his/her status in the group falls below a critical threshold level. ...The main advantage to the individual is supposed to be that depression promotes adjustment to failure or defeat. According to the social competition hypothesis of depression, when the goals of the depressed person are given up they are not replaced by new personal goals, but rather by the goals of other more powerful group members. The depressed person tries to adopt these new goals, so that their goals become identical with the goals of the group or of its powerful members and this can lead to acceptance and reconciliation.

Is depression good for you?

Dr. Paul Keedwell, an expert on mood disorders at the Institute of Psychiatry, Kings College, London, believes that depression may be good for you. (See Tom Geoghegan, *BBC News Magazine*, Feb. 28, 2008 http://news.bbc.co.uk/2/hi/uk_news/magazine/7268496.stm):

Pills aren't the answer to helping many people recover from depression.... But there's growing evidence that gloominess could be a positive experience.

What depressed the cavemen? It may strike us as a particularly modern malaise for a time-poor, fast-paced society but a new reappraisal of depression suggests it has always been around.

A leading psychiatrist says that depression is not a human defect at all, but a defence mechanism that in its mild and moderate forms can force a healthy reassessment of personal circumstances.

Dr. Paul Keedwell, an expert on mood disorders at the Institute of Psychiatry, King's College London, argues all people are vulnerable to depression in the face of stress to varying degrees, and always have been.

The fact it has survived so long—and not been eradicated by evolution—indicates it has helped the human race become stronger.

"There are benefits and that's why it has persisted. It's a tough message to hear while you are in depression but I think that there's a life afterwards," he says.

"I have received e-mails from ex-sufferers saying in retrospect it probably did help them because they changed direction, a new career for example, and as a result they're more content day-to-day than before the depression."

One woman left an abusive relationship and moved on, he says, and might not have done if depression had not provided the necessary introspection.

Similarly, unrealistic expectations are revised when depression sparks a more humble reassessment of strengths and weaknesses.

In Britain one in four men and one in five women are estimated to suffer depression during their lifetime, and one in 20 suffers it at any one time.

Creativity

Dame Kelly Holmes has spoken in the past about how the depression she suffered in 2003 made her a stronger person, a year before her double-gold performance at the Olympics. Alastair Campbell has said it was the making of him.

But there are other qualities depression generates, not just resilience, says Dr. Keedwell, author of *How Sadness Survived*.

"Psychological unease can generate creative work and the rebirth after depression brings a new love affair with life."

Aristotle believed depression to be of great value because of the insights it could bring. There is also an increased empathy in people who have or have had depression, he says, because they become more attuned to other people's suffering.

Depression can be traced all the way back to the Stone Age, say Dr. Keedwell, when close-knit communities of about 50 people would have identified it quickly. The rest of the group would have rallied round and changes followed, such as a new role for the individual.

Some remote communities are more aware of it. The Banda tribe in Uganda calls it "illness of thought" and those affected are allowed time out from the group, a concession not extended to many with the condition in the UK.

The high and rising incidence in the UK and US—compared to countries like Brazil and Mexico—could be due to the breakdown of family bonds and the fragmentation of society. And compared to past decades, there are increased expectations of success.

Severe depression

Dr. Keedwell says his theory does not cover severe depression, which is an illness accompanied by a catatonic lack of energy, cannot be worked through and requires the intervention of a GP.

Anti-depressants, which were reported this week to have little clinical benefit for many patients, have a part to play, says Dr. Keedwell, especially in severe depression. But an individual must address the social or emotional cause either on his own, with a loved one or with a professional.

"Don't beat yourself up about being depressed, in most cases it will run its course provided you take yourself out of the situation that caused it.

"I know that's an easy and glib thing to say, because I'm not a single mum living 12 floors up in a high-rise block. Sometimes it's not easy to escape but that's the fault of society, not the fault of depression."

The trouble with psychiatry

Here are excerpts from a review of Daniel Carlet's *Unhinged: The Trouble with Psychiatry* written by Gaetan Lion on Amazon.com (*Unhinged: The Trouble with Psychiatry—A Doctor's Revelations about a Profession in Crisis,* Daniel J. Carlat, New York: Free Press, 2010):

This is essentially a whistle blower reporting on the corruption of psychiatry by Big Pharma. ...There are several themes to Carlat's analysis of psychiatry devolution.

First, psychiatrists have given up on understanding their patients. They don't do psychotherapy anymore. They essentially just prescribe drugs (mainly anti-depressants). They now call themselves psychopharmacologists instead of psychotherapists. For psychotherapy, you have to go to a psychologist (who got a graduate degree in psychology, but did not go to med school, and is not allowed to prescribe drugs).

Second, psychiatrists overdiagnose their patients. Way too many children are overdiagnosed with ADHD and even bipolar disorder (the latter being often meaningless for young children). From 1994 to 2003, children and adolescents treated for bipolar disorder rose by 8,000%! The majority of cases are misdiagnosed. The psychological troubles are related to complex sociological problems the psychiatrists make no effort to understand. And, way too many adults are overdiagnosed with ADHD, social anxiety, and mild depression for what are often normal responses to the challenges of daily life.

Third, psychiatrists are overdrugging their patients. Psychiatrists too readily prescribe anti-depressants and stimulants to treat just about any small psychological discomfort that could better be resolved through just a few therapy sessions.

Fourth, the efficacy of most drugs is highly questionable because they are based on an unproven scientific hypothesis: the brain chemical imbalance theory (called "monoamine hypothesis"). Carlat states that chemical imbalance is a myth perpetrated by the profession. Depression is explained by a deficiency in the neurotransmitter called serotonin. The problem is that the causal link between serotonin level and depression has never been proven. Actually, several studies attempting to prove this link ultimately served to disprove it. Therefore, SSR anti-depressants aimed at boosting serotonin levels work no better than placebo. In 50% of drug trials, the drugs do not beat placebo. Another outstanding book on this subject is: *The Emperor's New Drugs: Exploding the Antidepressant Myth.*

Fifth, psychiatrists understand very little regarding the human brain. Its functioning at the neurobiological level remains a mystery. Additionally, "to a remarkable degree our choice of medication is subjective, even random" acknowledges Carlat. ...

All those themes have a common root: economic conflict of interest. About three decades ago, psychiatrists noted that they could make a lot more money by prescribing drugs instead of conducting therapy. A therapy session takes an hour. During this same hour, a psychiatrist can see three patients, quickly diagnose them and give them a prescription. As a result, psychopharmacology is far more lucrative and efficient than psychotherapy. The increased efficiency translated into lower claim cost per patient. Therefore, insurance coverage became more generous for drugs than for therapy. This only accelerated the transition to psychopharmacology.

Carlat suggests there are two major problems with this transition to psychopharmacology. First, it does not work that well. Many studies have confirmed that psychotherapy works often better than drugs and with no side effects. The relapse rate is lower as patients learn lifelong solving skills. And, second, psychopharmacology has turned psychiatry into the marketing arm of Big Pharma. Now, over 27 million Americans are on anti-depressants that work little better than placebo but with side effects. Big Pharma spends twice as much on marketing as research. Carlat states that all the "new" drugs work no better than the original ones of 50 years ago. They are just a lot more lucrative because they are under patent. Antidepressants often bring in between $1 billion to $5 billion in annual revenues.

The conflict of interest in psychiatry have reached a critical level whereby the credibility of the profession is being questioned. Dr. Carlat covers the practice of drug reps and leading psychiatrists receiving millions of dollars from Big Pharma to give speeches to other doctors pushing their drugs and even testing their drugs in clinical trials. Psychiatrists lead the pack of specialties receiving the most money from Big Pharma. How can a clinician objectively evaluate a drug when he is paid a fortune by the developer of that drug? This is an egregious conflict of interest resulting in poor science and perpetrating the ignorance of psychiatrists. How can they figure what really works since they can't trust the original studies. ...

Carlat's recommendations make sense. But, the psychiatry lobby will resist all such proposals to protect their income. Nevertheless at the risk of becoming ostracized by colleagues, Carlat is really courageous for stating what is necessary to restore integrity to his profession.

Chapter 39

Pharmacy economics 101

Many people seem to think that the pharmaceutical industry is fundamentally different from any other industry in America because it sells products that treat human illness. One of the biggest surprises customers have, in my experience, is when they discover that retail prescription prices can vary by as much as 30% or more for the same medication at various drugstores. Many people seem to think that pharmacy should be a uniquely benevolent enterprise and that pharmacists and doctors should be public servants who are unconcerned with the profit motive. The harsh reality of the marketplace in health care surprises many people. Otherwise very intelligent people are often shocked and indignant to discover that the same prescription can cost $30.00 at one drugstore and $45.00 at another.

Some people seem to think that the prices of prescription drugs should somehow be handled like a public utility. The prices charged by the local electric utility and water utility are tightly regulated by a public service commission. I think that explains why I've seen a look of disgust on the faces of so many customers when they are comparing prices for prescription drugs among various drugstores. Many customers feel that prescription drugs should be priced the same at every pharmacy just like residential customers pay the same for every kilowatt hour of electricity or thousand gallons of water from the local utilities. In reality, many customers have an attitude toward the pharmacist that implies, *You ought to be ashamed of yourself for charging more than the drugstore down the street!!* Many people seem to feel that it's fine for most consumer products to be subject to competition and market forces, whereas the retail prices of prescription drugs should be regulated by some governmental entity similar to that in some advanced countries with a national health service. Customers need to realize that, in some ways, the retail pricing of prescription drugs is much like the retail pricing of any commodity in the marketplace in that the price varies from store to store. (For customers with insurance coverage for prescription drugs, however, the price is usually the same from pharmacy to pharmacy.) Many customers have learned that it pays to compare prices from at least three or four different pharmacies before having their prescriptions filled.

I have had several occasions in which customers became extremely angry when I quoted them a price for their prescription. The customer would say, "I got a price quote of several dollars less at a drugstore nearby." Then I would say "We'll match that price" or "Company policy allows us to match our competitors' prices." The customer then goes into orbit and says, "If you're willing to match the price now, why didn't you quote me that price to begin with?" I usually try to explain to them that there is a very logical reason for this and that it does not involve any hanky-panky on the part of the pharmacist. The simple reason that we do not quote a lower price to begin with is that we have no idea what our competitors are charging for the vast majority of drugs.

Keep in mind that there are a few thousand drugs in the average pharmacy. There is absolutely no way that we would know the prices that our competitors charge for each of these drugs. Do customers think we have some kind of undercover link with our competitors' pharmacy computers? Pricing of prescription drugs is, in this regard, just like the pricing of the rest of the merchandise in the drugstore. We have no way of knowing what our competitors charge for Crest toothpaste, Prell shampoo, Bayer aspirin, Robitussin cough syrup, or Doan's pills, unless we actually visit our competitors' stores and write down the prices they charge for each and every item.

I worked in one store in which a customer gave me a long story about why he no longer patronized one of our competitors. During this conversation, he identified himself as a lawyer. He said that when he began comparing prescription prices, he found a competitor with lower prices. He then confronted his long-time pharmacist with this information. When his pharmacist told him that company policy allowed price matching, the lawyer told me that he (the lawyer) became extremely irate because he said the pharmacist should have been charging him the lower prices all along. I proceeded to try to explain to this lawyer that we don't know what our competitors charge for most of their drugs. I don't know if he understood this simple explanation. He told me that he was transferring all his prescriptions to our store. I did not tell him that I have had customers become very angry with me under precisely the same circumstances that caused him to leave our competitor. I was surprised that a lawyer did not understand that pharmacists have no way of knowing what our competitors charge for each and every drug in their pharmacy.

It is true that we may find out what competitors charge for maybe a dozen very common drugs. For example, we may have heard what our competitors charge for thirty Prevacid 30 mg capsules or thirty Prozac 20 mg capsules or certain birth control pills. That is only because we have been informed of this, by customers, when these customers are in the process of price checking. For example, a customer will call us from home or come to the pharmacy and ask, "How much do you charge for thirty Prozac 20 mg capsules?" After I quote a price, the customer either decides to get the capsules at our pharmacy or says something like, "Well I can get it for X dollars at (CVS, Walgreens, Wal-Mart, Rite Aid, etc.)." As likely as not, when our price is higher, the customer's attitude implies something like: *You ought to be ashamed of yourself for ripping off the public!* The customer does not understand that, at best, we know the prices of only a very few top-selling drugs at our competitors. With the exception of the dirt cheap prices some chains charge for many generic drugs (like a thirty-day supply for four dollars), pharmacists know the prices that our competitors charge on a tiny percent of drugs.

Of course, for most customers, the actual retail price of prescriptions is of little interest because they have either private insurance coverage for drugs or they're on some governmental program such as Medicaid. The number of customers who pay the full cash price for prescriptions diminishes each year. According to *Drug Topics*, "The percentage of prescriptions paid for with cash has dropped dramatically, from 63% in 1990 to just above 11% in 2005." (Sandra Levy, "Chain industry is alive and well: NACDS profile," *Drug Topics*, Nov. 20, 2006, p. 49)

I used to work in a town of approximately 100,000 people. My employer, a large chain with a few thousand stores, had several drugstores in this town. Believe it or not, my employer had different prices at the various locations in town based on the amount of competition in each specific neighborhood. (When I worked for Revco, there were six pricing "zones" or pricing structures based on local competition.) If there were discount drugstores nearby, then the prices at these stores were usually lower. If a store was located in a neighborhood in which there was very little competition, then the prices were usually higher at those stores. If you phone around to various drugstores in town, you need to keep in mind that you may not be quoted the same price at each outlet of the same chain drugstore. For example, Chain Drugstore X may charge a certain price for a drug at one location and may charge a few (or several) dollars less (or more) at another outlet of this same chain in another neighborhood of the same city based on the amount of local competition. If you live in a neighborhood or town with very few drugstores, it may pay you to get all your prescriptions filled during one of your trips to another neighborhood or town. If you live in a small town with few drugstores, it may pay you to fill all your prescriptions during one of your visits to a larger town that has lots of drugstores.

Savings of 10% to 30% are common if you are willing to compare prices at three or four drugstores. But keep in mind that low profit-margin drugstores are often just assembly-line operations that sling out prescriptions as quickly as the pharmacy staff can prepare them. If you have significant questions about your medications, you may be better off patronizing a store that charges a little more yet has adequate staffing so that the pharmacist has time to answer your questions. You may also want to keep in mind that some high-volume stores that have the best prices may increase profitability by understaffing. Understaffing increased the chances of errors. If you patronize a very busy pharmacy that seems to be in chaos (e.g., they "can't find" your prescriptions that you dropped off earlier) every time you're at that pharmacy, you may want to consider the possibility that the accuracy rate at that pharmacy is suspect.

In addition to shopping around for the best price, here's another way to save money. If you're uncertain whether you can tolerate a certain medication, ask for just a few pills. Keep in mind that you will usually pay a lot more per tablet or capsule when you ask for just a few. In most cases, the more pills you get, the less you pay per pill. But, if you ask for just a few pills, you are less likely to be stuck with a lot of expensive pills that you cannot tolerate. Many customers have a prescription filled for the entire amount ordered by the doctor and then return to the drugstore after a day or two, saying that they can't tolerate the medication. They ask for a refund. Some pharmacists will agree to give the customer a refund to keep the customer happy. But it's less of a hassle if you just request a few pills in the beginning—if you suspect you might not be able to tolerate the drug— rather than have to bring back a bottle full of pills and ask for a refund.

Many pharmacists refuse to accept medications returned by customers. State boards of pharmacy regulations usually prohibit pharmacists from dispensing this returned medication to other customers. Would you want your pharmacist to fill your prescription with pills that another customer has had at his house for a few days? Nevertheless, some pharmacists do indeed dispense these returned drugs to other customers, particularly if the customer who returned the drugs looks like he is unlikely to have handled the drugs improperly (admittedly a purely subjective judgment on the part of the pharmacist).

Many brand name drugs are incredibly expensive so it pays to be a wise consumer. Physicians have become accustomed to hearing complaints from patients about the high cost of drugs. Occasionally, a physician will ask the pharmacist what the patient will pay for the prescription the physician is calling in. I recall one phone call from a doctor who, feeling that his patient couldn't afford an expensive medication, had the following reaction when I stated the price: First, this physician said, "Wow, that's pretty expensive." Then he said jokingly, "Well, he'll probably think that the more he pays, the more it will help him!" It reminded me of Sigmund Freud's famous dictum that the act of a patient paying for a consultation increases the perception that that consultation has been effective. Patients think a free consultation certainly can't be worth much. Similarly, some pharmacy customers think inexpensive drugs can't be very effective. Some customers equate a higher price with more potency. They say things like, "Wow! That must be a really potent medication!" Many drugs that are off patent and that are available generically are amazingly inexpensive, prompting some customers to question whether they are effective.

"Me-too" or copy-cat drugs

Explaining the high cost of prescription drugs to customers is one part of my job I hate. There are frequently articles in the pharmacy magazines suggesting we should tell the customer that, yes, prescription drugs are expensive, but they sure are a lot cheaper than hospitalization. In some cases, this is certainly true. In many cases, it diverts attention from a far more complicated reality.

Pharmacists frequently rationalize the high cost of drugs with the explanation that drug companies need big profits to fund research. It is true that it takes a lot of money to bring a drug to market, but it is also true that most of the drugs brought to market are what's known as "me-too" or "copy-cat" drugs. Whenever there's a big hit on television, the next season the other networks make clones of the hit. The same thing happens with prescription and non-prescription drugs. After Upjohn made a fortune with the non-steroidal anti-inflammatory drug (NSAID) Motrin, more than a dozen other companies eventually came out with their own NSAID. Similarly, each company wants to have its own ACE inhibitor, calcium channel blocker, cholesterol-lowering statin, non-sedating antihistamine, beta blocker, H2 antagonist, SSRI-type antidepressant, PPI-type acid suppresser, fluoroquinolone antibiotic, triptan-type antimigraine, etc. For example, as of this writing, there are seven antimigraine triptans on the market: sumatriptan (Imitrex), zolmitriptan (Zomig), naratriptan

(Amerge), rizatriptan (Maxalt), almotriptan (Axert), eletriptan (Relpax), and frovatriptan (Frova).

The pharmaceutical industry often cites the figure $800 million to bring a new drug to market. The first time I heard the figure *one billion dollars* was in the Senate debate on the Medicare drug benefit on C-Span on June 19, 2003. Is it worth these huge sums to bring me-too drugs to the market?

More often than you realize, those high-priced new drugs at your local pharmacy have only marginal benefits, at best, over similar drugs that have been on the market for years. However, drug advertisements on TV make the latest me-too drugs look like they're as important as the discovery of insulin and penicillin. According to the *Associated Press* (Lauran Neergaard, "Few New Drugs Made Improvement," May 29, 2002):

Only 15 percent of new drugs approved in the last decade were novel chemicals that the Food and Drug Administration deemed a significant improvement over older drugs, a study says.

The vast majority instead were similar to existing medicines. Yet during the same time, consumer spending on prescription drugs more than doubled to $132 billion—and most of the increase was spent not on the most innovative drugs, but on the less important or copycats, says the study by the National Institute for Health Care Management.

The FDA and other groups have long cautioned that major pharmaceutical breakthroughs are rare. But the study to be released Wednesday—by an institute partly funded by managed care—is among the first to rank spending according to drugs' relative importance to health care.

The findings show patients must be smart consumers, said institute president Nancy Chockley. "We are all under the impression that 'new and improved' is always much better," yet that's not always true, she said.

...The institute reviewed 1,035 drugs that FDA approved between 1989 and 2000, and found that only 153 were both FDA-designated priority drugs and made of novel chemicals—in other words, a highly innovative drug.

The same copy-cat game is being played with non-prescription drugs. Drugstore shelves are full of what seems like an endless number of non-prescription products for colds, coughs, sore throat, constipation, vaginal yeast infection, athlete's foot, jock itch, poison ivy, allergies, dry skin, hemorrhoids, insomnia, arthritis, etc. Drugstore shelves are like an orgy of eye-catching packages, brightly colored, each screaming "BUY ME!" In many ways, I consider the packaging to be more impressive than the contents. In many cases, the differences between the products in each category are trivial.

The drug companies like to speak in terms of markets for each medical condition: the hypertension market, the arthritis market, the depression market, the anxiety market, the cholesterol-lowering market, the ulcer market, the diabetes market, the migraine market, the angina market, etc. Each market is quantified in terms of millions or billions of dollars. Drug companies speak of entering a market for arthritis just as they would enter a market for toothpaste or underarm odor. Each market is finite (unless it can be hyped beyond its natural boundaries) and each manufacturer wants a piece of the pie for each condition. In this market view of disease, depression, for example, is not viewed as a consequence of one's life circumstances, unloving parents, an abusive spouse, etc. The drug industry views depression through a purely economic lens, i.e., a multi-billion dollar market for drugs like Prozac, Paxil, Wellbutrin, Zoloft, etc.

Traditional conservative dogma states that price regulation will stifle innovation in the pharmaceutical industry. It is true that the profit motive can inspire a lot of people to try to develop new products. But, in the case of the drug industry, the profit motive mainly inspires them to look for an entry into a lucrative market. They want a piece of the pie for as many conditions as possible, especially when it's a popular condition like hypertension, elevated cholesterol, arthritis, depression, anxiety, ulcers, angina, migraine, etc. "A piece of the pie" usually means a "me-too" drug. Developing truly innovative drugs is far more costly and risky than developing copy-cats. Despite what you're led to believe in drug advertisements on television, the pharmaceutical industry today rarely develops truly miraculous drugs like penicillin and insulin. The drug industry has morphed into a marketing enterprise, hyping copy-cat drugs as if they were genuine breakthroughs. Prescription drugs are marketed the same today as automobiles, beer, and detergents.

A large number of pharmacy customers are happy to pay any-thing for prescription drugs, thinking they are getting the latest won-der drug when, very often, they're simply getting the latest me-too drug. In many cases, older and cheaper drugs may do as well or bet-ter than newer drugs. Furthermore, these older drugs may have a long track record of safety. But direct-to-consumer ads have the public salivating for the latest copy-cat drugs.

According to Marcia Angell, M.D., a former editor of *The New England Journal of Medicine* ("The Pharmaceutical Industry—To Whom Is It Accountable?" *NEJM*, June 22, 2000, pp. 1902-1904 http://www.nejm.com/content/2000/0342/0025/1902.asp):

The industry produces copy-cat drugs directed toward people who can be persuaded by a huge marketing budget that the next antihista-mine or statin or lifestyle drug is somehow better than the last.

Important new drugs do not need much promotion. Me-too drugs do. ...to rely on the drug companies for unbiased evaluations of their products makes about as much sense as relying on beer companies to teach us about alcoholism. The conflict of interest is obvious. The fact is that marketing is meant to sell drugs.

Is it correct that the U.S. pharmaceutical industry is highly innovative? Only partly. Some recently launched drugs do indeed fill important, previously unmet medical needs. But it is hard to escape the conclusion that many other new drugs add little to the therapeutic armamentarium except expense and confusion. Consider the welter of very similar drugs to lower cholesterol levels. Developing genuinely innovative drugs is difficult and chancy. It is easier to make "me-too" drugs or minor variants of established products. To be profitable, the variation need only be sufficient to secure a new patent, and the rest is marketing. Critics believe drug companies are doing far too much of that sort of thing. They also charge that many industry-sponsored clinical trials are designed more to find small advantages that can be highlighted in promotional campaigns than to find clinically meaningful effects.

Writing in the *Washington Post* ("Prescription for Profit," June 20, 2001, p. A27) Angell and another former editor of *The New England*

Journal of Medicine, Arnold S. Relman, M.D., say this about me-too drugs:

The pharmaceutical giants are now putting a major part of their resources into the development and marketing of "me-too" drugs—variants of drugs already on the market. Among many examples, Claritin is one of a number of similar antihistamines; Zoloft is like many other antidepressants; and Zocor is just one of a family of cholesterol-lowering drugs. "Me-too" drugs are relatively easy to develop but require massive promotion campaigns to attract customers to a particular brand and persuade physicians to prescribe one instead of another.

ABOUT THE AUTHOR

The author graduated from West Virginia University School of Pharmacy in 1975. Over the next twenty-five years, he worked for three of the largest drugstore chains in America. He worked as a pharmacist in West Virginia (primarily in Charleston, Huntington, and Summersville) and in North Carolina (primarily in Raleigh, Durham, Chapel Hill, Burlington, Oxford, and Henderson). He has worked as a staff pharmacist and as pharmacist-in-charge. He was the manager of the entire store several years ago in Burlington, North Carolina when the Revco chain had pharmacist store managers.

The author has spent the last several years researching and writing this book and writing articles/editorials for major national pharmacy magazines. He has written a total of seventeen editorials for *Drug Topics*. He has also written two articles for *American Druggist* which were subsequently reprinted in the physicians' newsmagazine *Medical Tribune*. He wrote a 25-page chapter on pharmacy errors for a book published in 2005 for lawyers and judges (*Drug Injury: Liability, Analysis, and Prevention*, Phoenix, Arizona: Lawyers and Judges Publishing Company). He was a major source for an article on pharmacy errors in the June 2005 issue of *Good Housekeeping*. Several of the author's editorials are available on the *Drug Topics* website (drugtopics.com) by entering "Dennis Miller" in the search field.

The author welcomes comments, suggestions, and corrections at dmiller1952@aol.com.

The author is not related to another pharmacist named Dennis Miller who wrote a book on manic depression.

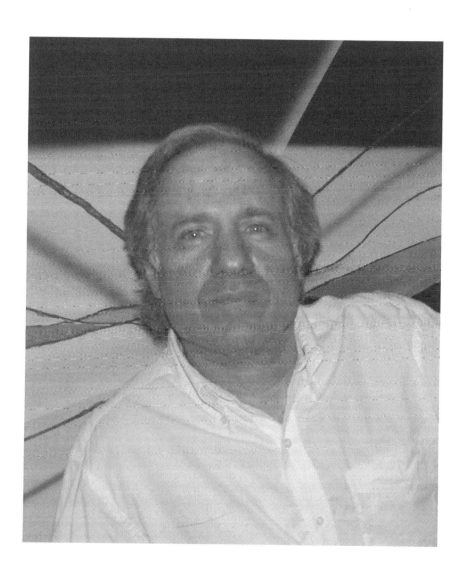

Made in the USA
Lexington, KY
13 January 2013